# NEUROLOGY SECRETS

SECRETS

## Fifth Edition

**Loren A. Rolak, MD**
Director, Marshfield Clinic Multiple Sclerosis Center, Marshfield, Wisconsin
Clinical Professor of Neurology, University of Wisconsin College of Medicine,
Madison, Wisconsin
Adjunct Professor of Neurology, Baylor College of Medicine, Houston, Texas

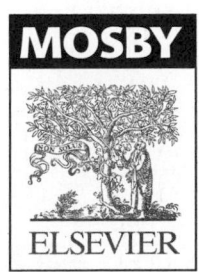

MOSBY

ELSEVIER

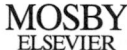

## MOSBY
ELSEVIER

1600 John F. Kennedy Boulevard
Suite 1800
Philadelphia, PA 19103-2899

NEUROLOGY SECRETS                                            ISBN: 978-0-323-05712-7

---

### NOTICE

Knowledge and best practice in this field are constantly changing. As new research and experience broaden our knowledge, changes in practice, treatment, and drug therapy may become necessary or appropriate. Readers are advised to check the most current information provided (i) on procedures featured or (ii) by the manufacturer of each product to be administered, to verify the recommended dose or formula, the method and duration of administration, and contraindications. It is the responsibility of the practitioner, relying on his or her own experience and knowledge of the patient, to make diagnoses, to determine dosages and the best treatment for each individual patient, and to take all appropriate safety precautions. To the fullest extent of the law, neither the Publisher nor the Editor assumes any liability for any injury and/or damage to persons or property arising out of or related to any use of the material contained in this book.

The Publisher

---

**Library of Congress Cataloging-in-Publication Data**
Neurology secrets / [edited by] Loren A. Rolak. – 5th ed.
        p. ; cm. – (Secret series)
    Includes bibliographical references and index.
    ISBN 978-0-323-05712-7
    1. Neurology–Miscellanea.   I. Rolak, Loren A.   II. Series: Secrets series.
    [DNLM: 1.  Nervous System Diseases–Examination Questions.  WL 18.2 N493 2011]
    RC346.N4559 2011
    616.8–dc22

                                                                        2010011617

Acquisitions Editor: James Merritt
Developmental Editor: Andrea Vosburgh
Publishing Services Manager: Hemamalini Rajendrababu
Project Manager: Nayagi Athmanathan
Marketing Manager: Marla Lieberman

Printed in Canada

Last digit is the print number: 9 8 7 6 5 4 3 2 1

Working together to grow
libraries in developing countries

www.elsevier.com | www.bookaid.org | www.sabre.org

ELSEVIER    BOOK AID    Sabre Foundation
            International

# CONTENTS

# CONTRIBUTORS

Tetsuo Ashizawa, MD
Professor and Chair, Department of Neurology, University of Florida, Gainesville, Florida;
Adjunct Professor, Department of Neurology, Baylor College of Medicine, Houston, Texas;
Adjunct Professor, Department of Neurology, The University of Texas Medical Branch,
Galveston, Texas

Sudhir S. Athni, MD
Adjunct Clinical Professor, Department of Family Practice, Mercer School of Medicine;
Staff Neurologist, Department of Internal Medicine, Neurology Division, Coliseum
Northside Hospital, Macon, Georgia

Suur Biliciler, MD
Assistant Professor of Neurology, The University of Texas Health Science Center at Houston,
Houston, Texas

Maria E. Carlini, MD
Clinical Assistant Professor of Medicine, Department of Infectious Disease, Baylor College of
Medicine, Houston, Texas

Igor M. Cherches, MD
Department of Neurology, Methodist Hospital; Department of Neurology, St. Luke's Hospital,
Houston, Texas

David Chiu, MD, FAHA
Associate Professor, Department of Clinical Neurology, Weill Cornell Medical College;
Medical Director, Eddy Scurlock Stroke Unit, The Methodist Hospital, Houston, Texas

Howard Derman, MD
Associate Professor, Department of Neurology, The Methodist Neurological Institute,
Houston, Texas

Rachelle Doody, MD, PhD
Effie Marie Cain Chair in Alzheimer's Disease Research, Director, Alzheimer's Disease and
Memory Disorders Center, Professor of Neurology, Department of Neurology, Baylor College of
Medicine; Department of Neurology, The Methodist Hospital, Houston, Texas

Everton A. Edmondson, MD
Private practice, Houston, Texas

Clifton L. Gooch, MD
Professor and Chairman, Department of Neurology, University of South Florida College of
Medicine, Tampa, Florida

Philip A. Hanna, MD
Associate Professor of Neurology, Department of Neurology (Movement Disorders),
New Jersey Neuroscience Institute, JFK Medical Center, Seton Hall University, Edison,
New Jersey

**Yadollah Harati, MD, FACP**
Professor of Neurology (Neuromuscular Disease), Chief, Neuromuscular Disease Section, Baylor College of Medicine, Houston, Texas

**Richard L. Harris, MD**
Professor of Medicine, Associate Dean of Graduate Medical Education, Baylor College of Medicine; Director, Infection Control, The Methodist Hospital, Houston, Texas

**Richard A. Hrachovy, MD**
Professor and Head, Peter Kellaway Section of Neurophysiology, Department of Neurology, Baylor College of Medicine; Medical Director, Neurophysiology Laboratory, St. Luke's Episcopal Hospital; Deputy Executive, Neurology Care Line, Michael E. DeBakey Veterans Affairs Medical Center, Houston, Texas

**Steven B. Inbody, MD**
Director, Consultative Neurology, Texas Medical Center, Houston, Texas

**Shahram Izadyar, MD**
Resident, Department of Neurology, Baylor College of Medicine, Houston, Texas

**Joseph Jankovic, MD**
Professor of Neurology, Distinguished Chair in Movement Disorders, Director, Parkinson's Disease Center and Movement Disorders Clinic, Department of Neurology, Baylor College of Medicine, Houston, Texas

**Yvonne Kew, MD, PhD**
Department of Neuro-Oncology, Baylor College of Medicine, Houston, Texas

**James M. Killian, MD**
Professor and Director, EMG Laboratory, Department of Neurology, Baylor College of Medicine, Houston, Texas

**Philip Kurle, MD**
Department of Neurology, University of Wisconsin Medical School, Madison, Wisconsin

**Justin Kwan, MD**
Assistant Professor of Neurology, Department of Neurology, Baylor College of Medicine, Houston, Texas

**Eugene C. Lai, MD, PhD**
Professor, Department of Neurology, Baylor College of Medicine, Houston, Texas

**Jonathan N. Levine, MD**
Department of Radiology, Baylor College of Medicine, Houston, Texas

**Brian Loftus, MD**
Chief Medical Officer, BetterQOL Inc; Neurologist, Bellaire Neurology, Bellaire, Texas

**Dennis R. Mosier, MD, PhD**
Assistant Professor, Department of Neurology, MDA Neuromuscular Clinic, Baylor College of Medicine; Neurology Service, Houston Veterans Affairs Medical Center, Houston, Texas

**James Owens, MD, PhD**
Assistant Professor, Departments of Pediatrics and Neurology, Baylor College of Medicine, Houston, Texas

**Salah U. Qureshi, MD**
Neuropsychiatry Fellow, Department of Neurology, Baylor College of Medicine; Mental Illness Research, Education, and Clinical Center Fellow, Department of Psychiatry, MEDVAMC, Houston, Texas

Loren A. Rolak, MD
Director, Marshfield Clinic Multiple Sclerosis Center, Marshfield, Wisconsin; Clinical Professor of Neurology, University of Wisconsin College of Medicine, Madison, Wisconsin; Adjunct Professor of Neurology, Baylor College of Medicine, Houston, Texas

David B. Rosenfield, MD
Professor, Department of Neurology, Weill Medical College of Cornell University; Director, EMG and Motor Control Laboratory; Director, Speech and Language Center, Department of Neurology, The Methodist Hospital Neurological Institute; Adjunct Professor, Department of Communication Sciences and Disorders, University of Houston; Adjunct Professor, Shepherd School of Music, Rice University, Houston, Texas

Paul Rutecki, MD
Department of Neurology and Neurosurgery, University of Wisconsin Medical School; William S. Middleton Veterans Affairs Hospital, Madison, Wisconsin

Pankaj Satija, MD
Assistant Professor, Department of Neurology, The Methodist Neurological Institute, Houston, Texas

Heike Schmolck, MD
Adjunct Assistant Professor, Department of Neurology, Des Moines University; Staff Neurologist/Behavioral Neurology, Department of Neurology, Mercy Medical Center/Ruan Neurology Clinic; Staff Neurologist, Department of Neurology, Lutheran Hospital, Des Moines, Iowa

Paul E. Schulz, MD
Associate Professor of Neurology, Neuroscience, and Translational Biology; Vice Chair for Education, Department of Neurology, Baylor College of Medicine; Department of Neurology, The Methodist Hospital; Director, Cognitive Disorders Clinic, Neurology Careline, The Michael E. DeBakey Veterans Administration Medical Center; Department of Neurology, St. Luke's Episcopal Hospital; Department of Neurology, Ben Taub County Hospital, Houston, Texas

Ericka P. Simpson, MD
Residency Education Director, Co-Director, ALS/MDA Clinics; Director, ALS Clinical Research, Department of Neurology, Methodist Neurological Institute, Houston, Texas

Shane Smyth, MD, MRCPI
Clinical Neuromuscular Fellow, Neuromuscular Disease Section, Baylor College of Medicine, Houston, Texas

Angus A. Wilfong, MD
Associate Professor, Departments of Pediatrics and Neurology, Baylor College of Medicine; Medical Director, Comprehensive Epilepsy Program, Departments of Neurology and Clinical Neurophysiology, Texas Children's Hospital, Houston, Texas

Merrill S. Wise, MD
Sleep Medicine Specialist, Methodist Healthcare Sleep Disorders Center, Memphis, Tennessee

Randall Wright, MD
Medical Director, Stroke Center, St. Luke's Community Hospital, The Woodlands, Texas; Chairman and Director, Neurovascular/Stroke Program, Department of Neurology, Conroe Regional Medical Center, Conroe, Texas; Staff Neurologist, Department of Neurology, Memorial Herman Hospital, The Woodlands, Texas

# PREFACE

The human brain is the most complex object in the universe. With its millions of neurons making trillions of connections, it is what gives each of us our individual personalities, thoughts, and emotions; it is what makes us uniquely human. More scientists are involved in studying the brain than in any other endeavor—there are more neuroscientists than there are astronomers, biologists, chemists, or any other group of specialists. Their studies have profoundly altered our conception of the human brain and the diseases that afflict it, and the treatment of neurologic disease has changed perhaps more than any other field of medicine. During the process of revising the 5th edition of *Neurology Secrets*, it became obvious how much the practice of neurology has advanced in just the past few years. The management of almost every neurologic disease has changed, and in many cases our understanding of basic sciences and disease processes has been fundamentally altered. This new edition, therefore, required the rewriting of many answers, the addition of new questions, and the deletion of old ones. To reflect the pace of change, appropriate websites have been added for further reference and updates.

Neurology is one of the most dynamic medical specialties, and this revised edition should enable the reader to continue asking the right questions and finding the right answers.

Loren A. Rolak, MD

# TOP 100 SECRETS

These secrets are 100 of the top board alerts. They summarize the concepts, principles, and most salient details of neurology.

1. The first step in treating patients with neurologic disease is to localize the lesion.

2. Myopathies cause proximal symmetric weakness without sensory loss.

3. Neuromuscular junction diseases cause fatigability.

4. Peripheral neuropathies cause distal asymmetric weakness with atrophy, fasciculations, sensory loss, and pain.

5. Radiculopathies cause radiating pain.

6. Spinal cord disease causes a triad of distal symmetric weakness, sphincter problems, and a sensory level.

7. A unilateral lesion within the brain stem often causes "crossed syndromes," in which ipsilateral dysfunction of one or more cranial nerves is accompanied by hemiparesis and/or hemisensory loss on the contralateral body.

8. Cerebellar disease causes ataxia and an action tremor.

9. In the brain, cortical lesions may cause aphasia, seizures, and partial hemiparesis (face and arm only), while subcortical lesions may cause visual field cuts, dense numbness of primary sensory modalities, and more complete hemiparesis (face, arm, and leg).

10. The brain is isolated from the rest of the body by the blood-brain barrier.

11. Learning and memory are possible because repetitive input to a synapse can cause persistent changes in neuronal function (long-term potentiation).

12. Some of the most common and important neurologic diseases are caused by abnormalities in neurotransmitters: Alzheimer's (acetylcholine), epilepsy ($\gamma$-aminobutyric acid, GABA), Parkinson's (dopamine), migraine (serotonin), and others.

13. Many genetic neurologic diseases have been shown to be caused by expansion of trinucleotide (triplet) repeat sequences.

14. Foot drop (weakness of the tibialis anterior muscle) can be caused by lesions to the common peroneal nerve or L5 nerve root.

15. If the facial nerve is damaged (such as from Bell's palsy), the entire side of the face is weak. If the cortical input to the facial nerve is damaged (such as from a stroke), only the lower half of the face will be weak.

16. A dilated or "blown" pupil implies compression of the third cranial nerve. This is often due to a serious lesion such as an aneurysm or brain herniation.

17. Collateral blood flow, often routed through the circle of Willis, sometimes protects against damage from strokes.

18. Noncommunicating hydrocephalus is often a medical emergency because the obstructed cerebrospinal fluid (CSF) will cause the intracranial pressure to rise.

19. The diagnosis of myopathies often is based on serum creatine kinase (CK) levels, electromyography (EMG) findings, and muscle biopsy.

20. Myotonic dystrophy is the most common muscular dystrophy in adults.

21. The possibility of respiratory failure is the most serious concern in the management of most patients with myopathies or neuromuscular junction diseases.

22. Drug toxicity should always be considered in the differential diagnosis of many neurologic conditions.

23. Neuroleptic malignant syndrome is a true medical emergency with a high mortality.

24. Patients with myasthenia gravis show a decremental response (fatigue) with repetitive stimulation of their muscles.

25. Up to 40% of myasthenic patients experience a transient exacerbation after starting high-dose steroids, usually within 5 to 7 days.

26. Lambert-Eaton myasthenic syndrome (LEMS) resembles myasthenia gravis with autonomic dysfunction and arises from an autoimmune attack on presynaptic voltage-gated calcium channels.

27. Myotonia, a delayed relaxation after muscle contraction, is most common in muscular dystrophies but can be seen in a host of other conditions.

28. On an EMG, muscle disease shows full contraction of all muscles but with short, small motor units.

29. On an EMG, nerve disease shows a dropout and reduction in muscle contraction, with prolonged, large motor units. There may be fibrillations and fasciculations.

30. The most common causes of peripheral neuropathy are diabetes and alcoholism.

31. The most common motor neuropathy is Guillain-Barré syndrome.

32. Nerve biopsy is seldom necessary for the diagnosis of peripheral neuropathy.

33. The most often overlooked cause of peripheral neuropathy is genetic.

34. The spinal fluid of patients with Guillain-Barré syndrome has high protein but low (normal) cell counts.

35. The most common motor neuron disease is amyotrophic lateral sclerosis (ALS).

36. Indications for surgery in patients with radiculopathies are intractable pain, progressive motor weakness or sensory deficits, or symptoms refractory to a reasonable degree of nonoperative therapy.

37. Neurogenic claudication (pseudoclaudication) presents typically as bilateral, asymmetric, lower extremity pain that is provoked by walking (occasionally standing) and relieved by rest.

38. Sudden damage to the spinal cord can cause spinal shock, which results in temporary flaccid paralysis, hyporeflexia, sensory loss, and loss of bladder tone.

39. Occlusion of the artery of Adamkiewicz may result in anterior spinal artery syndrome, causing bilateral weakness, loss of pain and temperature, and hyperreflexia below the lesion with preserved dorsal column functions (position and vibration).

40. Cauda equina syndrome is a neurosurgical emergency that presents with weakness and sensory loss in the lower extremities, prominent radicular pain, saddle anesthesia, and urinary incontinence.

41. Symptoms of brain stem ischemia are usually multiple, and isolated findings (such as vertigo or diplopia) are more often caused by peripheral lesions affecting individual cranial nerves.

42. Ménière's disease presents with the symptomatic triad of episodic vertigo, tinnitus, and hearing loss. It is caused by an increased amount of endolymph in the scala media. Pathologically, hair cells degenerate in the macula and vestibule.

43. The blood supply of the brain stem is derived from the vertebrobasilar system of the posterior circulation.

44. There are only two causes of coma: a process affecting the reticular activating system in the brain stem or a process affecting both cerebral hemispheres simultaneously.

45. Posterior fossa neoplasms account for 50% of the total number of neoplasms in children. In adults, they are much rarer.

46. Lesions of the cerebellar hemisphere impair movement on the ipsilateral side of the body because of a double-crossing of the pathways.

47. Loss of pigmented dopaminergic neurons in the substantia nigra is the pathologic hallmark of Parkinson's disease.

48. Sinemet (levodopa) remains the most valuable therapy for Parkinson's disease.

49. Essential tremor is the most common cause of tremor.

50. Torticollis is the most common form of focal dystonia.

51. Botulinum toxin is the treatment of choice for most focal dystonias.

52. Tardive dyskinesia is a serious side effect of many neuroleptic drugs.

53. Cardinal symptoms of autonomic insufficiency include orthostatic hypotension, bowel and bladder dysfunction, impotence, and sweating abnormalities.

54. Diabetic neuropathy is one of the most common causes of autonomic dysfunction.

55. Syncope is seldom a neurologic problem; loss of consciousness is almost always due to cardiovascular disease.

56. Traditionally, the diagnosis of multiple sclerosis requires two separate symptoms at two different times, or lesions disseminated in time and space.

57. Faulty interpretation of magnetic resonance imaging (MRI) scans is the most common error in misdiagnosing multiple sclerosis.

58. No treatment has yet been shown to prevent ultimate disability in multiple sclerosis.

59. Dementia must be differentiated from delirium and depression.

60. Dementia is a category, not a diagnosis. The clinician must determine the cause of dementia.

61. Seizures that persist or recur without regaining consciousness are called *status epilepticus*. To avoid permanent brain damage, these should be stopped within 1 hour of onset.

62. Alzheimer's disease and other dementias are treatable. Both cognitive and behavioral symptoms can be treated, and long-term therapy may slow decline and help maintain function.

63. Vascular dementia cannot be diagnosed by MRI or computed tomography (CT) scan alone. It also requires a clinical picture of cerebral ischemia.

64. A common cause of excessive daytime sleepiness is obstructive sleep apnea syndrome.

65. A patient's own assessment of his sleep quantity and quality is often unreliable. Polysomnographic evaluation (sleep laboratory testing) is the only reliable means for obtaining objective information regarding a suspected sleep disturbance.

66. The classic tetrad of narcolepsy is excessive daytime sleepiness, cataplexy, sleep paralysis, and hypnagogic hallucinations.

67. Gliomas are the most common primary brain tumors.

68. Astrocytomas are the most common spinal cord tumors.

69. Metastatic brain tumors are 10 times more common than primary brain tumors.

70. Cancer that metastasizes to the spine usually causes pain, a sensory level, paraplegia, and sphincter disturbances. It is usually treated by radiation therapy.

71. Many cancer patients die in pain because physicians fail to treat pain appropriately.

72. Dysarthria is a defect in the way speech sounds, which can arise from many causes, whereas aphasia is a defect in the use of language and results from damage to the dominant (usually left) cerebral cortex.

73. Antibiotics should be given immediately to patients with meningitis and not delayed while other tests are performed.

74. Mad cow disease is a variant of Creutzfeldt-Jakob disease caused by a prion—a protein that does not require DNA or RNA to replicate and produce infection.

75. Herpes simplex, the most common sporadic encephalitis, often produces focal neurologic damage and must be aggressively treated with acyclovir.

76. Patients with acquired immunodeficiency syndrome (AIDS) may develop problems from the virus itself, the drugs used to treat it, or opportunistic infections.

77. Most patients with a headache due to a serious underlying illness have an abnormal physical examination. The sudden onset of "the worst headache of my life" should raise concern about an intracranial hemorrhage.

78. The use of narcotic analgesics for treatment of headaches should be strongly discouraged.

79. The first-choice drugs for acute migraine therapy are the triptans.

80. The best treatment for tension headache is usually amitriptyline plus a nonsteroidal anti-inflammatory drug (NSAID).

81. Temporal arteritis should be considered in any elderly patient with new headaches.

82. The normal adult electroencephalogram (EEG), relaxed with eyes closed, is characterized by 9 to 11 cycles/sec activity in the back of the brain (occipital lobes) and is called the *alpha rhythm*.

83. Each different stage of sleep has a highly characteristic EEG pattern.

84. In most jurisdictions, a patient is considered to have died if he meets the criteria for brain death, even if his vital signs (e.g., pulse, blood pressure) are otherwise normal.

85. Strokes can be thrombotic, embolic, lacunar, or hemorrhagic.

86. The clinical features, etiology, and treatment of strokes are different depending on whether they involve the anterior circulation (carotid arteries) or posterior circulation (vertebral basilar arteries).

87. The most important modifiable risk factors for stroke are hypertension, smoking, heart disease, hyperlipidemia, and hyperhomocysteinemia. Other modifiable risk factors include diabetes, alcohol consumption, drugs of abuse, oral contraceptives, and obesity.

88. When administered properly, tissue plasminogen activator (tPA) is a beneficial therapy for acute ischemic stroke.

89. The role of anticoagulation in cerebrovascular disease is the prevention of stroke in patients at high risk for cardiac emboli.

90. The best way to prevent strokes is to control the risk factors.

91. Surgery is superior to medical therapy in symptomatic stroke patients with a 70% stenosis or more in their internal carotid arteries.

92. The most important complications of subarachnoid hemorrhage are rebleeding, vasospastic ischemia, hydrocephalus, seizures, and syndrome of inappropriate antidiuretic hormone secretion (SIADH).

93. Accurate seizure classification guides appropriate antiepileptic therapy. Each type of seizures requires its own specific anticonvulsant drug.

94. All partial seizures should be evaluated with an MRI scan.

95. A significant change in antiepileptic drug levels should alert you to either noncompliance or a new drug interaction. Noncompliance is probably the most common cause of status epilepticus.

96. The most common cause of antiepileptic drug treatment failure is drug side effects.

97. Patients whose seizures are refractory to two appropriate antiepileptic drugs should be evaluated at an epilepsy center for definitive diagnosis and surgical evaluation.

98. The most common cause of aphasia in adults is stroke.

99. Broca's aphasia is impaired comprehension, repetition, naming, and speech output due to a left frontal lobe lesion; Wernicke's aphasia is fluent speech full of nonsense words and phrases due to a left temporal lobe lesion.

100. The drug most often recommended by neurologists is acetaminophen!

# CLINICAL NEUROSCIENCE

*Dennis R. Mosier, MD, PhD*

# CHAPTER 1

## INTRODUCTION

1.  **Why is it important to understand the molecular and cellular mechanisms underlying normal and abnormal nervous system function?**
    The answer to this question could easily require a book. Several advantages to the practicing clinician are listed as follows:
    1. Enhancement of diagnostic possibilities and treatment options
    2. More appropriate selection of diagnostic tests and interpretation of test results
    3. Prediction of drug side effects and interactions
    4. Selection of optimal drug regimens
    5. Aid to critical review of novel concepts and therapies
    6. Understanding of the rationale for current clinical trials
    7. Provision of a background for communicating information to patients and families

2.  **Name several types of cellular alterations that can lead directly to neurologic disease.**
    The following is only a partial list:
    1. Altered volume regulation (e.g., cytotoxic edema)
    2. Anatomic alterations
        - Loss of neurons
        - Loss of axons
        - Loss of synaptic connections
    3. Inappropriate synaptic connections
    4. Deafferentation (e.g., loss of receptors in sensory end organs)
    5. Altered membrane excitability
    6. Failure of axonal conduction
    7. Disordered synaptic function
    8. Altered excitation-contraction coupling in muscle

## CELLULAR ANATOMY

3.  **Describe the major types of glial cells in the central nervous system (CNS) and their influence on neurologic disease.**
    1. **Astrocytes**—large glial cells that stabilize extracellular fluids and ions. Astrocytes proliferate in response to many CNS insults and may release neuronal growth factors and form barriers to the spread of infection.
    2. **Oligodendroglia**—myelin-forming glial cells. Myelin antigens may form targets for autoimmune attack in multiple sclerosis.
    3. **Ependymal cells**—neuroepithelial cells lining the ventricular system, choroid plexus, and central canal of the spinal cord.

4. **Microglia**—resident mononuclear phagocytic cells that become reactive in degenerative diseases and demyelinating disorders as well as in more acute CNS insults. They produce numerous cytokines (which regulate inflammatory processes), present antigens to T-cells, and secrete a number of cytotoxic factors (e.g., free radicals, low–molecular-weight neurotoxins).

4. **What are the components of the blood-brain barrier?**
   The blood-brain barrier is not a single barrier, but a composite of many systems that act to control the entry of substances from the blood to the brain:
   1. Capillary **endothelial cells** linked by tight junctions and expressing specialized uptake systems for particular metabolic substrates (e.g., glucose, amino acids)
   2. A prominent **basement membrane** between endothelia and adjacent cells
   3. Pericapillary **astrocytes** with end-feet adjacent to capillaries
   A similar system exists for the choroidal epithelium (blood-cerebrospinal fluid [CSF] barrier).

5. **Which regions of the brain lack a significant blood-brain barrier?**
   Brain regions that lack a significant blood-brain barrier tend to be midline structures located near ventricular spaces. They include the area postrema, median eminence of the hypothalamus, and neurohypophysis.

6. **Under what conditions is the integrity of the blood-brain barrier compromised?**
   - Inflammation or infection
   - Osmotic injury
   - Malignant hypertension
   - Neovascularization (particularly around tumors)
   - Cerebral ischemia and reperfusion
   - Seizure activity
   Compromise of the blood-brain barrier often can be demonstrated by contrast enhancement in radiographic studies or suspected when acute elevations of CSF protein are observed. Consequences of blood-brain barrier (or blood-CSF barrier) compromise include vasogenic edema, enhanced penetration of antibiotics or other drugs, and increased entry of potentially toxic substances from the systemic circulation.

## NERVE CONDUCTION

7. **What is an action potential?**
   The action potential, as classically defined, is an all-or-nothing, regenerative, directionally propagated, depolarizing nerve impulse. In axons, the rising (depolarizing) phase of the action potential is mediated by $Na^+$ currents, which depolarize the membrane. Repolarization of the membrane is influenced by two processes: (1) inactivation of $Na^+$ currents and (2) activation of $K^+$ currents, which hyperpolarizes the membrane. When $Na^+$ currents are inactivated, a new action potential cannot be initiated (absolute refractory period).

8. **What is saltatory conduction?**
   In myelinated axons, currents underlying the action potential flow from one node of Ranvier to another, propagating the action potential by depolarizing distant sites rather than adjacent membrane. This "jumping" of the impulse from node to node, which greatly increases the conduction velocity, is termed *saltatory conduction* (from Latin *saltare,* "to leap").

## SYNAPSES

9. **How are signals transmitted across chemical synapses?**
At a commonly studied excitatory chemical synapse, the neuromuscular junction, the following events occur:
   1. Depolarization of the presynaptic motoneuron terminal by an arriving action potential
   2. Activation of voltage-dependent calcium ($Ca^{2+}$) channels
   3. Entry of $Ca^{2+}$, which locally increases intra-terminal calcium concentrations
   4. Synchronized, quantal release of neurotransmitter from the presynaptic terminal (According to the vesicle hypothesis of release, neurotransmitter packaged in synaptic vesicles is released into the synaptic cleft by exocytosis.)
   5. Diffusion of neurotransmitter across the synaptic cleft
   6. Binding of neurotransmitter to specific receptors on the postsynaptic membrane
   7. Receptor-mediated opening of ion channels that mediate an excitatory postsynaptic potential (an endplate potential at the neuromuscular junction)
   8. Initiation of an action potential in the postsynaptic cell if the postsynaptic potential reaches the threshold of activation

10. **Can synapses undergo modification?**
Synapses are not static structures. They are constantly modified in the nervous system through alterations of connectivity (e.g., sprouting and new synapse formation or retraction of synaptic connections) and alterations in the efficacy of synaptic transmission (e.g., use-dependent facilitation, potentiation, or depression of the function of individual synapses). Induction of both types of synaptic modifications, often referred to as *synaptic plasticity*, may occur at central and peripheral synapses.

11. **Briefly describe the cellular processes thought to subserve learning and memory.**
In most models, the major biologic basis for learning and memory is thought to derive from changes in synaptic function:
   **Long-term potentiation** (LTP) is a long-lasting increase in the amplitude of a synaptic response following stimulation. LTP can be induced by weak but temporally contiguous stimulation of separate input pathways to the same postsynaptic neuron. However, the exact mechanism by which LTP produces memories is an area of considerable debate. Long-term changes in synaptic function may underlie not only normal processes, such as learning and memory, but also the establishment of chronic pain states and recovery from CNS insults.
   Ji RR, Kohno T, Moore KA, et al.: Central sensitization and LTP: Do pain and memory share similar mechanisms? Trends Neurosci 26:696-705, 2003.
   Feldman D: Synaptic mechanisms for plasticity in neocortex. Annu Rev Neurosci 32:542-551, 2009.

## NEUROTRANSMITTERS

12. **How is a chemical substance established as a neurotransmitter?**
As classically proposed, the following features should be demonstrated to establish that a given substance is acting as a neurotransmitter:
   1. Presence of the substance within neuron terminals.
   2. Release of the substance with neuronal stimulation.
   3. Application of the exogenous substance to the postsynaptic membrane (at physiologic concentrations) reproduces the effects of stimulation of the presynaptic neuron.

4. The concentration-response curve of the substance applied to the postsynaptic membrane is affected by drugs in the same way as normal postsynaptic responses are affected.
5. A local mechanism exists for inactivation of the substance (e.g., enzymatic degradation, uptake into nerve terminals or glia).

**13. What is Dale's principle?**

Dale's principle states that a given neuron contains and releases only one neurotransmitter and exerts the same functional effects at all of its termination sites. For example, a spinal motoneuron contains and releases only one neurotransmitter (acetylcholine), which generates the same effect (excitation) at both of its termination sites (neuromuscular junction and recurrent collateral synapse to the Renshaw cell). This useful generalization allows us to describe neurons in terms of their principal transmitters and functions (e.g., a glutamatergic excitatory neuron or a cholinergic inhibitory neuron). However, the assertions of Dale's principle are not universally true.

Gunderson V: Co-localization of excitatory and inhibitory transmitters in the brain. Acta Neurol Scand 188(Suppl):29-33, 2008.

**14. Discuss the anatomy and functions of the neurotransmitter acetylcholine (ACh).**

Acetylcholine is synthesized from acetyl coenzyme A and choline by the enzyme choline acetyltransferase.

At **peripheral synapses**, ACh acts as the principal neurotransmitter of:
■ Motoneurons innervating striated muscle
■ Preganglionic autonomic neurons innervating ganglia
■ Postganglionic parasympathetic neurons
■ Sympathetic sudomotor fibers

The functions of **central cholinergic synapses** are generally less well defined than at peripheral synapses. Central cholinergic pathways or nuclei include:
■ Pedunculopontine nuclei (modulation of sleep states)
■ Projections to the neocortex from basal forebrain nuclei (particularly the nucleus basalis of Meynert, which is thought to be involved early in Alzheimer's disease)
■ Local interneurons in the striatum (regulation of motor activity)

**15. Name and describe the two major types of ACh receptors.**

1. **Nicotinic ACh receptors** (nAchRs) are located at the skeletal neuromuscular junction, in autonomic ganglia, and in the brain. The nAChR at the neuromuscular junction is the major antigenic target in most cases of myasthenia gravis. Mutations in genes encoding subunits of neuronal nicotinic receptors have been linked to some inherited frontal lobe epilepsies.
2. **Muscarinic ACh receptors** (mAchRs) are located in parasympathetic sites and in the brain. Modulation of brain mAChRs can affect sleep-wake states and modify seizure thresholds. It is the main target of drugs to improve cognitive function in patients with dementing illnesses.

**16. What is the most abundant excitatory neurotransmitter in the CNS? By what mechanisms does it induce its effects?**

Glutamate, an excitatory amino acid neurotransmitter, is synthesized from $\alpha$-ketoglutarate by transamination and from glutamine by the enzyme glutaminase. After release from the presynaptic terminal, its most important effects are at N-methyl-D-aspartate (NMDA) receptors. These receptors are thought to be critically involved in processes underlying learning and memory and (if excessively stimulated) may contribute to $Ca^{2+}$-dependent processes that mediate neuronal injury.

17. **What is GABA? How does it exert its action(s)?**
γ -Aminobutyric acid (GABA) is a neurotransmitter synthesized from glutamate via the enzyme glutamic acid decarboxylase (GAD). GABA is metabolized via GABA transaminase. GABA receptors include $GABA_A$ and $GABA_B$ receptors. Receptors of the $GABA_A$ type (the majority of GABA receptors) act as chloride channels, exercising largely inhibitory effects. Many drugs act on GABA pathways. $GABA_A$ receptors are modulated by barbiturates and benzodiazepines; baclofen is an agonist for $GABA_B$ receptors. Vigabatrin (γ-vinyl GABA), a potent anticonvulsant, inhibits GABA transaminase. Of interest, anti-GAD antibodies have been reported in most patients with stiff-person syndrome, which presents with continuous, involuntary muscular activity.

18. **Discuss the synthesis, receptors, and termination of action of the neurotransmitter dopamine.**
Synthesis of catecholamines
1. Tyrosine → L-hydroxyphenylalanine (L-DOPA) via tyrosine hydroxylase (TH)
2. L-DOPA→ dopamine via DOPA decarboxylase
3. Dopamine → norepinephrine via dopamine β-hydroxylase (DBH)
4. Norepinephrine → epinephrine via phenylethanolamine N-methyltransferase (PNMT)
**Receptors.** Five types of dopamine receptors (D1 to D5) have been identified, each exhibiting a distinct pharmacologic profile as well as a unique neuroanatomic distribution.
**Termination of action.** The action of dopamine is terminated primarily by reuptake via specific transporters. Dopamine is also inactivated by catabolism. Intracellular dopamine is oxidatively deaminated by monoamine oxidase to homovanillic acid (HVA), and extracellular dopamine is methylated by catechol O-methyltransferase (COMT) to produce dihydroxyphenylacetic acid (DOPAC).

19. **List the major functions of dopamine in the nervous system.**
1. Motor control (via nigrostriatal projections)
2. Modulation of short-term or working memory (via projections from ventral tegmental area to prefrontal cortex)
3. Behavioral reinforcement (via mesolimbic projections)
4. Hypothalamic regulation of pituitary function (e.g., by inhibiting prolactin secretion)
5. Modulation of brain regions controlling emesis (e.g., area postrema of the medulla)
Salamone JD: Dopamine, effort, and decision making. Behav Neurosci 123:463-467, 2009.

20. **What is serotonin?**
Serotonin, or 5-hydroxytryptamine (5-HT), is produced from the amino acid tryptophan by the actions of two enzymes, tryptophan hydroxylase and an aromatic amino acid decarboxylase. The action of released 5-HT is terminated by reuptake into nerve terminals; its major metabolite is 5-hydroxyindoleacetic acid (5-HIAA), which is formed following oxidative deamination by monoamine oxidase.

21. **Where does serotonin act in the nervous system?**
Serotonergic neurons are found in the **raphe nuclei** of the brain stem. N-Acetylation of serotonin by cells of the **pineal gland** is followed by O-methylation to produce the hormone melatonin. Multiple receptor subtypes for 5-HT have been described. The $5\text{-HT}_{1B}$ and $5\text{-HT}_{1D}$ receptors, which are found on **trigeminal nerve terminals supplying cranial blood vessels** and meninges, modulate the vasodilatation associated with migraine headaches. $5\text{-HT}_3$ receptor antagonists, such as ondansetron, which have both peripheral and central actions, are effective in suppressing nausea and vomiting.
    Some of the most common and important neurologic diseases are caused by abnormalities in neurotransmitters: Alzheimer's (ACh), epilepsy (GABA), Parkinson's (dopamine), migraine (serotonin), and others.
    Dayan P, Huys QJ: Serotonin in affective control. Annu Rev Neurosci 32:578-591, 2009.

22. **What is denervation supersensitivity?**

 Two to three weeks after the loss of an innervating neuron, the postsynaptic membrane of an innervated cell develops increased sensitivity to the neurotransmitter that was released by the presynaptic terminal of the innervating neuron. This hypersensitivity underlies many phenomena observed in clinical neurology.

## KEY POINTS: NEURONS AND NEUROTRANSMITTERS

1. The brain is isolated from the rest of the body by a blood-brain barrier.

2. Learning and memory are possible because repetitive input to a synapse can cause persistent changes in neuronal function (long-term potentiation).

3. Most neurons contain a single neurotransmitter with a single mechanism of action, but there are exceptions to this rule.

### ION CHANNELS

23. **What is an ion channel? How does it work?**

 Ion channels, formed from membrane-spanning proteins, allow the selective and rapid flux of ions across cell membranes. Channels respond to (are gated by) specific stimuli, such as changes in the transmembrane voltage gradient (voltage-gated channels), chemical agonists (ligand-gated channels), or mechanical stretch or pressure.

24. **What are ion channelopathies? How do they present clinically?**

 Ion channelopathies, or disorders in which the clinical presentation results primarily from ion channel dysfunction, frequently present with brief exacerbations or episodes of clinical symptoms. In such disorders (e.g., periodic paralysis), interictal function is typically normal, and attacks are often triggered by specific factors (e.g., exercise, temperature changes, startle responses, and drugs). Therapies, in addition to symptom management and treatment of underlying causes of the ion-channel abnormality (e.g., autoimmunity), have been directed at identification and avoidance of triggering factors as well as use of drugs that ameliorate the specific ion-channel dysfunction observed at the molecular level.

 Ackerman MJ, Clapham DE: Ion channels—basic science and clinical disease. N Engl J Med 336:1575-1586, 1997.

25. **In which disorders affecting the nervous system have abnormalities of potassium channel function been suggested to play a critical role?**

 **Ataxia-myokymia syndrome** (EA-1), presenting as dominantly inherited myokymia and episodic ataxia, has been associated with mutations for a $K^+$ channel expressed in brain and peripheral nerve.

 1. Two of the **dominantly inherited long Q-T syndromes** (LQT1 and LQT2), which may present as syncopal seizures as well as syncope and sudden cardiac death, are associated with mutations in genes encoding $K^+$ channels.

 2. Recently, syndromes of dominantly inherited **benign familial neonatal convulsions**, which may be associated with an increased risk of adult epilepsy, have been linked to mutations, which encode $K^+$ channels expressed in the brain.

 3. Some cases of **Isaacs' syndrome**, which presents as acquired neuromyotonia, have been suggested to result from an antibody-mediated autoimmune attack on $K^+$ channels in motor nerves.

4. Some **snake toxins** (e.g., dendrotoxin from the African green mamba) exhibit potent $K^+$ channel–blocking activity.

Benarroch EE: Potassium channels: Brief overview and implications in epilepsy. Neurology 72:664-669, 2009.

26. **In which neurologic disorders is alteration or dysfunction of calcium channels believed to play a critical role?**
   ■ Lambert-Eaton myasthenic syndrome: autoimmune attack on voltage-gated $Ca^{2+}$ channel at motoneuron terminals
   ■ Hypokalemic periodic muscle paralysis: mutation in gene coding for the skeletal voltage-gated $Ca^{2+}$ channel
   ■ Familial hemiplegic migraine and episodic ataxia type 2: mutation in gene coding for $Ca^{2+}$ channel in brain

   Meola G, Hanna MG, Fontaine B: Diagnosis and new treatment in muscle channelopathies. J Neurol Neurosurg Psychiatry 80:360-365, 2009.

   Pietrobon D: Calcium channels and channelopathies of the central nervous system. Mol Neurobiol 25:31-50, 2002.

## NEURONAL INJURY AND DEATH

27. **What is the excitotoxicity hypothesis? Why is it important?**
   The excitotoxicity concept states that overstimulation of neurons (by chemical or electrical means) leads to cell injury or death. In the CNS, excitotoxicity is hypothesized to occur with processes (e.g., ischemia, seizure activity, and some neurodegenerative diseases) that lead to elevated concentrations of excitatory amino acids such as glutamate. Interaction of high levels of glutamate with NMDA receptors results in increased calcium entry, which may injure susceptible cells. Much of the damage induced by short-term ischemia in animal models of stroke can be blocked by antagonists of glutamate receptors. Riluzole, a drug that affects glutamate receptor function, has shown limited efficacy in patients with amyotrophic lateral sclerosis. Memantine, a drug with NMDA-receptor blocking activity, has shown benefit in patients with Alzheimer's disease.

   Dong X, Wang Y, Qin Z: Molecular mechanisms of excitotoxicity and their relevance to pathogenesis of neurodegenerative diseases. Acta Pharmacol 30:379-387, 2009.

28. **What are free radicals? What is their relationship to neuronal injury?**
   Free radicals are molecules with one or more unpaired electrons, such as superoxide anion ($O_2^-$) and hydroxyl radical (OH). Free radical–induced biochemical alterations have been documented in ischemic stroke as well as many neurodegenerative diseases. The challenge has been to establish whether these changes initiate cell injury, amplify other pathologic processes, or occur simply as late markers of cell injury. Two basic strategies are being tested to modify free radical–induced damage in neurologic illness: antioxidants, which reduce free radical production, and free-radical scavengers, which react with free radicals to trap unpaired electrons.

29. **Discuss the differences between necrotic and apoptotic neuronal death.**
   **Necrotic cell death** is generally triggered by an insult that overwhelms cellular homeostatic mechanisms and proceeds by cell swelling, disruption of organelles, and eventual lysis of dying cells. In contrast, the characteristic features of **apoptotic cell death** are chromatin condensation, DNA fragmentation, cell membrane blebbing, loss of the nuclear membrane, and eventual fragmentation of the cell into easily phagocytosed "apoptotic bodies."

   Apoptotic cell death is believed to be a major means of cell death induced by irradiation (tumor cells), glucocorticoids (lymphocytes), cell death mediated by cytotoxic T-lymphocytes, and growth-factor withdrawal. Early-onset forms of spinal muscular atrophy have been linked to mutations in neuronal apoptosis inhibitory protein (NAIP) genes. Enhanced susceptibility to apoptosis induced by normally sublethal insults has been documented in animal models of adult-onset neurodegenerative illnesses; the contribution of this form of cell death to the corresponding human disorders remains to be defined.

## REGULATORY PROTEINS

30. **What are adhesion molecules? How may they play a role in neurologic disease?**
Cell adhesion to other cells and to the extracellular matrix regulates many cellular functions, including neurite outgrowth during development, cell growth, cell recognition, immune responses, and responses to mechanical stress. Examples of specialized molecules involved in cell adhesion include the following:
1. ICAM-1 (an intercellular adhesion molecule) is up-regulated in endothelial cells after cerebral ischemia and may potentiate injury by facilitating invasion of neutrophils into ischemic brain tissue.
2. Merosin (an extracellular matrix component) is deficient in one form of congenital muscular dystrophy.
3. Mutations in the gene for L1CAM (L1-neural cell adhesion molecule) are associated with an X-linked syndrome of mental retardation, hydrocephalus, and agenesis of the corpus callosum.
4. Cell adhesion molecules with known signaling functions may serve as receptors for pathogenic organisms or regulate their entry. For instance, entry of the retrovirus HTLV-1 (a cause of tropical spastic paraparesis) into susceptible cells is inhibited by CD82 adhesion molecules.
   Finckh U, Schroder J, Ressler B, et al.: Spectrum and detection rate of L1CAM mutations in isolated and familial cases with clinically suspected L1-disease. Am J Med Genet 92:40-46, 2000.
   Pique C, Lagaudriere-Gesbert C, Delamarre L, et al.: Interaction of CD82 tetraspanin with HTLV-1 envelope glycoproteins inhibits cell-to-cell fusion and virus transmission. Virology 276:455-465, 2000.

31. **What is a neurotrophic factor?**
During development, the survival of many types of neurons requires one or more factors derived from the targets that the neurons innervate. The most famous of the neurotrophic factors, or factors that promote the survival and growth of neurons, is nerve growth factor (NGF). Although primary deficiency of neurotrophic factors has not been shown to cause any of the major human neurodegenerative diseases, growing evidence indicates that these factors can regulate neuronal properties even in the adult nervous system and may have survival-promoting effects on neurons injured by a variety of causes.

## MOLECULAR BIOLOGY

32. **What is the fundamental principle of molecular biology?**
The fundamental principle of molecular biology states that the flow of genetic information in cells is from DNA to RNA to protein. Synthesis of RNA from a DNA template is called *transcription*, whereas synthesis of protein from an RNA template is called *translation*. A notable exception to this principle is the replication of certain RNA viruses (retroviruses), in which DNA can be synthesized from an RNA template by reverse transcriptase.

**33. Distinguish among the terms *gene*, *allele*, *polymorphism*, and *mutation*.**
A **gene** is the nucleic acid sequence that carries the information to build a particular protein. **Alleles** are any of the alternative forms (sequence variants) of a gene. **Polymorphism** occurs when multiple alleles on any locus exist as stable components in a population. In common usage, a nondisease-causing genetic variant is termed a *benign polymorphism*. A **mutation** is a change in DNA sequence (which may or may not result in detectable effects). Obviously, alleles, including those that are now considered benign polymorphisms, resulted from mutations in the past.

**34. Name several types of genomic alterations that can lead to disease.**
1. Single base-pair substitutions: may alter a single amino acid or stop the DNA from being read
2. Insertion or deletion of one or more base pairs: may alter the reading frame (frameshift)
3. Repetition of sequences of base pairs (e.g., triplet repeat mutations)
4. Duplication of a gene or chromosome (e.g., PMP22 gene duplication in Charcot-Marie-Tooth disease 1A)
5. Chromosomal deletion or translocation
6. Imprinting due to differential activity of paternal and maternal copies of a gene
7. Alterations of a regulatory protein (e.g., a promoter region) that controls expression of one or more downstream genes
8. Alteration in a gene with widespread effects on DNA transcription (e.g., the MeCP-2 gene in Rett syndrome) may cause misregulation of a large number of distant genes
   Bernard G, Shevell M: The wobbly child: An approach to inherited ataxias. Semin Pediatr Neurol 15:194-208, 2008.

**35. What is the polymerase chain reaction?**
Polymerase chain reaction (PCR) is a process that is used to amplify a region of DNA, thus allowing it to be detected with high sensitivity. It requires knowledge of the DNA sequence on either side of a target region *(flanking sequence)*. DNA primers matching the flanking sequence are used to initiate copying of the target region DNA by a heat-stable DNA polymerase. The resulting DNA strands are then heated to separate them and allow the primers to copy again, synthesizing new strands. This cycle is repeated until the desired amplification (repeated copying) of the target region DNA is achieved.

**36. What are functional cloning and positional cloning?**
Two principal strategies have been used to isolate genes underlying human genetic disorders:
1. **Functional cloning** is based on identification of the protein that is altered in a disorder, with subsequent sequencing of the protein and design of cDNA probes to try to find the gene coding for the protein. This approach requires prior knowledge of the defective protein, which is not available for most inherited diseases.
2. The more recent approach is **positional cloning** (reverse genetics), in which the gene responsible for a disease phenotype is mapped to a chromosomal location, usually by analysis of markers linked to it or by identifying an associated genetic defect (chromosomal translocation or deletion). This candidate region is then physically mapped, cloned, and ultimately sequenced to identify genetic mutations associated with the disease phenotype. The task of identifying the function(s) of the altered protein product and the mechanism(s) by which it produces disease then begins. In many cases, the second task may prove more difficult than the task of isolating the disease gene.

**37. What are trinucleotide or triplet repeats? How have they been linked to neurologic diseases?**
In many genes, short blocks of repeated sequences (e.g., CAGCAG... or CTGCTG...) normally occur. Expansions of these trinucleotide or triplet repeat sequences beyond their normal size have recently been associated with a number of neurodegenerative disorders, including the following:

- Fragile X syndrome
- Myotonic dystrophy (DMPK or myotonic dystrophy protein kinase gene)
- Huntington's disease (Huntington gene)
- X-linked spinobulbar muscular atrophy (androgen receptor gene)
- Dentatorubral-pallidoluysian atrophy
- Spinocerebellar atrophies (notably SCA1 [ataxin-1 gene] and SCA6 [CACNL1A4, coding for a P/Q-type voltage-gated $Ca^{2+}$ channel])
- Friedreich's ataxia (frataxin gene)

For most of these disorders, longer repeat size is associated with an earlier age of onset and/or more severe phenotype. The length of expanded repeats is characteristically unstable, and often lengthens further with successive generations, producing the clinical phenomenon of **anticipation** (earlier onset and more severe phenotype with successive generations).

## FUTURE DIRECTIONS

38. **Discuss the prion hypothesis and its relevance to neurologic disease.**
The transmissible spongiform encephalopathies are caused by infectious proteins called *prions*. The prion hypothesis states that infectivity is transmitted solely by the altered protein and does not require reproduction using DNA or RNA. The infection instead is caused by a conformational change in a normal protein (PrP or prion protein) that is caused by some sort of interaction with the abnormal form of the same protein. The information necessary for replication is contained within the conformation of the protein itself. This represents a challenge to the fundamental principle of molecular biology that DNA is required for replication (see question 32). Human prion diseases include kuru, Creutzfeldt-Jakob disease, Gerstmann-Sträussler-Scheinker disease, fatal familial insomnia, and variant CJD or "mad cow" disease.

Lai E: Prion diseases. In Samuels MA, Feske SE (eds): Office Practice of Neurology. Philadelphia, Churchill-Livingstone, 2003, pp 512-514.

39. **What is a stem cell?**
Stem cells are cells with the potential to give rise to precursors of different cell types. Stem cells may be pluripotent (able to give rise to precursors of many different cell types) or unipotent (apparently committed to a particular lineage). They have the capacity, at least theoretically, to regenerate injured tissues. Increasing evidence has shown that neural stem cells exist not only during CNS development, but also in the adult CNS, and may be activated by injury. Moreover, bone marrow–derived hematopoietic stem cells recently were induced to differentiate along neuronal lines, thus providing another potential source of neuronal cells for transplantation.

Isaacson O: The production and use of cells as therapeutic agents in neurodegenerative diseases. Lancet Neurol 2:417-424, 2003.

## KEY POINTS: NEUROLOGIC DISEASES

1. Some neurologic diseases (HIV infection, prion diseases) seem to violate the fundamental principle of molecular biology that information flows from DNA to RNA to proteins.

2. Many genetic neurologic diseases have been shown to be caused by expansion of trinucleotide (triplet) repeat sequences.

3. Prion diseases, all of which are neurologic (including "mad cow" disease), represent an entirely unknown area of biology.

40. **Name several potential obstacles to successful neuronal transplantation in humans.**
   The following is only a partial list:
   1. Appropriate differentiation of neurons (e.g., from stem cells)
   2. Maintaining stability of neuronal phenotype over time
   3. Regulating neurotransmitter production and cell proliferation
   4. Making connections with both upstream and downstream targets
   5. Reintegration into functioning neural networks (i.e., "relearning")
   6. Protection from ongoing disease processes
   7. Ethical issues with cells derived from human embryos
   At present, it is unknown which of these obstacles will pose serious challenges to the success of neuronal transplants. However, the potential for improvement using cell transplants may be quite large, and a number of clinical trials are under way to evaluate the safety and efficacy of neuronal transplantation in a variety of CNS disorders.
   Freed CR, Greene PE, Breeze RE, et al.: Transplantation of embryonic dopamine neurons for severe Parkinson disease. N Engl J Med 344:710-719, 2001.

41. **Describe some of the challenges encountered in producing successful "gene therapy" for neurologic disorders.**
   1. Loss of function, which can be corrected with replacement of nonfunctioning genes, accounts for only a small percentage of genetic disorders. Disorders resulting from a toxic gain of function may require suppression of abnormal gene product or actual correction of the defective DNA sequences, a more formidable task.
   2. Most vectors for introducing DNA into cells are inefficient (i.e., only a minority of cells successfully express the introduced gene).
   3. Expression of proteins from viral vectors on cell surfaces may trigger host immune responses.
   4. Introduction of the normal protein itself may trigger host immune responses.
   5. Expression of introduced DNA may be transient.
   6. Vectors may introduce genes into nontarget cells.
   7. Integrated DNA sequences may be regulated abnormally.
   This is only a partial list. Despite these challenges, the promise of correcting genetic disorders at a fundamental level has spurred a high level of research aimed at bringing gene therapies to clinical trial. The recent results from replacement of the gene encoding for adenosine deaminase in T cells of patients with one form of severe immunodeficiency have further stimulated interest in extending gene therapeutic approaches to brain and neuromuscular disorders.

# WEBSITE

http://www.thalamus.wustl.edu/course

# BIBLIOGRAPHY

1. Hille B: Ionic Channels of Excitable Membranes, 3rd ed. Sunderland, MA, Sinauer, 2001.
2. Kandel ER, Schwartz JH, Jessell TM: Principles of Neural Science, 4th ed. New York, McGraw-Hill, 2000.
3. Mather JP: Stem Cell Culture (Methods in Cell Biology, vol. 86). San Diego, Academic Press, 2008.
4. Squire LR, Berg D, Bloom F, et al.: Fundamental Neuroscience, 3rd ed. New York, Academic Press, 2008.

# CHAPTER 2

# CLINICAL NEUROANATOMY

*Brian D. Loftus, MD, Sudhir S. Athni, MD, and Igor M. Cherches, MD*

## EMBRYOLOGY

1. **How is the neural tube formed?**
   Beginning around the eighteenth gestational day, a midline notochordal thickening anterior to the blastopore forms the neural plate. A midsagittal groove called the *neural groove* appears in the plate, and the sides elevate to form the neural folds. As the folds fuse, the neural tube is formed. Some cells at the edges of the fold do not fuse into the tube and become neural crest cells.

2. **What types of cells are derived from the neural crest cells?**
   Neural crest cells give rise to (1) unipolar sensory cells, (2) postganglionic cells of sympathetic and parasympathetic ganglia, (3) chromaffin cells of the adrenal medulla, (4) some microglial cells, (5) pia mater, (6) some arachnoid cells, (7) melanocytes, and (8) Schwann cells.

3. **What are the alar plate and the basal plate?**
   As the neural tube is formed, a longitudinal groove appears on each side and divides the neural tube into a dorsal half, or alar plate, and a ventral half, or basal plate. The **alar plate** gives rise to the prosencephalon; the sensory and coordinating nuclei of the thalamus; the sensory neurons of the cranial nerves; the coordinating nuclei including cerebellum, inferior olives, red nucleus, and quadrigeminal plate; and the posterior horn area (sensory) of the spinal cord. The **basal plate** stops at the level of the diencephalon and gives rise to the motor neurons of the cranial nerves and anterior horn (motor) area of the spinal cord.

4. **What is the process of formation of the ventricles, prosencephalon, mesencephalon, and rhombencephalon?**
   Around the end of the first gestational month, a series of bulges anterior to the first cervical somites appears. The first bulge is the prosencephalon, or forebrain. The cavity of this bulge forms the lateral ventricles and third ventricle. Secondary outpouchings from the forebrain are called *optic vesicles* and eventually form the retina, pigment epithelium, and optic nerve. The second bulge is the mesencephalon, or midbrain. The cavity of this bulge forms the cerebral aqueduct. The third bulge is the rhombencephalon, or hindbrain. This cavity gives rise to the fourth ventricle.

5. **Which structures arise from the prosencephalon, mesencephalon, and rhombencephalon?**
   The **prosencephalon** develops into the telencephalon, which includes the cerebral cortex and basal ganglia, and the diencephalon, which includes the thalamus and the hypothalamus. The **mesencephalon** gives rise to the midbrain. The **rhombencephalon** gives rise to the metencephalon (pons plus cerebellum) and myelencephalon (medulla). See Table 2-1.

TABLE 2-1. EMBRYONIC DIVISIONS OF THE CENTRAL NERVOUS SYSTEM

| Embryonic Divisions | Adult Derivatives | Ventricular Cavities |
| --- | --- | --- |
| **Forebrain (prosencephalon)** | | |
| Telencephalon | Cerebral cortex | Lateral ventricles |
| | Basal ganglia | |
| Diencephalon | Thalamus | |
| | Hypothalamus | |
| | Subthalamus | Third ventricle |
| | Epithalamus | |
| Midbrain (mesencephalon) | Tectum | Aqueduct |
| | Cerebral peduncles | |
| **Hindbrain (rhombencephalon)** | | |
| Metencephalon | Cerebellum | Fourth ventricle |
| | Pons | |
| Myelencephalon | Medulla | |
| Spinal cord | Spinal cord | No cavity |

## MUSCLE

6. **What is the histologic organization of skeletal muscle?**
   Skeletal muscle is composed of long, thin, cylindrical, multinucleated cells called
   *musclefibers* (or myofibrils). Each fiber has a motor endplate at its neuromuscular junction
   and is surrounded by connective tissue called *endomysium*. Groups of fibers, or a fascicle,
   are surrounded by a connective tissue layer called the *perimysium*. Fascicles are grouped
   together and surrounded by epimysium.

7. **What is found at the A band, H band, I band, and Z line?**
   The **A band** contains the thin filaments (actin) and the thick filaments (myosin). The **H band**
   is the portion of the A band that contains only myosin, and the **I band** is the portion that
   contains only actin. The actin is anchored at the **Z line** (Figure 2-1).

8. **How does the muscle contract?**
   When the sarcoplasmic reticulum is depolarized, calcium ions enter the cell and bind to
   troponin. This causes a conformational change that allows exposure of the actin-binding site
   to myosin. The myosin attaches to the actin-binding site and flexes, causing the actin filament
   to slide by the myosin filament. Adenosine triphosphate (ATP) is required to allow the
   myosin-actin crossbridge to release and the muscle to relax.

9. **What is meant by the term *motor unit*?**
   The motor unit is one motor nerve (lower motor neuron) and all muscle fibers that it innervates.

## THE MUSCLE STRETCH REFLEX

10. **What is the muscle stretch reflex?**
    The muscle stretch reflex is a reflex arc that responds to stretching of muscle fibers to
    keep the muscle in an appropriate state of tension and tone, ready to contract or relax as

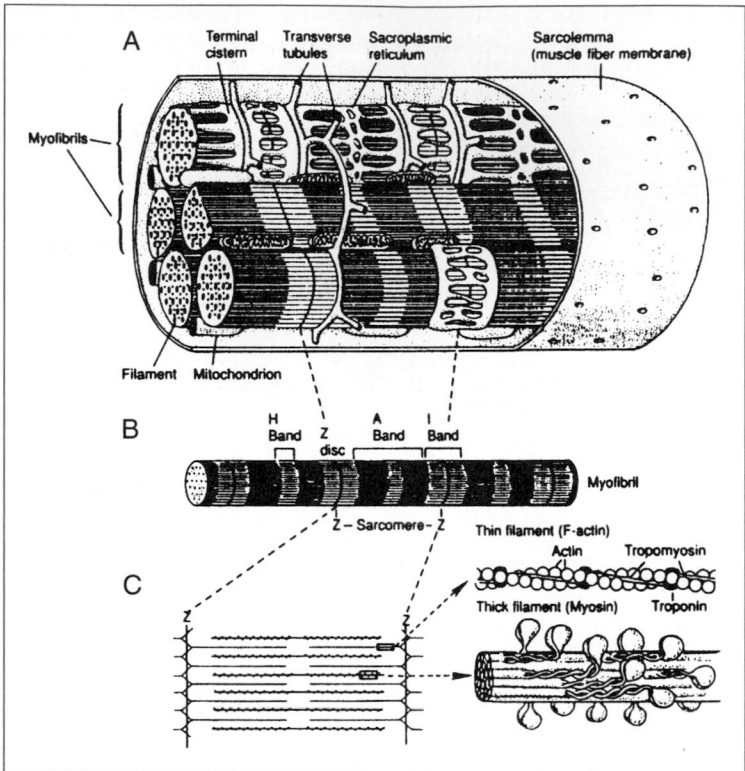

A

Terminal cistern | Transverse tubules | Sacroplasmic reticulum | Sarcolemma (muscle fiber membrane)

Myofibrils

Filament   Mitochondrion

B

H Band   Z disc   A Band   I Band

Myofibril

Z – Sarcomere – Z

Thin filament (F-actin)

Actin   Tropomyosin

C

Thick filament (Myosin)   Troponin

**Figure 2-1.** The histologic anatomy of the human skeletal muscle. From Kandel E, Schwartz JH, Jessell TM (eds): Principles of Neuroscience, 3rd ed. New York, Elsevier, 1991, p 549.

needed. The sensory input (afferent) of the reflex is from two structures in the muscle called *spindles* and *Golgi tendon organs*. The output (efferent) is the alpha motor neuron that contracts (tightens) the muscle. (The muscle fibers are sometimes referred to as *extrafusal fibers*.)

11. **What type of nerve fiber innervates the muscle?**
    An anterior horn motor neuron, called an *alpha motor neuron,* innervates the muscle. It is the final common pathway for muscle contraction.

12. **What is the function of the Ia nerve fiber?**
    The Ia nerve arises from annulospiral endings within the muscle spindle. When the muscle spindle is stretched (i.e., when the muscle is relaxed), the Ia sensory nerve, through the dorsal root, monosynaptically stimulates the alpha motor neuron, which fires and contracts (shortens) the muscle. Thus, the muscle stretch reflex maintains tone and tension in the muscle, by contracting it when it gets too relaxed.

13. **Is the Ia reflex monosynaptic or polysynaptic?**
    It is monosynaptic, but it initiates a polysynaptic inhibition of the antagonist muscle group.

14. **In the spinal cord, which nerve fibers synapse on the alpha motor neuron?**
    Both the corticospinal tract and afferent Ia sensory nerves regulate the alpha motor neuron by snapping on it in the anterior horn of the spinal cord. Renshaw cells are interneurons that are stimulated by the alpha motor neuron and then, by a feedback mechanism, inhibit the alpha motor neuron, causing auto inhibition.

15. **What is the role of the gamma efferent nerve?**
    The muscle spindle is kept tense and responsive by tiny muscle fibers inside it, called *intrafusal fibers*. The gamma efferent nerve fibers keep the muscle spindles "tight" by innervating and contracting the intrafusal fibers in the muscle spindle. This process ensures that the spindle remains sensitive to any stretch.

16. **Where does the Ib fiber originate?**
    The Ib fiber originates from the Golgi tendon organ, another structure that monitors muscle stretch and acts to inhibit muscle contraction (not shown in the diagram).

17. **Where does the Ib neuron synapse?**
    At the spinal cord level, the Ib sensory nerve polysynaptically inhibits the alpha motor neuron to prevent muscle contraction and also stimulates the gamma efferent nerve to the intrafusal fiber to reset the muscle spindle.

## LUMBOSACRAL PLEXUS AND LEG INNERVATION

18. **Which roots make up the lumbar plexus?**
    Roots of L1, L2, L3, L4, and sometimes T12 make up the lumbar plexus.

19. **What are the two largest branches of the lumbar plexus?**
    1. **Obturator nerve (L2, L3, L4).** It leaves the pelvis through the obturator foramen and supplies the adductors of the thigh.
    2. **Femoral nerve (L2, L3, L4).** It exits the pelvis with the femoral artery and supplies the hip flexors and knee extensors. Distally, it continues as the saphenous nerve to supply sensation to the medial anterior knee and medial distal leg, including the medial malleolus (Figure 2-2).

20. **What are the other branches of the lumbar plexus?**
    1. **Iliohypogastric nerve (L1)**—sensation to skin over hypogastric and gluteal areas; to abdominal muscles
    2. **Ilioinguinal nerve (L1)**—sensation to skin over groin and scrotum (labia)
    3. **Genitofemoral nerve (L1, L2)**—enters the internal inguinal ring and runs in the inguinal canal
    4. **Lateral femoral cutaneous nerve (L2, L3)**—sensation to skin over anterior and lateral parts of the thigh

21. **Which nerve is at risk during appendectomy (McBurney's incision)?**
    The iliohypogastric nerve may be cut as it passes between the external and internal oblique muscles. This results in weakness in the inguinal canal area, putting the patient at risk for direct inguinal hernia.

22. **What is meralgia paresthetica?**
    Meralgia paresthetica is numbness and tingling in the lateral thigh secondary to compression of the lateral femoral cutaneous nerve as it runs over the inguinal ligament. It commonly occurs in obese or pregnant patients. It can also be caused by placing hard objects in the pockets of low rider jeans.

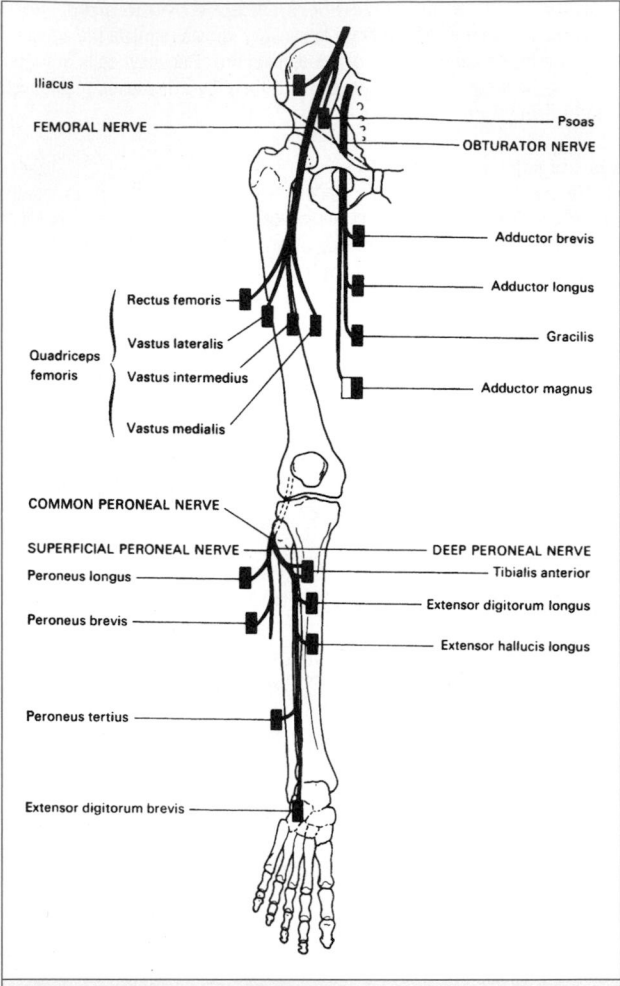

**Figure 2-2.** Diagram of the nerves and muscles on the anterior aspect of the lower limb. From Medical Research Council: Aids to the Examination of the Peripheral Nervous System, London, 1976.

23. **Which nerve supplies the gluteus maximus?**
    The inferior gluteal nerve (L5, S1, S2) supplies the gluteus maximus muscle.

24. **What is the largest nerve in the body?**
    The sciatic nerve (L4, L5, S1, S2, S3), the largest nerve in the body, is composed of the common peroneal nerve (L4, L5, S1, S2) in its dorsal division and the tibial nerve (L4, L5, S1, S2, S3) in its ventral division (Figure 2-3).

25. **What is the only nerve in the sacral plexus that emerges through the greater sciatic foramen, superior to the piriformis muscle?**
    The superior gluteal nerve (L4, L5, S1) supplies the gluteus medius and minimus, and tensor fascia lata (abduction and medial rotation of the thigh).

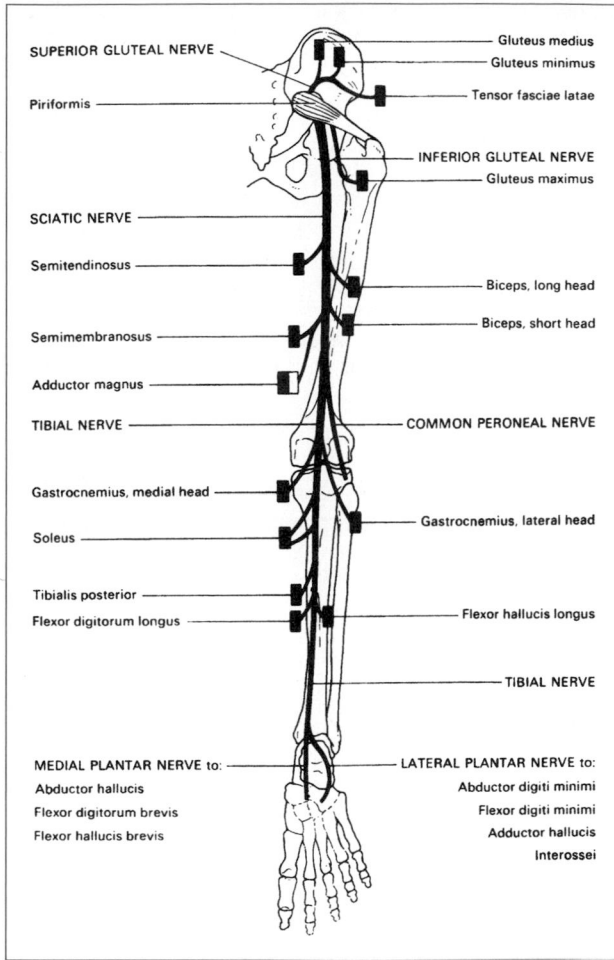

**Figure 2-3.** Diagram of the nerves and muscles on the posterior aspect of the lower limb. From Medical Research Council: Aids to the Examination of the Peripheral Nervous System, London, 1976.

26. **Which nerve supplies the inferior buttock and posterior thigh?**
    The posterior femoral cutaneous nerve (S1, S2, S3), which runs with the inferior gluteal nerve, supplies the inferior buttock and posterior thigh.

27. **Which nerve supplies the structures in the perineum?**
    The pudendal nerve (S2, S3, S4) supplies the perineum.

28. **What is the only muscle supplied by the sciatic nerve that receives innervation exclusively from the dorsal division (i.e., peroneal component) of the sciatic nerve?**
    The biceps femoris has only dorsal innervation. This point is important clinically in trying to differentiate lesions caused by damage to the common peroneal nerve versus the sciatic nerve itself.

29. **Which muscles are supplied by the tibial nerve?**
    The tibial nerve supplies plantar flexors and invertors of the foot.

30. **What are the two divisions of the common peroneal nerve?**
    1. **Deep peroneal nerve**—dorsiflexion of the foot and toes and sensation to a small area of skin between the first and second toes.
    2. **Superficial peroneal nerve**—evertors of the foot and sensation to the skin of the dorsal and lateral foot.

## BRACHIAL PLEXUS AND ARM INNERVATION

31. **The brachial plexus comprises which roots?**
    The brachial plexus comprises the ventral rami of C5, C6, C7, C8, and T1 (Figure 2-4).

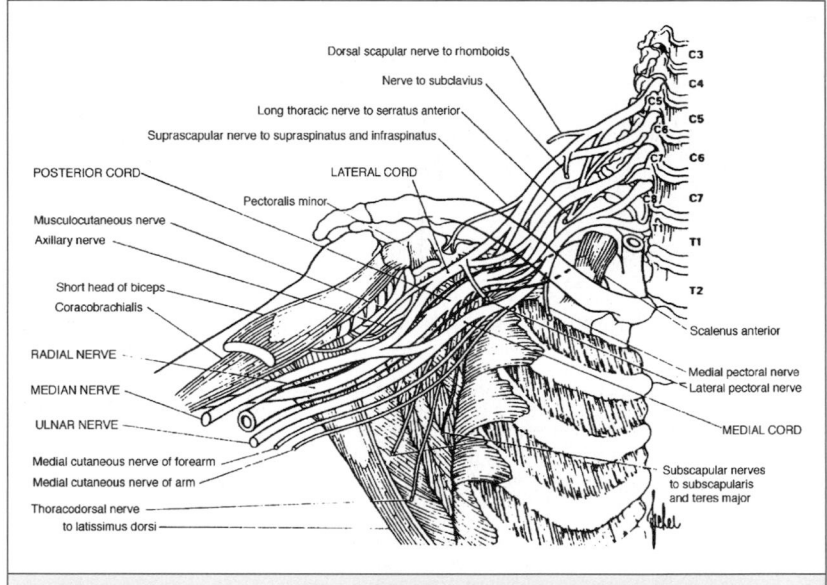

**Figure 2-4.** The brachial plexus. From Tindall B: Aids to the Examination of the Peripheral Nervous System. London, W.B. Saunders, 1990.

32. **Which nerves arise from the ventral rami of the roots before formation of the brachial plexus?**
    1. **Dorsal scapular nerve**, from C5 to rhomboid and levator scapula muscles; responsible for elevation and stabilization of the scapula.
    2. **Long thoracic nerve**, from C5, C6, C7 to serratus anterior; responsible for abduction of the scapula.
       Testing these nerves is useful in differentiating between root and plexus lesions. If there is a deficit in one of these nerves (clinically or electrically), the lesion is proximal to the plexus.

33. **Which roots form the three trunks of the brachial plexus?**
(1) Superior trunk, formed by C5 and C6; (2) middle trunk, formed by C7; and (3) lower trunk, formed by C8 and T1.

34. **Which nerves originate from the cervical roots before formation of the brachial plexus?**
Dorsal scapular nerve (C5) and long thoracic nerve (C5, C6, C7).

35. **What is the only nerve from the trunks of the brachial plexus?**
The suprascapular nerve (C5) comes off the upper trunk and supplies the supraspinatus (abduction) and infraspinatus (external rotation) of the shoulder.

36. **Which vascular structure is associated with the three cords of the brachial plexus?**
The lateral cord (C5, C6, C7), medial cord (C8, T1), and posterior cord (C5, C6, C7, C8) are named in relationship to the axillary artery.

37. **What are the nerves off the cords of the brachial plexus?**
Lateral cord
1. Lateral pectoral nerve (C5, C6, C7)—to pectoralis minor
2. Musculocutaneous nerve (C5, C6)—to brachialis and coracobrachialis (elbow flexion)
3. Median nerve (partial; C6, C7)—to pronator teres, flexor carpi radialis, part of flexor digitorum superficialis, part of palmaris longus
Medial cord
4. Medial pectoral nerve (C8, T1)—to pectoralis major (shoulder adduction)
5. Ulnar nerve (C8, T1)—ulnar wrist and long finger flexors
6. Median nerve (partial; C8, T1)—long finger flexors and small hand muscles
7. Medial brachial cutaneous nerve—skin over medial surface of arm and proximal forearm
8. Medial antebrachial cutaneous nerve—skin over medial surface of forearm
Posterior cord
9. Upper subscapular nerve (C5, C6)—to subscapularis (medial rotation of the humerus)
10. Thoracodorsal nerve (C6, C7, C8)—to latissimus dorsi (shoulder adduction)
11. Lower subscapular nerve (C5, C6)—to teres major (adducts the humerus)
12. Axillary nerve (C5, C6)—to deltoid (abduction of the humerus) and teres minor (lateral rotation of humerus)
13. Radial nerve (C5, C6, C7, C8, T1)—to extensor muscles of upper limb (Figures 2-5 and 2-6).

38. **What is Erb's palsy?**
Erb's palsy is an injury to the upper brachial plexus (C5, C6) resulting from excessive separation or stretch of the neck and shoulder (such as from a sliding injury or from pulling on an infant's neck during delivery). The result is decreased sensation in the C5 and C6 dermatomes and paralysis of scapular muscles. The arm may be held in adduction, with the fingers pointing backward, so-called waiter's tip position. Distal strength in the upper extremity remains intact.

39. **What is Klumpke's palsy?**
Klumpke's palsy results from maximal abduction of the shoulder, causing injury to the lower brachial plexus (C8, T1) and leading to weakness and anesthesia in a primarily ulnar distribution.

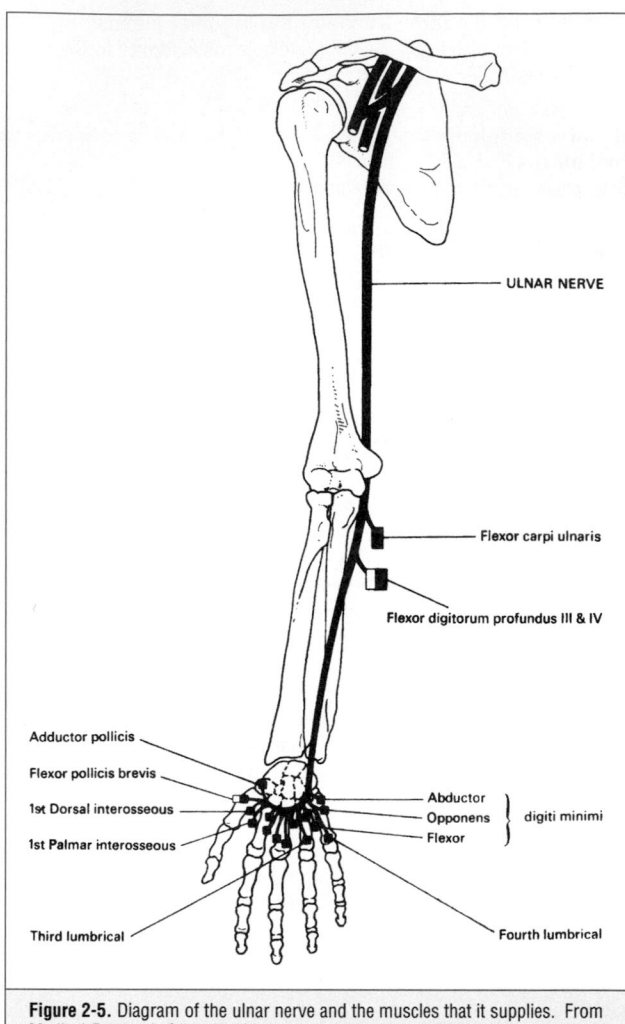

**Figure 2-5.** Diagram of the ulnar nerve and the muscles that it supplies. From Medical Research Council: Aids to the Examination of the Peripheral Nervous System. London, 1976.

40. **What is Parsonage-Turner syndrome?**
Parsonage-Turner syndrome is an acute brachial plexus neuritis, commonly also affecting the long thoracic, musculocutaneous, and axillary nerves. It causes patchy upper extremity weakness and numbness, usually accompanied by pain. Symptoms are bilateral in 20% of patients. This condition is associated with diabetes, systemic lupus erythematosus, and polyarteritis nodosa and may follow immunizations or viral infections. One-third of patients recover within 1 year and 90% within 3 years.

41. **What deficit results from poorly fitting crutches?**
Pressure from crutches results in a lesion of the posterior cord or the radial nerve, leading to weakness of the elbow, wrist, and digits.

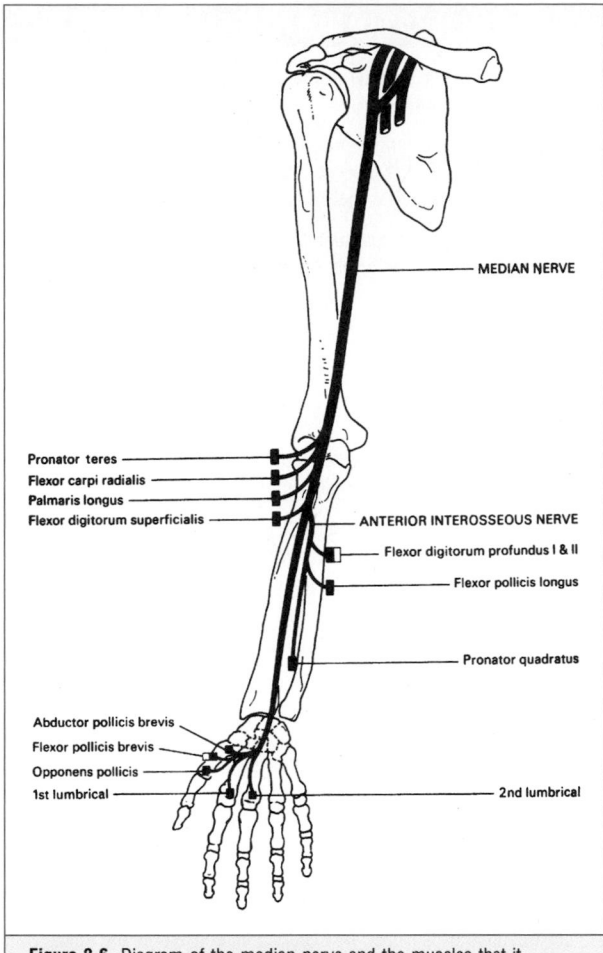

**Figure 2-6.** Diagram of the median nerve and the muscles that it supplies. From Medical Research Council: Aids to the Examination of the Peripheral Nervous System. London, 1976.

42. **Which nerve is commonly affected in shoulder dislocation or fracture of the humerus?**
    The axillary nerve is affected, resulting in a lesion that causes decreased abduction of the shoulder and anesthesia over the lateral part of the proximal arm.

43. **What is thoracic outlet syndrome (TOS)?**
    Classically, TOS consists of decreased upper extremity pulses, with tingling and numbness in the medial aspect of the arm secondary to compression of the medial cord of the brachial plexus and the axillary artery by a cervical rib or other structures.

## KEY POINTS: INNERVATION OF LEG AND ARM

1. Foot drop (weakness of the tibialis anterior muscle) can be caused by lesions to the common peroneal nerve or L5 nerve root.

2. Testing the dorsal scapular and long thoracic nerves is useful in trying to differentiate between root and plexus lesions. If there is a deficit in one of these nerves (clinically or electrically), the lesion is proximal to the plexus.

3. The median nerve is involved in carpal tunnel syndrome. There are typically no objective findings in the exam of a patient with this syndrome.

### ROOTS AND DERMATOMES

44. **What is found in the ventral nerve root?**
The ventral nerve root contains principally motor axons.

45. **What is found in the dorsal nerve root?**
The dorsal nerve root contains principally sensory axons.

46. **What synapse is found in the dorsal root ganglia?**
There is no synapse in the dorsal root ganglia. The dorsal root ganglia are made up of unipolar cell bodies for the sensory system.

47. **What are the dermatomes of the following landmarks: thumb, middle finger, little finger, breast nipple, umbilicus, medial knee, big toe, and little toe?**
Thumb—C6, middle finger—C7, little finger—C8, breast nipple—T4, umbilicus—T10, medial knee—L4, big toe—L5, little toe—S1.

48. **What are the common signs and symptoms of lumbar radiculopathies?**
Lumbar radiculopathies cause back pain with radiation below the knee. The pain increases with a Valsalva maneuver or leg stretch (such as the straight leg raising test). Weakness or numbness may develop in the distribution of the involved root. An S1 radiculopathy diminishes ankle reflexes, whereas an L4 radiculopathy decreases knee reflexes. Statistically, an L5 radiculopathy is more common than S1, followed by L4. This is because the intervertebral discs at these levels are under greatest pressure from the curvature of normal lumbar lordosis and thus are most vulnerable to herniation and compression of the spinal roots.

49. **What are the common signs and symptoms of cervical radiculopathies?**
Cervical radiculopathies usually involve the lower cervical roots (C6, C7, C8). Patients typically complain of pain in the back of the neck, frequently with radiation to the arm in a dermatomal distribution. Paresthesias are often present in one or two digits. Absent biceps, brachioradialis, or triceps reflexes suggest lesions of C5, C6, and C7, respectively, and these muscles also may lose strength.

## SPINAL CORD: GROSS ANATOMY

**50. How is the spinal cord organized?**
Sections of the spinal cord cut perpendicular to the length of the cord reveal a butterfly-shaped area of gray matter with surrounding white matter. The white matter consists mainly of longitudinal nerve fibers, carrying the ascending and descending tracts up and down the cord. Midline grooves are present on the dorsal and ventral surfaces (the dorsal median sulcus and ventral median fissure). The gray matter of the cord contains dorsal and ventral enlargements known as *dorsal horns* and *ventral horns*.

**51. In a given transverse section of the spinal cord, how is the gray matter subdivided?**
The gray matter can be subdivided into groups of nuclei. When the spinal cord is cut along its length, these nuclei appear to be arranged in cell columns or laminae. Rexed divides the cord into 10 laminae. Each lamina extends the length of the cord, with lamina I at the most dorsal aspect of the dorsal horn, lamina IX at the most ventral aspect of the ventral horn, and lamina X surrounding the central canal. Lamina II is also called the *substantia gelatinosa* and is the area of synapse for the spinothalamic tract. Lamina IX is the site of the cell bodies for the anterior horn motor cells.

**52. What are the major ascending tracts in the spinal cord?**
(1) Dorsal columns; (2) spinothalamic tract; (3) dorsal spinocerebellar tract (DSC); and (4) ventral spinocerebellar (VSC) tract.

**53. What are the major descending tracts in the spinal cord?**
(1) Intermediolateral columns; (2) lateral corticospinal tract; (3) lateral reticulospinal tract; (4) lateral vestibulospinal tract; (5) medial longitudinal fasciculus (MLF); and (6) ventral corticospinal tract.

**54. Going from rostral to caudal, what are the five divisions of the spinal cord?**
Cervical, thoracic, lumbar, sacral, and coccygeal are the five divisions of the spinal cord.

**55. In the adult, at what vertebral level does the spinal cord end?**
The spinal cord ends at vertebral level L1 to L2.

**56. How many spinal nerves exit from each region of the spinal cord?**
Spinal nerves exit the spinal cord in pairs: 8 cervical, 12 thoracic, 5 lumbar, 5 sacral, and 1 coccygeal. Each spinal nerve is composed of the union of the dorsal sensory root and the ventral motor root.

**57. What is the filum terminale?**
Although the spinal cord ends at the lower border of vertebral level L1, the pia mater continues caudally as a connective tissue filament, the filum terminale, which passes through the subarachnoid space to the end of the dural sac, where it receives a covering of dura and continues to its attachment to the coccyx.

**58. What is the cauda equina?**
The lumbar and sacral spinal nerves have very long roots, descending from their respective points in the spinal cord to their exit points in the intervertebral foramina. These roots descend in a bundle from the conus, termed the cauda equina for its resemblance to a horse's tail.

59. **Describe the blood supply of the spinal cord.**
    The one anterior spinal artery and the two posterior spinal arteries travel along the length of the cord to supply blood to the cord. These arteries originate from the vertebral arteries. Other arteries replenish the anterior and posterior spinal arteries and enter the spinal canal through the intervertebral foramina in association with the spinal nerves. They are called radicular arteries if they supply only the nerve roots, and radiculospinal arteries if they supply blood to both the roots and the cord. Each radiculospinal artery supplies blood to approximately six spinal cord segments, with the exception of the great radicular artery of Adamkiewicz, which usually enters with the left second lumbar ventral root (range T10 to L4) and supplies most of the caudal third of the cord.

## SENSORY: DORSAL COLUMNS AND PROPRIOCEPTION

60. **What type of information is carried in the dorsal columns?**
    The dorsal columns convey tactile discrimination, vibration, and joint position sense.

61. **What types of receptors are stimulated to sense this information?**
    Muscle spindles and Golgi tendon organs perceive position sense, Pacinian corpuscles perceive vibration, and Meissner corpuscles perceive superficial touch sensation needed for tactile discrimination. Pacinian and Meissner corpuscles are examples of mechanoreceptors.

62. **What type of peripheral nerve fiber is involved with transmission of dorsal column information?**
    Large, myelinated, fast-conducting nerve fibers carry dorsal column-type information.

63. **What is the pathway by which this information reaches the cerebral cortex?**
    Sensation on skin → afferent sensory nerve → dorsal column on ipsilateral side (fasciculus gracilis and cuneatus) → lower medulla → synapse in nucleus gracilis and cuneatus → arcuate fibers → cross to the contralateral side into the medial lemniscus → ascend to the ventral posterolateral (VPL) nucleus of the thalamus → synapse → through the posterior limb of the internal capsule → postcentral gyrus of the cortex.

64. **Where do dorsal column fibers decussate? At what locations do they synapse?**
    The dorsal columns decussate in the lower medulla, after synapsing in the nucleus gracilis and cuneatus. They also synapse in the VPL of the thalamus before going to the cortex.

## SENSORY: SPINOTHALAMIC

65. **What type of information is carried in the spinothalamic tract?**
    The spinothalamic tract conveys pain, temperature, and crude touch.

66. **What type of peripheral nerve fiber is involved with transmission of spinothalamic information?**
    Small, myelinated, and unmyelinated fibers carry spinothalamic-type information.

67. **What is the pathway by which this information reaches the cerebral cortex?**
    Sensation on skin → afferent sensory nerve → substantia gelatinosa of the ipsilateral dorsal horn → synapse → cross via the anterior white commissure → contralateral spinothalamic tract → ascend to the VPL nucleus of the thalamus → synapse → through the posterior limb of the internal capsule → postcentral gyrus of the cortex.

68. **Where do the spinothalamic fibers decussate? At what locations do they synapse?**
These fibers decussate at the level they enter the spinal cord, after synapsing in Rexed's lamina II (substantia gelatinosa). They also synapse in the VPL of the thalamus before going to the cortex.

69. **What types of receptors are stimulated to sense this information?**
Pain and temperature are perceived by naked terminals of A delta and C fibers and by many specialized chemoreceptors that are excited by tissue substances released in response to noxious and inflammatory stimuli. Substance P is thought to be the neurotransmitter released by A delta and C fibers at their connections with the interneurons in the spinal cord.

70. **Where in the internal capsule do the afferents travel from the VPL thalamic nucleus?**
The sensory tracts from the VPL travel in the posterior aspect of the posterior limb of the internal capsule.

71. **To which anatomic locations do the afferents from the VPL project?**
They project to the postcentral gyrus (Brodmann's area 3, 1, 2; also called *somatosensory I*), and to somatosensory II (the posterior aspect of the superior lip of the lateral fissure).

## SENSORY: SPINOCEREBELLAR

72. **Which pathway carries proprioception from the lower limbs to the cerebellum?**
Proprioception travels from the legs to the cerebellum in the dorsal columns.

73. **Where does cerebellar proprioception for the lower limb synapse?**
These fibers synapse in the midthoracic level of the spinal cord in the nucleus dorsalis of Clarke.

74. **Where is the spinocerebellar tract located?**
The spinocerebellar tract lies lateral to the corticospinal tract in the cord.

## MOTOR: CORTICOSPINAL

75. **Where do the motor fibers originate?**
The motor fibers originate from the precentral gyrus (Brodmann's area 4). Initiation of movement arises from the premotor cortex (Brodmann's area 6), which lies anterior to the precentral gyrus.

76. **Where do the motor fibers travel in the internal capsule?**
The corticospinal fibers travel in the anterior portion of the posterior limb of the internal capsule. The motor fibers to the face (corticobulbar fibers) travel in the genu of the internal capsule.

77. **Which cranial nerve exits the midbrain in close proximity to the corticospinal fibers?**
Cranial nerve III exits the midbrain in close proximity to the corticospinal fibers, which explains the symptoms of a common vascular syndrome. In Weber's syndrome, a stroke in this location causes an ipsilateral third nerve palsy with contralateral hemiparesis.

78. **Where do the motor fibers decussate?**
    The corticospinal tract decussates in the lower ventral medulla, and most fibers continue in the cord as the lateral corticospinal tract, with a small percentage descending in the ventral corticospinal tract.

79. **On what type of neurons in the spinal cord do the corticospinal fibers synapse?**
    In the spinal cord, the corticospinal fibers synapse on the alpha and gamma motor neurons in Rexed's lamina IX.

## MOTOR: OTHER TRACTS

80. **What is the reticulospinal tract?**
    The reticulospinal tract also originates in the precentral gyrus, but instead of descending uninterrupted to the spinal cord, these fibers synapse in the reticular formation of the brain stem as they descend to the spinal cord. They mainly have an inhibitory effect on the alpha and gamma motor neurons.

81. **What is the vestibulospinal tract?**
    The vestibulospinal tract is the efferent from the lateral vestibular nucleus. This tract descends the spinal cord, residing lateral to the spinothalamic tract, and coordinates motor and vestibular performance.

82. **What is the MLF?**
    The MLF is primarily an efferent of the lateral vestibular nucleus. This tract ascends to the sixth, fourth, and third cranial nuclei. Other major components of the MLF are interneurons originating from the paramedian pontine reticular formation (PPRF) (see question 150).

## BRAIN STEM: CRANIAL NERVES

83. **What are the three parts of the brain stem?**
    The brain stem consists of the midbrain, pons, and medulla.

84. **What is the reticular formation?**
    The reticular formation is a loosely organized longitudinal collection of interneurons that fill the central core of the brain stem, which is concerned with modulating awareness and behavioral performance.

85. **Name the 12 cranial nerves.**

    | | | | |
    |---|---|---|---|
    | I. Olfactory | IV. Trochlear | VII. Facial | X. Vagus |
    | II. Optic | V. Trigeminal | VIII. Auditory | XI. Spinal accessory |
    | III. Oculomotor | VI. Abducens | IX. Glossopharyngeal | XII. Hypoglossal |

86. **What are general somatic afferent nerves? Which cranial nerves carry them?**
    General somatic afferent fibers carry exteroceptive (pain, temperature, touch) and proprioceptive impulses. Cranial nerves for proprioception: III, IV, V, VI, XII; for pain, temperature, and touch: V, VII, IX, X.

87. **What are general visceral afferent nerves? Which cranial nerves carry them?**
General visceral afferent fibers carry impulses from the visceral structures, and cranial nerves IX and X contain these fibers.

88. **What are special somatic afferent nerves? Which cranial nerves carry them?**
Special somatic afferent fibers carry sensory impulses from the special senses (vision, hearing, equilibrium), and cranial nerves II and VIII contain these fibers.

89. **What are special visceral afferent nerves? Which cranial nerves carry them?**
Special visceral afferent fibers carry impulses from the olfactory and gustatory senses, and cranial nerves I (olfactory) and VII, IX, and X (gustatory) contain these fibers.

90. **What are general somatic efferent nerves? Which cranial nerves carry them?**
General somatic efferent fibers carry motor impulses to somatic skeletal muscles. In the head, the tongue and extraocular muscles are of this type. Cranial nerves III, IV, VI, and XII carry these fibers.

91. **What are general visceral efferent nerves? Which cranial nerves carry them?**
General visceral efferent fibers carry parasympathetic autonomic axons. The following cranial nerves carry general visceral efferent fibers:
    1. **Cranial nerve III** (Edinger-Westphal nucleus): the preganglionic fibers from the Edinger-Westphal nucleus terminate in the ciliary ganglion, and the postganglionic fibers innervate the pupil.
    2. **Cranial nerve VII** (superior salivatory nucleus): the preganglionic fibers from the superior salivatory nucleus terminate in the pterygopalatine and submandibular ganglion. The postganglionic fibers innervate the lacrimal gland (from the pterygopalatine ganglion) and the submandibular and sublingual gland (from the submandibular ganglion).
    3. **Cranial nerve IX** (inferior salivatory nucleus): the preganglionic fibers from the inferior salivatory nucleus terminate in the otic ganglion, and the postganglionic fibers innervate the parotid gland.
    4. **Cranial nerve X** (dorsal motor nucleus): the dorsal motor nucleus innervates the abdominal viscera.

92. **What are special visceral efferent nerves? Which cranial nerves carry them?**
Special visceral efferent fibers innervate skeletal muscle derived from the branchial arches. Cranial nerves V (muscles of mastication, first branchial arch), VII (muscles of facial expression, second branchial arch), IX (stylopharyngeus muscle, third branchial arch), X (muscles of the soft palate and pharynx, fourth branchial arch), and XI (muscles of the larynx/sternocleidomastoid (SCM)/trapezius, sixth branchial arch) carry them.

## MIDBRAIN

93. **What are the three anatomic subdivisions of the midbrain?**
The midbrain can be divided into the tectum, tegmentum, and cerebral crus (Figure 2-7).

94. **What is the quadrigeminal plate?**
The quadrigeminal plate is formed by the tectum and the superior and inferior colliculi.

95. **What is the substantia nigra?**
The substantia nigra, a motor nucleus in the basal ganglia system, lies anterior to the tegmentum but posterior to the crus (pyramidal tract) in the midbrain.

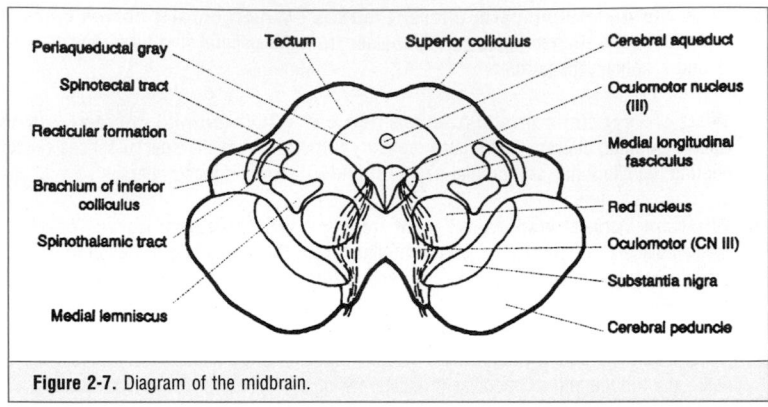

**Figure 2-7.** Diagram of the midbrain.

96. **Which disease affects the substantia nigra? What is the pathology?**
The primary efferent neurotransmitter from the substantia nigra is dopamine. Parkinson's disease damages the substantia nigra. Pathologically, the neurons lose their melanin and the nucleus becomes depigmented. Many neurons also contain inclusion bodies called Lewy bodies.

97. **What is the red nucleus?**
The red nucleus is a globular mass located in the ventral portion of the tegmentum of the midbrain. It is a relay center for many of the efferent cerebellar tracts. The crossed fibers of the superior cerebellar peduncle (SCP) pass through and around its edges.

98. **What is the Edinger-Westphal nucleus?**
The Edinger-Westphal nucleus, in the posterior midbrain, supplies parasympathetic fibers that terminate in the ciliary ganglion via cranial nerve III. It is mainly involved in pupillary constriction and the light accommodation reflex.

99. **What is the function of cranial nerve III?**
Cranial nerve III innervates all the extraocular muscles except for the lateral rectus and superior oblique. In innervates the medial rectus, superior rectus, inferior rectus, and inferior oblique muscles.

100. **Where does cranial nerve III originate and exit the brain stem?**
Cranial nerve III, the oculomotor nerve, exits the brain stem medially from the midbrain between the posterior cerebral artery and the superior cerebellar artery. This is important because the nerve can be affected by aneurysms of these arteries.

101. **What is the function of cranial nerve IV?**
Cranial nerve IV, the trochlear nerve, innervates the superior oblique muscle.

102. **What is the route of cranial nerve IV?**
Cranial nerve IV travels posteriorly and medially, crosses the midline, wraps around the midbrain, and exits the brain stem laterally between the posterior cerebral artery and superior cerebellar artery. It has the longest intracranial route (approximately 7.5 cm) of any cranial nerve. It then travels through the cavernous sinus and enters the orbit through the superior orbital fissure. Because it crosses the midline, the right trochlear nerve innervates the left superior oblique muscle.

103. **In a superior oblique palsy, which way would the patient tilt his or her head?**
If the left superior oblique muscle is weak, then tilting the head to the right would reduce the diplopia, and tilting the head to the left would worsen the diplopia. So a patient tilts his or her head away from the affected eye (Figure 2-8).

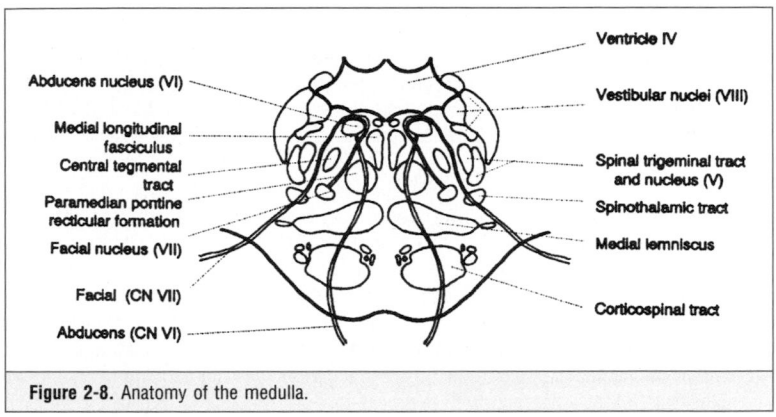

**Figure 2-8.** Anatomy of the medulla.

## PONS

104. **Which cranial nerves exit at the pontomedullary junction?**
Cranial nerve VI exits medially, and cranial nerves VII and VIII exit laterally (Figure 2-9).

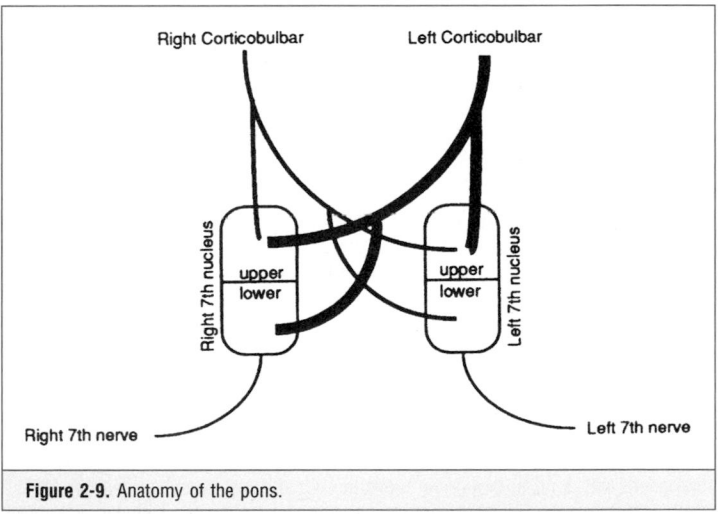

**Figure 2-9.** Anatomy of the pons.

105. **Where does cranial nerve V exit the brain stem?**
Cranial nerve V, the trigeminal nerve, exits the brain stem laterally at the mid-pons level. It divides into three main branches: V1 (ophthalmic), V2 (maxillary), and V3 (mandibular).

106. **What are the four subdivisions of the trigeminal nucleus?**
    1. Mesencephalic nucleus (which is a nucleus of unipolar cell bodies similar to the dorsal root ganglion, with no synapse)
    2. Chief sensory nucleus
    3. Descending spinal nucleus
    4. Motor nucleus

107. **What type of information does cranial nerve V carry?**
    The trigeminal nerve carries sensation (general somatic afferent) from the anterior two-thirds of the face, and motor innervation (special visceral efferent) to the muscles of mastication (medial/lateral pterygoid, masseter, temporalis), the mylohyoid, anterior belly of the digastric, tensor tympani, and tensor palati.

108. **What is the pathway by which sensation from the face reaches the cortex?**
    After cranial nerve V enters the brain stem, the afferent nerves split into two parts: those carrying dorsal column–type information and those carrying spinothalamic-type information. The former goes to the ipsilateral chief sensory nucleus of V (mid-pons) → synapse → enters the contralateral trigeminal lemniscus (which lies medial to the medial lemniscus) → ventral posteromedial nucleus (VPM) of the thalamus → synapse → through the posterior limb of the internal capsule to the postcentral gyrus. The pain-carrying fibers become the spinal tract of V → descend from mid-pons to lower medulla → synapse in the spinal nucleus of V → cross diffusely to form the contralateral trigeminal lemniscus (at mid-pons) → VPM nucleus of the thalamus → synapse → through the posterior limb of the internal capsule to the postcentral gyrus.

109. **What is the function of cranial nerve VI?**
    Cranial nerve VI, the abducens nerve, abducts the eye.

110. **What is the function of cranial nerve VII?**
    Cranial nerve VII, the facial nerve, innervates the muscles of facial expression (special visceral efferent); innervates the lacrimal, submandibular, sublingual, and parotid glands (general visceral efferent); supplies taste sensation to the anterior two-thirds of the tongue (special visceral afferent); and supplies sensation to the external ear (general somatic afferent).

111. **How does the nucleus for cranial nerve VII receive higher cortical input?**
    The innervation to the muscles of facial expression can be separated into the muscles of the upper part of the face and the muscles of the lower part of the face. The supranuclear input responsible for the movement of the upper facial musculature is a bilateral input from the cortex to the nucleus. The supranuclear input responsible for the movement of the lower facial musculature is only a contralateral input from the cortex to the facial nucleus (Figure 2-10).

112. **What is the difference between an upper motor neuron (central) and lower motor neuron (peripheral) facial weakness?**
    If the patient with a facial droop can move the upper facial muscles (i.e., wrinkle the forehead), the lesion is supranuclear on the contralateral side. The lesion is somewhere in the contralateral corticobulbar tracts above the facial nerve nucleus (e.g., in the crus or in the genu of the internal capsule). If the patient cannot voluntarily move any muscle involved in facial expression (either upper or lower facial musculature), the lesion is localized to the facial nucleus or the peripheral facial nerve on the ipsilateral side.

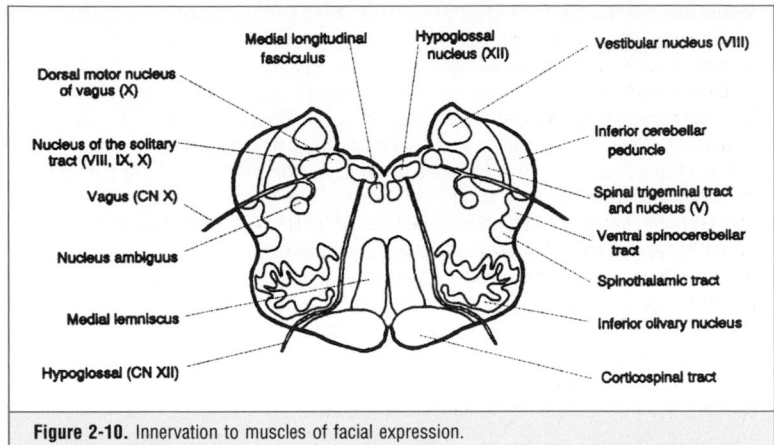

**Figure 2-10.** Innervation to muscles of facial expression.

**113. What is Möbius syndrome?**

Möbius syndrome is congenital absence of both facial nerve nuclei, resulting in a facial diplegia. Patients also may have associated absence of the abducens nuclei.

**114. What is the function of cranial nerve VIII?**

Cranial nerve VIII, the vestibulocochlear nerve, has two functionally distinct sensory divisions: the vestibular nerve and the cochlear (or auditory) nerve. The vestibular nerve responds to position and movement of the head, serving functions often identified as equilibrium. The cochlear nerve mediates auditory functions.

## MEDULLA

**115. What is the nucleus ambiguus?**

It is a cigar-shaped nucleus that lies in the depths of the medulla. It innervates the volitional muscles of the pharynx by way of both cranial nerves IX and X and the larynx (for phonation) via cranial nerve X. The larynx and pharynx have bilateral cortical input.

**116. What is the nucleus solitarius?**

It is the nucleus in the medulla that receives afferent information from the larynx (via cranial nerve X) and posterior pharynx and mediates the gag and cough reflexes (cranial nerves IX and X). Pain sensation from these areas enters the brain stem through cranial nerves IX and X but terminates in the descending spinal tract of the trigeminal nerve.

**117. What is the salivatory nucleus?**

The superior salivatory nucleus sends efferent autonomic fibers (general visceral efferent) through cranial nerve VII to innervate the lacrimal, submandibular, and sublingual glands as well as the mucous membranes of the nose and hard and soft palate. The inferior salivatory nucleus sends efferent autonomic fibers via cranial nerve IX to innervate the parotid gland.

**118. What is the gustatory nucleus?**

The gustatory nucleus is the nucleus in the medulla that receives afferent sensory information for the sensation of taste. Taste from the anterior two-thirds of the tongue is innervated by the chorda tympani (cranial nerve VII), the posterior one-third of the tongue is innervated by cranial nerve IX, and the epiglottis is innervated by cranial nerve X.

119. **Describe the function of cranial nerves IX and X (glossopharyngeal–vagal complex)**
Cranial nerve IX (the glossopharyngeal nerve) and cranial nerve X (the vagus nerve) are usually considered together because of their overlapping functions. Both cranial nerves travel together intracranially, and both exit the cranial vault through the jugular foramen. The nucleus ambiguus innervates the volitional muscles of the pharynx through both cranial nerves IX and X, and the larynx via cranial nerve X. Sensation from the larynx enters the medulla via cranial nerve X to terminate in the nucleus solitarius. Taste fibers from the posterior one-third of the tongue travel via cranial nerve IX, and taste from the epiglottis via cranial nerve X. They terminate in the gustatory nucleus. Cranial nerve IX also supplies parasympathetic innervation to the parotid, originating in the inferior salivatory nucleus. Branches of cranial nerve X, the vagus nerve, continue beyond the larynx to innervate the heart, lungs, and abdominal viscera, providing primarily parasympathetic input.

120. **What is the function of cranial nerve XI?**
Cranial nerve XI, the spinal accessory nerve, is a small nerve of about 3500 motor fibers that arises from the upper cervical and lower medullary anterior horn cells and supplies the SCM and trapezius muscles. It exits the cranial vault via the jugular foramen.

121. **What is jugular foramen syndrome?**
Because cranial nerves IX, X, and XI exit the cranial vault through the jugular foramen, jugular foramen syndrome is a constellation of symptoms arising from a lesion (typically a tumor) at the level of the jugular foramen that compromises the function of these cranial nerves. Symptoms include loss of taste to the posterior two-thirds of the tongue; paralysis of the vocal cords, palate, and pharynx; and paralysis of the trapezius and SCM muscles.

122. **If the left spinal accessory nerve is cut, which functions are lost?**
Because cranial nerve XI supplies the SCM and the trapezius, these muscles are weakened. Because the left SCM is involved in turning the head to the right, a lesion of the left cranial nerve XI results in an inability to turn the head to the right. The left trapezius also loses function, and the patient would not be able to shrug the left shoulder.

123. **If the left hypoglossal nucleus is injured, which way does the tongue deviate?**
Lesioning the nucleus is similar to lesioning the peripheral nerve. The left hypoglossal nerve innervates the left tongue muscles, which, if acting alone, pushes the tongue to the right. The right hypoglossal nerve innervates the right tongue muscles, which, if acting alone, pushes the tongue to the left. Usually, these muscles work together to push the tongue forward without deviation. If the left hypoglossal nucleus is lesioned, the right hypoglossal muscles act unopposed. The tongue thus deviates to the left, or, in other words, the tongue deviates toward the affected side.

## KEY POINTS: CRANIAL NERVE REFLEXES

1. Critical in establishing level of damage in coma

2. Critical to finding a cause (focal—structural lesion; nonfocal—metabolic)

3. Pupil reaction: (II in, III out)

4. Doll's eyes or cold water calorics: VIII in, III, IV, VI out

5. Gag: IX in, X out

6. Able to breathe: medulla function

## BREATHING

**124. What is Cheyne-Stokes breathing? Where is the lesion that causes it?**
Cheyne-Stokes breathing is a crescendo-decrescendo pattern of periodic breathing in which phases of hyperpnea regularly alternate with apnea. Cheyne-Stokes respirations are seen most often with lesions affecting both cerebral hemispheres.

**125. What is central neurogenic hyperventilation? What causes it?**
Central neurogenic hyperventilation is a sustained, rapid, deep hyperpnea. It is produced by lesions in the low midbrain to upper one-third of the pons.

**126. What is apneustic breathing? What causes it?**
Apneusis is a prolonged respiratory cramp, a pause at full inspiration. Apneustic breathing may occur after damage to the mid or caudal pons.

**127. What is cluster breathing? When does it occur?**
Cluster breathing, a disorderly sequence of breaths with irregular pauses between the breaths, may result from damage to the lower pons or upper medulla.

**128. What is ataxic breathing? Where is the lesion that causes it?**
It is a completely irregular pattern of breathing in which both deep and shallow breaths occur randomly. The respiratory rate tends to be slow. The lesion that causes it is in the central medulla.

## POSTURING

**129. What is decorticate posturing? What causes it?**
Decorticate posturing is a stereotyped response to noxious stimuli. In the upper extremity, it consists of flexion of the arm, wrist, and fingers; in the lower extremity, it consists of extension, internal rotation, and plantar flexion. Decorticate posturing most often occurs in comatose patients with lesions below the thalamus but above the red nucleus.

**130. What is decerebrate posturing? In whom does it occur?**
Decerebrate posturing is a stereotyped response to noxious stimuli. It consists of extension, adduction, and hyperpronation in the upper extremity and extension with plantar flexion in the lower extremity. Comatose patients with lesions below the red nucleus but above the vestibular nucleus may have decerebrate posturing.

## VESTIBULAR APPARATUS

**131. What are the five receptors of the vestibular apparatus, and what do they sense?**
Three semicircular canals that are oriented 90 degrees to each other sense rotational acceleration in all three planes. One horizontally oriented utricle and one vertically oriented saccule sense linear acceleration.

**132. Where does the vestibular information synapse?**
The vestibular nerve, carrying sensory data from the receptors, divides and synapses in four vestibular nuclei grouped together in the medulla: the superior, inferior, medial, and lateral vestibular nuclei.

**133.** **What is the output from these nuclei?**
The vestibulospinal tracts and the MLF are the two efferent tracts from the vestibular nuclei.

**134.** **Where do the vestibular nuclei project?**
Vestibular nuclei project to (1) the oculomotor nuclei (cranial nerves III, IV, and VI), (2) cranial nerve XI, (3) cervical nuclei for head and neck position, (4) fastigial nuclei of the cerebellum, and (5) reticular formations of the brain stem.

**135.** **What is the response of a normal person to cold water injected in the left ear?**
Injecting cold water in to the left ear causes slow eye movements toward the left, followed by a fast phase of nystagmus back to the right.

**136.** **What is the expected response of a comatose patient with an intact brain stem to cold water in the left ear?**
The patient will have slow eye deviation toward the left ear. The fast-phase nystagmus is absent.

## HEARING

**137.** **Which structures constitute the external ear, middle ear, and inner ear?**
The external ear is composed of the pinna, the external auditory canal, and the tympanic membrane. The middle ear is composed of the tympanic membrane, ossicles (malleus, incus, stapes), and oval window. The ossicles function as an impedance matching device between air and fluid during the travel of the sound wave. The inner ear is composed of part of the oval window, the cochlea, and the round window.

**138.** **Which compartments of the cochlea are filled with perilymph?**
- Scala vestibuli. It is separated from the scala tympani by Reissner's membrane.
- Scala tympani. It is separated from the scala media by the basilar membrane.
- Scala media. The third compartment is filled with endolymph and is located between Reissner's and the basilar membranes (Figure 2-11).

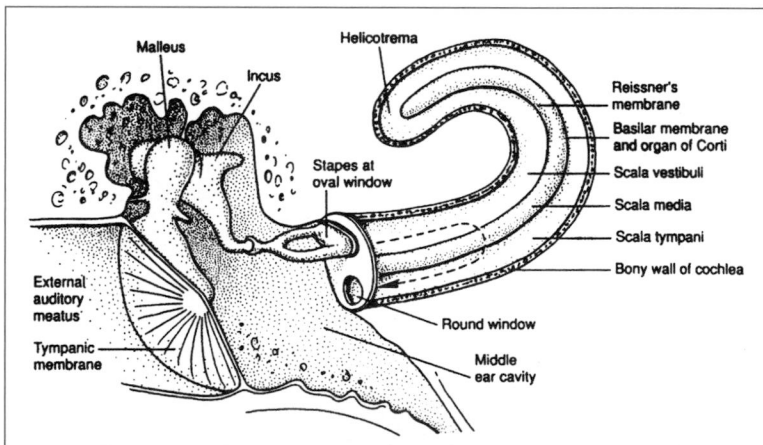

**Figure 2-11.** Anatomy of the hearing apparatus. From Kandel E., Schwartz JH, Jessell TM (eds): Principles of Neuroscience, 3rd ed. New York, Elsevier, 1991, p. 369.

**139.** **What is the pathway traveled by the cochlear fluid pressure wave initiated by a sound wave?**
The stapes transmits the pressure to the round window and from it to the perilymph of the scala vestibuli, which, in turn, sets up vibrations of Reissner's membrane, resulting in a wave in the scala media. The basilar membranes move next and transmit the pressure to the scala tympani and from there to the oval window.

**140.** **What is the arrangement of the neuroepithelial cells of the organ of Corti?**
1. The outer hair cells (arranged in three rows) rest on the basilar membrane, with their stereocilia inserted into the tectorial membrane; these cells are able to contract and initiate the flow of endolymph toward the inner hair cells.
2. The inner hair cells (one row) sit on the bone; they do not contract. These cells respond to the movement of endolymph and provide most of the afferent input to the spiral ganglion.

**141.** **How does the organ of Corti serve as an audiofrequency analyzer?**
The anatomic arrangement allows frequency analysis of sounds:
1. The basilar membrane responds to high frequencies at its base and to low frequencies at its apex.
2. The hair cells in the base of the cochlear duct have short and fat stereocilia, which are stimulated by high frequencies.
3. The hair cells in the apex of the cochlea have long and thin stereocilia, which respond best to low frequencies.

**142.** **What is the anatomy of the auditory pathway?**
Spiral ganglion → auditory nerve (cranial nerve VIII) → dorsal and ventral cochlear nuclei at the junction of the medulla and pons → trapezoid body (at this point 50% of the axons cross over to the other side) → superior olivary nucleus → lateral lemniscus → inferior colliculus → medial geniculate body → transverse gyrus of Heschl (area 41, partly buried in the sylvian fissure).

**143.** **At what level is there crossing of information between the left and right ascending tracts?**
The crossing of axons occurs on every level from the trapezoid body to the medial geniculate body.

**144.** **To produce unilateral deafness, where could the lesion be?**
The lesion must be at the cochlear nucleus or more peripheral because of multiple crossovers above the cochlear nucleus.

**145.** **What is a Weber's test?**
A vibrating tuning fork is placed in the middle of the forehead. In patients with conduction deafness, the sound is localized to the affected ear (bone > air conduction). In patients with sensorineural deafness, the signal is localized to the healthy ear.

**146.** **What is Rinne's test?**
A vibrating tuning fork is placed on the mastoid bone; when the patient can no longer hear it, it is removed and placed next to the ear. Thus, bone conduction is compared with air conduction. In conduction deafness, bone > air conduction. In sensorineural deafness, air > bone conduction.

**147.** **What is the innervation of the external ear canal?**
The external ear canal is supplied by cranial nerves V3, VII, IX, and X.

148. **Damage to which structures results in hyperacusis?**
    1. Facial nerve (VII)—innervates the stapedius muscle, which retracts the stapes from the round window.
    2. Trigeminal nerve (V)—supplies the tensor tympani, which inserts into the malleus and tenses the tympanic membrane, thus preventing it from vibrating.

149. **What is the pathway for the feedback loop?**
    When auditory input reaches the superior olive, it sends signals to the olivocochlear bundle through the VIII nerve; the signals then terminate on the outer hair cells or afferent fibers in the spiral ganglia.

## EYE MOVEMENTS

150. **What is the paramedian pontine reticular formation (PPRF)?**
    The PPRF is a collection of cells lying in the pons adjacent to the nucleus of cranial nerve VI, and is an important center for horizontal gaze. Efferent fibers from the PPRF project to the ipsilateral abducens (VI) nucleus, and to the contralateral oculomotor (III) nucleus through the MLF, stimulating both eyes to move horizontally.

151. **What is the difference between saccades and smooth pursuit movements?**
    Saccades are fast conjugate eye movements that are under voluntary control. Saccades are generated in the contralateral frontal lobe (Brodmann's area 8). Smooth pursuits are slow involuntary movements of eyes fixed on a moving target. Pursuit movements to one side are generated in the ipsilateral occipital lobe (Brodmann's areas 18 and 19).

152. **What is the pathway for saccades?**
    Fibers from the frontal eye field (Brodmann's area 8) pass through the genu of the internal capsule, decussate at the level of the upper pons, and synapse in the PPRF.

153. **What is the pathway for smooth pursuit?**
    The pathway for smooth pursuit is not clearly defined but appears to arise in the anterior occipital lobe (Brodmann's areas 18 and 19) and travel to the ipsilateral PPRF.

154. **What is the brain stem area for vertical gaze?**
    Near the superior colliculus, there are subtectal and pretectal centers that control vertical eye movements and project to cranial nuclei III, IV, and VI.

155. **What are the pathways for voluntary vertical eye movements?**
    Vertical movements are driven symmetrically from both frontal lobes. When activated bilaterally, fibers from Brodmann's area 8 project via the frontopontine tract to act upon bilateral cranial nuclei III, IV, and VI, which then innervate their respective muscles.

## CEREBELLUM

156. **Describe the anatomic divisions of the cerebellum.**
    The cerebellum is anatomically divided into the two hemispheres, the midline vermis and the flocculonodulus.

157. **What are the functions of each cerebellar "lobe"?**
    The hemispheres are involved in appendicular control, the vermis is involved in axial control, and the flocculonodular lobe is involved in vestibular balance.

**158. What are the three layers of the cerebellar cortex?**
1. Outermost molecular cell layer
2. Middle Purkinje cell layer
3. Innermost granular cell layer

**159. What types of cells are located in each of these layers?**
The molecular layer contains (1) stellate cells, (2) basket cells, (3) dendrites of Purkinje cells, (4) dendrites of Golgi type II cells, and (5) axons of granule cells. The Purkinje layer contains the cell bodies of Purkinje cells. The granular layer contains (6) granule cells, (7) Golgi type II cells, and (8) glomeruli (synaptic complexes that contain mossy fibers, axons and dendrites of Golgi type II cells, and dendrites of granule cells).

**160. What is the afferent fiber from the inferior olives? Through which peduncle does it reach the cerebellum?**
The afferent fiber from the inferior olives is the climbing fiber. It enters the cerebellum through the inferior cerebellar peduncle.

**161. What is Mollaret's triangle?**
Mollaret's triangle is a physiologic connection between the red nucleus, inferior olives, and dentate nucleus of the cerebellum. A lesion in this pathway can cause palatal myoclonus.

**162. What are the deep nuclei of the cerebellum (medial to lateral)?**
Medial to lateral, the cerebellar deep nuclei are fastigial, globus, emboliform, and dentate.

**163. What are the primary inputs and outputs of the cerebellum?**
Cerebellar function can be conceptualized as a feedback loop, with input arriving from an origin, synapsing in a cerebellar nucleus, and then projecting back, often to the same origin (Table 2-2).

### TABLE 2-2. CEREBELLAR CONNECTIONS

| Cerebellar Peduncle | Connected to | Tracts that Run in the Peduncle |
| --- | --- | --- |
| Superior (SCP) | Midbrain | DRT and VSC |
| Middle (MCP) | Pons | CPC |
| Inferior (ICP) | Medulla | All other tracts to/from the cerebellum |

| Origin | Inflow Tract | Inflow Peduncle | Cerebellar Nucleus | Outflow Peduncle | Outflow Tract | Destination |
| --- | --- | --- | --- | --- | --- | --- |
| Precentral gyrus | CPC | MCP | Dentate | SCP | DRT | Precentral gyrus |
| Spinal cord | SC | ICP | Fastigial | ICP | — | Vestibular nucleus |
| Vestibular nucleus | VC | ICP | Vestibular | ICP | LVS (MLF) | Spinal cord |

SCP, superior cerebellar peduncle; MCP, middle cerebellar peduncle; ICP, inferior cerebellar peduncle; DRT, dentatorubrothalamic; VSC, ventral spinocerebellar; CPC, corticopontocerebellar; SC, spinocerebellar; VC, vestibulocerebellar; LVS, lateral vestibulospinal; and MLF, medial longitudinal fasciculus.

164. **What type of fiber originating in the cerebellar cortex is inhibitory on the deep cerebellar nuclei?**
Purkinje fibers originate in the cerebellar cortex and synapse on the deep nuclei as an inhibitory neuron.

165. **Where does the dentatorubrothalamic tract synapse?**
These fibers synapse in the ventrolateral (VL) nucleus of the thalamus before ascending to the cortex.

## BASAL GANGLIA

166. **What are the basal ganglia?**
The basal ganglia are a collection of nuclei, largely concerned with motor control, composed primarily of the corpus striatum, and the lenticular complex. (See Figure 10-1.)

167. **What are the parts of the corpus striatum?**
The corpus striatum is composed of the putamen and caudate.

168. **What is the lenticular complex?**
The lenticular complex, or lentiform nucleus, is composed of the globus pallidus and putamen.

169. **Which structure is the lateral border of the caudate?**
The anterior limb of the internal capsule is the lateral border of the caudate.

170. **What is the major outflow of the basal ganglia?**
The major outflow of the basal ganglia projects from the medial globus pallidus as a fiber bundle known as the lenticular fasciculus (Forel's field H2). Another bundle from the medial globus pallidus loops around the internal capsule as the ansa lenticularis. It then merges in Forel's field H with the lenticular fasciculus and with fibers from the dentatorubrothalamic tract. These fibers then continue as the thalamic fasciculus (Forel's field H1) and synapse in the thalamic nuclei: centromedian, ventral lateral, and ventral anterior. These thalamic nuclei then relay information up to the motor cortex.

171. **Is there any other output from the medial globus pallidus?**
Yes. Apart from the lenticular fasciculus and the ansa lenticularis, a third fiber tract leaves the medial globus pallidus as the pallidotegmental tract and descends onto the pedunculopontine nucleus in the midbrain, where neurons help to regulate posture. This is the only descending tract from the basal ganglia.

172. **Is there any output from the basal ganglia that does not originate in the medial globus pallidus?**
The only other output is a small tract (pallidosubthalamic fibers) that leaves the lateral globus pallidus to synapse in the subthalamic nucleus.

173. **What is the major input to the basal ganglia?**
The major input is from the motor cortex and the thalamic nuclei. The basal ganglia function, simplistically, as a feedback loop: cerebral cortex → basal ganglia → thalamus → cerebral cortex.

## THALAMUS

**174. Which structure lies lateral to the thalamus and medial to the thalamus?**
The posterior limb of the internal capsule is the lateral border of the thalamus. The third ventricle lies medial to the thalamus.

**175. What is the anatomy of the thalamus?**
The intermedullary lamina divides the thalamus into anterior, medial, and lateral groups. The lateral group is further divided into ventral and dorsal tiers. Each group contains specific nuclei:

- Anterior group: Anterior nucleus
- Medial group: Dorsomedial (DM) nucleus
- Lateral group:
  - Dorsal tier
  - Lateral dorsal (LD) nucleus
  - Lateral posterior (LP) nucleus
  - Pulvinar
- Ventral tier
  - Ventral anterior (VA) nucleus
  - VL nucleus
  - VPL nucleus
  - VPM nucleus
  - Lateral geniculate (LG)
  - Medial geniculate (MG)

Other nuclei that are often considered part of the thalamus include (1) reticular nucleus—a small group of neurons that projects to other thalamic nuclei and may help regulate cortical activity; (2) midline nuclei—diffuse neurons connected to the hypothalamus; and (3) centromedian (CM)—an intralaminar nucleus that is part of the reticular formation that activates the cortex.

**176. What are the inputs to and from the main thalamic nuclei?**
See Table 2-3.

**177. What is the limbic lobe?**
The limbic lobe is not a true lobe of the brain but rather a functional collection of structures that regulate higher activities such as memory and emotion. It is commonly said to include (1) cingulate gyrus, (2) parahippocampal gyrus, (3) hippocampal gyrus, and (4) uncus.

**178. What is Papez's circuit?**
This is a route by which the limbic system communicates between the hippocampus, thalamus, hypothalamus, and cortex. It forms a circuit from the hippocampal formation → fornix → mammillary body → mammillothalamic tract → anterior group of thalamus → cingulate gyrus → cingulate bundle → hippocampus (Note: the amygdala is not part of the classic Papez circuit).

## OLFACTION

**179. What are the olfactory receptor cells?**
The receptor cells are bipolar neurons that pass from the olfactory mucosa through the cribriform plate to the olfactory bulb. Collectively, the central processes of the olfactory receptor cells constitute cranial nerve I.

**TABLE 2-3. CONNECTIONS OF THE THALAMIC NUCLEI**

| Thalamic Nucleus | Principal Input | Principal Output | Function |
|---|---|---|---|
| LP | Parietal lobe | Parietal lobe | Sensory integration |
| LD | Cingulate gyrus | Cingulate gyrus | Emotional expression |
| Pulvinar | Association areas of cortex | Association areas of cortex | Sensory integration |
| DM | Amygdala, olfactory, and hypothalamus | Prefrontal cortex | Limbic |
| MG | Auditory relay nuclei (from inferior colliculus) | Auditory cortex-area 41, 42 | Hearing |
| LG | Optic tract | Visual cortex-area 17 | Vision |
| Anterior | Mammillary body | Cingulate gyrus | Limbic |
| VA | Globus pallidus | Premotor cortex | Motor |
| VL | Cerebellum | Premotor and motor cortices | Motor |
| VPM | Trigeminal lemniscus | Postcentral gyrus | Somatic sensation (face) |
| VPL | Medial lemniscus and spinothalamic | Postcentral gyrus | Somatic integration (body) |
| CM | Reticular formation, globus pallidus, hypothalamus | Basal ganglia (striatum) | Sensory integration, smell, limbic |

*LP,* lateral posterior nucleus; *LD,* lateral dorsal nucleus; *DM,* dorsomedial nucleus; *MG,* medial geniculate; *LG,* lateral geniculate; *VA,* ventral anterior nucleus; *VL,* ventrolateral nucleus; *VPM,* ventral posteromedial nucleus; *VPL,* ventral posterolateral nucleus; CM, centromedian.

180. **What is the anatomy of the olfactory pathway?**
    1. In the olfactory bulb, the axons of receptor cells synapse on dendrites of mitral and tufted cells (forming a glomerulus).
    2. The axons of mitral and tufted cells compose the olfactory tract, which soon divides into medial and lateral stria. Medial stria fibers cross to the contralateral side via the anterior commissure, while the lateral stria fibers terminate in the anterior perforated substance, amygdaloid complex, and lateral olfactory gyrus (which is the primary olfactory cortex).
    3. From the lateral olfactory gyrus (prepiriform area), fibers project to the entorhinal cortex, the medial dorsal nucleus of the thalamus, and the hypothalamus.

181. **What is unique about the projection of olfactory information to the cerebral cortex?**
    Unlike other sensory modalities, olfaction reaches the cortex without relay through the thalamus.

**182. What are the most common causes of anosmia?**
1. Rhinitis/nasal congestion
2. Smoking
3. Head injury
4. Craniotomy
5. Subarachnoid hemorrhage
6. Meningiomas of the olfactory groove
7. Zinc and vitamin A deficiency
8. Hypothyroidism
9. Congenital disorders (Kallmann's syndrome)
10. Dementing diseases (Alzheimer's, Parkinson's)
11. Multiple sclerosis

## VISION

**183. What is the arrangement of cones and rods in the retina?**
The 6 million cones are concentrated toward the center, and the 120 million rods are in the periphery of the retina. In the fovea, located centrally within the macula, each cone is served by a single ganglion cell, resulting in very high resolution. In the periphery, many rods project to a single ganglion cell, giving high sensitivity but lower resolution.

**184. What are the primary functions of rods?**
Rods are concerned with night vision and are most sensitive between the blue and green wavelengths.

**185. What are the primary functions of cones?**
Cones are concerned with color vision and daytime vision. The three types of cones are tuned, via visual pigments, to different frequencies in the blue, green, and red wavelength ranges.

**186. What is the afferent pathway for the pupillary light reflex?**
Retinal ganglion cells concerned with the light reflex travel with the optic nerve and tract and then break away to project down to the midbrain pretectal nucleus. From the pretectal nucleus, fibers project bilaterally, decussating via the posterior commissure to each Edinger-Westphal nucleus.

**187. Which nucleus mediates pupil constriction?**
The Edinger-Westphal nucleus, or preganglionic parasympathetic nucleus of cranial nerve III, mediates pupillary constriction.

**188. What is the pathway for pupillary dilatation?**
This pathway has three neurons. First-order fibers descend from the ipsilateral hypothalamus through the brain stem and cervical cord to T1 to T2. They synapse on ipsilateral preganglionic sympathetic fibers, exit the cord, travel up the sympathetic chain as second-order neurons to the superior cervical ganglion, and then synapse on postganglionic sympathetic fibers. The third-order neurons travel via the internal carotid artery to the orbit and innervate the radial smooth muscle of the iris.

**189. What is Horner's syndrome?**
Horner's syndrome is an interruption of the sympathetic supply to the eye, resulting in the classic triad of ptosis, miosis, and anhydrosis.

190. **Describe the pharmacologic tests to diagnose Horner's syndrome.**
Instill 2% cocaine solution in both eyes, which dilates the pupils by preventing the reuptake of the sympathetic neurotransmitter norepinephrine. If one eye fails to dilate, a diagnosis of Horner's syndrome can be made because failure to dilate indicates an interruption of the sympathetic supply (norepinephrine) to that eye. To further localize the lesion, one can use amphetamine in the affected eye, which displaces norepinephrine from the nerve terminal and dilates the pupil. If the pupil dilates in response to this test, the lesion affects the third-order neuron, causing denervation hypersensitivity. Otherwise, the lesion is in the first- or second-order neurons.

191. **What is the anatomy of the lesion that causes an afferent pupillary defect?**
An afferent pupillary defect means the pupil will not react to light. The lesion must be prechiasmal and almost always involves the optic nerve.

192. **What is the test for an afferent pupillary defect (Marcus Gunn pupil)?**
The swinging flashlight test determines an afferent pupillary defect. Shine a light into the normal eye and the pupil constricts (the affected eye also constricts consensually). Quickly move the light onto the opposite affected eye, and the pupil dilates. Removing the light from the normal pupil causes it and the affected pupil, responding consensually, to dilate. The affected pupil thus seems to dilate when the swinging light hits it.

193. **What is the value of the pupillary reflex for diagnosing third-nerve palsies?**
Because the parasympathetic fibers travel along the outside of the third nerve, they are usually damaged by nerve compression, resulting in pupillary dilatation. Third-nerve palsies that cause pupillary dilatation are usually masses (e.g., tumors, aneurysms), whereas palsies that do not involve the pupil are usually medical (e.g., ischemia, vasculitis).

194. **What is the pathway for pupillary constriction that occurs with convergence?**
The pathway begins in the occipital lobe (Brodmann's area 18) and projects to the Edinger-Westphal nucleus bilaterally. The details of how pupils constrict during convergence are poorly understood.

195. **What is an Argyll Robertson pupil?**
An Argyll Robertson pupil, one form of light-near dissociation, is an irregular pupil that does not constrict to light but does constrict to accommodation. This finding is quite specific for central nervous system (CNS) syphilis. Light-near dissociation with a regular pupil can be found in many diseases and is not specific for CNS syphilis.

196. **What is the pathway of the optic nerve?**
The ganglion cells from the nasal half of the retina travel in the optic nerve, where they decussate in the optic chiasm and join the contralateral optic tract to the lateral geniculate body. The ganglion cells from the temporal half of the retina travel in the optic nerve, stay in the ipsilateral optic tract, and project to the lateral geniculate body. Thus, the contralateral visual field is projected from each eye to the lateral geniculate body.

197. **What thalamic nucleus is concerned with vision?**
The lateral genicular body is the thalamic nucleus that handles vision.

198. **What is the pathway of the optic radiation?**
Second-order neurons from the lateral geniculate body project to the calcarine cortex (Brodmann's area 17). The superior visual field fibers wrap around the temporal horn on their way to the inferior lip of the calcarine fissure. The macular area is served by the most medial area of the calcarine cortex.

# VISUAL FIELDS

**199. Where is the lesion that causes a field defect in only one eye?**
If only one eye is affected, the lesion must be prechiasmal.

**200. Where are the lesions that cause left homonymous hemianopsia, bitemporal hemianopsia, and binasal hemianopsia?**
Left homonymous hemianopsia can arise from the right optic tract, right lateral geniculate body, right optic radiations, or the right occipital cortex. **Bitemporal hemianopsia** is caused by midline chiasmal lesions such as pituitary lesions (from below) or craniopharyngeal tumors (from above). **Binasal hemianopsia** can be caused only by simultaneous lesions on the lateral optic nerves or chiasm, such as bilateral internal carotid artery aneurysms.

**201. What is a junctional scotoma?**
A junctional scotoma results from a lesion at the junction of the optic nerve and chiasm. It causes an ipsilateral central scotoma and a superior temporal defect in the other eye. It occurs because some optic nerve fibers from the inferior temporal retina travel forward for a few millimeters in the contralateral nerve when they decussate in the chiasm; they are thus affected by a lesion in that nerve.

**202. Where is the lesion that causes superior quadrantanopsia?**
Superior quadrantanopsia usually results from damage to the inferior optic radiations. This may occur in Meyer's loop, which is the bundle of inferior optic radiations that swings forward into the temporal lobe.

**203. What visual field results from a right occipital lobe infarction?**
A right occipital lobe infarction causes a left homonymous hemianopsia with macular sparing.

# CORTEX

**204. What are the layers of the cerebral cortex?**
The layers of the cerebral cortex are
I. Molecular layer
II. Outer granular layer
III. Outer pyramidal layer
IV. Inner granular layer
V. Inner pyramidal or ganglion layer
VI. Multiform layer
   Afferent fibers activated by various sensory stimuli terminate in layers IV, III, and II. These signals are then transmitted to adjacent superficial and deep layers through multiple interconnections. All the efferent fibers originate in layer V (Figures 2-12 and 2-13).

**205. What is the columnar organization of the cortex?**
Cortical neurons are arranged in cylindrical columns, each containing 100 to 300 neurons, which are heavily interconnected up and down through the cortical layers. Throughout the somatosensory system, cells responding to one modality are grouped together in the columns. All neurons in the column receive input from the same area and therefore comprise an elementary functional module of cortex.

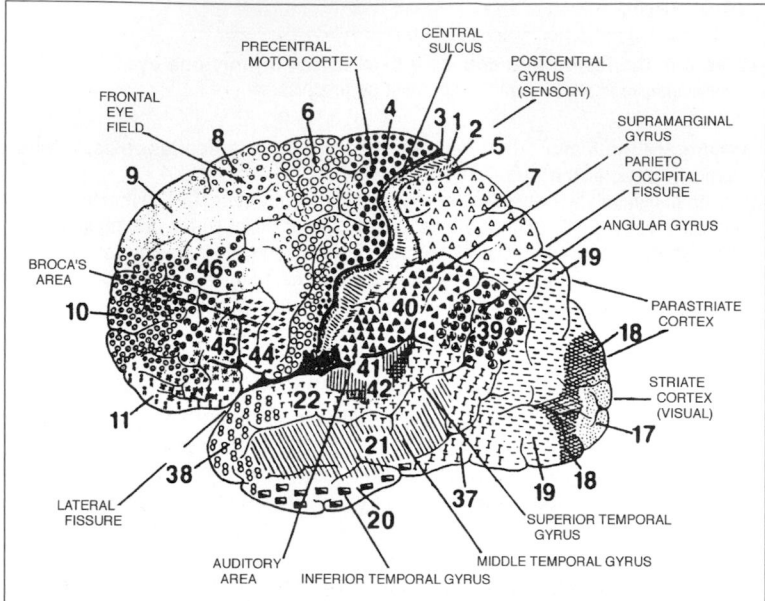

**Figure 2-12.** The superficial anatomy of the cerebral cortex showing Brodmann's areas. From Garoutte B: Survey of Functional Neuroanatomy, 2nd ed. Greenbrae, CA, Jones Medical Publications, 1992, p. 144, with permission.

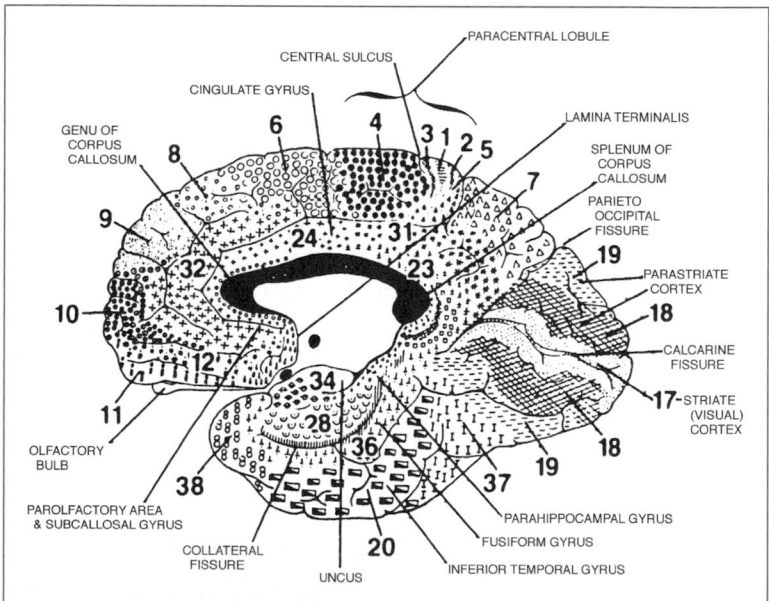

**Figure 2-13.** The superficial anatomy of the cerebral cortex showing Brodmann's areas. From Garoutte N: Survey of Functional Neuroanatomy, 2nd ed. Greenbrae, CA, Jones Medical Publications, 1992, p. 144, with permission.

**206. What is the line of Gennari?**
The fourth layer of the occipital cortex in area 17 is divided by a greatly thickened band of myelinated fibers, which is grossly visible and is called the *line of Gennari*. This stripe also gives the name of *striate cortex* to that area of the brain. Brodmann's areas 18 and 19 lack the line of Gennari.

**207. In what cortical cell layer are the Betz cells located?**
Betz cells give rise to efferent motor tracts (corticospinal fibers) and lie in cortical layer V.

**208. What is the function of the frontal lobe?**
The frontal lobes (both right and left) are involved in voluntary eye movements, somatic motor control, planning and sequencing of movements, and emotional affect. The left frontal lobe is crucial for motor control of speech (Broca's area).

**209. What is the function of the temporal lobe?**
The temporal lobes (both right and left) handle auditory and visual perception, learning and memory, emotional affect, and olfaction. The dominant temporal lobe influences comprehension of speech (Wernicke's area). The nondominant temporal lobe mediates prosody and spatial relationships.

**210. What is the function of the parietal lobe?**
The parietal lobes (both right and left) handle cortical sensation, motor control, and visual perception. The dominant parietal lobe also handles ideomotor praxis. The nondominant parietal lobe controls spatial orientation.

**211. What is the function of the occipital lobe?**
The occipital lobes (both right and left) mainly handle visual perception and involuntary smooth pursuit eye movements.

**212. In which lobe is visual-spatial information processed?**
Visual-spatial information is mainly processed in the nondominant parietal lobe.

**213. Where is language processed?**
Language is primarily processed in Broca's area (posterior inferior frontal gyrus, Brodmann's area 44) and Wernicke's area (posterior part of the superior temporal gyrus, posterior part of Brodmann's area 22) in the dominant hemisphere.

**214. Where is the lesion that causes achromatopsia (inability to match colors and hues)?**
Achromatopsia results from a lesion of the dominant occipital lobe (Brodmann's area 18) and is a feature of the syndrome of alexia without agraphia.

## CIRCULATION

**215. What is meant by the terms *anterior* and *posterior circulation*?**
*Anterior circulation* refers to the common carotid and its distal ramifications, including the internal carotid, middle cerebral, and anterior cerebral arteries. The *posterior circulation* refers to the vertebral and basilar arteries and their branches, including the posterior cerebral artery.

**216. Which vessels make up the circle of Willis?**
1. The **anterior circulation**, which is composed of the middle cerebral arteries, anterior cerebral arteries, and the anterior communicating artery, which connects the two anterior cerebral arteries.
2. The **posterior circulation**, which is composed of the posterior cerebral arteries.
3. The **posterior communicating artery**, which connects the middle cerebral with the posterior cerebral arteries, thus forming a true circle.

**217. If the right anterior cerebral artery is occluded proximally, how does the circle of Willis protect the patient from becoming symptomatic?**
If the occlusion is slow enough for the blood flow to accommodate, the right anterior cerebral artery receives blood from the contralateral internal carotid via the left anterior cerebral and anterior communicating arteries.

**218. What regions are supplied by the anterior cerebral artery, middle cerebral artery, and posterior cerebral artery?**
The **anterior cerebral artery** supplies the medial (midline) cerebral hemispheres, superior frontal lobes, and superior parietal lobes. The **middle cerebral artery** supplies the inferior frontal, inferolateral parietal, and lateral temporal lobes. The **posterior cerebral artery** supplies the occipital lobes and medial temporal lobes.

**219. What is the first intracranial branch off of the internal carotid artery?**
The ophthalmic artery.

**220. What is the blood supply to the deep brain nuclei?**
The basal ganglia are supplied by small lenticulostriate arteries arising from the middle cerebral artery, whereas the thalamus is supplied by perforating thalamogeniculate arteries from the posterior cerebral artery. The blood supply of the thalamus comes from the posterior circulation.

**221. What is the name of the artery that supplies the genu of the internal capsule?**
The recurrent artery of Heubner, which is one of the named anteromedial lenticulostriate arteries, supplies the genu of the internal capsule.

**222. Which artery is the first branch off of the basilar artery?**
The anterior inferior cerebral artery (AICA).

**223. What is the blood supply to the brain stem?**
The brain stem receives its blood supply exclusively from the posterior circulation, including the vertebrals and basilar artery. The medulla receives its blood supply from the vertebrals via medial and lateral perforating arteries. The pons and midbrain receive their blood from the basilar via the medial and lateral perforating arteries.

**224. What is the blood supply to the cerebellum?**
The cerebellum receives its blood supply from the three cerebellar vessels:
1. Posterior inferior cerebellar artery (PICA), off of the vertebrals.
2. Anterior inferior cerebellar artery (AICA), the first branch off of the basilar.
3. Superior cerebellar artery (SCA), the last branch off of the basilar.

**225. Which nerves exit the brain stem area between the posterior cerebral artery and superior cerebellar artery?**
Cranial nerve III exits between the vessels medially, whereas cranial nerve IV exits between them laterally. Aneurysms of these blood vessels may thus damage these cranial nerves.

## KEY POINTS: INNERVATION OF FACE AND HEAD

1. If the facial nerve is damaged (such as from Bell's palsy), the entire side of the face is weak. If the cortical input to the facial nerve is damaged (such as from a stroke), only the lower half of the face will be weak.

2. The most common cause of loss of smell is shearing of olfactory neurons from a sudden blow to the head.

3. A dilated or "blown" pupil implies compression of the III nerve.

4. Collateral blood flow, often routed through the circle of Willis, sometimes protects against damage from strokes.

5. Noncommunicating hydrocephalus is often a medical emergency because the obstructed cerebrospinal fluid (CSF) will cause the intracranial pressure to rise.

### CEREBROSPINAL FLUID

**226. What anatomic structure or structures produce CSF?**
The majority of CSF is produced by the choroid plexus. A small amount of CSF is also produced by the blood vessels in the subependymal region and pia.

**227. Where is the choroid plexus located?**
The choroid plexus is located within the ventricular system, mainly in the lateral and fourth ventricles.

**228. What is the rate of CSF production?**
The rate is approximately 25 cc/hr (approximately 500 cc/day).

**229. How much CSF does an average adult normally have?**
The average male adult has approximately 100 to 150 cc of CSF.

**230. What is communicating hydrocephalus? Noncommunicating hydrocephalus?**
Communicating hydrocephalus occurs when there is dilatation of the ventricles due to obstruction of CSF flow outside the ventricular system (i.e., distal to the foramen of Magendie), so the CSF communicates with the subarachnoid space. Noncommunicating hydrocephalus occurs when there is dilatation of the ventricles due to an obstruction of CSF flow within the ventricular system at or above the foramen of Magendie.

**231. What is the route of CSF from production to clearance?**
Choroid plexus → lateral ventricle → interventricular foramen of Monro → third ventricle → cerebral aqueduct of Sylvius → fourth ventricle → two lateral foramina of Luschka and one medial foramen of Magendie → subarachnoid space → arachnoid granulations → dural sinus → venous drainage.

**232. What space is invaded by a lumbar puncture?**
During a lumbar puncture, the needle enters the subarachnoid space.

**233. What is the ideal spinal level to do a lumbar puncture?**
The ideal level for a lumbar puncture is below the conus medullaris at approximately vertebral level L4 to L5.

## WEBSITE

http://www.biostr.washington.edu/

## BIBLIOGRAPHY

1. Garoutte B: Survey of Functional Neuroanatomy, 2nd ed. Greenbrae, CA, Jones Medical Publications, 1992.
2. Gilman S, Newman SW: Manter and Gatz's Essentials of Clinical Neuroanatomy and Neurophysiology, 10th ed. Philadelphia, F.A. Davis, 2002.
3. Haines D: Neuroanatomy, 7th ed. New York, Lippincott Williams and Wilkins, 2007.
4. Kandel E, Schwartz JH, Jessell TM (eds): Principles of Neuroscience, 3rd ed. New York, Appleton & Lange, 1991.
5. Patten JP: Neurological Differential Diagnosis, 2nd ed. London, Springer, 1996.
6. Posner JP, Saper CB, Schiff N, et al.: Plum and Posner's Diagnosis of Stupor and Coma, 4th ed. London, Oxford University Press, 2007.
7. The Guarantors of Brain: Aids to the Examination of the Peripheral Nervous System, 4th ed. London, W.B. Saunders, 2000.

# CHAPTER 3

# APPROACH TO THE PATIENT WITH NEUROLOGIC DISEASE

*Loren A. Rolak, MD*

1. **What is the first question to be answered in any patient with neurologic disease?**
   Where is the lesion? The neurologist, unlike most physicians, approaches patients from an anatomic perspective, leaving issues of physiology and etiology to be addressed later. The first step in evaluating patients with neurologic symptoms is to localize the lesion to a specific part of the nervous system.

2. **What is the best way to localize a lesion?**
   The history and physical examination accurately localize most lesions of the nervous system. The brain is unique among organs for its high degree of specialization. Because each part of the peripheral nerves, spinal cord, and brain has such specialized functions, damage to each region produces unique clinical effects. Identification of specific signs and symptoms, therefore, permits localization, sometimes within a millimeter, to discrete parts of the nervous system. Pioneer neurologists of the past century referred to the brain as "eloquent"—it speaks directly to the clinician.

3. **What are the most important regions for anatomic localization?**
   For clinical purposes, the great complexity of neuroanatomy can be simplified to a few major regions. Lesions should be localized to one of the following regions:
   1. Muscle
   2. Neuromuscular junction
   3. Peripheral nerve
   4. Root
   5. Spinal cord
   6. Brain stem
   7. Cerebellum
   8. Subcortical brain
   9. Cortical brain

4. **How are symptoms localized to these neuroanatomic regions?**
   The history is the most important part of the neurologic evaluation of a patient. Although precise localizing information can be gleaned from the neurologic physical examination, asking the proper questions during the history accurately localizes most neurologic lesions.
   A helpful system for diagnosis is to begin distally and ask patients questions about each part of the neurologic anatomy, working proximally through the muscle, neuromuscular junction, peripheral nerve, root, spinal cord, cerebellum, brain stem, and subcortex and ending with the cortex of the brain. By sequentially asking about each of these areas, the patient can be "examined" thoroughly. If localization of the lesion is still not clear after a careful history directed at each anatomic region, do not begin the physical examination yet—go back and take a better history.

5. **Which clinical features of muscle disease can be elicited by history?**
   Muscle disease (myopathy) causes proximal symmetric weakness without sensory loss. Questions, therefore, should elicit these symptoms.
   1. **Proximal leg weakness:** Can the patient get out of a car, off the toilet, or up from a chair without using the hands?

2. **Proximal arm weakness:** Can the patient lift or carry objects, such as grocery bags, garbage bags, young children, school books, or briefcases?
3. **Symmetric weakness:** Does the weakness affect both arms or both legs? (Although generalized processes such as myopathies are often slightly asymmetric, weakness confined to one limb or one side of the body is seldom caused by a myopathy.)
4. **Normal sensation:** Is there numbness or other sensory loss? (Although pain and cramping may occur in some myopathies, actual sensory changes should not occur with any disease that is confined to the muscle.)

6. **After a history of muscle disease is elicited, what findings can be expected on physical examination?**
The examination should show proximal symmetric weakness without sensory loss. The muscles are usually normal in size, without atrophy or fasciculations, and muscle tone is usually normal or mildly decreased. Reflexes are also normal or mildly decreased.

7. **Which clinical features of neuromuscular junction disease can be elicited by history?**
Fatigability is the hallmark of diseases affecting the neuromuscular junction, such as myasthenia gravis. Because strength improves with rest, fatigability does not usually manifest as a steadily progressive decline in function; rather, it presents as waxing and waning weakness. When the muscles fatigue, the patient must rest, leading to recovery of strength, which permits further use of the muscles, causing fatigue, which necessitates rest and recovery again. This cycle of worsening with use and recovery with rest produces a variability or fluctuation in strength that is highly characteristic of neuromuscular junction diseases.

8. **After a history of neuromuscular junction problems is elicited, what findings can be expected on physical examination?**
Examination should show fatigable proximal symmetric weakness without sensory loss. Repetitive testing weakens the muscles, which regain their strength after a brief period of rest. The weakness is often extremely proximal, involving muscles of the face, eyes (ptosis), and jaw. The muscles are normal in size, without atrophy or fasciculations, with normal tone and reflexes. There is no sensory loss.

9. **Which clinical features of peripheral neuropathies can be elicited by history?**
Unlike myopathies and neuromuscular junction disease, weakness caused by peripheral neuropathies is often distal rather than proximal. It is also often asymmetric and accompanied by atrophy and fasciculations. Sensory changes almost always accompany neuropathies. The history should elicit the following symptoms:
1. **Distal leg weakness:** Does the patient trip, drag the feet, or wear out the toes of shoes?
2. **Distal arm weakness:** Does the patient frequently drop things or have trouble with the grip?
3. **Asymmetric weakness:** Are symptoms confined to one localized area? (Some neuropathies cause a symmetric stocking-and-glove weakness and numbness, especially those due to metabolic conditions such as diabetes. However, most neuropathies are asymmetric.)
4. **Denervation changes:** Is there a wasting or shrinkage of the muscle (atrophy) or quivering and twitching within the muscle (fasciculations)?
5. **Sensory changes:** Has the patient felt numbness, tingling, or paresthesias?

10. **After a history of peripheral neuropathy is elicited, what findings can be expected on physical examination?**
Examination should reveal distal, often asymmetric weakness with atrophy, fasciculations, and sensory loss. Muscle tone may be normal but is often decreased. Reflexes are usually diminished. Because involvement of autonomic fibers is common in peripheral neuropathies, trophic changes, such as smooth, shiny skin, vasomotor changes (e.g., swelling or temperature dysregulation), and loss of hair or nails, may occur.

11. **Which clinical features of root diseases (radiculopathies) can be elicited by history?**
Pain is the hallmark of root disease. Otherwise, radiculopathies often resemble peripheral neuropathies because of their asymmetric weakness with evidence of denervation (atrophy and fasciculations) and sensory loss. The weakness, while asymmetric, may be either proximal or distal, depending on which roots are involved. (The most common radiculopathies in the legs affect the L5 and S1 roots, causing distal weakness, whereas the most common radiculopathies in the arms affect the C5 and C6 roots, which innervate proximal regions.) The history, therefore, should elicit symptoms similar to a neuropathy with the added component of pain. The pain is usually described as sharp, stabbing, hot, and electric, and it typically shoots or radiates down the limb.

## KEY POINTS: PERIPHERAL NERVOUS SYSTEM

1. The first step in treating patients with neurologic disease is to localize the lesion.

2. Myopathies cause proximal symmetric weakness without sensory loss.

3. Neuromuscular junction diseases cause fatigability.

4. Peripheral neuropathies cause distal asymmetric weakness with atrophy, fasciculations, sensory loss, and pain.

5. Radiculopathies cause radiating pain.

12. **After a history of a radiculopathy is elicited, what findings can be expected on physical examination?**
As is the case with a peripheral neuropathy, the physical examination shows asymmetric muscle weakness with atrophy and fasciculations. Tone is normal or decreased, and the reflexes in the involved muscles are diminished or absent. Weakness is confined to one myotomal group of muscles, such as those innervated by the C6 root in the arm or the L5 root in the leg. Similarly, sensory loss occurs in a dermatomal distribution. Maneuvers that stretch the root often aggravate the pain, such as straight leg raising or neck rotation.

13. **Which clinical features of spinal cord disease can be elicited by history?**
Spinal cord lesions usually cause a triad of symptoms:
    1. **A sensory level is the hallmark of spinal cord disease.** Patients usually describe a sharp line or band around their abdomen or trunk, below which there is a decrease in sensation. The symptom of a sensory level is essentially pathognomonic for spinal cord disease.
    2. **Distal, symmetric, and spastic weakness.** The muscle, neuromuscular junction, nerves, and roots make up the peripheral nervous system, but the spinal cord is in the central nervous system and so has special motor properties. Damage to the spinal cord produces upper motor neuron lesions, affecting the pyramidal (or corticospinal) tract. The weakness is distal more than proximal. In actual clinical practice, almost all processes affecting the cord are symmetric. Upper motor neuron lesions cause spasticity, but this increase in tone may cause few noticeable symptoms—it is best extracted from the history by asking about stiffness in the legs.
    3. **Bowel and bladder problems.** Sphincter dysfunction commonly accompanies cord lesions because of involvement of the autonomic fibers within the cord.

14. **Which questions should be asked during the history to elicit the symptoms of spinal cord disease?**
    1. **Distal leg weakness:** Does the patient drag the toes or trip?
    2. **Distal arm weakness:** Does the patient drop things or have trouble with the grip?
    3. **Symmetric symptoms:** Does the process involve the arms and/or legs approximately equally?
    4. **Sensory level:** Is a sensory level present? Patients often describe it as a band, belt, girdle, or tightness around the trunk or abdomen.
    5. **Sphincter dysfunction:** Is there retention or incontinence of bowel or bladder? (The bladder is usually involved earlier, more often, and more severely than the bowel in spinal cord lesions.)

15. **After a history of spinal cord disease is elicited, what findings can be expected on physical examination?**
    The physical examination in a patient with spinal cord disease usually shows a sensory level below which all sensory modalities are diminished. The sensory (and motor) tracts in the spinal cord are somatotopically organized; distinctive anatomic layering and lamination to the pathways result in greatest damage to fibers from the legs and lower part of the body in the majority of spinal cord lesions. Because most leg fibers lie laterally and are easily compressed, spinal disease usually affects the legs more than the arms. In addition, the level of the symptoms detected clinically does not always correspond to the true anatomic site of the damage. For example, a mass pressing on the spinal cord may cause a sensory level and weakness any place below the actual anatomic level of the lesion.
    The patient also may have urinary retention or incontinence and may lose superficial reflexes, including the anal wink, bulbocavernosus, and cremasteric reflexes. The examination shows evidence of the following upper motor neuron damage:
    1. Distal weakness greater than proximal weakness
    2. Greater weakness of the extensors and antigravity muscles than of the flexors
    3. Increased tone (spasticity)
    4. Increased reflexes
    5. Clonus
    6. Extensor plantar response (positive Babinski sign)
    7. Absent superficial reflexes
    8. No significant atrophy or fasciculations

16. **Which clinical features of brain stem disease can be elicited by history?**
    Cranial nerve symptoms characterize brain stem disease. The brain stem is essentially the spinal cord with embedded cranial nerves. Thus, brain stem lesions cause many of the symptoms of spinal cord disease accompanied by symptoms of cranial nerve impairment.
    Like the spinal cord, the brain stem contains "long tracts," or pathways that extend from the brain down through the spinal cord. The major long tracts are the pyramidal (corticospinal) tract for motor function, the spinothalamic tract carrying pain and temperature sensations up to the thalamus, and the dorsal columns carrying position and vibration sense up to the thalamus. Because of the decussation of these tracts, lesions in the brain stem do not produce a horizontal motor or sensory level as they do in the spinal cord but rather produce a vertical motor or sensory level—that is, hemiparesis or hemianesthesia affecting one side of the body.
    Lesions affecting the cranial nerves in the brain stem often produce symptoms referred to as the "Ds" (Table 3-1).

17. **Which questions elicit symptoms of combined cranial nerve and long tract dysfunction?**
    1. **Long tract signs:** Does the patient have hemiparesis or hemisensory loss?
    2. **Cranial nerve signs:** Does the patient have diplopia, dysarthria, dysphagia, dizziness, deafness, or decreased strength or sensation over the face?

| TABLE 3-1. SYMPTOMS OF CRANIAL NERVE DAMAGE | |
|---|---|
| Cranial Nerve | Symptoms |
| III | Diplopia |
| IV | Diplopia |
| V | Decreased facial sensation |
| VI | Diplopia |
| VII | Decreased strength and drooping of the face |
| VIII | Deafness and dizziness |
| IX | Dysarthria and dysphagia |
| X | Dysarthria and dysphagia |
| XI | Decreased strength in neck and shoulders |
| XII | Dysarthria and dysphagia |

3. **Crossed signs:** Because the long tracts cross, but the cranial nerves generally do not, brain stem lesions often produce symptoms on one side of the face and the opposite side of the body. For example, a lesion in the pons that affects the pyramidal tracts and the facial (VII) nerve will cause weakness of that side of the face and the opposite, crossed side of the body. Brain stem disease often produces bilateral or crossed findings.

18. **After a history of brain stem disease is elicited, what findings can be expected on physical examination?**
Examination of the cranial nerves may reveal ptosis; pupillary abnormalities; extraocular muscle paralysis; diplopia; nystagmus; decreased corneal and blink reflexes; facial weakness or numbness; deafness; vertigo; dysarthria; dysphagia; weakness or deviation of the palate; decreased gag reflex; or weakness of the neck, shoulders, or tongue.
Long tract abnormalities may include hemiparesis, which shows an upper motor neuron pattern of distal extensor weakness with hyperreflexia, spasticity, and a positive Babinski sign. Hemisensory loss may occur to all modalities.

19. **Which clinical features of cerebellar disease can be elicited by history?**
Cerebellar disease causes incoordination, clumsiness, and tremor because the cerebellum is responsible for smoothing out and refining voluntary movements. Questions, therefore, should focus on the following symptoms:
1. **Clumsiness in the legs:** Does the patient have a staggering, drunken walk? (Most laymen describe cerebellar symptoms in terms of alcohol and drunkenness, probably because drinking alcohol impairs the cerebellum. The characteristic ataxic, wide-based, staggering gait of the person intoxicated by alcohol is a reflection of cerebellar dysfunction.)
2. **Clumsiness in the arms:** Does the patient have difficulty with targeted movements, such as lighting a cigarette or placing a key in a lock? (Cerebellar tremor is worse with voluntary, intentional movements that require accurate placement.)
3. **Brain stem symptoms:** Are brain stem symptoms present? (Because the cerebellar inflow and outflow must pass through the brain stem and the blood supply to the cerebellum arises from the same vessels that supply the brain stem, cerebellar disease is almost always accompanied by some brain stem abnormalities as well, and vice versa.)

20. **After a history of cerebellar disease is elicited, what findings can be expected on physical examination?**
The patient's gait is staggering, wide-based, and ataxic, causing difficulties especially with tandem walking. Fine coordinated movements of the legs are impossible, such as sliding a heel

down a shin or tracing patterns on the floor with the foot. The cerebellar tremor is most visible in the upper extremities, which waver and wobble with attempts to touch a specific target, such as the examiner's finger or the patient's own nose. Rapid alternating movements are irregular in rate and rhythm.

21. **How can the history determine whether disease of the brain is subcortical or cortical?**
The history can differentiate subcortical from cortical disease by focusing on the following four major areas:
1. The presence of specific cortical deficits
2. The pattern of motor and sensory deficits
3. The type of sensory deficits
4. The presence of visual field deficits

22. **What specific deficits are seen with cortical lesions?**
The most useful symptom of cortical disease in the dominant (usually left) hemisphere is aphasia. The history, therefore, should focus on any difficulties with language functions, including not only speech but also writing, reading, and comprehension. A lesion affecting the left side of the brain that does not affect language function is unlikely to be cortical.

In the nondominant (usually right) hemisphere, cortical dysfunction is more subtle, but usually causes visual–spatial problems. Patients with nondominant cortical lesions often have neglect and denial, including inattention to their own physical signs and symptoms. This finding can be difficult to elicit on history, however, and sometimes depends on the physical examination. Note also that seizures are almost always cortical in origin.

23. **How does the pattern of motor and sensory deficits differentiate cortical from subcortical involvement?**
The motor homunculus in the primary and supplemental motor strips is spread upside down over a vast expanse of gray matter. Neurons controlling the lower extremities reside between the two hemispheres, in the interhemispheric fissure, whereas neurons moving the trunk, arms, and face are draped upside down over the superficial cortex. Cortical lesions, therefore, often involve the face, arm, and trunk, but spare the legs, which are protected in the interhemispheric fissure. Cortical lesions thus cause an incomplete hemiparesis, affecting the face and arm but not the leg.

Of course, fibers to the leg descend and merge with those to the face and arm as the pyramidal tract forms deep within the brain, subcortically, to run in the internal capsule, cerebral peduncles, and the pyramids themselves. Therefore, even a small subcortical lesion can affect all of these conjoined fibers. Subcortical lesions thus cause a complete hemiparesis, affecting face, arm, and leg.

The sensory homunculus has a similar somatotropic arrangement that results in an analogous pattern of localization.

24. **How does the type of sensory deficit differentiate cortical from subcortical lesions by history?**
Most of the primary sensory modalities reach "consciousness" in the thalamus and do not require the cortex for their perception. A patient with severe cortical damage can still feel pain, touch, vibration, and position. A history of significant numbness or sensory loss, therefore, suggests a subcortical lesion.

Cortical sensory loss is more refined and usually involves complicated sensory processing such as two-point discrimination, accurate localization of perceptions, stereognosis, and graphesthesia. These symptoms can be difficult to elicit by history alone.

25. **How do visual symptoms differentiate cortical from subcortical disease by history?**
Visual pathways run subcortically for most of their length. Visual impulses in the optic nerves may cross in the chiasm and run through the optic tracts, lateral geniculate bodies, and optic radiations before synapsing in the occipital cortex. Cortical lesions, such as those affecting the motor strip, sensory strip, or language areas, are too superficial to affect these visual fibers and thus do not cause visual field deficits. Subcortical lesions often affect the visual fibers, producing visual field cuts. Therefore, a history of visual field loss suggests a subcortical lesion. (Of course, a strictly cortical lesion in the occipital lobes produces visual symptoms, but it does not affect motor, sensory, or other functions and so does not cause confusion with the typical picture of a subcortical lesion.)

## KEY POINTS: CENTRAL NERVOUS SYSTEM

1. Spinal cord disease causes a "triad" of distal symmetric weakness, sphincter problems, and a sensory level.

2. Brain stem disease causes abnormalities of cranial nerves plus long tracts.

3. Cerebellar disease causes ataxia and an action tremor.

4. In the brain, cortical lesions may cause aphasia, seizures, and partial hemiparesis (face and arm only), while subcortical lesions may cause visual field cuts, dense numbness of primary sensory modalities, and more complete hemiparesis (face, arm, and leg).

26. **After a history of cortical or subcortical disease is elicited, what findings can be expected on physical examination?**
Physical examination findings parallel the historical deficits.
1. **Cortical dysfunction:** The patient may show aphasia, visual-spatial dysfunction, or seizures.
2. **Motor involvement:** Physical examination shows upper motor neuron weakness affecting the face and arm in a cortical lesion and the face, arm, and leg in a subcortical lesion.
3. **Sensory dysfunction:** In subcortical disease, the examination shows problems with primary sensory modalities, such as decreased pinprick and vibration, but in cortical disease, it shows relatively normal sensation with impaired higher sensory processing, such as graphesthesia and stereognosis.
4. **Visual dysfunction:** Patients with subcortical disease may have visual field cuts, but patients with cortical disease do not.

27. **How accurate are the history and physical examination for diagnosing neurologic disease?**
The clinical examination is highly accurate in localizing neurologic disease. Once a lesion has been localized to one of the broad anatomic regions, an etiology usually suggests itself. For example, if a lesion can be localized to the peripheral nerve, it is usually easy to develop a differential diagnosis for peripheral neuropathies (such as diabetes, alcoholism) and a diagnostic plan (e.g., blood testing, nerve conduction studies). The anatomy usually implies an etiology.
Organized questioning and examination of the nervous system in this fashion are excellent ways to approach the neurologic patient.

## WEBSITES

1. http://www.neuroguide.com
2. http://www.neuroland.com

## BIBLIOGRAPHY

1. Brazis P, Masdeu JC, Biller J: Localization in Clinical Neurology. Philadelphia, Lippincott Williams & Wilkins, 2006.
2. Campbell W: Dejong's The Neurologic Examination, 6th ed. Philadelphia, Lippincott Williams &Wilkins, 2005.
3. Caplan L: The Effective Clinical Neurologist, 2nd ed. Boston, Butterworth-Heinemann, 2001.
4. DeMyer WE: Technique of the Neurological Examination, 5th ed. New York, McGraw-Hill, 2003.

# CHAPTER 4

# MYOPATHIES

*Yadollah Harati, MD, FACP, and Suur Biliciler, MD*

## INTRODUCTION

1. **What is a myopathy?**
   A myopathy is a disorder in which there is a primary functional or structural impairment of skeletal muscle.

2. **What signs and symptoms are suggestive of a myopathy?**
   1. Proximal symmetric weakness, which may be acute, subacute, or chronic
   2. Reduced, preserved, or enlarged muscle bulk
   3. Muscle pain or discomfort with palpation (myalgia)
   4. Muscle stiffness or cramps
   5. Asthenia and fatigue
   6. Myoglobinuria

3. **Define *myoblast, myotube, myofiber,* and *myofibril*.**
   A myoblast is a postmitotic, mononucleated cell capable of fusion and contractile protein synthesis. Myotubes are long, cylindrical, multinucleated (syncytial) cells formed from the fusion of myoblasts. When their central nuclei are shifted to a subsarcolemmial position in the later stages of development, they are called *myofibers*. The appearance of central nuclei within an otherwise normal adult muscle is a useful sign of muscle regeneration. Each adult myofiber is packed with numerous myofibrils, largely composed of hexagonal arrangements of thick and thin contractile filaments. Myosin is the major constituent of the thick filaments, whereas actin is the contractile protein of the thin filaments.

4. **Describe the embryonic origin of skeletal muscle.**
   Muscles develop from mesodermal cell populations arising in the somite. The connective tissues around the muscles have a different embryologic origin and are derived from the somatopleural mesoderm.

5. **What is a motor unit?**
   A motor unit consists of a motor neuron, its single axon, the associated neuromuscular junctions and terminal axon branches, and the many muscle fibers that they supply. All muscle fibers belonging to a single motor unit are of the same histochemical and physiologic type.

6. **What are the general categories of myopathies?**
   - Inflammatory myopathies (e.g., polymyositis, dermatomyositis, inclusion body myositis)
   - Muscular dystrophies (e.g., Duchenne, myotonic, limb-girdle)
   - Congenital myopathies (e.g., central core, centronuclear myopathy)
   - Metabolic myopathies (e.g., myophosphorylase deficiency, phosphofructokinase deficiency)
   - Mitochondrial myopathies (e.g., Kearns-Sayre syndrome)
   - Toxic myopathies (e.g., alcohol, zidovudine)
   - Endocrine myopathies (e.g., hypothyroidism, hypoadrenalism)
   - Infectious myopathies (e.g., trichinosis, AIDS)

7. **How do we grade functional weakness?**

   The most widely used system was developed by the Medical Research Council (MRC) of Great Britain. The MRC system grades strength from 0 to 5. The addition of a plus (+) or minus (−) further quantifies strength:

   0 No movement
   1 Trace movement
   2 Able to move, but not against gravity
   3 Able to move full range against gravity
   4 Able to move against some resistance
   5 Normal strength

   In addition, the clinician may observe the patient performing the following maneuvers to look for subtle weakness:

   1. Arise from a chair with arms folded.
   2. Walk the length of the examining room on toes, on heels, and tandem.
   3. Hop on either foot.
   4. Perform deep knee bends.
   5. Climb a step.
   6. Horizontally abduct arms and reach the vertex of the head.
   7. Lift up the head from a table.
   8. Arise from supine position with hands overhead.
   9. Lift head and shoulders, and extend the neck while in a prone position.

   Medical Research Council: Aids to the Examination of the Peripheral Nervous System. London: W.B. Saunders, 2000.

8. **What is Gower's sign?**

   This term describes the maneuver of rising from a supine position in the presence of marked proximal weakness. The patient must roll to a prone position, push off the floor, lock the knees, and push the upper body upward by "climbing up" the legs with the hands. Although Gower's sign is usually seen in children with myopathies, it may be present in any patient with marked proximal weakness.

## DIAGNOSIS

9. **What are the most valuable tests for evaluating patients with suspected muscle disease?**

   A diagnosis often can be established by supporting the clinical findings with results from three key tests: (1) serum creatine kinase (CK) levels, (2) electromyography (EMG), and (3) muscle biopsy.

10. **Which myopathies are associated with elevated serum CK levels?**

    CK catalyzes the reversible reaction of adenosine triphosphate (ATP) and creatine to form adenosine diphosphate (ADP) and phosphocreatine. It is elevated in many myopathies due to myofiber disruption or degeneration. However, CK levels may be normal in some patients with an ongoing myopathy. Examples include profound muscle wasting and selected conditions such as hyperthyroidism. Serum CK is especially high in limb-girdle muscular dystrophies (dysferlinopathies and sarcoglycanopathies), Duchenne and Becker muscular dystrophies, inflammatory myopathies, and rhabdomyolysis.

11. **What conditions other than myopathies are associated with an elevated CK level?**
    - Exercise
    - Increased muscle bulk

- Muscle trauma (needle injection, EMG, surgery, edema, vigorous exercise, or contusion)
- Viral illnesses
- African American race
- Drug use (including alcohol and cholesterol-lowering agents)
- Eating licorice
- Hypothyroidism
- Hypoparathyroidism
- Malignant hyperthermia
- Neurogenic disease (e.g., amyotrophic lateral sclerosis)
- Benign hereditary CK elevation
  Typically CK levels are increased less than threefold in these conditions, whereas CK levels greater than fivefold often suggest an underlying myopathic etiology.

12. **After unaccustomed exercise, normal people often have pain and soreness of muscles. Does the type of exercise play any role in the extent of muscle pain and damage?**
Yes. In the face of a markedly elevated CK level in a healthy person engaged in exercises, it is important to ask about the type of exercise. Activities that involve **concentric** contractions of muscles (shortening of muscles) produce less muscle pain and damage than activities involving **eccentric** contraction (lengthening of muscles). An example of concentric contraction is the shortening of the muscle that occurs in the flexed leg during climbing stairs. Eccentric contraction is the lengthening of the muscle in the extended leg that supports the body during walking downstairs. Elevation of CK level by 10- to 100-fold after even 30 minutes of vigorous eccentric leg exercises has been observed. Because such exercises may be especially damaging to an already diseased muscle, physical therapists should be made aware of any disease state.

13. **What is the approach to evaluating a persistent but incidental elevation of serum CK?**
Perform an EMG if symptoms of weakness, myalgia, cramps, or tenderness are present. If the EMG findings are suggestive of a myopathy, a muscle biopsy may be considered. If both the examination and EMG are normal, have the patient rest for three to four days and recheck serum CK early in the morning. If levels are still high, a muscle biopsy might be beneficial. If serum CK is within normal limits, then follow the patient clinically. A muscle biopsy in this setting rarely yields any useful information.

14. **When is a muscle biopsy indicated? How is the muscle site chosen?**
Muscle weakness with associated laboratory or electrophysiologic evidence of a myopathy is an indication to pursue a muscle biopsy. Selection of the most appropriate muscle for biopsy is important, and several factors need to be considered, including availability of normative data for the site. Although affected muscles are ideal to biopsy, moderately affected muscles are better than severely affected muscles because fibrosis and fatty replacement of the muscle, which are characteristic of end-stage muscle disease, may not provide adequate information. In addition, muscles affected by other conditions (e.g., radiculopathy or trauma) should be avoided if possible. In general, the biceps or deltoid muscles in the upper extremity or the vastus lateralis muscle in the lower extremity are selected. Because upper extremity muscles are more vascular, they may have a higher diagnostic yield when a vasculitic process is suspected.

15. **What minimum number of stains is typically used to evaluate a myopathy? What morphologic features of a myopathy may be seen on biopsy?**
Both the hematoxylin and eosin (H&E) and the modified Gomori trichrome stains provide useful general information about the muscle structures and cellular details. In addition, the modified Gomori trichrome stain allows visualization of the mitochondrial activity and

collection by staining red (ragged red fibers). The ATPase stain defines the fibers by their histochemical type. Reduced nicotinamide adenine dinucleotide trazolium reductase (NADH-TR) also differentiates type 1 and type 2 fibers and provides information about the oxidative activity of muscle fibers.

Morphologic features of a myopathy include muscle fiber necrosis, phagocytosis and regeneration, increased central nuclei, fiber hypertrophy and rounding, variation in fiber size and shape, and increased endomysial connective tissue (Figure 4-1).

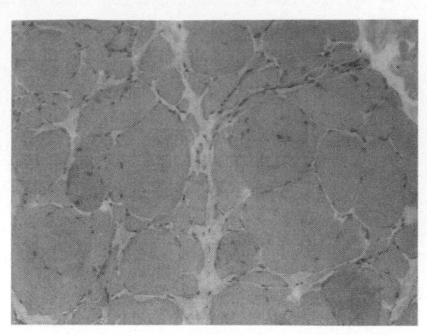

**Figure 4-1.** Note hypertrophic fibers, increased variation in fiber size and shape, and increased nuclei in a patient with limb-girdle muscular dystrophy (hematoxylin and eosin stain).

16. **How many fiber types are recognized by muscle histochemistry?**
Type 1 fibers are slow-twitch, red fibers; type 2 fibers are fast-twitch, white fibers. The two major subtypes of type 2 fibers are types 2A and 2B. The histochemical and physiologic properties of each fiber type are determined by the anterior horn cell that innervates it.

17. **What are ragged red fibers?**
Ragged red fibers are muscle fibers with an accumulation of subsarcolemmal and intermyofibrillar material that stains red with modified Gomori trichrome stain (Figure 4-2). This red-stained material is actually mitochondria that are abnormal in number, size, and structure when viewed by electron microscopy. Although ragged red fibers are typically seen in mitochondrial myopathies, they may occur in other conditions such as inclusion body myositis. They are a nonspecific finding in an otherwise normal biopsy, especially if the biopsy is from an elderly patient, because their frequency increases with age.

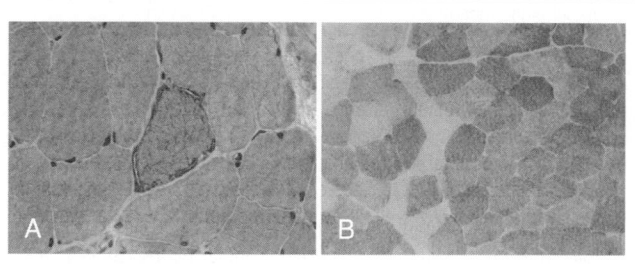

**Figure 4-2.** (A) A ragged red fiber in a patient with progressive ophthalmoplegia (modified trichrome stain). (B) Note COX-negative fibers corresponding with ragged red fibers (cytochrome C oxidase stain).

18. **What are tubular aggregates?**
Tubular aggregates are clusters of tubular proliferation arising from the sarcoplasmic reticulum, usually affecting type 2 fibers. They have a red appearance with modified Gomori trichrome stain, stain dark with NADH-TR, and do not react to succinyl dehydratase (SDH),

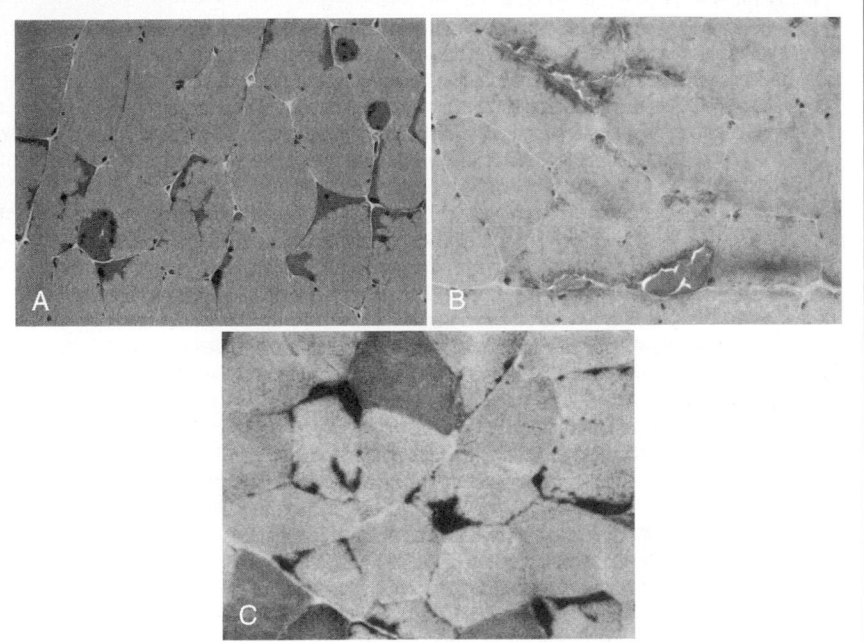

**Figure 4-3.** Tubular aggregates. (A) Hematoxylin and eosin stain. (B) Modified trichrome stain. (C) NADH-TR stain.

ATPase, and myophosphorylase (Figure 4-3). They can be a minor pathologic feature in hypokalemic periodic paralysis, myotonia congenita, or other myotonic disorders, congenital myasthenic syndromes, muscle disorders associated with cramps, as well as exposure to certain medications and alcohol.

## INFLAMMATORY MYOPATHIES

19. **What are the most common causes of muscle pain?**
Most muscle pains are caused by a nonmuscular condition, such as vascular insufficiency, joint disease, or neuropathy. The vast majority of myopathies are painless. Myopathies that may be associated with pain include inflammatory myopathies, metabolic myopathies, mitochondrial myopathies, and some muscular dystrophies (limb-girdle, Becker muscular dystrophy [BMD]). In general, in patients with a normal exam and a normal serum CK level, muscle pain is usually not myopathic in origin.

20. **How are the polymyositis (PM) and dermatomyositis (DM) syndromes classified?**
1. Adult polymyositis and dermatomyositis
2. Childhood and juvenile dermatomyositis
3. Dermatomyositis associated with other diseases (connective tissue disorders, malignancy)
4. Polymyositis associated with other diseases (connective tissue diseases, malignancy)

**21. What are the clinical features of PM and DM?**

The history and pattern of weakness (subacute proximal weakness greatest in the upper extremities and neck flexors) are similar in DM and PM, and both are responsive to immunosuppression. Pharyngeal weakness is also common in both (about 30% of cases). Tendon reflexes might be depressed on examination. Females predominate in all age groups. Approximately 5% of patients develop symptomatic systemic involvement, including fever, weight loss, cardiac arrhythmias and conduction abnormalities, and pulmonary involvement. The presence of anti-Jo-1 antibody is a marker for interstitial lung disease. Anti-Mi2 (a chromodomain helicase DNA-binding protein) antibody positive DM cases have a better prognosis and less interstitial lung disease. Higher titers of polymyositis-scleroderma (PM-Scl) antibodies can be associated with scleroderma in either of the myopathies. Both PM and DM also have been associated with malignancies, in particular lung, GI, breast, and ovarian cancers. Most experts agree that patients should be screened with routine blood work, chest radiograph, mammography, and pelvic and rectal exams. Patients age 50 years and older with DM are at higher risk of developing cancer and should be watched closely. Although EMG findings vary according to the stage of the disease, fibrillation and sharp wave potentials are present in most patients (including the paraspinous muscles).

Unique to DM are cutaneous manifestations that typically present at the same time as the weakness. The characteristic heliotrope rash involves the eyelids, cheeks, nose, neck and upper chest (V sign), shoulders (shawl sign), elbows, knees, medial malleoli, and buttocks. Gottron's papules are often seen on the knuckles. Skin may become scaly and atrophic, and the nail beds may appear shiny and red. Rash worsens with exposure to sunlight. Although PM is an adult disease, DM occurs in both children and adults. The skin manifestations and gastrointestinal vasculitis that might result in hemorrhage and perforation are much more common in children.

**22. What is inclusion body myositis (IBM)?**

IBM is now considered the most common cause of acquired chronic myopathy in patients age 50 years and older. It is similar to polymyositis immunopathologically, although it has a distinct clinical phenotype. Characteristically, the painless weakness and atrophy are gradual and insidious in onset and more commonly involve the quadriceps, finger flexors, and foot dorsiflexors. Dysphagia is common. There is early loss of patellar reflexes, and a mild neuropathy may be present. CK levels are either normal or only mildly elevated. One-third of cases appear stable or show improvement for periods of 6 months or more. Electrodiagnostic evaluation reveals mixed myopathic and neurogenic changes. Muscle biopsy shows varying degrees of inflammation, cytoplasmic "rimmed" vacuoles and eosinophilic inclusion bodies, and small angular atrophic and denervated fibers. The vacuoles contain filaments and several proteins ($\beta$-amyloid, desmin, ubiquitin, tau, transglutaminanes 1 and 2). The vacuolated fibers are rarely invaded by inflammatory cells. Mitochondrial dysfunction (cytochrome oxidase negative fibers and multiple mDNA deletions) is seen in 50% of IBM cases. Despite the evident inflammation, IBM is resistant to conventional immunotherapies. Cricopharyngeal myotomy might be beneficial in cases of dysphagia and might delay the need for a percutaneous endoscopic gastrostomy.

Askanas V, Engel WK: Inclusion body myositis: Muscle fiber molecular pathology and possible pathogenic significance of its similarity to Alzheimer's and Parkinson's disease brains. Acta Neuropathol 116:583-595, 2008.

Karpati G, O'Ferrall EK: Sporadic inclusion body myositis: Pathogenic considerations. Ann Neurol 65:7-11, 2009.

Oh TH, Brumfield KA, Hoskin TL, et al.: Dysphagia in inflammatory myopathy: Clinical characteristics, treatment strategies, and outcome in 62 patients. Mayo Clinic Proc 82:441-447, 2007.

23. **What are the major pathologic changes on light microscopy in the muscle biopsies of patients with PM, DM, and IBM?**

Both PM and DM have the following (Figures 4-4 to 4-6):
1. Inflammatory infiltrate
   - Perivascular (more in DM)
   - Endomysial or perimysial
2. Fiber necrosis, phagocytosis
3. Perifascicular atrophy (especially in DM of childhood)
4. Variation and rounding of muscle fibers; occasional angular and atrophic fibers
5. Capillary loss or necrosis (more in DM)
6. Eosinophilic cytoplasmic inclusions and rimmed vacuoles, denervation changes, and interstitial infiltration (especially in IBM)

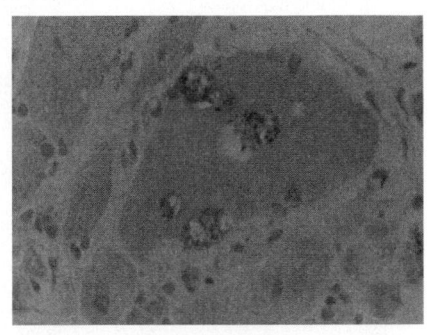

**Figure 4-4.** Inclusion body myositis, rimmed vacuoles (hematoxylin and eosin stain).

24. **What does the muscle biopsy in Figure 4-6 signify?**

This is the typical finding of perifascicular atrophy. The muscle fibers at the periphery of the muscle fascicles are smaller, whereas the fibers in the deepest part of the fascicle are of normal size. This type of atrophy is generally recognized to be a conspicuous feature of childhood dermatomyositis and, to a lesser extent, adult dermatomyositis. Even in the absence of inflammation, this biopsy is characteristic. The pattern of atrophy is probably due to capillary changes and involves mainly muscle fibers near the perimysial connective tissue because these fibers are less likely to have collateral circulation.

**Figure 4-5.** Polymyositis, endomysial inflammation showing rounding of fibers (hematoxylin and eosin stain).

## MYOTONIA

25. **Define *myotonia*.**

Myotonia is the phenomena of impaired relaxation of muscle after forceful voluntary contraction and most commonly involves the hands and eyelids. Myotonia is due to repetitive depolarization of the muscle membrane. Patients may complain of muscle stiffness or tightness resulting in difficulty releasing their handgrip after a handshake, unscrewing a bottle top, or opening their eyelids if they shut their eyes forcefully. Myotonia classically improves with repeated exercise, while in contrast, paramyotonia is typically worsened by exercise. Exposure to cold makes both myotonia and paramyotonia worse.

26. **What are the inherited myotonic disorders?**
    - Myotonic dystrophy (type 1 myotonic dystrophy)
    - Proximal myotonic myopathy (PROMM; type 2 myotonic dystrophy)
    - Myotonia congenita (Thomsen disease, Becker's disease*)
    - Paramyotonia congenita
    - Periodic paralysis (hypokalemic, normo/hyperkalemic)
    - Chondrodystrophic myotonia* (Schwartz-Jampel syndrome)

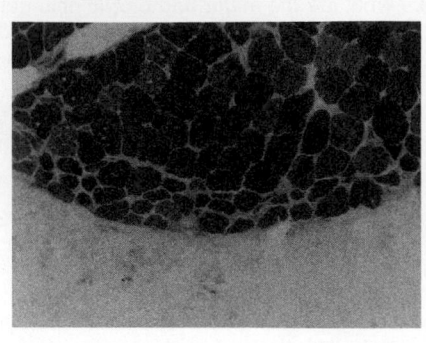

**Figure 4-6.** ATP 9.6. Dermatomyositis—perifascicular atrophy.

27. **What is the most common muscular dystrophy in adults? How does it present?**
    Myotonic dystrophy type 1 (MyD), which has an estimated prevalence of 13.5 per 100,000 live births in Western countries, is most common in adults. MyD is a multisystem disorder with an autosomal dominant pattern of inheritance, but severity and degree of systemic involvement vary considerably. The most common form of the disease presents in the second decade of life, but there is also a congenital form. In contrast to other major dystrophies, muscle weakness is usually secondary in nature. The first symptom is usually myotonia; hand weakness and gait difficulties are also common presenting complaints.
    The characteristic appearance of a patient with MyD is important to recognize. Facial weakness and temporalis muscle atrophy give rise to a narrow, hatchet-faced appearance. In addition, patients develop frontal baldness, ptosis, and neck muscle atrophy early in the disease.

28. **What systems are involved in MyD?**
    - **Cardiac.** Conduction problems are a major cause of morbidity and mortality. About 90% of patients have electrocardiogram (ECG) abnormalities, and complete heart block and sudden death are well recognized. Prophylactic pacemaker implantation is needed in patients with conduction block.
    - **Respiratory.** Excessive daytime sleepiness is common because of a combination of weakness of the diaphragm and intercostal muscles, decreased response to hypoxia, alveolar hypoventilation, hypercapnia, and abnormalities of brain stem neuroregulatory mechanisms.
    - **Gastrointestinal.** Smooth muscle involvement results in many symptoms, including abdominal pain, dysphagia, emesis, diarrhea, and bowel incontinence.
    - **Central nervous system** symptoms include impaired intelligence, apathy, reluctance to seek or follow medical advice, and personality disorders.
    - **Skeletal muscle** symptoms include atrophy, weakness, and myotonia.
    - **Endocrine.** Testicular atrophy and insulin resistance are common; overt diabetes is uncommon.
    - Other symptoms include frontal balding, cranial hyperostosis, air sinus enlargement, and minor sensory neuropathy.

---

*Autosomal recessive inheritance, while all other conditions are of autosomal dominant inheritance.

**29. What are the characteristics of the *MyD* gene?**

The mutation in MyD is an expansion of a trinucleotide (CTG) repeat in the protein kinase gene on the long arm of chromosome 19. In normal people, the number of repeats is less than 37, whereas in MyD, it ranges from 50 to a few thousand. The size of the expanded repeat closely correlates with the severity and age of onset of MyD and generally increases in successive generations within a family, providing a molecular basis for the clinical observed phenomenon known as *anticipation* (progressively earlier onset of the disease in successive generations).

Mutant transcripts cause muscle dysfunction by interfering with biogenesis of other mRNAs. The toxic effects of mutant RNAs are mediated partly through sequestration of splicing regulator Musclebind-like 1 (Mbnl1), a protein that binds the expanded RNA. Another gene that is prominently affected encodes the Clcn1 (chloride channel 1) protein, which results in loss of channel function, thus leading to myotonia.

Osborne RJ, Lin X, Welle S, et al.: Transcriptional and post-transcriptional impact of toxic RNA in myotonic dystrophy. Human Mol Genet 18:1471-1481, 2009.

**30. What is PROMM (myotonic dystrophy type 2)?**

Muscle weakness is usually proximal and facial weakness is minimal. Myotonia is usually absent on examination but is present on EMG testing. There is no congenital form. Systemic involvement closely resembles MyD type 1. The mutation is due to a CCTG expansion in a specific zinc-finger gene (ZNF9) localized to chromosome 3q. Anticipation is less marked when compared to MyD. PROMM should be considered in any atypical progressive disorder with proximal muscle weakness.

## PERIODIC PARALYSIS

**31. What are the periodic paralysis (PP) disorders?**

They are muscle channelopathies that consist of hyperkalemic (potassium sensitive) PP, Hypokalemic PP, and Andersen-Tawil syndrome (ATS). All are inherited in an autosomal dominant fashion. Most cases in hyperkalemic PP are caused by mutations in the sodium channel gene *SCN4A*, while most of the hypokalemic PPs are due to mutations in the calcium channel gene *CACNA1S* on chromosome 1q31. ATS is secondary to mutations in the potassium channel gene *KCNJ2* on chromosome 17q23. They have a distinct clinical presentation with attacks of weakness that can be mild or severe and focal or generalized. Over time, patients might develop fixed weakness. ATS patients have dysmorphic features (e.g., hypertelorism, high-arched palate) and cardiac arrhythmias. During attacks, serum CK is usually elevated with serum potassium levels being variable (high, low, or normal). Between attacks, EMG may show myotonia in hyperkalemic PP patients, while muscles are electrically silent in all types during an episode of weakness.

Saperstein DS: Muscle channelopathies. Semin Neurol 28:168-184, 2008.

**32. What is the treatment for periodic paralysis?**

Acetazolamide and dichlorphenamide, both of which are carbonic anhydrase inhibitors, are effective in some patients with each form of periodic paralysis. In patients with hypokalemic PP, potassium-sparing diuretics such as sprionolactone and triamterene might be used in addition to oral potassium supplements and a low-carbohydrate and low-sodium diet. Beta-adrenergic agents or ingestion of a high-carbohydrate, low-potassium diet may alleviate the attacks in hyperkalemic PP. Antiarrhythmics, beta-blockers, or cardioverter-defibrillators should be considered in ATS.

## OTHER MUSCULAR DYSTROPHIES

33. **Describe the salient features of the Duchenne muscular dystrophy gene.**
The gene is large (2.3 Mb), located in the short arm of the X chromosome, and codes for a structural protein called *dystrophin*. It is by far the largest gene characterized to date, consisting of 2.3 million base pairs and occupying approximately 1% of the human X chromosome. Dystrophin is a protein located in the subsarcolemmal region of the muscle fiber. It is expressed predominantly in skeletal, cardiac, and smooth muscle and in kidney, cerebral cortex, and lung. Mutations within the gene cause Duchenne muscular dystrophy (DMD); Becker's muscular dystrophy (BMD); exercise intolerance with myalgias, cramps, and myoglobinuria; minimal limb girdle weakness or quadriceps myopathy; asymptomatic elevation of CK level; cardiomyopathy with mild muscle weakness; and fatal X-linked cardiomyopathy without muscle weakness. Between 50% and 70% of cases of dystrophin mutations arise from intragenic deletions involving one or many exons. Duplication of the gene accounts for 10% of mutations. Rarely, intronic mutations can also cause clinically overt disease.
    Baskin B, Banwell B, Khater RA, et al.: Becker muscular dystrophy caused by an intronic mutation reducing the efficiency of the splice donor site of intron 26 of the dystrophin gene. Neuromuscul Disord 19:189-192, 2009.

34. **What organs other than skeletal muscle are involved in DMD?**
About 90% of patients have ECG abnormalities, but symptomatic involvement occurs in less than 1% of patients. Although the heart may be enlarged with minimal fibrosis, the myocardial muscle fibers do not undergo necrosis or other myopathic changes. There is also an increased incidence of gastrointestinal hypomotility that may lead to intestinal pseudo-obstruction and gastric dilatation. Finally, pachygyria and smaller-than-normal brains have been noted in some patients with DMD. In addition, an association between mental retardation and mutations causing central exon deletions has been observed.

35. **Which dystrophies are associated with contractures?**
    ■ Dystrophinopathies
    ■ Limb-girdle muscular dystrophy 1G and 2A
    ■ Emery-Dreifuss muscular dystrophy

36. **What is fascioscapulohumeral muscular dystrophy (FSHD)?**
FSHD is the third most common inherited disease of muscle.
It has autosomal dominant inheritance.
There is a decrease in the number of DNA repeat sequence (D4Z4), which is located on chromosome 4q35. Age of onset varies from the first to the fifth decade. There is progressive weakness of facial and shoulder girdle muscles that is frequently asymmetric. With shoulder elevation, the scapula rides into the trapezius muscle (the trapezius hump sign; Figure 4-7). Deltoids are initially well preserved, while biceps muscles are atrophied (Popeye appearance). In addition, there is leg weakness, especially of the tibialis anterior muscles, resulting in weak dorsiflexion. FSHD might be associated with sensorineural hearing loss or visual loss (Coat's disease). Serum CK may be raised. Muscle biopsy reveals myopathic changes

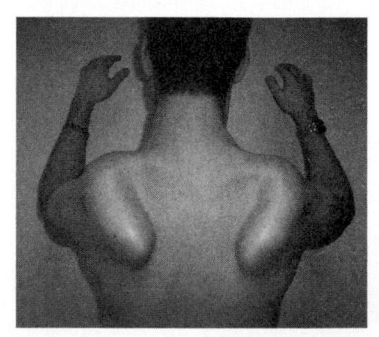

**Figure 4-7.** Patient with FSH showing scapular winging.

and sometimes few foci of endomysial and perivascular inflammation. In such cases, it can be misdiagnosed as an inflammatory myopathy.

37. **What are the characteristic features of myofibrillar myopathies?**

■ **Clinical features:** These autosomal dominantly inherited conditions have several subsets, including desminopathy, αβ-crystallinopathy, myotilinopathy, zaspsopathy, and filaminopathy. Symptoms include slowly progressive weakness (which is more distal than proximal), paresthesias, muscle wasting, stiffness, aching, and cramps. Respiratory failure may be the presenting feature. Cardiomyopathies and peripheral neuropathy are frequently encountered. EMG usually reveals myopathic motor unit potentials, abnormal electrical irritability, and/or denervation changes. Serum CK could be normal or elevated less than fifteenfold above the upper limit of normal. Diagnosis is established by muscle biopsy.

■ **Pathologic features:** The major abnormalities are myofibrillar disorganization that starts at the Z-disk followed by accumulation of myofibrillary degeneration products and expression of ectopic proteins (desmin, αβ-crystallin, dystrophin, myotilin, sarcoglycans, neural cell adhesion molecule [NCAM], plectin, gelsolin, ubiquitin, filamin C, Xin, and amyloid deposits). Abnormal fiber regions either have absent or decreased oxidative enzyme activity.
Selcen D: Myofibrillar myopathies. Curr Opin Neurol 21:585-589, 2008.
Selcen D, Ohno K, Engel AG: Myofibrillar myopathy: Clinical, morphological and genetic studies in 63 patients. Brain 127:439-451, 2004.

## CONGENITAL MYOPATHIES

38. **What are the most important congenital myopathies?**
The following congenital myopathies are generally classified based on the observed morphologic abnormalities in muscle biopsies:
1. Central-core disease
2. Nemaline myopathy
3. Centronuclear (AD) and X-linked myotubular myopathy
4. Congenital fiber type disproportion
5. Reducing-body myopathy
6. Myopathy associated with tubular aggregates
7. Fingerprint-body myopathy
8. Sarcotubular myopathy
9. Myopathy with apoptotic changes
10. Multicore myopathy in type 1 fibers
11. Trilaminar myopathy
12. Zebra body myopathy
13. Multiminicore disease
14. Hyaline body (myosin storage) myopathy
15. Cap disease
16. Broad A band disease
17. Cylindrical spirals myopathy
18. Lamellar body myopathy
19. Congenital myopathy with mosaic fibers
20. Myopathy with muscle spindle excess

39. **Is there a relationship between malignant hyperthermia (MH) and central-core disease (CCD)?**
Central-core disease is a congenital myopathy. Malignant hyperthermia is a reaction to general anesthetics characterized by abnormal calcium homeostasis in skeletal muscles. Both conditions are transmitted by an autosomal dominant pattern of inheritance, and the genes for

both diseases are located next to each other on chromosome 19 (19 q12 to q13.2). More than 100 mutations in the ryanodine receptor type 1 gene (RYR1) have been associated with MH susceptibility, central-core disease, or both. RYR1 mutations may account for up to 50% to 70% of MH-susceptible cases. CACNA1S (calcium channel, voltage-dependent, L type α-1s subunit), located on chromosome 1q32 encoding the α1 subunit of the voltage-gated dihydropyridine receptor, is another candidate gene for MH but not for CCD.

Patients with CCD and their family members must be cautioned about the possibility of MH reactions to anesthetics. Genetic confirmation might be challenging because most of the mutations are private and are distributed throughout the RYR1 gene.

Levano S, Vukcevic M, Singer M, et al.: Increasing the number of diagnostic mutations in malignant hyperthermia. Hum Mutat 30:590-598, 2009.

Nishio H, Sato T, Fukunishi S, et al.: Identification of malignant hyperthermia-susceptible ryanodine receptor type 1 gene (RYR1) mutations in a child who died in a car after exposure to a high environmental temperature. Leg Med (Tokyo) 11:142-143 2009.

## METABOLIC MYOPATHIES

40. **What features are suggestive of a metabolic myopathy?**
Clinical features suggestive of a metabolic myopathy include acute, recurrent, and usually reversible exercise-related muscular pain, stiffness, or cramps and myoglobinuria. Some disorders are associated with fixed or progressive weakness.

41. **How are metabolic myopathies classified?**
According to the metabolic pathway that is impaired:
**Glycogen** is metabolized to either lactic acid or pyruvate, providing energy during both high-intensity activity and anaerobic states. During aerobic conditions, pyruvate enters the TCA cycle to generate more energy through oxidative metabolism.

**Lipid** metabolism is a source of energy at rest and with sustained submaximal exercise. Long-chain fatty acids are transported into the mitochondria with the help of carnitine, where carnitine palmitoyltransferase (CPT) catalyzes the reaction, forming acyl carnitine esters that are oxidized to acetyl-CoA and ATP. Acetyl-CoA then enters the TCA cycle.

**Phosphocreatine** and the **purine** nucleotide cycle are utilized during brief high-intensity exercise. Phosphocreatine restores the level of ATP from ADP, and CK is the enzyme that catalyzes the transfer of the phosphoryl group in these reactions.

The **mitochondria** produce enzymes that mediate the oxidation of pyruvate, glucose, and fatty acids under aerobic conditions by producing a hydrogen ion gradient.

42. **What is acid-maltase deficiency? Give the differential diagnosis.**
Acid-maltase deficiency (type II glycogenosis) is an autosomal recessive disorder caused by a deficiency of the lysosomal enzyme alphaglycosidase (acid maltase), a lysosomal hydrolase that degrades glycogen to glucose. The gene encoding for acid maltase is located on chromosome 17q21 to 23. It can present at any age and has three different forms: infantile (Pompe's disease), childhood, and adult onset. Infantile form presents with cardiomegaly, macroglossia, hepatomegaly, and hypotonia. Juvenile form presents with slowly progressive weakness. Some cases might have calf hypertrophy and might be misdiagnosed as muscular dystrophy. Organomegaly is uncommon in both juvenile and adult forms. The adult patient usually becomes symptomatic in the third or fourth decade of life with insidious painless limb-girdle weakness and is frequently misdiagnosed as polymyositis, motor neuron disease, myotonic dystrophy, or limb-girdle muscular dystrophy. The respiratory muscles are disproportionately affected. The CK level is usually mildly elevated (2 to 10 times normal), and lactate production is normal. The EMG shows abundant complex repetitive discharges, myopathic changes, and spontaneous activity. In addition, myotonic and pseudomyotonic

potentials can be prominent, especially in the paraspinal muscles. If the discharges are not overt, the EMG findings resemble polymyositis. Therefore, a muscle biopsy may be necessary to make the diagnosis. Characteristic findings are those of a vacuolar myopathy. The vacuoles themselves contain PAS-positive material with a prominent acid phosphatase activity. Similar vacuoles also occur in chloroquine myopathy. For definite diagnosis, enzyme activity is first measured in dried blood spots, followed by confirmatory testing of acid maltase activity in cultures of fibroblasts, muscle tissue, or by genetic testing. Enzyme replacement therapy with recombinant alpha-glucosidase has shown significant clinical response in infantile form and modest response in juvenile and adult forms. A high-protein, low-carbohydrate diet combined with exercise might result in slight benefit.

Bembi B, Cerinin E, Danesino C, et al.: Diagnosis of glycogenosis type II; review. Neurology 2: (23 Suppl 2):S4-S11, 2008.

Katzin LW, Amato AA: Pompe disease: A review of the current diagnosis and treatment recommendations in the era of enzyme replacement therapy. J Clin Neuromuscul Dis 9:421-431, 2008.

Kishani PS, Corzo D, Nicolino M, et al.: Recombinant human acid [alpha]-glucosidase: major clinical benefits in infantile-onset Pompe disease. Neurology 68:88-89, 2007.

Slonim AE, Bulone L, Goldberg T, et al.: Modification of the natural history of adult-onset acid maltase deficiency by nutrition and exercise therapy. Muscle Nerve 35:70-77, 2007.

43. **What is McArdle's disease? How is it treated?**
Myophosphorylase deficiency (McArdle's disease; glycogen storage disease type V) is an autosomal recessive myopathy, and heterozygotes are usually asymptomatic. The myophosphorylase gene is located at 11q13. It is characterized by muscle cramps and stiffness with exercise and intermittent myoglobinuria. Absence of myophosphorylase blocks carbohydrate metabolism, and lipids must be used for energy metabolism at rest and during exercise. Because this source of energy is insufficient for intense exercise, symptoms develop. A "second-wind" phenomenon in which the symptoms disappear after a brief rest and do not recur with resumed mild exercise has been described. Resting causes a metabolic shift to fatty acid oxidation and enables the individual to continue with the exercise. This shift occurs more efficiently in patients who undertake regular aerobic exercise. With advancing age, a small proportion of patients may develop fixed proximal muscle weakness. Definite diagnosis is made by muscle histochemistry and the finding of absent functional myophosphorylase or by DNA analysis.

Treatment begins with counseling about the risks of exercise-induced rhabdomyolysis. Patients should be instructed to adjust their lifestyles to avoid strenuous exercise and to seek prompt medical attention and treatment if myoglobinuria develops. Treatments aimed at bypassing the biochemical block by supplying the muscle with a glycolytic intermediate (i.e., glucose, fructose) appear to increase work capacity in some patients, but their long-term use results in undesirable weight gain and usually proves disappointing.

The main differential diagnosis is phosphofructokinase (PFK) deficiency or Tarui's disease. Increased bilirubin concentration and reticulocyte count reflecting hemolytic anemia in PFK are useful in distinguishing this condition from McArdle's disease.

Auinlivan R, Beynon RJ, Martinuzzi A: Pharmacological and nutritional treatment for McArdle disease. Cochrane DataBase Sys Rev 6:CD003458, 2008.

44. **What are the clinical features of primary carnitine deficiency?**
Carnitine plays an essential role in the metabolism of fatty acids by muscle fiber. Carnitine deficiency is of autosomal recessive inheritance, and the gene abnormality is located on chromosome 5q31.1. It can present with progressive hypertrophic and dilated cardiomyopathy with lipid myopathy between the ages of 1 and 7, or may become overt earlier, between 3 months and 2.5 years of age, with recurrent episodes of hypoglycemic hypoketonemic encephalopathy. Treatment is with high-dose oral L-carnitine supplementation. Muscle strength and heart function return to normal, and hypoglycemic episodes disappear with treatment.

**45. What is the most common disorder of lipid metabolism in muscle?**

Carnitine palmitoyltransferase 2 (CPT2) deficiency is the most common disorder of lipid metabolism in muscle and a major cause of hereditary recurrent myoglobinuria, which is precipitated by fasting, cold, strenuous exercise, and fever. It has three phenotypes: (1) juvenile-adult onset, which is the myopathic form; (2) infantile hepatocardiomuscular form, which is life threatening; and (3) fatal neonatal form, which presents shortly after birth with respiratory distress, seizures, cardiohepatomegaly, dysmorphic features, and neuronal migration deficits.

The juvenile-adult form is the most frequent type, and usually has a benign course. Between episodes of myoglobinuria, muscle strength and serum CK are normal. There is no fasting hypoglycemia. Lactic acid production is normal during exercise. the most severe complication is acute renal failure due to rhabdomyolysis. Avoidance of fasting, restriction of fat and long-chain fatty acids with increased intake of dietary carbohydrates, and limitation of long-duration exercise prevents recurrent episodes of muscle breakdown.

## MITOCHONDRIAL MYOPATHIES

**46. What symptoms are classic for a mitochondrial myopathy?**

Although the degree of impairment varies, most mitochondrial myopathies are associated with nonfluctuating, insidiously progressive ptosis and ophthalmoplegia. Actual diplopia is rare. Other involved organ systems include the following:

- Cardiac (conduction abnormalities and cardiomyopathy)
- Gastrointestinal (pseudo-obstruction)
- Endocrine (diabetes, goiter, short stature)
- Central nervous system (ataxia, deafness, seizures, cerebrovascular ischemia, neuropathy)
- Skin (lipomas)
- Eye (retinitis pigmentosa, cataracts)
- Ear (deafness)

**47. What are the most important myopathies due to point mutations in tRNA genes of mitochondrial DNA?**

1. Myoclonic epilepsy with ragged red fibers (MERRF)
2. Mitochondrial encephalomyopathy with lactic acidosis (MELAS)
3. Some myopathies with cardiomyopathy

**48. What are POLG (DNA polymerase γ) gene–associated mitochondrial disorders?**

1. Childhood myocerebrohepatopathy spectrum disorders
2. Alpers syndrome (most common autosomal recessive disease caused by mutations in the POLG gene)
3. Ataxia neuropathy spectrum (ANS) disorders; includes spinocerebellar ataxia with epilepsy (SCAE) and mitochondrial recessive ataxia syndrome without ophthalmoplegia (MIRAS)
4. Myoclonus epilepsy myopathy sensory ataxia (MEMSA)
5. Autosomal recessive progressive external ophthalmoplegia (arPEO)*
6. Autosomal dominant progressive external ophthalmoplegia (adPEO)*

Wong LJC, Naviaux RK, Brunetti-Pierri N: Molecular and clinical genetics of mitochondrial diseases due to POLG mutations. Hum Mutat 29:E150-E172, 2008.

---

*Includes sensory ataxic neuropathy with dysarthria and ophthalmoparesis (SANDO).

## CONTINUOUS MUSCLE ACTIVITY SYNDROMES

**49. What is myokymia?**
Myokymia is the continuous undulation of a group of muscle fibers caused by the successive spontaneous contraction of motor units. On EMG, they appear as groups of 2 to 10 potentials, firing at 5 to 60 Hz and recurring regularly at 0.2- to 1-second intervals. Myokymia, frequently observed in facial muscles, occurs in a number of brain stem diseases, especially multiple sclerosis, radiation-induced nerve damage, Guillain-Barré syndrome, chronic peripheral nerve disorders, timber rattlesnake envenomation, gold therapy, and Isaacs' syndrome.

**50. What is neuromyotonia?**
Neuromyotonia is the continuous muscle rippling and stiffness resulting from bursts of discharges from the peripheral nerve. It is neurogenic in origin and is due to an immune-mediated neurogenic hyperexcitability. On EMG, bursts of spontaneous motor unit activity firing at 40 to 300 Hz and lasting for several seconds are observed. Antibodies against voltage-gated potassium channels are found in many cases. Myotonia differs from neuromyotonia in that myotonia is thought be of myogenic origin. This theory is supported by the failure of curare to inhibit myotonia.

Gonzalez G, Barros G, Russi ME, et al.: Acquired neuromyotonia in childhood: A case report and review. Pediatr Neurol 38:61-63, 2008.

Maddison P: Neuromyotonia. Clin Neurophysiol 117:2118-2127, 2006.

**51. What is Isaacs' syndrome?**
Isaacs' syndrome has been described under several other names, including myokymia with impaired muscle relaxation, neuromyotonia, pseudomyotonia, quantal squander, armadillo disease, and continuous muscle fiber activity. Complaints include hyperhidrosis, muscle stiffness, intermittent cramping, and difficulty with chewing, speaking, and even breathing. Either myokymia or neuromyotonia can be observed. If CNS dysfunction such as encephalitis is also present, then it is called *Morvan's fibrillary chorea.*

EMG studies of Isaacs' syndrome show spontaneous and continuous long, irregularly occurring trains of variably formed discharges that originate along the course of the motor axon. Antibodies specific for voltage-gated potassium channels (VGKC) of presynaptic terminals have been reported as a serologic marker of this syndrome. Antibodies against neuronal ganglionic acetylcholine receptor are also found in some of these patients. Successful symptomatic treatment has been achieved with phenytoin (300 to 400 mg/day) or carbamazepine (200 mg, 3 or 4 times/day). Some patients may respond favorably to plasma exchange or intravenous immunoglobulin. Isaacs' syndrome can be associated with thymoma, small cell lung cancer, and Hodgkin's lymphoma, or other autoimmune disorders.

Takahashi H, Mori M, Sekguchi Y, et al.: Development of Isaacs' syndrome following complete recovery of voltage-gated potassium channel antibody-associated limbic encephalitis. J Neurol Sci 275:185-187, 2008.

Toothaker TB, Rubin M: Pareneoplastic neurological syndromes: A review. Neurologist 15:21-33, 2009.

Vernino S, Lennon VA: Ion channel and striational antibodies define a continuum of autoimmune neuromuscular hyperexcitability. Muscle Nerve 26:702-707, 2002.

**52. What is "stiff-person syndrome"?**
Stiff-person, or stiff-man, syndrome (SPS) is a fluctuating motor disturbance characterized by sudden muscular rigidity with superimposed spasms. The classical form predominantly affects the axial and proximal limb muscles and is aggravated by emotional, somatosensory, or acoustic stimuli. Many patients have associated autoimmune endocrinopathies; the most common is insulin-dependent diabetes mellitus. Patients might also have associated

dysautonomia. Antibodies directed against the GABA-synthesizing enzyme glutamic acid decarboxylase (GAD) are present in the serum and cerebrospinal fluid (CSF). EMG discloses a continuous low-frequency firing of normal motor unit potentials that persists at rest. A significant symptomatic improvement is achieved by oral administration of benzodiazepines, primarily diazepam (10 to 100 mg/day). Baclofen and valproic acid also may help the symptoms. Immune modulation by corticosteroids, plasmapheresis, or IVIG may result in improvement in some patients. Improvement of paroxysmal symptoms is reported with levetiracetam, vigabatrin, tiagabine, rituximab, propofol, and focal botulinum injections. The use of tricyclic antidepressants might worsen stiffness.

Espay AJ, Chen R: Rigidity and spasms from autoimmune encephalomyelopathies: Stiff-person syndrome. Muscle Nerve 34:677-690, 2006.

Hattan E, Angle MR, Chalk C: Unexpected benefit of propofol in stiff-person syndrome. Neurology 70:1641-1642, 2008.

Rüegg SJ, Steck AJ, Fuhr P: Levetiracetam improves paroxysmal symptoms in a patient with stiff-person syndrome. Neurology 62:338, 2004.

53. **What are variants of SPS?**
   - Stiff-limb syndrome (SLS) is the focal form of SPS that presents with stiffness in one limb, usually the arm. Some patients may develop dementia and ataxia. SLS might progress to classical SPS.
   - Progressive encephalomyelitis with rigidity and myoclonus (PERM) presents with axial and lower limb stiffness followed by myoclonus, long tract, and brain stem signs (i.e., ataxia, deafness, oculomotor impairment, dysarthria, dysphagia).
   - Paraneoplastic SPS may be associated with small cell lung cancer, breast cancer, thymoma, and Hodgkin lymphoma. Patients are negative for anti-GAD autoantibodies, but often test positive for anti-amphiphysin autoantibodies. In rare cases, anti-gephyrin and anti-Ri autoantibodies might be detected.

   Dalakas MC: Stiff person syndrome advances in pathogenesis and therapeutic interventions. Curr Treat Options Neurol 11:102-110, 2009.

   Espay AJ, Chen R: Rigidity and spasms from autoimmune encephalomyelopathies: Stiff-person syndrome. Muscle Nerve 34:677-690, 2006.

## TOXIC MYOPATHIES

54. **What are the most common myotoxic drugs?**
   1. Statins and fibrates (myalgias, elevated CK, rhabdomyolysis, drug-induced dermatomyositis)
   2. Chloroquine (vascular myopathy)
   3. Alcohol (rhabdomyolysis)
   4. Fluoroquinolones (ofloxacin, norfloxacin, levofloxacin, ciprofloxacin—tendinopathy, tendon ruptures, rhabdomyolysis)
   5. D-Penicillamine (drug-induced dermatomyositis)
   6. Protease inhibitors (saquinavir, ritonavir, indinavir, nelfinavir, amprenavir—rhabdomyolysis, risk is increased with concurrent use of statins)
   7. Nucleoside-analogue reverse transcriptase inhibitors (zidovudine, stavudine, didanosine, zalcidabine, lamivudine—associated mitochondrial myopathy and ragged red fibers)

55. **What is statin myopathy?**
   Statin myopathy is characterized by myalgias and elevated CK levels, which might lead to rhabdomyolysis. The exact pathophysiology underlying myopathy is unknown. Proposed

mechanisms are decreased sarcolemmal cholesterol, mitochondrial dysfunction from reduction of coenzyme Q (CoQ), and depletion of key isoprenoids that control myofiber apoptosis. Treatment with CoQ is still controversial. Drug-drug interactions should be considered at the initiation of statin therapy, because hepatic CYP 3A4 competitors such as antifungal agents, HIV protease inhibitors, anticoagulants, erythromycin, and cyclosporine might increase the plasma levels of statins, increasing the possibility of myotoxicity.

Tolerable myalgias and mildly elevated CK levels should not lead to discontinuation of statins given its benefits on the cardiovascular system.

Baker SK, Samjoo IA: A neuromuscular approach to statin-related myotoxicity. Can J Neurol Sci 35:8-21, 2008.

Klopstock T: Drug induced myopathies. Curr Opin Neurol 21:590-595, 2008.

56. **What neuromuscular conditions are associated with HIV infection?**
    1. HIV polymyositis
    2. Inclusion body myositis
    3. Nemaline myopathy
    4. Diffuse infiltrative lymphocytosis syndrome
    5. HIV-wasting syndrome
    6. Vasculitic processes
    7. Myasthenic syndromes and chronic fatigue
    8. Mitochondrial myopathy due to antiretroviral drugs
    9. Lactic acidosis, hepatic steatosis, and myopathy
    10. HIV-associated lipodystrophy syndrome
    11. HAART-related immune restoration inflammatory syndrome

    Authier FJ, Chariot P, Gherardi R: Skeletal muscle involvement in human immunodeficiency virus (HIV) infected patients in the era of highly active antiretroviral therapy (HAART). Muscle Nerve 32:247-260, 2005.

    Louthrenoo W: Rheumatic manifestations of HIV infection. Curr Opin Rheumatol 20:92-99, 2008.

    Robinson-Papp J, Simpson DM: Neuromuscular complications of human immunodeficiency virus infection. Phys Med Rehabil Clin N Am 19:81-96, 2008.

57. **A patient with AIDS who is taking AZT complains of myalgia and weakness. What is wrong?**
    The exact diagnosis in this setting is often difficult. Myalgia and increased CK are frequently encountered in patients with AIDS, and some patients have a symmetric and predominantly proximal muscle weakness. EMG findings are those usually seen in polymyositis. Many patients have typical muscle biopsy findings of polymyositis (necrotic fibers with perimysial, endomysial, and perivascular lymphocytic inflation). AZT is also associated with myopathy, which is characterized chiefly by muscle wasting and proximal weakness and tends to occur in patients treated with high doses of the drug for more than 6 months. Muscle biopsy, however, may show changes suggestive of a mitochondrial disorder. Numerous ragged red fibers, indicative of abnormal mitochondria, may be seen. Rods (nemaline) and cytoplasmic bodies also may be seen. Both myopathy and biopsy abnormalities improve with discontinuation of AZT. It is thought that AZT inhibits mitochondrial DNA polymerase, which causes depletion of mitochondrial DNA and thus results in myopathy.

58. **What is steroid myopathy?**
    There are two forms of steroid myopathy. The more common form produces progressive, painless weakness. Typically the myopathy is related to chronic use, but inhaled corticosteroids can cause diaphragmatic weakness within 2 weeks of initial exposure. Chronic steroid myotoxicity can be prevented in part by exercise, and symptoms improve if the dose

is reduced or discontinued. CK is not elevated, and EMG may be normal or show minimal myopathic changes. Muscle biopsy shows type 2 fiber atrophy.

The second form of steroid myopathy, which is still a subject of controversy, is related to high-dose exposure, usually in association with depolarizing neuromuscular blocking agents, sepsis, hyperglycemia, and/or malnutrition. It is characterized by acute, severe paralysis that can affect all muscles, including respiratory muscles. This syndrome has been given many names, including acute quadriplegic myopathy, thick filament myopathy, and critical illness myopathy. EMG may show an acute axonal neuropathy in addition to myopathic changes, which can confound the diagnosis. Symmetric proximal weakness and atrophy develop over days. The cause of myopathy is extensive loss of thick myofilaments with preservation of thin filaments and Z disks in the atrophic muscle fibers. Between 30% and 50% of patients may have elevated CK levels. With supportive care, the prognosis for recovery is variable (weeks to 1 year), but there may be considerable mortality.

Hermans G, De Jonghe B, Bruyninckx F, et al.: Clinical review: Critical illness polyneuropathy and myopathy. Crit Care 12:238, 2008.

Hermans G, Schrooten M, Van Damme P, et al. Benefits of intensive insulin therapy on neuromuscular complications in routine daily critical care practice. Critical Care 13(1)R5, 1–12, 2009.

## KEY POINTS: MYOPATHIES

1. Myopathies usually cause proximal symmetric weakness, with or without other symptoms.

2. The diagnosis of myopathies often rests upon CK levels, EMG findings, and muscle biopsy.

3. Muscles contain both slow (type 1 red) and fast (type 2 white) fibers.

4. Myotonic dystrophy is the most common muscular dystrophy in adults.

5. The possibility of respiratory failure is the most serious concern in the management of most patients with myopathies.

6. Drug toxicity should always be considered in the differential diagnosis.

## CLINICAL FEATURES

59. **Which myopathies cause respiratory failure?**
    - Some muscular dystrophies (Duchenne, Becker, limb-girdle, Emery-Dreifuss, myotonic,* congenital)
    - Acid-maltase deficiency*
    - Carnitine deficiency
    - Nemaline myopathy*
    - Mitochondrial myopathy
    - Centronuclear myopathy*
    - Polymyositis/dermatomyositis

60. **Which myopathies are associated with dysphagia?**
    - Oculopharyngeal muscular dystrophy
    - Inclusion body myositis
    - Myotonic muscular dystrophy

_____

*Respiratory failure may be the presenting feature.

- Mitochondrial myopathy
- Polymyositis and dermatomyositis
- Duchenne muscular dystrophy

61. **Which myopathies are associated with cardiac disease?**
   - **Arrhythmias:** Kearns-Sayre disease; Anderson's syndrome; polymyositis; muscular dystrophies: myotonic; limb-girdle type 1B, 2C-F, 2G, 2I; and Emery-Dreifuss
   - **Congestive heart failure:** muscular dystrophies: Duchenne; Becker's; Emery-Dreifuss; myotonic; limb-girdle 1B, 2C-F, 2G, 2I; nemaline myopathy; acid-maltase deficiency; carnitine deficiency; polymyositis

62. **Which myopathies are associated with ptosis or ophthalmoplegia?**
   Ptosis usually without ophthalmoplegia:
   - Myotonic dystrophy
   - Congenital myopathies
   - Centronuclear myopathy
   - Nemaline myopathy
   - Central core myopathy
   - Myofibrillary (desmin subtype) myopathy
   Ptosis with ophthalmoplegia:
   - Oculopharyngeal muscular dystrophy
   - Oculopharyngodistal myopathy
   - Chronic progressive external ophthalmoplegia (mitochondrial myopathy)

63. **Which myopathies are characterized by predominant distal weakness?**
   - Late adult-onset distal myopathy type 1 (Welander)
   - Late adult-onset distal myopathy type 2 (Markesbery) and tibial muscular dystrophy (Udd)
   - Early adult-onset distal myopathy type 1 (Nonaka)
   - Early adult-onset distal myopathy type 2 (Miyoshi)
   - Early adult-onset distal myopathy type 3 (Laing)
   - Late adult-onset distal dystrophinopathy
   - Myofibrillary myopathy
   - Childhood-onset distal myopathy
   - Myotonic dystrophy
   - Facioscapulohumeral dystrophy
   - Scapuloperoneal myopathy
   - Oculopharyngeal dystrophy
   - Emery-Dreifuss humeroperoneal dystrophy
   - Inflammatory myopathies: inclusion body myositis
   - Metabolic myopathy: Debrancher deficiency, acid-maltase deficiency
   - Congenital myopathy: nemaline myopathy, central core myopathy, centronuclear myopathy
   Guglieri M, Straub V, Bushby K, et al.: Limb-girdle muscular dystrophies. Curr Opin Neurol 21:576-584, 2008.

## WEBSITES

1. http://www.mdausa.org/disease
2. www.worldmusclesociety.org

## BIBLIOGRAPHY

1. Carpenter S, Karpati G: Pathology of Skeletal Muscles, 2nd ed. New York, Oxford University Press, 2001.
2. Engel AG, et al.: Myology, 3rd ed. New York, McGraw-Hill, 2004.
3. Harati Y, Nawasipirong O: Cramps and myalgias. In Jankovic J, Tolosa E (eds): Movement Disorders, Baltimore, Williams & Wilkins, 2003.
4. Ktirsi B, Kaminski HJ, Preston DC, et al.: Neuromuscular Disorders in Clinical Practice, Boston, Butterworth-Heinemann, 2002.
5. Mendell JR, Griggs RC, Logigan EL, et al.: Evaluation and Treatment of Myopathies. London, Oxford University Press, 2009.

# NEUROMUSCULAR JUNCTION DISEASES

*Clifton L. Gooch, MD, and Tetsuo Ashizawa, MD*

## ANATOMY AND PHYSIOLOGY

1. **What happens in the motor nerve terminal (presynaptically) during neuromuscular transmission?**

   When a wave of depolarization (the action potential) travels down the motor nerve and reaches its tip (the presynaptic nerve terminal), voltage-gated calcium channels in the neuronal membrane open, allowing influx of calcium ions ($Ca^{2+}$). This triggers the fusion of acetylcholine (ACh)-filled vesicles with the membrane and the release of acetylcholine into the space between the nerve and muscle membranes (the synaptic cleft) (Figure 5-1).

2. **What happens in the muscle (postsynaptically) during neuromuscular transmission?**

   The binding of two acetylcholine molecules to each ACh receptor (AChR) in the muscle (postsynaptic) membrane opens an $Na^+$ channel within the receptor, allowing $Na^+$ influx, which generates subthreshold depolarizations known as *miniature endplate potentials (MEPPs)*. The MEPPs in each muscle fiber summate to form the endplate potential (EPP) for that fiber. When a sufficient number of receptors are activated simultaneously, the EPP becomes large enough to trigger an action potential, which then propagates along the muscle sarcoplasmic membrane to the T-tubule system, leading to the release of $Ca^{2+}$ from the sarcoplasmic reticulum and muscle contraction.

3. **What happens in the synaptic cleft during neuromuscular transmission?**

   After acetylcholine molecules bind to and activate AChRs, they are released back into the synaptic cleft. Acetylcholinesterase (AChE) in the cleft then decomposes acetylcholine into choline and acetic acid within a fraction of a millisecond, and choline reuptake by the presynaptic nerve terminal provides material for the synthesis of new acetylcholine via the enzyme choline acetyl transferase.

4. **What is the structure of the nicotinic AChR?**

   The human AChR consists of five subunits: two alpha, one beta, one epsilon (or gamma in fetal form), and one delta subunit. Acetylcholine binds to the extracellular domain of the alpha subunit. Two acetylcholine molecules must bind with the receptor (one on each alpha subunit) to open its $Na^+$ channel (Figure 5-2).

   Ashizawa T, Oshima M, Ruan KH, et al.: Autoimmune recognition profile of the alpha chain of human acetylcholine receptor in myasthenia gravis. Adv Exp Med Biol 303:255-261, 1991.

5. **What is the "safety margin" for neuromuscular transmission?**

   In the normal subject, the amount of acetylcholine released from the presynaptic nerve terminal decreases with each repeated nerve depolarization at a slow rate. This means fewer receptors are activated at the muscle endplate, generating fewer MEPPs and a lower EPP. However, the number of receptors is still high enough that this slight decline in acetylcholine output does not drive the EPP below the depolarization threshold for the muscle fiber, and full contraction still occurs. This functional redundancy is known as the *safety margin* for neuromuscular transmission.

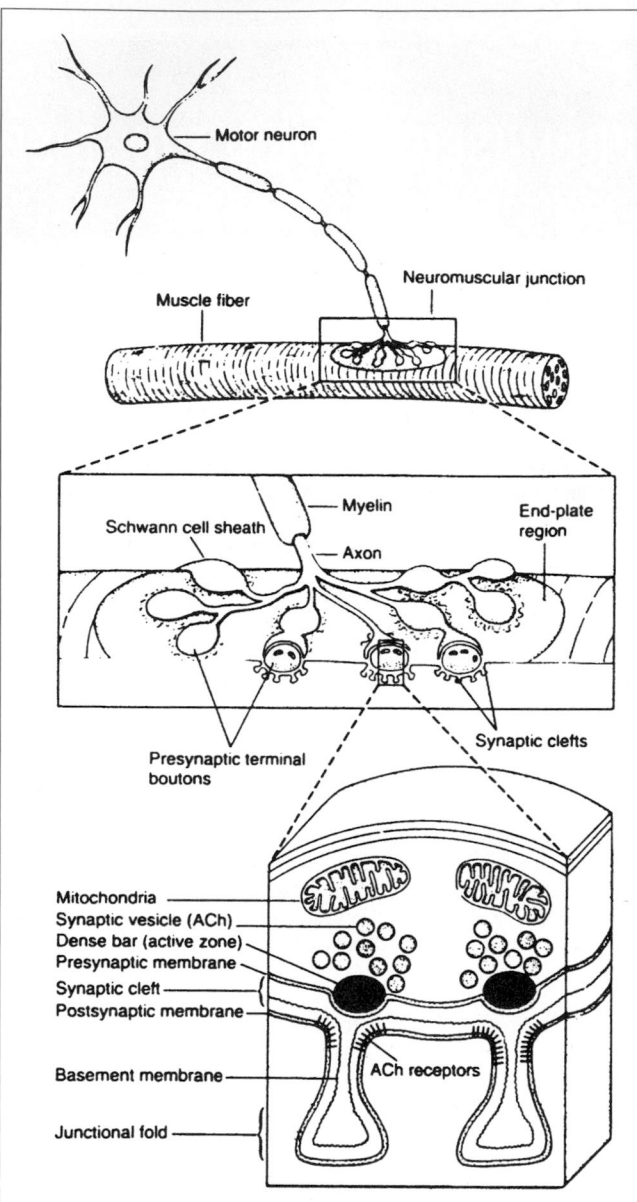

**Figure 5-1.** The neuromuscular junction. From Kandel ER, Schwartz JH, Jessel TM (eds): Principles of Neural Science, 3rd ed. New York, Elsevier, 1991, p 136.

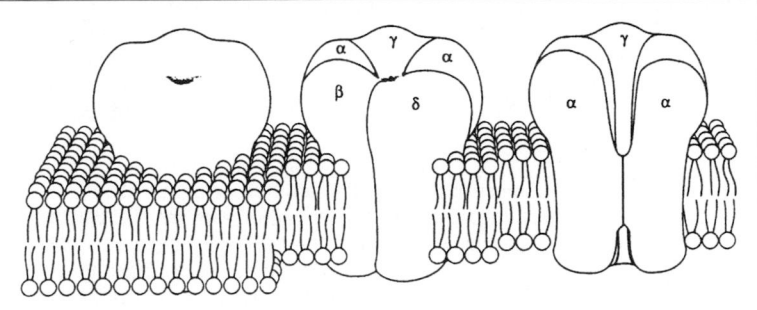

**Figure 5-2.** Diagram of the molecular structure of the AChR at the neuromuscular junction. From Kandel ER, Schwartz JH, Jessel TM (eds): Principles of Neural Science, 3rd ed. New York, Elsevier, 1991, p 146.

## MYASTHENIA GRAVIS

6. **What autoimmune diseases primarily affect the neuromuscular junction (NMJ)?**
   Myasthenia gravis (MG), in which most antibodies are directed against the AChR on the postsynaptic muscle membrane, and Lambert-Eaton myasthenic syndrome (LEMS), in which antibodies are directed against the voltage-gated calcium channel in the nerve terminal, primarily affect the neuromuscular junction.

7. **How is the safety margin for neuromuscular transmission altered in MG?**
   In MG, antibodies decrease the number of functional AChRs. Because fewer AChRs are available for activation, the safety margin for neuromuscular transmission is lowered. Fewer MEPPs are generated when acetylcholine output falls and the EPP is lower. With repeated activation of the nerve and further declines in acetylcholine output, the EPP eventually falls below the threshold necessary to trigger depolarization and contraction of the muscle fiber (blocking of neuromuscular transmission). With continued activation of the nerve, this happens at an increasing number of NMJs and many muscle fibers fail to activate, causing weakness. With extrinsic repetitive electrical stimulation of the nerve at low frequencies, the size of the electrical response accompanying muscle contraction (the compound motor action potential or CMAP) decreases due to this same phenomenon. After a period of rest, acetylcholine content is restored, and these abnormalities may improve.

8. **What are the clinical manifestations of MG?**
   Patients with MG often have variable degrees of weakness and easy fatigability of voluntary skeletal muscle. This weakness may or may not be noticeable with simple activity, but appears or worsens after sustained exercise and typically improves after a short rest. Weakness and fatigability of extraocular muscles (diplopia), bulbar muscles (dysarthria, dysphagia), and limb muscles is often easily detectable on clinical examination. The most critical manifestation is respiratory weakness, a potentially fatal complication, which can develop over hours in severe cases.

9. **What is the epidemiology of MG (i.e., incidence, sex differences, age of onset, inheritance, mortality, and natural history)?**
   The incidence of MG is approximately 1 in 20,000. It affects more women than men by a ratio of 3:2 and has a bimodal age distribution (affecting more women in the third decade and more men in the fifth decade), although it may appear at any age from birth to late adulthood.

Five to seven percent of cases are familial, but no Mendelian inheritance pattern has been identified. Prior to the advent of effective immunomodulatory therapy and artificial ventilation, 20% to 30% of MG patients died due to respiratory failure, 20% experienced persistent symptoms, 25% experienced spontaneous improvement, and a final 25% experienced spontaneous remission. In the modern era, MG is eminently treatable, and death in the properly treated compliant patient is rare.

10. **What is the scientific evidence that AChR antibodies cause MG?**
Myasthenia gravis is the prototypic antireceptor antibody disease and is one of the best understood of any of the autoimmune diseases at the basic science level. Animals immunized with AChRs develop serum antibodies against the receptor and exhibit both the clinical and electrophysiologic features of human MG. This model is known as *experimental autoimmune myasthenia gravis* or EAMG. Passive transfer of human MG IgG to animals also causes EAMG, and immunocytochemical studies have demonstrated IgG at the postsynaptic membrane of motor endplates in myasthenic skeletal muscle. AChR antibodies decrease the number of available AChRs in cultured muscle cells in vitro.

11. **What is the clinical evidence that AChR antibodies cause MG?**
More than 90% of patients with MG have circulating antibodies against nicotinic AChR. Removal of the antibodies by plasmapheresis often improves the symptoms and signs of MG. Decreased titers after therapy also may correlate with improved symptoms. Favorable responses to immunotherapy are also consistent with autoimmune, antibody-mediated injury.

12. **What is the thymus gland? What is a myoid cell?**
The thymus gland is a small gland located in the fat pad beneath the sternum. It plays a critical role in the maturation of immunologically active cells and in the development of immune self-tolerance in the healthy patient. Myoid cells are muscle-like cells found mainly within the medulla of the thymus. Myoid cells express nicotinic AChRs, and given their location within this critical site for the development of the global immune response, these cells may play a pivotal role in autosensitization against the receptor in MG.

13. **What evidence suggests that the thymus gland has a major role in the pathogenesis of MG?**
1. Removal of the thymus improves MG in the majority of patients.
2. The majority of patients with MG have an abnormal thymus, demonstrating either hyperplasia or thymoma.
3. Thymic myoid cells express AChRs proximate to the site of T-lymphocyte maturation (which includes immune self-tolerance).
4. AChRs in the thymic myoid cells in MG express the fetal gamma subunit, making them potential targets for antibody sensitization.
5. Thymic B-lymphocytes from patients with MG produce more anti-AChR antibodies than other antibodies.
6. Thymic cells selectively increase the production of antiacetylcholine antibodies when added to myasthenic B-lymphocytes in the laboratory.
7. MG thymus tissue transplanted to immunodeficient mice produces anti-AChR antibodies, which deposit at skeletal muscle endplates.
   Cizeron-Clairac G, LePense R, Frenkian-Cuvelier M, et al.: Thymus and myasthenia gravis. J Neuroimmunol 201:57-63, 2008.

14. **What is the role of thymectomy in the treatment of MG?**
Although prospective, randomized, controlled trials have not been performed, the beneficial effects of thymectomy in patients with MG (with or without thymic tumor) have been demonstrated in a plethora of studies. Over 75% of patients experience some benefit, which

may include a reduced requirement for immunomodulatory therapy, a greater likelihood of successful taper of immunosuppressant medication with continued control, and a greater chance of permanent symptomatic remission. The extended trans-sternal approach (sternal split with removal of the thymus and visual exploration of the mediastinum for removal of ectopic thymic tissue) appears to confer the best balance between benefit and risk, and is extremely safe in experienced hands. Benefits in children and patients over 60 years of age are less clear, and these groups may be at greater risk for the procedure. The congenital myasthenic syndromes do not appear to be immune-mediated and do not respond to thymectomy.

**15. What is the association between thymoma and MG?**

Approximately 15% of patients with MG have a thymoma, most of which are epithelial rather than lymphocytic in origin. Ninety percent are benign and easily treated with resection, whereas 10% are malignant, carrying an average survival of 5 to 10 years. Benign thymic hyperplasia is seen in about 50% of patients with MG.

Magg L, Andreetta F, Antozzi C, et al.: Thymoma-associated myasthenia gravis: Outcome, clinical and pathological correlations in 197 patients on a 20 year experience. J Neuroimmunol 201:237-244, 2008.

**16. What diagnostic tests can help identify a thymoma in patients with MG?**

Imaging studies are the gold standard for the diagnosis of thymoma in patients with MG, and all MG patients should undergo either a computed tomography (CT) or magnetic resonance imaging (MRI) scan of the chest. The sensitivity and specificity of chest CT for the identification of thymoma are 85% and 99%, respectively. Other adjunctive studies may also suggest thymoma, and antiskeletal muscle antibodies have a sensitivity of 94% in patients with MG and a thymic mass. Antiskeletal muscle antibody titers fall with successful treatment of the thymoma and rise with recurrence, making them useful screening tools for patient follow-up.

**17. What is transient neonatal MG?**

Approximately 12% of neonates born to mothers with MG are "floppy" babies who have difficulty with breathing and sucking. This "transient neonatal myasthenia" likely results from the transfer of maternal AChR antibodies to the infant through the placenta. It typically lasts for several weeks and then spontaneously resolves but should not persist for more than 12 weeks. Neither the severity of maternal disease or titers of maternal antibody reliably correlate with the development of neonatal MG; severely affected mothers may have normal infants, and mothers in clinical remission may have affected infants. Regardless, physicians caring for a myasthenic mother must be aware of this disorder and must be prepared to provide respiratory support to the newborn, if needed.

**18. What are the congenital myasthenic syndromes?**

The congenital myasthenic syndromes are a group of extremely rare disorders typically caused by genetic mutations affecting the structure and/or function of the NMJ. They manifest as extraocular, facial, bulbar, and/or limb weakness and fatigability beginning in early life and persisting into adulthood. These syndromes have been characterized by site of dysfunction within the NMJ and are the subject of ongoing investigation, with new syndromes described each year. Patients with these disorders do not respond to thymectomy or other immunotherapies. The presynaptic disorders involve defective release or synthesis of acetylcholine and account for 8% of the congenital syndromes. The synaptic basal lamina disorders are due to mutations in the collagen tail of AChE, and account for 16%. The postsynaptic disorders are caused primarily by mutations in various AChR subunits, altering receptor number and/or receptor ion channel kinetics. They account for the majority of cases (76%) (Table 5-1).

**TABLE 5-1.    THE CONGENITAL MYASTHENIC SYNDROMES**

| | |
|---|---|
| Presynaptic | Familial infantile congenital MG + episodic apnea |
| | Decreased synaptic vesicles and reduced ACh quantal release |
| | Congenital Lambert-Eaton–like episodic ataxia 2 |
| | Reduced quantal release |
| Synaptic basal<br>lamina defects | AChE deficiency at NMJs |
| Postsynaptic | |
| Kinetic AChR<br>abnormalities | Reduced numbers of AChRs at NMJs |
| | Slow AChR channel syndromes with increased response to ACh |
| | Fast-channel syndromes with reduced response to ACh |
| | Normal numbers of AChRs at NMJs with reduced response to ACh |
| | Fast-channel syndrome: AChR ε subunit dysfunction |
| | Fast-channel syndrome: AChR α subunit dysfunction |
| | High conductance and fast closure of AChRs |
| | Increased numbers of AChRs at NMJs |
| | Slow-channel syndrome: AChR β subunit dysfunction |
| Nonkinetic AChR<br>abnormalities | Reduced numbers of AChRs at NMJs due to AChR mutations |
| | Usually ε subunit abnormality |
| | Rarely, α, β, ε subunit abnormalities |
| Other postsynaptic<br>defects | Rapsyn mutations causing reduced numbers of AChRs at NMJs |
| | Plectin deficiency |
| | Weakness + episodic apnea, and bulbar dysfunction |

Ach. acetylcholine; AChR, acetylcholine receptor; AChE, acetylcholinesterase; NMJ, neuromuscular junction.
Washington University Neuromuscular Online Reference:
http://www.neuro.wustl.edu/neuromuscular/synmg.html
From Nogajski JH, Kiernan MC, Ouvrier RA, Andrews PI: Congenital myasthenic syndromes. J Clin Neurosci 16:1-11, 2009.

19. **What are the most common diagnostic tests for MG?**
The diagnosis of MG is a clinical one but may be supported by several different tests. Electrophysiologic tests are often the first step after clinical examination, and typically include repetitive nerve stimulation (RNS) studies, which have a sensitivity of 40% to 90% depending on disease severity. A more advanced test, single-fiber electromyography (SFEMG), is the single most sensitive assay in MG with a sensitivity of 90% to 95% even in mildly symptomatic patients. The AChR binding antibody assay (using serum samples) has a 90% sensitivity in generalized disease and 70% in pure ocular disease, but the blocking and modulating AChR antibody assays are less sensitive, particularly in pure ocular disease. Administration of the short-acting AChE inhibitor, edrophonium (the Tensilon test) may transiently improve strength and can also aid in diagnosis but must be properly performed in a patient having clearly discernible weakness on examination to serve as a gauge for response.

20. **What is repetitive nerve stimulation (RNS), and what does it show in MG?**
RNS involves the repeated transcutaneous electrical stimulation of all the motor fibers within a nerve, which generates successive impulses. These impulses travel down the nerve, across the NMJ, and into the muscle, from which consecutive electrical responses (CMAPs) are recorded. In MG, progressive failure of transmission across an increasing number of NMJs with repeated stimulation results in activation of fewer muscle fibers, and progressively smaller CMAP. This decrement in CMAP size with low-frequency (2 to 3 Hz) RNS confirms NMJ dysfunction. Decrement may be transiently repaired and CMAP amplitude transiently restored by brief voluntary exercise of the tested muscle between rounds of RNS (repair of decrement and postexercise facilitation). Decrement may also improve with anticholinesterase inhibitor administration.

21. **What is single-fiber electromyography (SFEMG), and what does it show in MG?**
SFEMG is a technique that enables the recording of single muscle fiber discharges, either during volitional contraction or during electrical stimulation of the axon branch to the muscle fiber. Mathematical analysis of consecutive SFEMG signals enables quantitation of the variability in transmission time across the NMJ from discharge to discharge, a value known as *jitter*. In MG, LEMS, and other NMJ disorders, jitter is increased and may be associated with intermittent failure of transmission across certain NMJs ("blocking" of neuromuscular transmission). SFEMG is the single most sensitive test for MG and is positive in 95% of generalized cases, and 90% of pure ocular cases. Increased jitter also occurs in myopathic and neuropathic diseases, so careful routine electromyography and nerve conduction studies are imperative to rule out these causes before SFEMG can be interpreted.

## KEY POINTS: CAUSES AND DIAGNOSIS OF MYASTHENIA GRAVIS

1. Myasthenia gravis (MG) is caused by different sets of antibodies directed against the AChR and its associated functional proteins.

2. The thymus plays a major role in the immunopathogenesis of MG, and its removal improves chances for remission and response to medical therapy.

3. Diagnostic tests for MG include RNS, AChR antibody assays, the Tensilon test, and single-fiber EMG.

4. Fifteen percent of MG patients have a thymoma, and 10% of thymomas in MG patients are malignant; therefore, every MG patient requires CT or MRI of the chest.

5. Single-fiber EMG has the greatest sensitivity of any test for MG (90% to 95%) and is particularly useful in mild or pure ocular cases when other assays are more likely to be negative or indeterminate.

22. **How is the edrophonium (Tensilon) test performed?**
The patient must have readily observable weakness (e.g., ptosis) or weakness that is easily quantified on examination. The test must be performed in a controlled setting, with emergency resuscitation equipment and trained personnel available, because there is a small risk of precipitating cardiac arrhythmia. Both a syringe containing normal saline (the placebo) and a syringe containing edrophonium (10 mg) must be prepared. The placebo is always administered first, and the same protocol should be used for both IV preparations. A test dose

of 1 mg is given, and the patient is observed for side effects over 5 min (i.e., flushing, palpitations, tearing). In some patients, clinical effect appears at this small dose. In most of them, however, the remaining 10 mg will be required. Each minute for the next 5 minutes after administration, the patient should be observed and tested for improvement, and the results documented. Unequivocal improvement occurring only with edrophonium and not with placebo supports the diagnosis of MG.

23. **What is the Mary Walker phenomenon?**
Fatigue and weakness of the forearm muscles develop in myasthenic patients when the forearm muscles are exercised with a cuff around the upper arm, inflated above systolic pressure to occlude circulation (ischemic exercise). After the cuff is deflated, myasthenic symptoms in the rest of the body may worsen within minutes in some patients. This phenomenon is named after Mary Walker, the physiologist who first described it in 1938, and is also present in the myasthenic dog. Although its mechanism is not clear, it may be due to transient lactic acidosis, because lactic acid binds calcium and reduces available ionized and serum calcium. Experimentally, lactate infusions increase weakness in patients with MG much more than in controls.
　　Walker MB: Myasthenia gravis: A case in which fatigue of the forearm muscles could induce paralysis of the extraocular muscles. Proc Roy Soc Med 31:722, 1938.

24. **What is pyridostigmine? Why is it the most widely used anticholinesterase medication in MG?**
Pyridostigmine (Mestinon) is slightly longer-acting (with a half-life of 4 hours) and has fewer cholinergic side effects than neostigmine bromide and other anticholinesterase preparations. Unlike physostigmine, pyridostigmine has no unwanted CNS effects because it does not cross the blood-brain barrier. However, some cases of MG may be refractory to pyridostigmine but respond to other anticholinesterases. A long-acting preparation, Mestinon Timespan 180 mg, may alleviate difficulty in swallowing medication in the morning when taken before bedtime but is not as useful for therapy while awake. A parenteral preparation is also available (2 mg parenteral dose = 60 mg oral dose).

25. **What is a cholinergic crisis?**
Overdosing with anticholinesterase may result in excessive acetylcholine in the synaptic cleft, causing a depolarizing block of AChRs. The end result is defective neuromuscular transmission causing symptoms similar to those of a myasthenic crisis. Fasciculations are also common. Establishing an airway, supporting respiration, and withholding anticholinesterase medications are the mainstays of treatment. This complication is rarely seen today because lower doses of anticholinesterase are typically utilized due to successful primary immunomodulatory therapy.

26. **What are the chronic adverse effects of anticholinesterases on NMJ?**
Chronic excess ACh may also damage the muscle end plate, cause simplification of the postsynaptic folds and loss of AChRs, similar to the endplate changes seen in MG. These changes may be superimposed on the primary damage caused by MG itself. However, as with cholinergic crises, this complication is rarely seen today because successful primary immunotherapy makes the chronic use of high doses of anticholinesterases unnecessary in most patients.

27. **Which drugs may worsen MG?**
Many routinely used drugs have adverse effects on the NMJ, which may not be significant in normal patients but can seriously worsen MG. The list is extensive, and the practitioner should be certain that a given drug does not have these effects before starting therapy in a myasthenic patient. The list includes many antibiotics, particularly the aminoglycosides;

CHAPTER 5 NEUROMUSCULAR JUNCTION DISEASES  **91**

cardiac drugs, particularly the beta-blockers (even Timoptic eye drops); chloroquine; phenytoin; lithium; magnesium; and excess doses of the anticholinesterases (cholinergic crisis). Of course, neuromuscular blocking agents worsen symptoms and may prolong recovery and weaning from ventilation postoperatively, especially the depolarizing agents. Rarely, drugs such as D-penicillamine may precipitate MG in previously unaffected patients (Table 5-2). A more complete list can be found on the website for the Myasthenia Gravis Foundation of America (MGFA) at www.myasthenia.org.

**TABLE 5-2.  DRUGS THAT ADVERSELY AFFECT NMJ FUNCTION**

| Antibiotics | Neuromuscular Blockers | Other Drugs |
| --- | --- | --- |
| Aminoglycosides | Cardiac drugs | Phenytoin |
| Neomycin | Quinine | Chloroquine |
| Streptomycin | Quinidine | Trimethadione |
| Kanamycin | Procainamide | Lithium carbonate |
| Gentamicin | Trimethaphan | Magnesium salts |
| Tobramycin | Lidocaine | Meglumine diatrizoate |
| Other peptide antibiotics | Beta-adrenergic blockers | Methoxyflurane |
| Polymyxin B | | Oxytocin |
| Colistin | | Aprotinin |
| Other antibiotics | | Propanidid |
| Oxytetracycline | | Diazepam |
| Rolitetracycline | | Ketamine |
| Lincomycin | | D-Penicillamine |
| Clindamycin | | Carnitine |
| Erythromycin | | |
| Ampicillin | | |

28. **What is drug-induced autoimmune MG?**
Approximately 1% of patients taking D-penicillamine for the treatment of diseases such as rheumatoid arthritis or Wilson's disease develop clinical myasthenia. The disease is six times more common in women, first striking the ocular muscles and then becoming generalized. Patients have autoantibodies against AChRs, which usually slowly disappear (along with MG symptoms) after discontinuation of the drug. Trimethadione, an anticonvulsant, also may induce myasthenia. These patients have high titers of antimuscle antibodies and antinuclear factor, and symptoms suggestive of systemic lupus erythematosus.

29. **Which temporizing therapies can rapidly improve MG?**
Both plasma exchange (PE) and IVIG induce improvement in most MG patients within 1 to 2 weeks. Typical courses of therapy might include six exchanges every other day over 2 weeks, or 400 mg/kg/day of IVIG for 5 days. Improvement usually peaks at 2 to 4 weeks and then gradually abates at 6 to 8 weeks. These therapies seem to have equivalent efficacy in general, though some patients may respond better to one or the other. There are no data suggesting that combined therapy is any more beneficial than treatment with either agent alone. They are helpful when rapid improvement is needed (i.e., myasthenic crisis), to prepare symptomatic patients for steroid induction, and for surgical procedures such as thymectomy.

In rare instances, patients refractory to chronic oral therapies may require indefinite courses of treatment with these temporizing therapies on a regular schedule.

Richman DP, Agius MA: Treatment of autoimmune myasthenia gravis. Neurology 61:1652-1661, 2003.

30. **What are the side effects of PE and IVIG?**
PE induces fluid shifts and can cause electrolyte imbalance, anemia, and thrombocytopenia. In addition, PE often requires a central line, which carries some placement and infection risk. IVIG can rarely precipitate renal failure, especially in diabetics, and may cause aseptic meningitis, resulting in headache. It increases blood viscosity, and may increase cardiac and stroke risk in elderly subjects. It also causes transient myelosuppression, though this is usually mild. Unlike PE, IVIG may be protective against infection.

31. **What drugs are effective as chronic immunosuppressives in MG?**
Oral prednisone is the single most effective treatment for MG, resulting in dramatic improvement in 90% of cases within 4 weeks. Azathioprine and mycophenolate are also often effective as sole agents but take longer to begin to work (3 to 6 months). They have a primary role as adjunctive therapy for patients in whom steroids cannot be effectively tapered, and may be drugs of first choice in patients with mild, nonprogressive disease. Methotrexate, cyclophosphamide, and Cytoxan may also be of benefit.

## KEY POINTS: TREATMENT OF MYASTHENIA GRAVIS

1. Steroids, PE, IVIG, and other immunosuppressive drugs can dramatically improve and successfully control MG.

2. Up to 40% of MG patients experience a transient exacerbation after starting high-dose steroids, usually within 5 to 7 days.

32. **What is a steroid-induced exacerbation?**
In addition to the usual side effects of corticosteroids, patients with MG may become acutely weaker 1 to 3 weeks (average 5 to 7 days) after initiation of oral prednisone therapy (steroid-induced exacerbation) for 24 to 48 hours. Pretreatment with PE and/or IVIG or, alternatively, gradually increasing doses of oral prednisone, from 25 mg orally every other day to 100 mg orally every other day, may alleviate this phenomenon. Consequently, respiratory functions should be carefully monitored during the acute phase of steroid induction.

33. **What is the usual chronic course of patients treated with steroids?**
Patients may be successfully tapered to very low doses over approximately 12 months in most cases, especially when thymectomy has been performed. However, a significant minority of patients will experience an exacerbation (usually mild) as steroids are tapered below a certain point. This is treated by slight, recurrent increases in dosage. However, should a second attempt at steroid taper fail, the introduction of an adjunctive agent, such as azathioprine, is often necessary before taper can be successfully resumed. Excessively rapid steroid tapers are responsible for many severe exacerbations in patients with MG.

Graves M, Katz JS: Myasthenia gravis. Curr Treat Options Neurol 6:163-171, 2004.

**34. What is a myasthenic crisis?**
Myasthenic crisis is an acute exacerbation of MG with severe weakness and/or bulbar and/or respiratory dysfunction. The maintenance of adequate ventilation is paramount, and patients should be hospitalized with close monitoring of pulmonary functions, especially forced vital capacity and $FEV_1$, which often decline before blood gases deteriorate. Early intubation with mechanical ventilatory support is lifesaving in a myasthenic crisis.

**35. After respiratory function is secured, how is a myasthenic crisis treated?**
A thorough work-up for intercurrent infection or other acute disease is needed, along with careful review of the patient's medication list and recent history (for potential agents contributing to NMJ dysfunction or recent changes in MG treatment regimen). Temporizing therapy with plasmapheresis or IVIG should be instituted as soon as possible, followed by chronic immunosuppressive therapy if not contraindicated by other intercurrent illness. If infection is present, IVIG is the temporizing therapy of choice. Anticholinesterases are problematic. If cholinergic crisis is suspected (i.e., very high daily doses used), anticholinesterases should be discontinued with careful respiratory monitoring.

**36. What is the value of the edrophonium test to differentiate myasthenic crisis from cholinergic crisis?**
The edrophonium (Tensilon) test improves myasthenic crisis but aggravates cholinergic crisis. However, interpretation of the result is often difficult and misleading because one group of muscles may deteriorate while others may improve. Securing respiratory function and discontinuing all anticholinesterase drugs in a monitored hospital environment is a safer and more practical solution.

**37. What is anti-MuSK antibody syndrome?**
A new population of antibodies has been identified in MG patients in recent years, directed against muscle-specific kinase (MuSK). MuSK is a tyrosine kinase, which has an important role in regulating and maintaining AChRs and their functional clusters at the NMJ. Anti-MuSK antibodies may be found in 40% to 60% of patients with clinical MG who are seronegative for antibodies directed against the AChR, and passive transfer of these antibodies produces physiologic effects at the NMJ similar to that caused by anti-AChR IgG (i.e., reduced MEPP amplitude). Initial clinical studies suggest that these patients have a syndrome of generalized myasthenia, often with prominent neck, shoulder, or respiratory muscle weakness with little or delayed ocular muscle involvement. Responses to cholinesterase inhibitors are variable, but PE is effective, and most patients also respond to other immunotherapies including oral steroids, azathioprine, cyclosporine, and mycophenolate. The benefits of thymectomy remain unclear at present.

## LAMBERT-EATON MYASTHENIC SYNDROME

**38. What are the primary manifestations of Lambert-Eaton myasthenic syndrome (LEMS)?**
In LEMS, weakness and fatigability of proximal muscles, especially in the thighs and pelvic girdle, with depressed or absent tendon reflexes are the primary manifestations. Muscle strength and/or reflexes may increase for a short while after exercise (postexercise facilitation and facilitation of reflexes). Although ptosis may be present in LEMS, extraocular and bulbar muscles are minimally involved. Mild autonomic dysfunction may be prominent in LEMS, manifesting primarily as dryness of the mouth.

39. **Which tumor is associated with LEMS?**
   About 50% to 66% of patients with LEMS have cancer, usually small-cell carcinoma of the lung, at the time of presentation or will ultimately be diagnosed with it, usually within 2 years. Although immunologic evidence suggests that this tumor may play an important role in the pathogenesis of LEMS, a substantial minority of patients with LEMS never develop malignancy.

40. **What experimental evidence suggests an autoimmune pathogenesis of LEMS?**
   Passive transfers of IgG from patients with LEMS to animals produce electrophysiologic defects characteristic of LEMS. The LEMS IgG contains autoantibodies against voltage-gated calcium channels.

41. **Describe the autoimmune pathophysiology involved in LEMS.**
   The primary antigen for the LEMS antibodies is found both at the presynapse and in small-cell carcinoma of the lung. LEMS antibodies cross-react with N-type and L-type voltage-gated $Ca^{2+}$ channels and with synaptotagmin in the presynapse. This decreases the number of voltage-gated $Ca^{2+}$ channels, which reduces activation of the cascade, thus leading to the release of acetylcholine (ACh) vesicles. Decreased ACh release decreases depolarization at the muscle end plate, and threshold for activation of the muscle fiber is not reached.

42. **Explain the mechanism of incremental response after high-frequency RNS in patients with LEMS.**
   Decreased $Ca^{2+}$ influx into the presynaptic nerve terminal (due to antibody attack) results in insufficient release of acetylcholine. When the nerve is stimulated at sufficiently high frequencies (either by extrinsic high-frequency RNS or by brief volitional exercise), recurrent depolarization of the nerve terminal causes such a high rate of calcium influx that it overwhelms the nerve cell's mechanisms for calcium clearance, temporarily increasing intracellular calcium levels and normalizing the release of acetylcholine. This manifests as a dramatic increase in compound muscle action potential size. However, low-frequency RNS results in decrement, which may be confused with the decrement of MG.

43. **What are the morphologic changes at the NMJ in LEMS?**
   In the normal subject, freeze-fracture technique shows submicroscopic bumps arrayed in parallel rows in the portion of the presynaptic membrane where calcium channels are clustered. These "active zone protein particles" correspond with the voltage-gated calcium channels, and show reduced numbers and disruption of their normal parallel arrays in patients with LEMS.

44. **What is the treatment for LEMS?**
   Release of acetylcholine from the presynaptic nerve terminal is facilitated by guanidine hydrochloride, 4-aminopyridine (4-AP), and 3,4-diaminopyridine (3,4-DAP). The aminopyridines, particularly 4-AP, decrease the seizure threshold. Anticholinesterases may improve symptoms in some patients. In paraneoplastic cases, successful treatment of the underlying neoplasm is the best therapy and may cause full remission of symptoms. Although improvement after IVIG also has been reported and other immunomodulatory therapies have been utilized (i.e., PE, oral steroids), the results of these interventions are often disappointing.
   Weimer MG, Wong J: Lambert-Eaton myasthenic syndrome. Curr Treat Options Neurol 11:77-84, 2009.

45. **What precautions must be taken for surgical procedures that require general anesthesia in patients with MG and LEMS?**
   Delayed recovery from neuromuscular blocking agents must be anticipated in both LEMS and MG. Nondepolarizing, short-acting neuromuscular blockers at minimal necessary doses are

preferred. Intravenous steroids equivalent to oral maintenance doses should be given until oral steroids can be resumed. An additional bolus during surgery may also be helpful. Anticholinesterase therapy is usually unnecessary during surgery but is started postoperatively as needed when the patient regains consciousness. The differences between parenteral and oral doses of anticholinesterase should be recognized. Maintain normal serum electrolytes, calcium, phosphorus, and magnesium. Avoid unnecessary medications to minimize drug-related complications, especially those that may worsen neuromuscular transmission (see Question 27, Table 5-2).

## KEY POINTS: OTHER NMJ DISEASES

1. Antibodies against the presynaptic voltage-gated calcium channel cause LEMS, which is paraneoplastic in 60% of cases.

2. MG and LEMS both cause decrement on low-frequency RNS, but LEMS also causes dramatic increment on high-frequency RNS (often greater than 100%).

3. Botulism can often be distinguished from the aggressive onset of MG by the presence of dilated, minimally reactive pupils.

### OTHER NEUROMUSCULAR JUNCTION DISEASES

46. **What are the clinical characteristics of botulism?**
    Two to 48 hours after ingesting improperly prepared or preserved foods contaminated with *Clostridium botulinum,* ocular and bulbar muscle paralysis begins, with difficulty in convergence of the eyes, diplopia, ptosis, weakness of the jaw muscles, dysphagia, and dysarthria. Nausea, vomiting, and diarrhea may precede these symptoms. Constipation, urinary retention, and nonreactive dilation of the pupils may occur because of autonomic dysfunction. Respiratory failure and total limb paralysis may ensue without sensory loss or mental status changes. Infantile botulism may result in poor sucking and difficulty with feeding, weak cry, loss of head control, and bilateral ptosis, with subsequent generalized flaccid paralysis. The course depends on the amount of toxin absorbed, ranging from death within 4 to 8 days without respiratory support to mild symptoms with complete recovery.

47. **What is the infectious process in botulism?**
    Botulinum toxin is an exotoxin of *C. botulinum.* The presence of common bacteria inhibits the growth of *C. botulinum,* but infection occurs when the victim ingests improperly prepared canned or bottled foods in which the common bacteria are killed, but the more resistant *Clostridium* spores are spared. In infants, the intestinal bacterial flora may not effectively inhibit the growth of *C. botulinum.* Human botulism is usually caused by exotoxin produced by types A, B, and E, which interfere with acetylcholine release.

48. **What is the pharmacologic action of black widow spider venom?**
    Black widow spider venom promotes rapid release of acetylcholine from the presynaptic nerve terminal, depleting its stores. The venom also inhibits choline uptake. Clinically, this causes painful muscle spasms with severe gastrointestinal symptoms, followed by weakness.

49. **What is the pharmacologic action of curare?**
    Curare is a classic antagonist of nicotinic AChRs and competes with acetylcholine for the binding site, which is effective as a neuromuscular blocking agent (nondepolarizing blocker) for general anesthesia.

50. **Which snake venom causes a neuromuscular disorder?**
Alpha-bungarotoxin, a potent toxin produced by the Banded Krait of Taiwan *(Bungarus multicinctus),* binds to the AChR at multiple sites on the alpha subunit, blocking acetylcholine binding in a manner similar to MG.

51. **What is the importance of alpha-bungarotoxin in experimental studies of MG?**
Because of its high affinity for the receptor, it is a useful marker for basic scientific investigation. Envenomation and clinical disease have become rare as the numbers of these snakes have steadily declined, potentially endangering their survival as a species in the wild.

# WEBSITES

1. http://www.myasthenia.org
2. http://www.neuro.wustl.edu/neuromuscular/synmg.html

## BIBLIOGRAPHY

1. Amato A, Russell J: Neuromuscular Disorders, New York, McGraw-Hill, 2008.
2. Antel J, Birnbaum G, Hartung H-P, Vincent A, eds. Clinical Neuroimmunology, 2nd ed. Boston, Blackwell Science, 2005.
3. Ciafaloni E, Sanders DB: Advances in myasthenia gravis. Curr Neurol Neurosci Rep 2:89-95, 2002.
4. Gooch CL, Swenson MR: The treatment of myasthenia gravis: A stepwise approach. Adv Immunother 10:19-23, 2003.
5. Newsome-Davis J: Therapy in myasthenia gravis and Lambert-Eaton myasthenic syndrome. Semin Neurol 23:191-198, 2003.

# CHAPTER 6

# PERIPHERAL NEUROPATHIES AND MOTOR NEURON DISEASES

*Yadollah Harati, MD, FACP, Justin Kwan, MD, and Shane Smyth, MD, MRCPI*

1. **What are the most common diseases affecting the peripheral nerve?**
   The most important neuropathies can be classified by the mnemonic DANG THE RAPIST:

   **D**iabetes      **T**rauma      **R**heumatic (collagen vascular)
   **A**lcohol      **H**ereditary      **A**myloid
   **N**utritional      **E**nvironmental toxins and drugs      **P**araneoplastic
   **G**uillain-Barré      **I**nfections
        **S**ystemic disease
        **T**umors

2. **How does a nerve's size and structure contribute to its speed of conduction? How are the peripheral fibers classified?**
   The larger the fiber, the less the electrical resistance and the faster the speed of conduction. Myelin increases a nerve's diameter and also insulates the current between nodes of Ranvier, increasing the overall conduction velocity. In myelinated nerves, the conduction velocity can be estimated to be 6 m/sec/micrometer (e.g., a nerve that is 10 micrometers in diameter will conduct at approximately 60 m/sec). In unmyelinated nerves, the velocity is approximately 1.7 m/sec/micrometer.

   Peripheral nerve fibers are classified according to diameter and conduction velocity (Table 6-1). The nomenclature can be somewhat confusing. Stated simply, there are three types of fibers: A, B, and C. A and B are myelinated fibers, and C are unmyelinated fibers. B and C are relatively straightforward: B fibers are myelinated preganglionic efferent fibers of the autonomic nervous system (conduction velocity 3 to 15 m/sec); C fibers are small, unmyelinated fibers (conduction velocity 1 to 2 m/sec) that comprise the postganglionic efferent nerves of the autonomic nervous system. C fibers also convey afferent "slow pain" sensation in somatic nerves.

   A fibers are myelinated fibers found in somatic nerves. There are three types: $\alpha$, $\beta$, and $\delta$ (conduction velocities 80 to 120 m/sec, 35 to 75 m/sec, and 5 to 30 m/sec, respectively). $\alpha$ fibers form a subset of muscle afferent nerves that supply the muscle spindle and are sensitive to the rate of change in fiber length. $\beta$ fibers also form a subset of afferent nerves supplying the muscle spindle and respond to the overall length of the muscle spindle fiber. $\beta$ fibers are also the fastest cutaneous afferent fibers and supply the hair and skin follicles. $\delta$ fibers convey "fast pain" sensation from skin and muscle. The motor neurons to muscle (also A fibers) are divided into $\alpha$ motor neurons supplying the muscle itself and $\gamma$ motor neurons to the muscle spindle. Both types are usually activated simultaneously, contracting the muscle spindle fibers in concert with the extrafusal fibers and thus allowing the spindle fibers to maintain sensitivity during contraction.

   The A $\alpha$, $\beta$, and $\delta$ muscle afferent fibers may alternatively be categorized as types I, II, and III, respectively. Type IV is an alternative categorical name for afferent C fibers. Finally, type I is subdivided into Ia and Ib, where Ia are the afferent A$\alpha$ fibers from the muscle spindle, and Ib are the afferent A$\alpha$ fibers serving the Golgi tendon organ at the junction between muscle and tendon. These latter fibers convey afferent information about the degree of muscle tension and may also prevent excessive muscular contraction.

**TABLE 6-1.  PERIPHERAL NERVE FIBERS**

| Classification | Alternate Classification | Myelinated? | Type | Conduction Velocity |
|---|---|---|---|---|
| A | | Yes | Somatic nerves | |
| α | I | Yes | Subset of afferent nerves supplying the muscle spindle | 80-120 m/sec |
| | | | Sensitive to the rate of change in fiber length | |
| | | | Also efferent motor neurons | |
| | Ia | | Afferent fibers from the muscle spindle | |
| | Ib | | Afferent fibers serving the Golgi tendon organ at the junction between muscle and tendon | |
| β | II | Yes | Subset of afferent nerves supplying the muscle spindle | 35-75 m/sec |
| | | | Respond to the overall length of the muscle spindle fiber | |
| | | | Fastest cutaneous afferent fibers, supplying the hair and skin follicles | |
| δ | III | Yes | Convey "fast pain" sensation from skin and muscle | 5-30 m/sec |
| B | | Yes | Preganglionic efferent fibers of the autonomic nervous system | 3-15 m/sec |
| C | IV, afferent | No | Postganglionic efferent nerves of the autonomic nervous system | 1-2 m/sec |
| | | | Convey afferent "slow pain" sensation in somatic nerves | |

3. **What are the patterns of peripheral nerve damage?**

   The nerve can be damaged by injury to the myelin, axon, cell body, or vasa nervorum. Three basic pathologic mechanisms underlie nerve injury (Figure 6-1):

   1. **Wallerian degeneration** develops after injury to the axon and myelin, as in transection of the nerve. Distal to the transection, the axon and then myelin degenerate, followed within 3 to 5 days by failure to generate and conduct a nerve action potential. The axon may regrow within the architecture provided by the basement membrane of Schwann cells, but the degree and efficiency of regrowth depend on good approximation of the nerve ends.

   2. **Segmental demyelination** develops after damage to the myelin sheath or Schwann cell. Because the muscle is not denervated, no atrophy develops, whereas in wallerian degeneration, the axon is also damaged and the muscle degenerates. Prognosis for complete recovery is good.

   3. **Neuronal (axonal) degeneration** develops when damage to the cell body of the neuron results in distal dying of the axon and subsequent loss of myelin. Once the distal nerve dies, the muscle is denervated; hence, muscle atrophy develops. The denervated muscle fibers are re-innervated by surrounding nerves, but recovery may not be complete.

4. **What are the electrophysiologic mechanisms that correlate with weakness in peripheral neuropathy?**

   Conduction block, denervation with loss of motor units, and failure of neuromuscular transmission. One or more of the above are needed. Slowing of motor conduction velocity in itself, even if severe, does not result in weakness.

5. **What is conduction block?**

   Conduction block is a focal abnormality across a nerve segment that results in failure to conduct an action potential, although distal to the block conduction is preserved. It is typically caused by focal disruption of the myelin sheath (although the underlying axon is often at risk of degeneration). The compound muscle action potential (CMAP) will drop as the motor nerve is stimulated distal, and then proximal to the site of injury. What constitutes conduction block electrophysiologically is not absolutely defined, but in general a CMAP drop of 30% to 50% is typical.

6. **What is the significance of conduction block in peripheral neuropathy?**

   Conduction block occurs only in certain limited settings of acute reversible ischemic injury, compression-induced demyelination, and acquired demyelinative neuropathies. It generally does not occur in hereditary neuropathies with one major exception—hereditary neuropathy with liability to pressure palsy (HNPP). It is clinically important because it implies a potentially reversible defect-causing weakness.

7. **Which peripheral neuropathies may have cranial nerve involvement?**

   See Table 6-2.

8. **Which neuropathies begin proximally rather than distally?**

   Most neuropathies begin distally, but a few may begin proximally: Guillain-Barré syndrome, chronic inflammatory demyelinating neuropathy, diabetes (diabetic lumboradiculoplexus neuropathy/diabetic amyotrophy), porphyric neuropathy, idiopathic acute brachial plexus neuropathy (Parsonage-Turner syndrome), and Tangier disease.

9. **Which neuropathies begin in the arms rather than the legs?**

   Most neuropathies present with symptoms in the feet. Once the symptoms in the lower limbs proceed to the middle of the calf, the neuropathies begin to appear in the hands. Although this pattern generally holds, some neuropathies may start in the upper limbs:

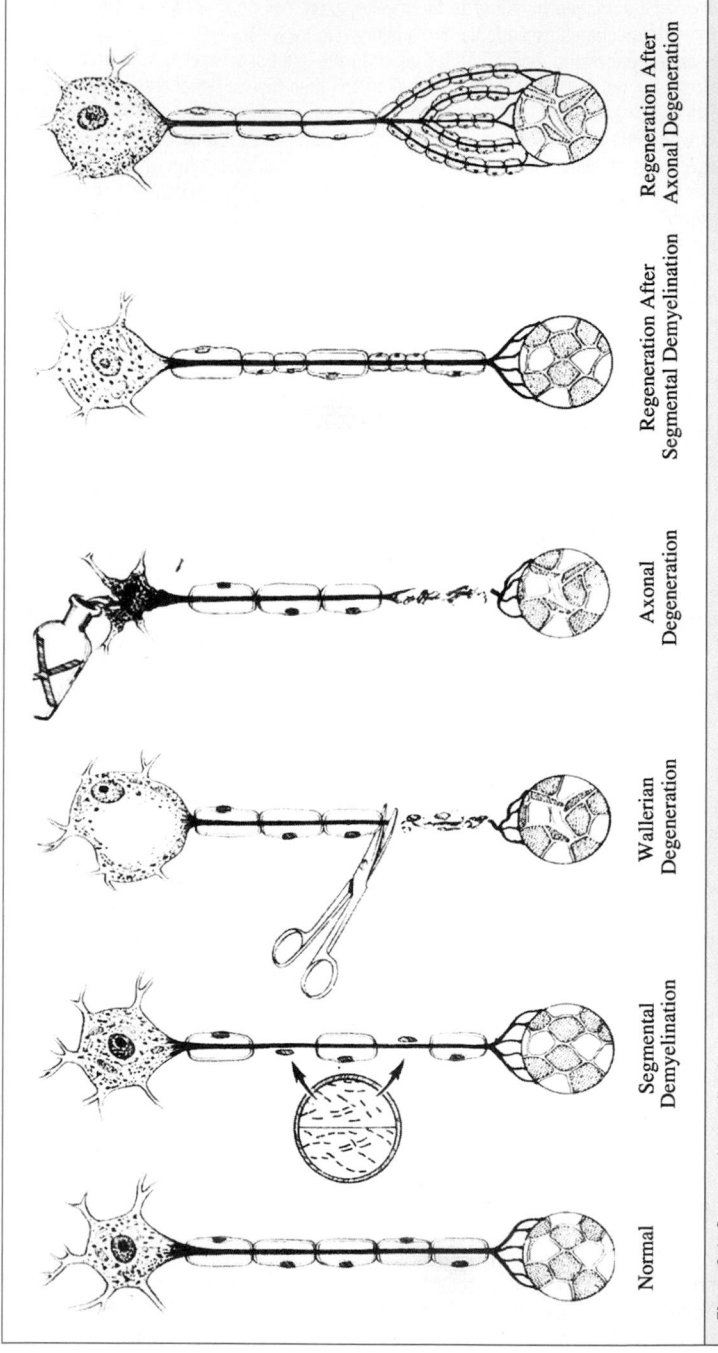

**Figure 6-1.** Segmental remyelination may follow segmental demyelination. The remyelinated segments are shorter and have a smaller diameter. Axonal regeneration is associated with the formation of clusters of small and thin myelinated fibers.

Normal

Segmental Demyelination

Wallerian Degeneration

Axonal Degeneration

Regeneration After Segmental Demyelination

Regeneration After Axonal Degeneration

**TABLE 6-2.  NEUROPATHIES WITH CRANIAL NERVE INVOLVEMENT**

| Neuropathy | Most Commonly Involved Cranial Nerves | Less Commonly Involved Cranial Nerves |
|---|---|---|
| Diphtheria | IX | II, III |
| Sarcoid | VII | I, III, IV, VI |
| Diabetes | III | IV, VI, VII |
| Guillain-Barré syndrome (GBS) | VI, VII | |
| Miller-Fisher variant of GBS | III, IV | |
| Sjögren syndrome | V | |
| Polyarteritis nodosa | VII, III | VIII |
| Wegener granulomatosis | VIII | |
| Lyme disease | VII, V | All but I |
| Porphyria | VII, X | III, IV, V, XI, XII |
| Refsum's disease | I, VIII | |
| Primary amyloidosis | VII, V, III | VI, XII |
| Syphilis | III | IV, V, VII, VIII |
| Arsenic | V | |

*Pupil is usually not affected.

1. Compression/entrapment syndromes (e.g., carpal tunnel syndrome, ulnar neuropathy at the elbow)
2. Diabetes
3. Vasculitic neuropathy
4. Guillain-Barré syndrome
5. Multifocal motor neuropathy
6. Lead toxicity (classically with wrist drop from a radial neuropathy)
7. Porphyria
8. Sarcoidosis
9. Leprosy
10. Charcot-Marie-Tooth disease (rare)
11. Tangier disease
12. Inherited recurrent focal neuropathies
13. Some forms of familial amyloid polyneuropathy (FAP)

**10. Which neuropathies are often predominantly motor?**
Guillain-Barré syndrome, diphtheric neuropathy, dapsone-induced neuropathy, porphyria, and multifocal motor neuropathy are often predominantly motor.

**11. Which neuropathies are often predominantly sensory?**
1. Drug toxicity: pyridoxine, doxorubicin, cisplatin, thalidomide, metronidazole
2. Autoimmune: Miller-Fisher syndrome, sensory variants of acute and chronic inflammatory demyelinating polyneuropathy, IgM paraproteinemia, paraneoplastic syndrome, Sjögren syndrome
3. Infectious: diphtheria, HIV, Lyme disease
4. Deficiency: vitamin E, pyridoxine
5. Inherited: neuropathies associated with abetalipoproteinemia and spinocerebellar degeneration

12. **What are the causes of multiple mononeuropathy (mononeuritis multiplex)?**
    1. Trauma or compression
    2. Diabetes
    3. Vasculitis, with or without connective tissue diseases; also virus-associated (HIV, hepatitis B and C)
    4. Leprosy
    5. Lyme disease
    6. Sarcoidosis
    7. Sensory perineuritis
    8. Tumor infiltration
    9. Lymphoid granulomatosis
    10. Demyelinating idiopathic and paraproteinemic neuropathies (MMN, MADSAM)
    11. Hereditary neuropathy with liability to pressure palsies (HNPP)

13. **What nutritional deficiencies can cause myelopathy and neuropathy?**
    1. Vitamin B12 deficiency
    2. Copper deficiency
    3. Vitamin E deficiency
    4. Folate deficiency

14. **What are the clinical features of copper deficiency?**
    The main neurologic symptom of copper deficiency is gait difficulty. Examination shows predominantly large fiber sensory loss in the distal legs, spasticity in the lower extremities, hyperreflexia, and extensor plantar response. Nerve conduction studies and needle EMG show an axonal sensorimotor neuropathy. Somatosensory evoked potential study shows impairment of central conduction. Anemia is a known associated laboratory finding, but the neurologic symptoms can be present in the absence of hematologic abnormalities.
    Kumar N: Nutritional neuropathies. Neurol Clin 25:209-255, 2007.
    Kumar N, Gross JB, Ahiskig JE: Copper deficiency myelopathy produces a clinical picture like subacute combined degeneration. Neurology 63:33-39, 2004.

15. **What are the risk factors for copper deficiency?**
    1. Zinc overdose
    2. Gastric bypass surgery
    3. Malabsorption syndrome
    4. Total parenteral nutrition without adequate copper supplementation
    5. Gastrectomy and small bowel resection
    6. Nephrotic syndrome
    Goodman BP, Bosch EP, Ross MA, et al.: Clinical and electrodiagnostic findings in copper deficiency myeloneuropathy. J Neurol Neurosurg Psychiatry 80:524-527, 2008 (epub 2008 May 21).

16. **In which conditions are the peripheral nerves palpably enlarged?**
    1. Hereditary motor and sensory neuropathies (HMSN) or Charcot-Marie-Tooth disease (demyelinative type) and Dejerine-Sottas syndrome (HMSNIII)
    2. Amyloidosis
    3. Refsum's disease
    4. Leprosy
    5. Acromegaly
    6. Neurofibromatosis

17. **Define an "onion-bulb" formation.**
    An onion-bulb formation is the pathologic hallmark of the hypertrophic neuropathies, in which repeated segmental demyelination and remyelination have occurred (Figure 6-2). When viewed

in transverse sections, onion-bulb formations are multiple concentric layers of intertwined, attenuated Schwann cell processes surrounding the remaining nerve fibers. The Schwann cell processes are separated from each other by layers of collagen fibers. The onion-bulb formations may be seen in any condition with chronic segmental demyelination and remyelination but are frequently seen in Charcot-Marie-Tooth disease, Dejerine-Sottas syndrome, Refsum's disease, and chronic relapsing idiopathic (inflammatory) demyelinating neuropathy.

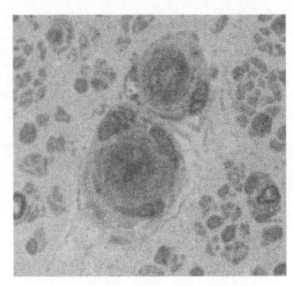

**Figure 6-2.** Semithin section. Note proliferation of Schwann cells with onion-bulb formation.

18. **Which nerves are commonly used for biopsy?**

The most common and best nerve to use is the sural nerve, a purely sensory nerve located lateral to the lateral malleolus. The nerve can be biopsied at this level or at a higher level between the heads of the gastrocnemius muscles. Superficial peroneal and radial cutaneous nerves offer advantages in certain situations; the radial cutaneous nerve or medial antebrachial cutaneous nerves are often biopsied in upper limb-predominant neuropathies (e.g., some cases of leprosy). The superficial peroneal nerve has the advantage of allowing sampling of muscle (the peroneus brevis muscle) via the same incision when both muscle and nerve specimens are required (e.g., in cases of suspected vasculitis). The intermediate cutaneous nerve of the thigh also has been biopsied in patients with proximal diabetic neuropathy.

19. **What are the indications for sural nerve biopsy?**

Sural nerve biopsy is most helpful when the underlying condition is multifocal and asymmetric. Examples include many of the disorders associated with multiple mononeuropathies, especially vasculitis and leprosy. It may be obtained in chronic demyelinating neuropathies with the aim of confirming the diagnosis when the clinical and electrophysiologic findings have been inconclusive, especially in patients who may be candidates for therapies with potentially harmful side effects. Nerve is one of a number of tissues useful in diagnosing amyloidosis. Genetic studies and enzyme assays have decreased the need for nerve biopsy in some inherited neuropathies, but it is still useful in unrecognized cases, for example, of HNPP and metachromatic leukodystrophy. Metabolic and toxic causes of peripheral neuropathies are not usually diagnosed by sural nerve biopsy. Nerve biopsy may be of value as a final resort in patients with progressive, disabling peripheral neuropathy of undetermined etiology. With teased nerve fiber preparation, segmental demyelination, remyelination, or axonal degeneration is identified. In segmental demyelination, the diameter of demyelinated segments is reduced. In remyelination, the internodal length varies. Axonal degeneration causes breakdown of myelin into "ovoids and balls" (Figure 6-3).

20. **Acronyms in peripheral nerve disease: What do the following acronyms stand for?**
   - **AIDP:** acute inflammatory demyelinating polyneuropathy (the most common subset of Guillain-Barré syndrome)
   - **CIDP:** chronic immune-mediated demyelinating polyneuropathy
   - **DADS:** distal acquired demyelinating symmetric neuropathy
   - **AMAN:** acute motor axonal neuropathy (a Guillain-Barré syndrome variant)
   - **AMSAN:** acute motor and sensory axonal neuropathy (a Guillain-Barré syndrome variant)
   - **MMN:** multifocal motor neuropathy (Often "MMN-CB," it means with conduction block, although this does not always occur in this condition. MMN is sometimes incorrectly referred to as Lewis-Sumner syndrome.)

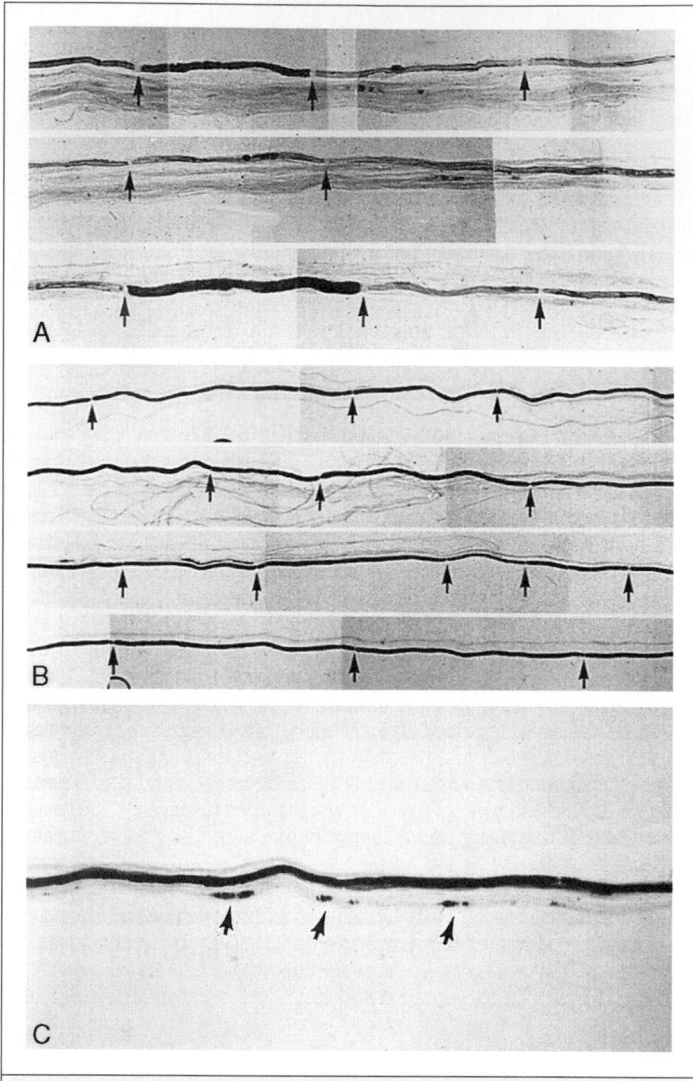

**Figure 6-3.** Teased nerve fiber preparation. **A**, Segmental demyelination.
**B**, Remyelination. **C**, Axonal degeneration.

- **MADSAM:** multifocal acquired demyelinating sensory and motor neuropathy (It is also known as Lewis-Sumner syndrome. It resembles MMN, but in contrast to this condition, it has sensory involvement and may be steroid responsive.)
- **MAMA:** multifocal acquired motor axonapathy (It is debated whether or not this is a distinct entity. It resembles MMN, but with axonal features on electrodiagnostic testing, and is rarely if ever associated with anti-GM1 antibodies.)
- **GALOP:** gait disorder antibody late-age onset polyneuropathy (A syndrome occurring in a subset of patients with neuropathy and anti-sulfatide antibodies. There is usually an M

protein and antibodies to a central meylin antigen Galopin. The syndrome appears to respond to cyclophosphamide or IVIG. Some texts list the "GA" of GALOP as standing for gait ataxia.)

- **POEMS:** polyneuropathy organomegaly endocrinopathy M-protein skin changes (This is a syndrome occurring in some patients with osteosclerotic myeloma.)
- **CANOMAD:** chronic ataxic neuropathy with ophthalmoplegia, M-protein, agglutination, disialosyl antibodies (These patients have distal sensory loss and sensory ataxia. There may be motor weakness and relapses of sensory or motor cranial neuropathies. A variety of anti-ganglioside antibodies have been found in these patients.)
- **BAD:** brachial amyotrophic diplegia (This is probably a variant of ALS. It involves progressive lower motor neuron weakness of the arms. Rarely, it may be the presentation of more typical ALS that becomes evident over time.)

## MISCELLANEOUS NEUROPATHIES

21. **What is the most common cause of peripheral neuropathy in the world?**
   Diabetes mellitus. It is estimated that between 20 and 30 million people worldwide are affected by symptomatic diabetic neuropathy, and this figure may double in the next 20 to 30 years. Leprosy was once the most common cause of neuropathy worldwide, but its incidence has dramatically decreased since 1982 when the World Health Organization implemented a shorter course of multiple drug therapy, allowing many more affected patients to complete treatment.
   Ooi WW, Srinivasan J: Leprosy and the peripheral nervous system: Basic and clinical aspects. Muscle Nerve 30:393-409, 2004.
   Said G: Diabetic neuropathy—a review. Nat Clin Prac Neurol 3:331-340, 2007.

22. **What are the clinical forms of diabetic neuropathy?**
   - Symmetric polyneuropathies (the most common form): sensory or sensorimotor polyneuropathy
   - Autonomic neuropathy
   - Focal neuropathies: asymmetric lower limb motor neuropathy (diabetic amyotrophy), compression mononeuropathies, isolated trunk radiculopathies, cranial neuropathies

23. **Which diabetic neuropathies are painful?**
   - Third cranial nerve neuropathy
   - Acute thoracoabdominal neuropathy
   - Acute distal sensory neuropathy
   - Acute lumbar radiculoplexopathy
   - Chronic distal small-fiber neuropathy

24. **What are the risk factors for developing diabetic peripheral neuropathy?**
   1. Duration of diabetes
   2. Degree of glycemic control
   3. Older age
   4. Male sex
   5. Excessive alcohol consumption
   6. Nicotine use
   7. Dyslipidemia
   8. Angiotensin-converting enzyme D allele
      Harati Y: Diabetic neuropathies: Unanswered questions. Neurol Clin 25:303-317, 2007.

25. **How does the global importance of leprous neuropathy compare to its importance in the United States? Is it true that armadillos spread leprosy?**
    The global registered prevalence of leprosy at the beginning of 2007 was 224,717 cases. In 2006, the number of new cases detected worldwide was 259,017. Over the last 5 years, the global number of new cases detected has fallen by an average of 20% per year. Despite the 10-fold decline in the global prevalence of leprosy to about 1 million, it is still the most common cause of neuropathy in developing countries. In contrast, the prevalence of leprosy in the United States is low (<10,000). In 2006, the number of new cases in the U.S. was 137. The yearly incidence in the past decade (100 to 200) fluctuated in previous decades, depending on the extent to which immigrants and refugees from endemic areas entered the U.S. About 85% of cases detected in the U.S. are in immigrants. Leprous neuropathy does occur rarely in native U.S. citizens, however. Although they represent a minority of cases (10% to 20%) in most regions of the U.S., native citizens are affected more commonly in the endemic southern border areas of Texas, Louisiana, and Florida as well as Hawaii.

    As regards armadillos, the WHO website says: "Up to 5% of armadillos in Louisiana have been found to have clinical disease with about 20% having serological evidence of *M. leprae* infection. The epidemiological significance of the armadillo is generally considered to be negligible in spite of occasional cases reported among individuals giving history of handling armadillos."

26. **How does one recognize and diagnose hereditary neuropathy with liability to pressure palsy (HNPP)?**
    HNPP, also called recurrent pressure-sensitive neuropathy or tomaculous neuropathy, is readily identified in cases of recurrent compression-induced mononeuropathies and in patients with autosomal dominant familial patterns, demyelinative features, and "sausage-shaped" swellings or tomaculi on nerve biopsy (Figure 6-4). However, a traumatic or compression-induced mechanism is not always obvious, and the pathologic evidence of numerous tomaculi may be the only diagnostic clue in sporadic cases presenting with a generalized polyneuropathy. Demonstrating *PMP22* gene deletion confirms the diagnosis. Clinical heterogeneity is becoming apparent with increased use of this genetic study. In addition, some patients have also been found to have subclinical CNS demyelination based on MRI and electrophysiologic testing.

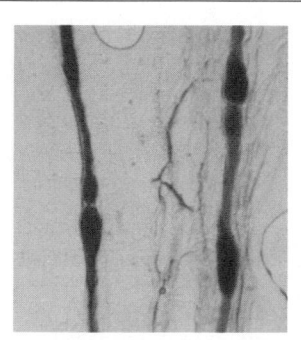

**Figure 6-4.** Teased nerve fiber preparation. Note focal areas of sausage-like (tomacula) thickening of the myelin sheaths.

27. **Which clinical features aid in the early diagnosis of carpal tunnel syndrome?**
    1. Pain, paresthesias, or numbness worse at night or during activities that maintain wrist extension or flexion (e.g., driving) or require repetitive wrist motion.
    2. Numbness often involving only partial median nerve innervation (e.g., thumb and index finger) rather than entire first three and one-half digits. Pain but not numbness may occur above the wrist.
    3. Symptoms of intermittent hand weakness before overt weakness of thenar muscles and lateral lumbricals.
    4. Provocative tests such as Tinel's sign and Phalen's test lack sufficient sensitivity and specificity to be reliable in the clinical setting. However, a recent review listed the "flick sign" as having the greatest sensitivity and specificity in confirming carpal tunnel

syndrome. This is when the patient demonstrates a flicking motion of the wrist and hand when describing attempts to relieve their symptoms.
Hui AC, Wong SM, Griffith J: Carpal tunnel syndrome. Pract Neurol 5:210-217, 2005.

28. **What are the three most common neurogenic causes of winging of the scapula?**
   1. **Long thoracic nerve palsy.** The long thoracic nerve innervates the serratus anterior muscle. Serratus anterior weakness leads to the most pronounced winging, which is accentuated with forward flexion of the arms and decreased with the arms at rest. The superior (medial) angle of the scapula is displaced closer to the midline, whereas the inferior angle swings laterally and away from the thorax.
   2. **Spinal accessory nerve palsy.** The spinal accessory nerve innervates the trapezius muscle. Trapezius muscle weakness leads to mild winging of the scapula at rest, which is accentuated by arm abduction to 90° and decreased by forward flexion to 90°. The superior (medial) angle of the scapula is displaced away from the midline, but the inferior angle is medially rotated. The shoulder is lower on the affected side because of atrophy of the trapezius muscle.
   3. **Dorsal scapular nerve palsy.** The dorsal scapular nerve innervates the rhomboid muscle. Weakness of this muscle produces minimal winging at rest, which is accentuated by slowly lowering the arm from the forward overhead position and decreased by elevation of the arms overhead. The superior (medial) angle is displaced away from the midline, and the inferior angle is laterally displaced.

   In addition, there are many nonneurogenic causes of winging of the scapula, including myopathies and muscular dystrophy (e.g., fascioscapulohumeral muscle dystrophy [FSH]).

29. **What are the different types of Lyme neuropathies?**
   Lyme disease is a multisystem illness caused by a tick-borne spirochete, *Borrelia burgdorferi*. Meningitis is the most common neurologic abnormality in Lyme disease. It may also cause many varieties of peripheral neuropathies, including cranial neuropathies (especially Bell's palsy), radiculitis, plexopathies, multiple mononeuropathies, a Guillain-Barré–like illness, and, more frequently, a symmetric sensory-motor neuropathy. In endemic areas, Lyme disease accounts for about two-thirds of pediatric cases of facial palsy and as many as one-fourth of adult cases. Involvement of other cranial nerves usually occurs in the setting of lymphocytic meningitis. Radiculitis may be indistinguishable from a compression-induced radiculopathy. Such radiculopathies usually occur in the lower limbs, and cerebrospinal fluid (CSF) pleocytosis is common. Unilateral or bilateral lumbosacral or brachial plexopathies are rarely observed. The symmetric distal sensory-motor neuropathy is usually mild and occurs in many patients with chronic Lyme disease. This neuropathy can start 6 months to 8 years after the infection and is more common in Europe, where it may be accompanied by acrodermatitis chronica atrophicans (a late manifestation of Lyme disease found very rarely in the United States, characterized by atrophic discolored skin in the extremities or digits, often with sensory complaints). The nerve pathology is consistent with axonal degeneration. A recent study did not demonstrate a higher prevalence of *B. burgdorferi* antibodies in patients with cryptogenic distal polyneuropathy when compared to patients with neuropathy of known causes. The authors concluded that, at least in Europe, Lyme disease was unlikely to be a cause of idiopathic distal polyneuropathy in the absence of other findings of the disease.
   Mygland A, Skarpass T, Ljøstad U: Chronic polyneuropathy and Lyme disease. Eur J Neurol 13:1213-1215, 2006.
   Said G: Infectious neuropathies. Neurol Clin 25:115-137, 2007.

30. **Which kinds of peripheral neuropathies are associated with HIV infection?**
   Up to 50% of patients with HIV infection develop a peripheral neuropathy, which may take one or a combination of the following forms:

1. Distal symmetric neuropathy (most common form)
   - Painful sensory type
   - Sensory-motor type (mild or minimal motor involvement)
   - Diffuse inflammatory lymphocytosis syndrome (symmetric or asymmetric, sensory-motor)
2. Inflammatory demyelinating polyneuropathy (both acute and chronic forms, usually with elevated CSF cell counts)
3. Mononeuropathy multiplex (in HIV infection; has also been associated with CMV, varicella, and hepatitis C infections)
4. Polyradiculopathy (cytomegalovirus [CMV], herpes zoster, syphilis, lymphomatous)
5. Cranial neuropathy
6. Autonomic neuropathy
7. Nutritional, vitamin deficiency neuropathy
8. Drug-induced neuropathy (associated with both nucleoside reverse transcription inhibitors [NRTIs] and protease inhibitors)
9. Neuropathies associated with immune reconstitution (there have been reports of Guillain-Barré syndrome in patients who have started highly active anti-retroviral therapy [HAART], but it is likely to be a rare occurrence in HIV infection).
10. HIV-associated neuromuscular weakness syndrome (This is a syndrome recently described in association with NRTI therapy. Patients develop progressive motor weakness, sometimes resulting in respiratory failure and death; it is also associated with vomiting, high lactate levels, and hepatomegaly. There have been findings of both an axonal sensorimotor polyneuropathy and an inflammatory myopathy.)

Ferrari S, et al: Human immunodeficiency virus-associated peripheral neuropathies. Mayo Clinic Proc 81:213-219, 2006.

31. **What are the most important industrial agents causing peripheral neuropathy?**
    1. **Acrylamide**. Direct skin exposure to the monomer of acrylamide has the highest risk for neurotoxicity. It is now a rare cause of neuropathy because the monomer is no longer a commercial product in North America. The neuropathy is caused by impairment of axoplasmic transport mechanisms, particularly retrograde transport.
    2. **Carbon disulfide**. Low-level prolonged inhalation of carbon disulfide, used in the production of cellophane films and rayon fibers, results in distal sensory and motor axonopathy and CNS dysfunction (memory impairment and extrapyramidal signs).
    3. **Dimethylaminopropionitrile (DMAPN)**. Inhalation of DMAPN, used in the manufacturing of polyurethane foam, results in urologic dysfunction (urinary hesitancy, decreased urine stream, incontinence, and sometimes impotence) followed by distal symmetric and predominantly sensory polyneuropathy, with a characteristic sensory loss in the sacral dermatomes.
    4. **Ethylene oxide**. At high levels of exposure, ethylene oxide causes a symmetric, distal polyneuropathy, sometimes with encephalopathic symptoms. Prolonged low-level exposure among hospital sterilizer workers and patients receiving long-term hemodialysis is claimed to cause a subclinical neuropathy. Withdrawal from exposure results in gradual improvement.
    5. **Hexacarbons (n-hexane, methyl n-butyl ketone)**. Industrial use of hexacarbon solvents in a poorly ventilated environment and the practice of inhalant abuse by teenagers (glue sniffing) are the major causes of hexacarbon neuropathy. High-level exposure, especially in glue sniffers, can result in a subacute motor neuropathy leading to quadraparesis mimicking Guillain-Barré syndrome. The neurotoxic effect is caused by the interruption of the retrograde axoplasmic flow, resulting in symmetric distal sensory neuropathy with loss of ankle reflexes and focally swollen axons (giant axons) on nerve pathology. There may be worsening of symptoms for up to 4 months after exposure to hexacarbon is discontinued.

6. **Organophosphates.** Intoxication most commonly occurs during accidental exposure to pesticides. Ingestion of tri-o-cresyl phosphate in contaminated food, drinks (Jamaica ginger extract), and cooking oil causes a delayed-onset distal predominantly sensory axonopathy. Central and peripheral axonal degeneration and neuropathic symptoms occur 2 to 3 weeks after exposure. Clinical features of cholinergic toxicity usually precede the onset of neuropathy, but they may be minimal and unrecognized.

Berger AR, Scaumburg HH: Human toxic neuropathy caused by industrial agents. In Dyck PJ, Thomas PK (eds): Peripheral Neuropathy, 4th ed. Philadelphia, W.B. Saunders, 2005, pp 2505-2525.

32. **Describe the association between neuropathy and neoplastic disease.**
Peripheral neuropathy is common in cancer patients due to a variety of causes including nutritional deficiencies and toxic effects of chemotherapy drugs. Vincristine may cause a painful sensory neuropathy after some weeks, and ultimately may cause distal symmetric weakness. Autonomic dysfunction may also occur. When the drug is stopped, the motor weakness usually recovers over time, but many patients have permanent sensory symptoms. Cisplatin is associated with a toxic sensory ganglionopathy resulting in ataxia with loss of proprioception, and reflexes and sensory symptoms may continue long after the drug is discontinued. A dorsal root sensory ganglionopathy may also be a pareneoplastic condition, most commonly associated with small cell lung cancer, and accounts for 20% of cases of sensory ganglionopathies (the remainder being largely idiopathic or associated with Sjögren's syndrome). Subacute autonomic neuropathy may also represent a paraneoplastic disorder. Autonomic dysfunction may be widespread, resulting in panautonomic failure, or may be more limited (e.g., isolated gastrointestinal dysmotility). The most common paraneoplastic neuropathy is probably a distal sensorimotor axonal neuropathy indistinguishable from an idiopathic, non-paraneoplastic neuropathy with the same features. Small cell lung cancer tends to be the most common tumor associated with these syndromes, but many tumors are potential culprits. Paraneoplastic neuropathies may occur in isolation or as part of a more generalized paraneoplastic neurologic syndrome (e.g., with limbic encephalitis and ataxia). The most common associated antibodies are anti-Hu (ANNA-1) and anti-CV2 (CRMP-5), with less common antibodies including amphiphysin, anti-Ri (ANNA-2), ANNA-3, and N-type calcium channel antibodies.

Apical lung tumors may directly invade the lower brachial plexus, and some tumors rarely metastasize to nerves. Brachial plexopathy may be a late complication of radiation therapy for cancer, classically with myokymic potentials on EMG. Peripheral nerves themselves may be associated with tumors, for example, schwannomas and neurofibromas. Malignant lymphomas and leukemias may rarely infiltrate peripheral nerves. Finally, a paraneoplastic vasculitic neuropathy has also been described.

33. **Define critical-illness polyneuropathy.**
Critical-illness polyneuropathy (CIP) develops in 50% to 70% of patients with systemic inflammatory response syndrome (SIRS), a condition that develops in 20% to 50% of patients in major ICUs. SIRS is associated with sepsis and/or trauma with associated organ failure and is theorized to lead to CIP through disturbances in the microcirculation of peripheral nerves. CIP may coexist with critical-illness myopathy (CIM) in the same patient. Attention typically is brought to the neuropathy by difficulty in weaning the patient from the ventilator as a result of respiratory muscle weakness. Severe cases, with lengthy hospitalization, have limb weakness, sensory loss, and depressed stretch tendon reflexes. However, because clinical examination is often difficult in such patients, reliance on diagnostic interventions has increased. Electrophysiologic testing and nerve and muscle biopsies show findings consistent with axonal polyneuropathy and help to distinguish CIP from Guillain-Barré syndrome, disorders of neuromuscular transmission, and myopathy. Initially, most patients who survived their critical illness were reported to recover from CIP, but more recent studies indicate that recovery may be slow and often incomplete, even after 1 to 2 years. It typically has a much worse prognosis than CIM.

Bolton CF: Neuromuscular manifestations of critical illness. Muscle Nerve 32:140-163, 2005.
Guarneri B, Bertolini G, Latronico N: Long-term outcome in patients with critical illness myopathy of neuropathy: The Italian multicentre CRIMYNE study. J Neurol Neurosurg Psychiatry 79:838-841, 2008.

34. **What is the outcome of the evaluation of patients with "peripheral neuropathy of undetermined etiology" when referred for a second opinion to a peripheral nerve expert at a tertiary referral center?**
In 42% of such patients, a hereditary neuropathy is found, in 21% an inflammatory neuropathy is identified by nerve biopsy, and in 13% other conditions are discovered. In 24% of the cases, even after extensive evaluation, no etiology for the neuropathy is identified.

35. **How are the inherited neuropathies classified?**
Most neuropathies that are initially labeled as idiopathic, and for which a cause is ultimately found, are inherited. As a group, they are probably underdiagnosed. They may be classified according to the pattern of inheritance (e.g., autosomal dominant: CMT1A-D, CMT2A-E; autosomal recessive: CMT4A-C; X-linked: CMTX); the gene involved (e.g., *PMP22*: CMT1A and HNPP; *MPZ*: CMT1B); the conduction velocity (e.g., demyelinating: CMT1A, CMT1B; axonal: CMT2; or with conduction velocities in the intermediate range: CMTX); or by the type of nerves involved (e.g., motor: HMN; sensory: HSN; autonomic: HAN; or combinations of all three: HMSN, HSAN). In addition, peripheral neuropathy forms part of several of the inherited ataxic syndromes (e.g., Friedreich's ataxia, spinocerebellar ataxias 3, 4, 10, and 18, among others) and accompanies many of the complicated hereditary spastic paraplegias. Finally, there are many inherited multisystem disorders that include peripheral neuropathy as part of the syndrome (e.g., Fabry's disease, Tangier disease, acute intermittent porphyria, and some of the leukodystrophies). The term *hereditary motor and sensory neuropathy* (HMSN) is broadly interchangeable with CMT.

Jani-Acasadi A, Krajewski K, Shy ME: Charcot-Marie-Tooth neuropathies: Diagnosis and management. Semin Neurol 28:185-194, 2008.

36. **How are the vasculitic neuropathies classified? What is their presentation and how are they treated?**
Vasculitic neuropathies can be classified into either systemic vasculitic neuropathies (SVN) or nonsystemic vasculitic neuropathies (NSVN), where the vasculitis is largely restricted to the peripheral nervous system (Figure 6-5). Vasculitis itself can be primary (e.g., Churg-Strauss syndrome, microscopic polyangitis, polyarteritis nodosa) or secondary (e.g., associated with

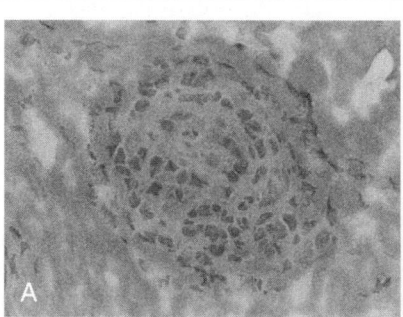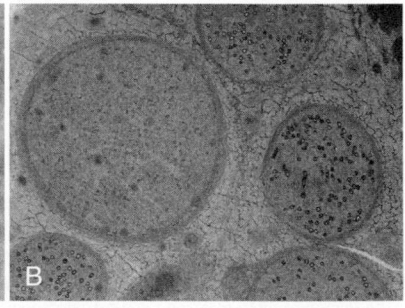

**Figure 6-5. A**, Modified trichrome. Inflammatory infiltrate with destruction of the blood vessel wall and obliteration of the lumen in a patient with vasculitic neuropathy. **B**, Semithin section. Differential involvement between and within nerve fascicles in a patient with vasculitic neuropathy. In most nonangiopathic/nonischemic neuropathies, involvement is more homogenous.

connective tissue disorders such as rheumatoid arthritis; Sjögren's syndrome; infections such as hepatitis B, CMV, or HIV; or other causes such as medications). The classic presentation from a neuropathy point of view involves acute or subacute painful sensory loss and weakness in the distribution of multiple peripheral nerves (a mononeuritis multiplex pattern). The stepwise progression and asymmetric multifocal involvement may become less evident as affected nerve territories become more confluent. Rare patients do have a distal symmetric sensory or sensorimotor neuropathy, and a plexopathy or polyradiculoneuropathy pattern may also occur. The diagnosis should be called into question when pain or sensory symptoms are absent. In order of frequency, the most common nerves affected are the peroneal, sural, tibial, ulnar, median, radial, femoral, and sciatic. In SVN, there may be constitutional symptoms (fever, weight loss, malaise) that generally are absent in NSVN. Treatment for the SVN usually involves induction therapy with steroid and cyclophosphamide (intravenous pulsed or oral daily doses) transitioning after several months to methotrexate or azathioprine to maintain remission. NSVN in contrast to SVN usually runs a more indolent course and may remit without treatment. However, steroids and occasional immunosuppressants may be necessary. For vasculitides associated with viral infections, treatment is aimed at the underlying infection (e.g., peglyated interferon and ribavirin for hepatitis C associated with cryoglobulinemia). Steroids and plasma exchange are occasionally used, but immunosuppression is generally avoided.

Gorson KC: Vasculitic neuropathies: An update. The Neurologist 13:12-19, 2007.

Lacomis D, Zivkovic, SA: Approach to vasculitic neuropathies. J Clin Neuromuscul Dis 9:265-276, 2007.

## IMMUNE-MEDIATED NEUROPATHIES

37. **Where are immune-mediated peripheral neuropathies most likely to cause initial nerve damage?**
Immune-mediated peripheral neuropathies are most likely to cause initial nerve damage in areas where the blood-nerve barrier is deficient (i.e., motor roots, dorsal root ganglion, and motor-nerve terminals). The blood-nerve barrier serves to protect nerve fibers and endoneurial content from the vascular compartment. Where this barrier is incomplete, circulating cellular and humoral immune components have access to the nerve.

38. **What is the relationship between connective tissue disease and trigeminal sensory neuropathy?**
Trigeminal sensory neuropathy, a slowly progressive cranial neuropathy with unilateral or bilateral facial numbness or paresthesia, may be the presenting manifestation of connective tissue disease (e.g., Sjögren's syndrome). The trigeminal sensory neuropathy is thought to be caused by vasculitis or fibrosis of the gasserian ganglion. Alternatively, the pervious blood-nerve barrier of this ganglion may allow autoantibodies access to react with peripheral nerve components.

39. **What is POEMS syndrome?**
**P**olyneuropathy
**O**rganomegaly
**E**ndocrinopathy
**M**-protein
**S**kin changes
POEMS syndrome is an expanded variant of osteosclerotic myeloma with peripheral neuropathy. Not all features of the syndrome are required to make the diagnosis. Patients typically have a chronic progressive sensory-motor polyneuropathy, peripheral edema, ascites, hypertrichosis, diffuse hyperpigmentation and thickening of the skin, hepatomegaly, splenomegaly, lymphadenopathy, gynecomastia, impotence, amenorrhea, and digital clubbing.

Increased serum level of vascular endothelial growth factor (VEGF) is frequently observed in POEMS syndrome. Treatment results in a decrease in the level of VEGF, which correlates with symptomatic improvement.

40. **How are monoclonal gammopathy and neuropathy associated?**
Approximately 10% of peripheral neuropathies are associated with serum monoclonal gammopathy (M-protein). Two-thirds of such cases are initially classified as monoclonal gammopathy of uncertain significance (MGUS), but the remaining one-third, in decreasing frequency, are identified as multiple myeloma, amyloidosis, macroglobulinemia, lymphoma, and leukemia. Of the patients with MGUS and neuropathy, the risk of ultimately developing an identifiable cause of the paraprotein (e.g., a hematologic malignancy) is 25%. Hence, it is important to follow these patients indefinitely. IgG forms the most common M-protein (74%) in patients with MGUS without neuropathy, but in patients with MGUS and neuropathy, IgM is more common (48% versus 37% IgG and 15% IgA). Neuropathies associated with MGUS are a heterogeneous group that includes symmetric polyneuropathy, mononeuritis multiplex, isolated mononeuropathy, and cranial nerve palsies. Neuropathies associated with IgM are the best characterized, and of these, the DADS phenotype is the most common and best described (see Question 41). Neuropathies associated with IgG and IgA are less well characterized. A variety of immunomodulating and immunosuppressant therapies have been tried in these neuropathies, often with modest but sometimes significant benefit. However, studies have often been conflicting.
Kwan JY: Paraproteinemic neuropathy. Neurol Clin 25:47-69, 2007.

41. **What is DADS, and how does it relate to anti-MAG neuropathy?**
Most length-dependent sensory or sensorimotor neuropathies are axonal in nature. DADS (distal acquired demyelinating symmetric neuropathy) represents a similar phenotype but with demyelinating features on electrodiagnostic studies (typically prolonged distal motor latencies). The syndrome is associated with an IgM paraprotein (usually with a kappa light chain) in about two-thirds of patients. When this paraprotein is present in association with DADS, several features are typical. Patients are usually males in their sixties or seventies with predominantly large fiber sensory loss in their distal lower extremities. Motor involvement occurs to a lesser extent as the disease progresses. Patients have significant gait ataxia and may manifest hand tremors. In about 50% of patients with DADS and IgM paraprotein, the paraprotein reacts against myelin-associated glycoprotein (MAG), which is thought to interfere with Schwann cell-axon interactions. In general, patients with DADS and IgM paraprotein are poorly responsive to the usual immunomodulatory treatments for demyelinating neuropathy, regardless of whether or not anti-MAG antibodies are present. There have been reports of significant benefit in some patients given fludarabine, cladribine, or rituximab.

DADS without an IgM paraprotein is a phenotype that can represent many different (largely untreatable) neuropathies such as hereditary and demyelinating neuropathies or diabetic neuropathies with conduction velocities that fall within the demyelinating range.
Nobile-Orazio E: IgM paraproteinemic neuropathies. Curr Opin Neurol 17:599-605, 2004.
Saperstein DS: Chronic acquired demyelinating polyneuropathies. Semin Neurol 28:168-184, 2008.

## CHRONIC IMMUNE-RELATED DEMYELINATING POLYRADICULONEUROPATHY

42. **What are the chronic acquired demyelinating polyneuropathies?**
   - CIDP (chronic inflammatory demyelinating polyradiculopathy)
   - CIDP variants: CIDP with CNS demyelination, and CIDP in patients with hereditary neuropathy (i.e., Charcot-Marie-Tooth disease)

- Multifocal acquired demyelinating sensory and motor neuropathy (Lewis-Sumner syndrome)
- Sensory predominant demyelinating neuropathy
- CIDP associated with systemic disorders: Hepatitis B and C, inflammatory bowel disease, HIV, bone marrow and organ transplants, collagen vascular disease, thyrotoxicosis, lymphoma, melanoma, nephrotic syndrome, diabetes mellitus

**43. What are the cardinal features of CIDP?**
- Symmetric proximal and distal weakness in all extremities (legs more than arms)
- Sensory impairment
- Progression over 8 weeks or a relapsing course
- Hyporeflexia or areflexia in all extremities
- Elevated cerebrospinal fluid (CSF) protein without pleocytosis
- Electrodiagnostic evidence of demyelinating neuropathy
- Pathologic evidence of demyelinating neuropathy on sural nerve biopsy

**44. What are the electrodiagnostic findings that suggest a demyelinating neuropathy?**
Findings on nerve conduction studies consistent with a demyelinating neuropathy are prolonged F-wave latency or absent F waves, slowed conduction velocity, prolonged distal latency, and presence of conduction block and/or temporal dispersion.

Saperstein DS: Chronic acquired demyelinating polyneuropathies. Semin Neurol 28:168-184, 2008.

**45. What immunosuppressive therapies are used in CIDP?**
The most common treatments for CIDP are corticosteroids, plasma exchange therapy, and high-dose intravenous immunoglobulin (IVIG). Randomized controlled studies have demonstrated efficacy in CIDP for all three therapies. Other immunosuppressives considered for CIDP include cyclophosphamide, cyclosporine, mycophenolate mofetil, interferon-$\beta$, interferon-$\alpha$, methotrexate, etanercept, rituximab, FK-506, and azathioprine. The efficacy of these immunosuppressive agents in CIDP has not been confirmed in sufficiently powered randomized controlled studies.

**46. What is the role of corticosteroids in the treatment of CIDP?**
Corticosteriods are an effective treatment for CIDP, and a trial of corticosteroids should be considered in all patients with this condition. Most patients who respond to prednisone demonstrate a positive effect within 8 weeks of therapy, but higher doses (1 mg/kg/day) may be required. Intermittent high-dose (1000 mg) intravenous methylprednisolone or oral prednisone has been used successfully in some patients and is probably a safer alternative to chronic oral corticosteroids.

Joint task force of the EFNS and PNS: European Federation of Neurological Societies/ Peripheral Nerve Society guidelines on management of chronic inflammatory demyelinating polyradiculoneuropathy. J Periph Nerv Syst 10:220-228, 2005.

Lopate G, Pestronk A, Al-Lozi M: Treatment of chronic inflammatory demyelinating polyneuropathy with high-dose intermittent intravenous methylprednisolone. Arch Neurol 62:249-254, 2005.

Muley SA, Praful K, Parry GJ: Treatment of chronic inflammatory demyelinating polyradiculopathy with pulsed oral steroids. Arch Neurol 65:1460-1464, 2008.

**47. What is the role of plasma exchange (PE) in CIDP?**
The efficacy of plasma exchange therapy in CIDP has been confirmed in two double-blind randomized controlled studies. With careful monitoring, benefit usually can be demonstrated within 6 weeks. Approximately 20% to 30% of patients with CIDP become refractory to all

other therapies and are dependent on long-term intermittent PE or intravenous gammaglobulin. PE is most commonly used in (1) the subgroup of patients with disability requiring treatment with immediate effectiveness while prednisone therapy is initiated; (2) patients with intermittent acute exacerbations; and (3) patients who are refractory or intolerant of other immunosuppressive therapies or in whom such therapies present substantial risks (e.g., diabetic or immunocompromised patients).

Hahn AF, Bolton CF, Pillay N, et al.: Plasma exchange therapy in chronic inflammatory demyelinating polyneuropathy: A double-blind, sham-controlled, cross-over study. Brain 119:1055-1066, 1996.

48. **Discuss the role of intravenous immunoglobulin (IVIG) in CIDP.**
The usefulness of IVIG in refractory and untreated CIDP has been confirmed by controlled studies. IVIG usually is administered intravenously at a dose of 0.4 gm/kg/day for 3 to 5 days or 1 gm/kg/day for 2 days. Benefits can be remarkable but are often short-lived (2 to 9 weeks), and stabilization of CIDP has been shown with regularly repeated infusions. The two factors that predict the need for continuing IVIG therapy for more than 2 years are the presence of profound weakness when the therapy is initiated and an incomplete recovery with residual deficits after 6 months of treatment. IVIG may offer advantages over chronic immunosuppressive or chronic plasmapheresis therapy in its ease of use and relative safety. In a controlled, cross-over study of 20 patients with CIDP, IVIG proved to be as effective as PE for short-term therapy.

Hughes RA, Donofrio P, Bril V, et al.: Intravenous immune globulin (10% caprylate-chromatography purified) for the treatment of chronic inflammatory demyelinating polyradiculoneuropathy (ICE study): A randomised placebo-controlled trial. Lancet Neurol 7:136-144, 2008.

49. **What distinguishes multifocal motor neuropathy (MMN) with conduction block (CB) from CIDP and motor neuron disease?**
MMN with CB is a presumed immune-mediated, chronic asymmetric motor neuropathy. The presence of weakness, atrophy, and fasciculations with normal sensation and asymmetric hypoactive reflexes identifies it as a lower motor neuron syndrome. Hyperreflexia does not typically occur, and there are no pathologic reflexes. Bulbar involvement is rare. Unlike CIDP, motor deficits usually start and are most prominent in the distal upper limbs. There is also a distinct predilection for more restricted and multifocal involvement of motor nerves. Motor conduction block in at least two nerves outside of the common entrapment sites with normal sensory nerve conduction study in the same segment defines MMN electrophysiologically. Effective treatments include high-dose IVIG (first choice) and cyclophosphamide. IVIG may result in fairly rapid, although temporary, improvement in association with partial resolution of CB. Long-term management usually requires repeat treatment at intervals immediately before expected relapse. There is no correlation between the presence of CB and elevated anti-GM1 antibodies titer with responsiveness to IVIG.

Olney RK, Lewis RA, Putnam TD, et al.: Consensus criteria for the diagnosis of multifocal motor neuropathy. Muscle Nerve 27:117-121, 2003.

Slee M, Selvan A, Donaghy M: Multifocal motor neuropathy: The diagnostic spectrum and response to treatment. Neurology 69:1680-1687, 2007.

## GUILLAIN-BARRÉ SYNDROME

50. **What is the typical presentation of Guillain-Barré syndrome (GBS)?**
A typical patient with GBS reports a numb or tingling sensation in the arms and legs, followed by rapidly progressive ascending symmetric muscle weakness. Symptoms often begin 1 to 3 weeks after a viral upper respiratory or gastrointestinal infection, immunization, or surgery.

Paralysis is maximal by 2 weeks in more than 50% of patients and by 1 month in more than 90%. A patient with a severe case of GBS may present with flaccid quadriplegia and an inability to breathe, swallow, or speak (due to oropharyngeal and respiratory paresis). Ten to 20% of patients require artificial respiration. Over 50% of patients develop facial weakness, and 10% have extraocular muscular paralysis. Hyporeflexia or areflexia is invariably present. Preservation of reflexes in a severely weakened patient should seriously challenge the diagnosis of GBS. The patient may have mild impairment of distal sensation, but significant sensory loss is not seen. Many patients also have autonomic dysfunction. Tachycardia (100 to 120 bpm) is the most common manifestation, but dangerous dysrhythmias may occur. Pain is present in 50% of patients. Miller-Fisher syndrome, Bickerstaff brainstem encephalitis, and the pharyngeal-cervical-brachial variant of GBS probably form a continuous spectrum of disease.

Burns TM: Guillain-Barré syndrome. Semin Neurol 28:152-167, 2008.

Nagashima T, et al.: Continuous spectrum of pharyngeal-cervical-brachial variant of Guillain-Barré syndrome. Arch Neurol 64:1519-1523, 2007.

51. **What are the two main pathologically distinct presentations of GBS?**
    1. Acute inflammatory demyelinating polyradiculoneuropathy (AIDP) due to an immune attack on Schwann cell membrane or myelin sheath.
    2. Acute (motor or motor-sensory) axonal neuropathy (AMAN or AMSAN) due to an immune attack against the axolemma/axoplasm. This presentation is distinguished from severe cases of AIDP, in which secondary axonal damage may occur. AMAN is much more common in Asia and occurs mainly in children. AMSAM may occur anywhere and affects adults preferentially. AMSAM has a much worse prognosis than AMAN, with only 20% of patients with the former ambulating at 1 year.

52. **What are the early immunopathologic events in AIDP?**
    Pathologic studies indicate that binding of complement-fixing antibodies to target antigen may be the primary event leading to complement activation and disruption of compact myelin. What previously had been observed as early lymphocytic infiltration of roots and nerves with macrophage-mediated myelin stripping and finally segmental demyelination may actually be a secondary event.

53. **What are the typical laboratory findings in GBS?**
    About 1 week after the onset of symptoms, CSF protein content begins to rise in most patients and peaks in 4 to 6 weeks. The CSF cell count does not increase. CSF pleocytosis should bring to mind HIV, CMV, Lyme disease, sarcoid, lymphomatous or carcinomatous polyradiculopathy. Nerve conduction velocities are slowed in AIDP, but may be normal within the first two weeks of onset. Conduction block accounts for most of the initial weakness, but after 2 to 3 weeks, axonal damage may contribute to weakness with EMG evidence of muscle denervation. Conduction block and slowed velocities are less likely to be found in early AIDP than prolonged distal CMAP duration and temporal dispersion. Absent H-reflex, abnormal F waves, and "sural sparing" are also more sensitive electrophysiologic findings in early AIDP. Sural sparing refers to the phenomenon of intact sural sensory responses but absent upper extremity sensory responses.

    Gordon PH, Wilbourn AJ: Early electrodiagnostic findings in Guillain-Barré syndrome. Arch Neurol 58:913-917, 2001.

54. **What is the significance of *Campylobacter jejuni* infection in GBS?**
    Most patients (75%) with GBS and a preceding *C. jejuni* infection present with AIDP and often the axonal form. Not all patients with serologic evidence of *C. jejuni* have gastrointestinal (GI) symptoms before the onset of GBS. Cross-reactivity between antigens from *C. jejuni* and various peripheral nerve gangliosides may explain the pathogenetic connection between the infection and GBS.

55. **What are the predictors of severe disease and poorer outcome in patients with GBS?**
    1. Old age
    2. Rapid onset of severe tetraparesis
    3. Need for early artificial ventilation
    4. Severely decreased compound muscle action potentials (<20% of normal)
    5. Acute motor-sensory axonal form of the disease
       There are conflicting data as to whether evidence of preceding *C. jejuni* infection or presence of anti-GM1 antibodies is a predictor of disease severity or outcome. The vast majority of patients with poor outcome required mechanical ventilation, and among this group predictors of poor outcome include increased age (highly predictive), upper limb paralysis, duration of ventilatory assistance, presence of inexcitable nerves, and delayed transfer to a tertiary center. Mortality is greatest in the elderly and those with comorbid illnesses. Of the complications occurring during ICU admission, one study found that the development of ileus and risk of bowel perforation was most strongly associated with mortality. Recovery in ventilated patients with GBS may be prolonged, and final judgment about outcome may require 2 or more years of follow-up. Relatively independent of many variables at the time of disease onset, many patients with GBS complain of pain, fatigue, and poor quality of life several years after their illness.
       Dhar R, Stitt L, Hahn AF: The morbidity and outcome of patients with Guillain-Barré syndrome admitted to the intensive care unit. J Neurol Sci 264:121-128, 2008.
       Rudolph T, Larsen JP, Farbu E: The long-term functional status in patients with Guillain-Barré syndrome. Eur J Neurol 15:1332-1337, 2008.

56. **What percent of patients with GBS suffer a relapse or second episode?**
    Based on several series of GBS patients, the incidence of recurrence lies somewhere between 1% and 6%, and recurrences may occur months to years after the initial episode. A recent study found that patients with Miller-Fisher syndrome, younger age, and milder disease were more likely to suffer a recurrence. There also appeared to be a trend toward shorter intervals between subsequent episodes and a more severe deficit with each recurrence.
       Kuitwaard K, van Koningsveld R, Ruts L, et al.: Recurrent Guillain-Barré syndrome. J Neurol Neurosurg Psychiatry 80:56-59, 2009.

57. **How is GBS treated?**
    PE and IVIG started within 2 weeks of the illness equally improve the degree and rate of recovery. The Quality Standards Subcommittee of the AAN (2003) recommends treatment with PE for nonambulant patients within 4 weeks of symptom onset; it should also be considered for ambulant patients within 2 weeks of symptom onset. Although PE initially was studied in moderate-to-severe disease, for which at least four exchanges are needed, the French Cooperative Group suggests that mild disease also benefits from at least two exchanges (mild disease defined as able to walk unaided but not run; moderate = unable to walk; severe = ventilated). The same group did not show increased benefit with six exchanges over four for patients with moderate to severe disease. Despite initial concerns about early relapse in about 10% of patients treated with IVIG, such patients responded to retreatment; furthermore, similar fluctuations and relapses have been reported with PE. Efficacy of the two treatments appears to be equal in all subsets of GBS, except perhaps IgG anti-GMI-positive patients, who usually present with AMAN and for whom IFIG may be somewhat superior. Because IVIG offers the advantages of greater ease and convenience as well as greater safety of administration at similar costs, it is now considered the treatment of first choice. There is no added benefit from combining the two treatments. Immunoabsorption is an alternative to plasma exchange and obviates the need to use human blood products. Corticosteroids are not indicated in GBS. Good supportive care is an essential part of GBS management (e.g., monitoring for and management of autonomic

dysfunction, respiratory failure, and cardiovascular instability). Forty percent of hospitalized patients with GBS require inpatient rehabilitation, and patients may also require long-term follow up for lingering symptoms (e.g., severe fatigue or sensory disturbances).

The prognosis in Miller-Fisher syndrome and Bickerstaff brain stem encephalitis is usually excellent, and therefore the role of IVIG or plasma exchange in the recovery from these conditions remains uncertain.

Burns TM: Guillain-Barré syndrome. Semin Neurol 28:152-167, 2008.

Hughes RA, et al: Supportive care for patients with Guillain-Barré syndrome. Arch Neurol 62:1194-1198, 2005.

## MOTOR NEURON DISEASES

58. **What is the most common condition affecting the motor neurons?**
Amyotrophic lateral sclerosis (ALS) is the most common adult-onset progressive degenerative disorder of the upper and lower motor neurons. It produces muscular weakness, spasticity, Babinski's sign, and hyperreflexia (upper motor neurons) as well as flaccidity, atrophy, fasciculations, and hyporeflexia (lower motor neurons). The deficits are strictly motor without significant signs of sensory loss, dementia, cerebellar, or extrapyramidal disease. Motor neurons controlling eye movements and sphincter function are usually spared as well. The reason for this selectivity is uncertain, although evidence suggests that cell-specific differences in protective regulatory calcium-binding proteins may be important. The disease, which usually begins in the sixth decade of life with a range spanning most of adulthood, generally progresses to death within 3 to 5 years from aspiration or respiratory failure.

## KEY POINTS: PERIPHERAL NEUROPATHIES

1. The most common causes of peripheral neuropathy are diabetes and alcoholism.

2. The most common motor neuropathy is Guillain-Barré syndrome.

3. Nerve biopsy is seldom necessary for the diagnosis of peripheral neuropathy.

4. Peripheral neuropathy is a common complication of HIV infection.

5. The most often overlooked cause of peripheral neuropathy is genetic.

6. The spinal fluid of patients with Guillain-Barré syndrome has high protein but low (normal) cell counts.

7. The most common motor neuron disease is ALS.

59. **How is ALS diagnosed?**
ALS is a clinical diagnosis. Efforts to identify a biochemical marker have been unsuccessful; advances in treatment will further drive the need for a method of earlier diagnosis. At the time of this writing, the most useful study is electrodiagnostic testing, which shows widespread denervation and re-innervation (fibrillation, fasciculations, and polyphasic high-amplitude muscle potentials). Craniospinal axis imaging studies to exclude underlying structural

compromise are important. Muscle biopsy shows neurogenic atrophy and re-innervation (small, angular fibers and fiber type grouping). Although serum CK levels may be mildly elevated, other laboratory studies are usually normal.

60. **What causes ALS?**

The exact cause of ALS is unknown. Approximately 8% to 10% of patients have a family history of the disease, usually in an autosomal dominant pattern. A genetic defect in an enzyme involved in free-radical metabolism, superoxide dismutase type 1 (SOD1), localized to chromosome 21, accounts for 15% to 20% of familial ALS. The role of mutant SOD1 in causing ALS remains unclear, but a toxic gain of function has been proposed as a potential mechanism. Mutations in at least seven other genetic loci are known to cause familial ALS. Other possible contributory factors leading to motor neuron demise include oxidative stress, toxic aggregates, mitochondrial dysfunction, impaired axonal transport, glutamate-induced excitotoxicity, and microglial activation.

Pasinelli P, Brown RH: Molecular biology of amytrophic lateral sclerosis: Insights from genetics. Nat Rev Neurosci 7:710-723, 2006.

61. **What is the differential diagnosis of ALS?**

Other conditions that may affect the pyramidal tract and lower motor neurons or mimic some of their clinical features include cervical cord/foramen magnum lesions (tumor, syringomyelia, syringobulbia, spondylosis), thyrotoxicosis, hyperparathyroidism, dysproteinemia, paraneoplastic conditions, and hexosaminidase A deficiency.

62. **Are ALS patients cognitively normal?**

Traditionally, cognition was felt to be spared in patients with ALS. More recent data show that most patients have subtle frontal/subcortical deficits. Up to 50% of patients who have ALS have cognitive impairment when detailed neuropsychologic evaluations are performed. Frontal executive dysfunction (i.e., verbal fluency and attention) is the most common finding. Other symptoms may range from mild behavioral impairment to severe cognitive impairment fulfilling the diagnostic criteria for frontotemporal dementia (FTD).

Phukan J, Pender NP, Hardiman O: Cognitive impairment in amyotrophic lateral sclerosis. Lancet Neurol 11:994-1003, 2007.

Ringholz GM, Appel SH, Bradshaw M, et al.: Prevalence and patterns of cognitive impairment in sporadic ALS. Neurology 65:586-590, 2005.

Strong MJ: The syndromes of frontotemporal dysfunction in amyotrophic lateral sclerosis. Amyotroph Lateral Scler 9:323-338, 2008.

63. **What other conditions primarily affect the lower motor neuron (anterior horn cell)?**

The differential diagnosis of deficits primarily confined to the anterior horn cell (AHC) includes several inherited diseases such as X-linked bulbospinal muscular atrophy and proximal spinal muscular atrophy. The latter includes infantile (Werdnig-Hoffmann disease), juvenile (Kugelberg-Welander disease), and adult forms. Acquired lower motor neuron syndromes include poliomyelitis, postpolio syndrome, progressive muscular atrophy, and AHC degeneration in other conditions (e.g., Creutzfeldt-Jakob disease).

64. **What causes spinal muscular atrophy (SMA)?**

SMA is an autosomal recessive disorder most commonly caused by mutations in the *SMN1* gene on chromosome 5q13.

Sumner CJ: Molecular mechanisms of spinal muscular atrophy. J Child Neurol 8:979-989, 2007.

65. **What are the clinical subtypes of SMA?**

SMA subtypes are usually defined by the highest level of motor function achieved by the patient.

- SMA type 1 (Werdnig-Hoffman disease) is the most severe and common phenotype, accounting for 50% of patients diagnosed with SMA. Children with SMA type 1 are never able to sit independently, and most patients die by 2 years of age from respiratory failure. The diagnosis is usually made before 6 months of age.
- SMA type 2 represents intermediate severity, and the age of onset is between 7 and 18 months. Patients are able to sit but unable to walk independently.
- SMA type 3 (Kugelberg-Welander disease) is variable in its prognosis for motor function. Some patients require a wheelchair for mobility during childhood, while others are able to ambulate independently and only have minor weakness.
- SMA type 4 is the mildest form of the disease and patients are diagnosed during the second and third decade of life. These patients have very mild weakness.

Lunn MR, Wang CH: Spinal muscular atrophy. Lancet 371:2120-2133, 2008.

### 66. What causes Kennedy's disease?

Kennedy's disease, or X-linked spinal and bulbar muscular atrophy (SBMA), is caused by an expansion of trinucleotide (CAG) repeats in the androgen receptor gene on chromosome Xq11-12. Normal individuals can have 11 to 33 CAG repeats; patients with Kennedy's disease have two to three times the normal number of CAG repeats. Longer repeat length correlates with earlier disease onset.

### 67. What is primary lateral sclerosis?

Primary lateral sclerosis is a rare, adult-onset, slowly progressive acquired motor neuron disease in which only signs of corticospinal tract dysfunction are seen. The diagnosis of PLS requires the presence of symptoms for more than 4 years and the absence of motor neuron findings, family history of similar disorder, and sensory signs on examination. Laboratory evaluation for other causes of myelopathy and craniospinal imaging should be normal. Electrodiagnostic tests show normal nerve conduction study, and the EMG should not satisfy the El Escorial criteria for ALS.

Gordon PH, Cheng B, Katz IB, et al.: The natural history of primary lateral sclerosis. Neurology 66:647-653, 2006.

Singer MA, Statland JM, Wolfe GI, et al.: Primary lateral sclerosis. Muscle Nerve 35:291-302, 2007.

### 68. Who was Lou Gehrig?

Lou Gehrig, whose name has been given to ALS, played first base for the New York Yankees from 1923 to 1939, usually batting after Babe Ruth in the lineup. He had a lifetime batting average of .340 with 23 grand slams (a record) and was the first modern player to hit four home runs in one game. He is best known as "Ironman"—a name undiminished despite the recent breaking of his record of playing 2130 consecutive games. A kind, conscientious, thoughtful, hard-working, shy, and courteous man, Lou Gehrig, who died of ALS, was a true sports hero.

## WEBSITES

1. http://www.neuro.wustl.edu/neuromuscular
2. http://www.neuropathy.org
3. http://www.genetests.org

## BIBLIOGRAPHY

1. Aminoff MJ: Electrodiagnosis in Clinical Neurology, Philadelphia, Churchill Livingstone, 2005.
2. Bertorini TE: Clinical Evaluation and Diagnostic Test for Neuromuscular Disorders, Boston, Butterworth-Heinemann, 2002.
3. Dyck PJ, Thomas PK: Peripheral Neuropathy, Philadelphia: Saunders, 2005.
4. Gries FA, Cameron N, eds. Textbook of Diabetic Neuropathy, New York, Thieme, 2003.
5. Harati Y: Peripheral Neuropathies, An Issue of Neurologic Clinics, Philadelphia: Saunders, 2007.
6. Harati Y, Bosch EP: Disorders of peripheral nerves. In: Neurology in Clinical Practice, Boston: Butterworth Heinemann, 2007.
7. Mendell JR, Cornblath DR, Kissell JT: Diagnosis and Management of Peripheral Nerve Disorders, Oxford, Oxford University Press, 2001.
8. Mitsumoto H, Przedborski S, Gordon PH: Amyotrophic Lateral Sclerosis (Neurological Disease and Therapy). Oxford, Informa Healthcare 2005.

# RADICULOPATHY AND DEGENERATIVE SPINE DISEASE

*Randall Wright, MD, and Steven B. Inbody, MD*

# CHAPTER 7

## BASIC ANATOMY

1. **Describe the difference between the dorsal and ventral rami of the spinal cord.**
   Nerve roots are attached to each segment of the spinal cord. Those that exit from the posterior lateral sulcus are called the *dorsal roots,* whereas the ventral roots emerge anterior over a wider area. Short mixed spinal nerves are formed when a pair of dorsal roots and ventral roots unite beyond the dorsal root ganglion. This mixed spinal root then divides into the thin dorsal root ramus and the thicker ventral root ramus. The dorsal root rami are the central processes of the unipolar cells located in the dorsal root ganglion. These fibers innervate the paraspinal muscles and overlying skin and also carry sensory information. The ventral root rami are essentially extensions of the anterior horn motor neurons, and innervate the muscles of the cervical, brachial, or lumbosacral plexus. In addition to motor fibers, the ventral ramus also contains axons originating from sensory and sympathetic ganglia (Figure 7-1).

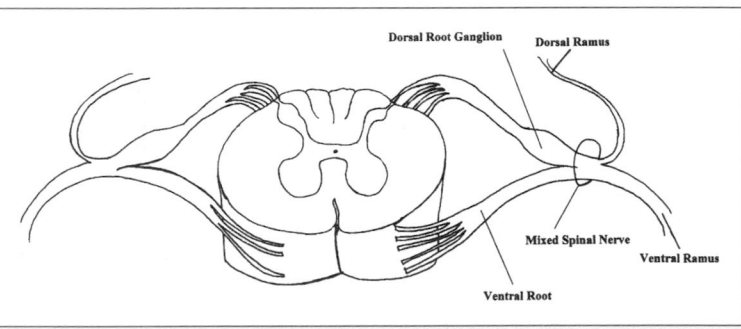

**Figure 7-1.** Anatomy of the spinal cord and its roots. Figure by Randall J. Wright, MD.

2. **How many spinal nerve pairs exit the spinal cord?**
   There are 31 pairs of spinal nerves (8 cervical, 12 thoracic, 5 lumbar, 5 sacral, and 1 coccygeal). Because there are only 7 cervical vertebrae, the first seven cervical nerves exit **above** the same numbered cervical vertebrae. The eighth cervical nerve exits above the T1 vertebrae, and the rest of the spinal nerves (T2 to L5) exit below their same numbered vertebrae. Think of it as "the heavenly seven cervical nerves arise above the vertebral body" (Figure 7-2).

3. **Where do the lumbar nerve roots exit, and which root is most likely to be injured in a disc herniation?**
   The lumbar nerve roots exit beneath the corresponding vertebral pedicle through the respective foramen. For example, the L5 nerve root exits beneath the L5 vertebral pedicle through the L5/S1 foramen. Since most disc herniations occur posterolaterally, the root that gets compressed is actually the root that exits the foramen **below** the herniated disc. So, a disc

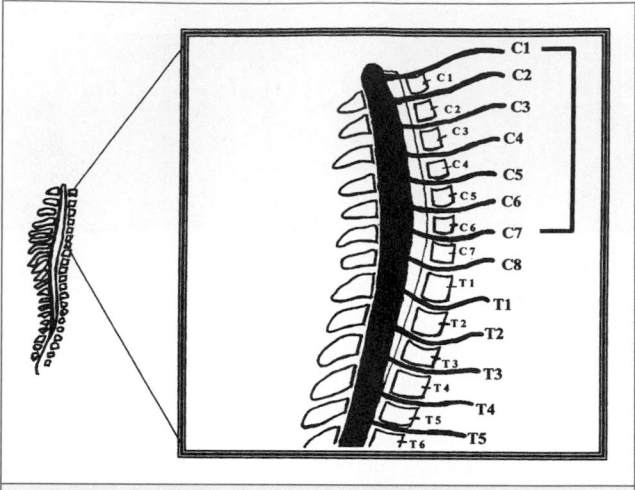

**Figure 7-2.** The first seven cervical nerves ("heavenly seven") exit above their corresponding vertebral bodies. Figure by Randall J. Wright, MD.

protrusion at L4/L5 will compress the L5 root, and a protrusion at L5/S1 will compress the S1 root. Ninety-five percent of disc herniations occur at the L4/5 or L5/S1 disc spaces. Herniations at higher levels are uncommon.

4. **Which anatomic structures are potential pain generators?**
   Back pain may originate from many spinal structures. These structures include: the vertebral body periosteum, intervertebral discs, paravertebral musculature and fascia, ligaments, facet joints, the annulus fibrosus, spinal nerve roots, dorsal root ganglia, and even paravertebral blood vessels. The most common causes for pain result from musculoligamentous injuries and age-related degenerative processes of the intervertebral discs and facet joints. Disc herniations and spinal stenosis are other common causes.

5. **What is the distinction among spondylosis, spondylolisthesis, and spondylolysis?**
   **Spondylosis** is a nonspecific degenerative process of the spine, often due to osteoarthritis with osteophyte formation. **Spondylolisthesis** refers to anterior subluxation of one vertebral body on another. **Spondylolysis** is a defect in the pars interarticularis that allows the vertebra to slip upward. All three of these conditions may cause pain when symptomatic and can be confirmed radiographically.

6. **What is the difference between a disc bulge, protrusion, and herniation?**
   A **bulging disc** occurs when dehydration leads to gradual flattening of the disc and an increase in the circumference of the intact annular ring, which then extends beyond the margins of the vertebral body. **Disc protrusion** occurs when the gelatinous disc material protrudes focally into tears or fissures within the intact annular shell, causing a focal outpouching of the still intact annular fibers. **Disc herniation** refers to extrusion of nuclear material through the disrupted annular shell.

7. **What are the most common causes of spinal stenosis?**
   A variety of conditions can cause spinal stenosis. It may result from minor developmental anatomic changes in the diameter of the spinal canal (e.g., shorter than normal pedicles,

thickened lamina). These conditions are rarely symptomatic but may predispose to degenerative changes that do become symptomatic. Such changes include degeneration of facets posteriorly and the disc anteriorly. Osteophyte formation may occur, thus narrowing both the nerve root and central canals. Degeneration of the intravertebral disc may also cause narrowing of the nerve root and central canals. Other causes of spinal stenosis include degenerative spondylolisthesis and postoperative spinal stenosis.

8. **What are the differences between radicular and referred pain?**
The key feature of radicular pain is hot, electric sensations that radiate in the territory of the affected nerve root. The pain will be sharp, shooting, and burning. The pain radiates down the limb but never up. Sensory loss is rarely complete due to overlapping of other roots.

   **Referred pain** is a phenomenon that occurs when irritated or injured tissues (e.g., muscle, facet joint, or periosteum) cause pain that is perceived in a dermatomal distribution. This pain may be shooting but is typically not hot or electrical as in radicular pain.

9. **Which spinal disorders cause both axial pain (back or neck) and disturbances in neurologic function of the limb (leg or arm)?**
Three syndromes are recognized in which spinal disorders cause both back or neck pain and neurologic dysfunction. The following examples are from the lumbar spine:
   1. **Herniated disc causing a single nerve root compression** (leg pain > back pain). Clinical features include positive straight leg–raising test and radicular pain in the limb disproportionate to pain in the spine. Loss of strength, reflex, and sensation occurs in the territory of the compressed root.
   2. **Lateral recess syndrome** (leg pain ≥ back pain). Single or multiple nerve roots on one or both sides become compressed. Pain in the limb is usually equal to or greater than that in the spine. Symptoms are brought on by either walking or standing and are relieved with sitting. Testing by straight-leg raising may be negative.
   3. **Spinal stenosis** (leg pain < back pain). Multiple nerve roots are involved, and the pain in the spine is significantly greater than that in the limb. Symptoms develop with standing or walking. Impairment in bowel and bladder dysfunction as well as sexual dysfunction may occur.

## LUMBAR SPINE DISEASE

10. **What are the clinical features of lumbar disc disease?**
Acute lumbosacral disc herniation may cause a continuum of pain ranging from an isolated dull ache to severe radicular pain due to neurocompression in the foramen or lateral recess. A rare complication is cauda equina syndrome due to a massive central herniation. Pain is often sudden in onset and exacerbated with the Valsalva maneuver. Concomitant paraspinal spasm is often present. Ninety-five percent of disc herniations occur at the L4/5 or L5/S1 disc spaces. Herniations at higher levels are uncommon.

11. **What are the signs of an L4 radiculopathy?**
Compression of the L4 root produces pain and paresthesias radiating to the hip, anterior thigh, and medial aspects of the knee and calf. Sensation is impaired over the medial calf. Weakness occurs in the quadriceps and hip adductors. The knee jerk is diminished.

12. **What are signs of an L5 radiculopathy?**
L5 root compression produces pain radiating to the posterolateral buttock, lateral posterior thigh, and lateral leg. Sensory loss is most likely in a triangular wedge involving the great toe, second toe, and adjacent skin on the dorsum of the foot. Weakness occurs in the muscles innervated by the L5 root (gluteus medius, tibialis anterior and posterior, peronei, and extensor

hallucis longus). This results in difficulty in ankle dorsiflexion, eversion, inversion, and hip abduction. It is most easily identified by weakness in the extensor hallucis longus (extension of the big toe). The ankle reflex is usually normal.

**13. What are the signs of an S1 radiculopathy?**
S1 root compression causes pain to radiate to the posterior buttock, posterior calf, and lateral foot (classic sciatica). Sensory loss occurs along the lateral aspect of the foot, especially in the third, fourth, and fifth toes. Weakness may occur in the gluteus maximus (hip flexor) and plantar flexors. The ankle jerk is usually diminished (Figure 7-3).

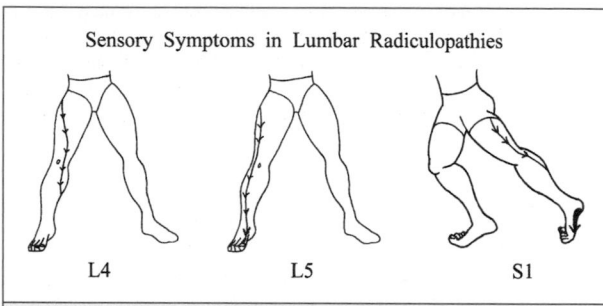

**Figure 7-3.** Pain from L4 compression radiates to the anterior thigh and medial portion of the lower leg. L5 compression causes radiating pain to the lateral aspect of the leg and big toe. S1 compression causes pain in the lateral foot. Figure by Randall J. Wright, MD.

**14. What are the clinical features of lumbar stenosis?**
Most patients are age 50 years and older and have had symptoms referable to lumbar spinal stenosis for more than 1 year. Neurogenic intermittent claudication or pseudoclaudication is the most common presenting and constant symptom in lumbar spinal stenosis. Symptoms are usually bilateral, with one leg more involved than the other, but they may be unilateral. The whole lower extremity is generally affected. Pain is provoked by walking and, in many patients, merely by standing. It is typically dull in character and is quickly relieved by sitting or leaning forward. In some patients, the pain is accompanied by numbness of the affected leg and the feeling that it "may give out" on them.

Daffner SD, Wang JC: The pathophysiology and non-surgical treatment of lumbar spinal stenosis. Instr Course Lect 58:657-668, 2009.

# KEY POINTS: CLINICAL FEATURES OF LUMBAR STENOSIS

1. Presence of intermittent neurogenic claudication (pseudoclaudication).
2. Pain is provoked by walking or standing and is relieved with rest (lying, sitting, or flexing).
3. Symptoms are usually bilateral but may be asymmetric.
4. Often there is no objective sensory loss.
5. Leg weakness and urinary incontinence are seldom present.
6. Unlike vascular claudication, pain may persist if the patient stops walking without flexing the spine.

15. **What is the mechanism for neurogenic claudication in lumbar spinal stenosis?**
Symptoms are related to the increase in lordotic posture provoked by standing or walking. Myelographic studies have shown that in lordosis, the cross-sectional area of the spinal canal narrows because of anterior encroachment by bulging discs, posterior encroachment by shortening and thickening of the ligamentum flavum, and lateral approximation of the articular facets. In flexion (as in sitting), all of these encroachments reverse, with a resultant increase in the cross-sectional area of the spinal canal. This may explain why some patients with neurogenic claudication may be able to ride a stationary bike (in the sitting position), while patients with vascular claudication may still have pain.

16. **What is the differential diagnosis of low back pain?**
The most common alternate diagnoses include focal hip pathology, vertebral compression fractures, metastasis from malignancy, ankylosing spondylitis, and vertebral osteomyelitis. Rare causes of low back pain include abdominal aortic aneurysm, pelvic disorders, abdominal visceral pathology, and other neuropathic disorders (e.g., inflammatory polyneuropathies or mononeuropathies).

## THORACIC SPINE DISEASE

17. **Describe the clinical presentation of a thoracic disc herniation.**
Less than 1% of protruded discs occur in the thoracic spine. Over 75% of herniated thoracic discs develop below T8, with the highest incidence at the T11 to T12 level. The protrusion is usually central. Most patients have a degenerative process as the main causative factor; trauma accounts for only 10% to 20% of protruded discs. Pain (radicular or midline) is the most common initial symptom, followed by numbness. Motor weakness involving the lower extremities is an initial symptom in 28% of patients. Bladder involvement is a rare initial symptom but may be seen in 30% of patients at presentation.

18. **What is the differential diagnosis of thoracic pain?**

| | |
|---|---|
| Malignant or benign tumors of the spine | Thoracic compression fractures |
| Ankylosing spondylosis | Intra-abdominal processes (gallbladder disease, gastric ulcer, pancreatitis) |
| Thoracoabdominal neuropathy (diabetes) | |
| Intercostal neuralgia | Cardiac etiology (i.e., aortic aneurysm) |
| Herpes zoster | Intramedullary lesion such as a demyelinating process |

## CERVICAL SPINE DISEASE

19. **What are the differentiating signs and symptoms between a C6, C7, and C8 radiculopathy?**
Compression of the cervical roots typically occurs from either osteophyte or disc herniation. Compression of the C6 nerve root results in radicular pain involving the shoulder, upper arm, and lateral side of the forearm and thumb. Weakness may occur in the deltoids, biceps, and pronator teres. Paresthesias may be felt in the thumb and index fingers. The bicep and brachioradialis reflexes may be diminished. Compression of the C7 nerve root results in radicular pain in the shoulder, chest, and forearm, as well as the index and middle fingers. Weakness may occur in the triceps and flexor carpi radialis. Paresthesias may occur in the index and middle fingers. The triceps reflex is typically diminished. C8 nerve root compression causes a similar pattern of pain as C7 radiculopathies, but paresthesias may occur in the fourth and fifth fingers. Weakness may occur in the intrinsic muscles of the hand and finger extensors (Figure 7-4).

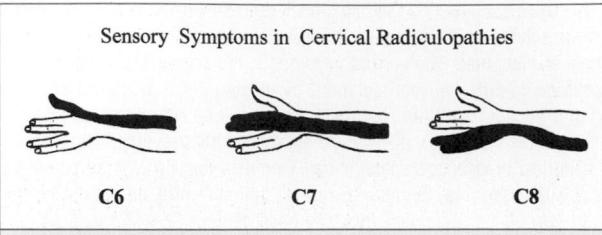

Sensory Symptoms in Cervical Radiculopathies

C6          C7          C8

**Figure 7-4.** Compression of the C6 nerve root causes radicular pain in the lateral side of the forearm and thumb. C7 compression causes pain in the index and middle fingers. C8 compression causes symptoms in the fourth and fifth fingers. Figure by Randall J. Wright, MD.

## KEY POINTS: SENSORY SYMPTOMS

1. The first seven cervical nerves exit **above** the same numbered cervical vertebrae.

2. L5 radiculopathies cause radiating pain along the posterior thigh to the dorsum of the foot and big toe.

3. Indications for surgery in patients with radiculopathies are intractable pain, progressive motor weakness or sensory deficits, or symptoms refractory to a reasonable period of nonoperative therapy.

4. Neurogenic claudication (pseudoclaudication) presents typically as bilateral, asymmetric, lower extremity pain that is provoked by walking (occasionally standing) and is relieved by rest.

5. Compression of the C6 nerve root causes radicular pain in the lateral side of the forearm and thumb, C7 compression causes pain in the index and middle fingers, and C8 compression causes symptoms in the fourth and fifth fingers.

20. **What is Spurling's sign?**
    Named after the neurosurgeon who popularized the posterior approach for cervical disc surgery, this maneuver is the cervical equivalent to the lumbar straight-leg raise. Reproduction of the patient's pain occurs when the examiner exerts downward pressure on the vertex of the head while tilting the head (and occasionally extending it a little) toward the symptomatic side. This causes narrowing of the intervertebral foramen, which is painful.
    Spurling RG, Scoville WB: Lateral rupture of the cervical intervertebral disc: A common cause of shoulder and arm pain. Surg Gynecol Obstet 78:350-358, 1944.

21. **What is the differential diagnosis for cervical pain?**
    Diseases that most closely mimic cervical disc disease include brachial plexus lesions and shoulder dysfunction due to tendinitis, subacromial bursitis, or rotator cuff disease. Neoplastic or infectious processes also need to be excluded.

### DIAGNOSTIC EVALUATION

22. **Which tests are useful in evaluating back pain?**
    1. **Plain radiograph**s provide information about bony alignment and degenerative changes.
    2. **Dynamic flexion/extension films** provide information about osseous instability.

3. **Magnetic resonance imaging (MRI)** is sensitive for identifying intrinsic cord lesions, spinal root compression, spinal cord tumors, infections (abscesses), and herniated discs (Figure 7-5).

4. **Computed tomography (CT) myelography** is especially valuable for evaluating nerve root compression (Figure 7-6).

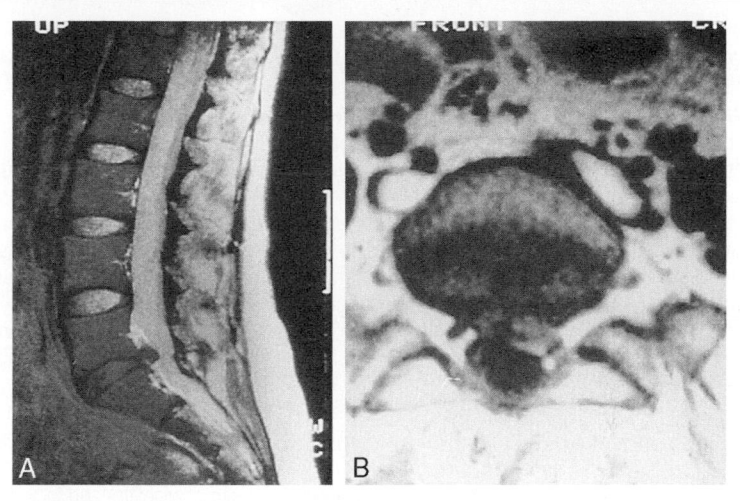

**Figure 7-5.** MRI scan shows a herniated disc at L5 and sagittal (left) and axial (right) views.

23. **Discuss the role of electromyography (EMG) in the evaluation of radiculopathy.**

Electromyography (EMG) provides neurophysiologic confirmation of the radiographic lesion. EMG evidence of altered innervation suggests significant nerve root compromise. The most widely accepted EMG evidence of radiculopathy is the presence of positive sharp waves and fibrillation potentials. EMG changes are first seen in the muscles closest to the site of nerve injury, underscoring the importance of examination of the paraspinous muscles. A disadvantage of EMG is the delay in the appearance of reliable abnormalities until 7 to 10 days after a root injury. The sequence of EMG changes begins with positive sharp waves in paraspinal muscles between days 7 and 10, followed by paraspinous fibrillation potentials and positive sharp waves in limb muscles between days 17 and 21.

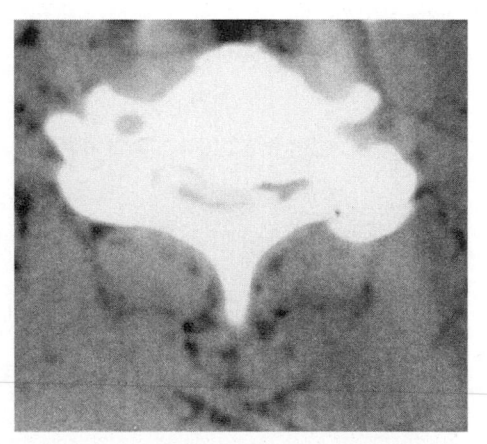

**Figure 7-6.** CT scan shows compression of the cervical spinal cord caused by severe cervical spondylosis.

Preston DC, Shapiro BE: Electromyography and Neuromuscular Disorders, 2nd ed. Boston, Butterworth-Heinemann, 2005.

24. **What is the role of the H-reflex in an S1 radiculopathy?**
    The H-reflex is an evoked potential study performed by submaximal electrical stimulation of the S1 root and measuring the nerve conduction velocity proximally. Its absence indicates proximal (root) injury. It is the electrodiagnostic equivalent of the ankle jerk. The H-reflex may demonstrate abnormalities within 1 or 2 days after nerve root injury.

## NONOPERATIVE TREATMENT OF SPINAL PAIN

25. **What is the rationale for nonoperative treatment of spine-related pain?**
    The natural history of nonspecific spinal pain has been demonstrated to be benign. Approximately 90% of patients experience improvement within 3 months. Recent studies temper these results by suggesting that 75% of patients have one or more relapses, and 72% may still have at least some residual pain at 1 year. Patients with radiculopathy, whether due to soft disc herniation or spondylitic compression, usually improve with time. However, spinal stenosis usually stays stable or worsens with time. About 15% of patients with spinal stenosis improve, 70% remain stable, and 15% worsen after 4 years.
    Chou R, Atlas SJ, Stanos SP, et al.: Non-surgical interventional therapies for low back pain: A review of the evidence for an American Pain Society clinical practice guideline. Spine 34: 1078-1093, 2009.

26. **Is bed rest and exercise helpful in treating acute and chronic back pain?**
    Studies suggest that empiric bed rest in the acute phase of back pain is not as helpful as we once thought. It has not been found to increase the speed of recovery and in some instances may even delay recovery. However, in patients who report symptomatic relief from bed rest, 1 or 2 days of rest can be recommended. In the acute phase, back exercises have not been found to be helpful, but their role is very important in treating chronic back pain. In general, rapid return to normal activities with neither bed rest nor exercise seems to be the best recommendation for most patients in the acute phase of back pain. However, patients should be told to avoid heavy lifting, twisting of the trunk, and bodily vibrations during the acute phase of their back pain. Chronic back pain responds well to intense exercise programs.
    Deyo R, Weinstein J: Low back pain. N Engl J Med 344:363-370, 2001.

27. **Which categories of medication may be of help during acute phases of pain?**
    **Nonsteroidal anti-inflammatory drugs** help relieve pain from mild musculoskeletal inflammation. Severe inflammation or nerve root swelling may be treated with a brief, tapering schedule of glucocorticoids. **Muscle relaxants** have been found helpful in some patients with muscle spasms and in helping to facilitate sleep (due to their sedative side effects). **Antidepressants** (e.g., tricyclics) and **antiepileptics** (e.g., Neurontin) may be helpful in treating neuropathic pain and also helping with sleep. Short-term pain relief with **opiate-based medications** can be beneficial in limited cases. For best results, pain medications should be given on a scheduled basis rather than on an as-needed basis.

## OPERATIVE TREATMENT OF THE SPINE

28. **What is the role of surgery to treat cervical radiculopathies?**
    Over 95% of patients with cervical radiculopathies due to a herniated disc improve with nonsurgical interventions. Surgery is indicated when symptoms fail to improve or progressive

neurologic deficits develop. The goal of surgery for cervical radiculopathy is adequate decompression of the nerve roots, using either an anterior or posterior approach. The anterior approach is recommended for medial or central disc herniation or when fusion is contemplated. A posterior approach is necessitated by a posterolateral disc or osteophytes that are otherwise inaccessible.

## KEY POINTS: INDICATIONS FOR SURGERY IN PATIENTS WITH RADICULOPATHIES

1. Intractable pain that has been refractory to conservative therapy

2. Severe or progressive motor weakness or sensory deficits

3. Symptoms refractory to a reasonable period of nonoperative therapy

4. Of note, outcomes are much better when signs and symptoms correlate with radiographic findings.

29. **Which surgical procedures are recommended for cervical radiculopathy?**
    1. **Anterior cervical discectomy (ACD)** is indicated when patients have minimal neck pain, normal cervical lordosis, and single-level pathology to avoid the potential complications of fusion. There is a 5% risk of laryngeal nerve injury with ACD.
    2. **Anterior cervical discectomy and fusion (ACDF)** is indicated for patients with symptoms of instability or more than one operative level. It is limited to levels C3 to C7. It allows for safe removal of osteophytes.
    3. **ACDF with internal fixation.** Plating is recommended for multilevel fusions with documented instability or history of prior fusion failure. It allows early mobilization without bracing.
    4. **Posterior cervical discectomy.** Usually reserved for either multiple cervical discs or osteophytes, cervical stenosis superimposed on disc herniation, and in situations where the risk of laryngeal nerve injury that is associated with ACD is unacceptable (e.g., professional singers and speakers).
    5. **Posterior keyhole laminotomy.** Used to decompress only individual nerve roots (not spinal cord). Useful in monoradiculopathy with posterolateral soft disc fragments and in cases in which the anterior approach is either difficult (patients with thick necks) or the risks are unacceptable (professional singers or speakers).
    Narayan P, Haid RW: Treatment of degenerative cervical disc disease. Neurol Clin 19:217-229, 2001.

30. **What is the most common postoperative complication of spinal surgery?**
    Arachnoiditis is commonly seen in the cauda equina after lumbar surgery, myelography using oil-based dye, and even intrathecal injections. It results in the adhesion and clumping of the nerve roots to each other. This results in radicular type pain, paresthesias, weakness, and sphincter dysfunction. MRI may show thickening and clumping of the nerve roots, adherence of roots to the thecal sac with enhancement, and loculations of spinal fluid. Surgical debridements, and epidural and intrathecal steroid injections, have been attempted as treatment, but none have shown efficacy. In fact, these techniques may even worsen the condition. Thus, treatment is mainly symptomatic.
    Bradley WG, Daroff R, Fenichel G, et al.: Neurology in Clinical Practice, Vol. II, 3rd ed. Philadelphia, Butterworth-Heinemann, 2003, pp 1981-1982.

31. **What are the most common causes of the failed (surgical) back?**
    1. The diagnosis was wrong. Therefore, even if the surgical treatment was technically flawless, the patient must be regarded as having never been treated and requires a thorough reassessment with generation of a new treatment plan.
    2. The diagnosis was correct, but the treatment was technically flawed, inappropriate, or incompetent.
    3. Whether or not the diagnosis was correct, something new has happened—perhaps an immediate or late consequence of treatment or an unrelated but intercurrent complication. This situation usually occurs when two or more pain-generating mechanisms coexist. For example, in disc herniation removal of disc material improves radicular symptoms but fails to address the mechanical pain produced by spinal instability after the herniation.
    4. A complication of diagnosis or treatment has arisen; for example, development of arachnoiditis, injury to a nerve root, or disc space infection.
    5. No counseling has been given. Physicians must negotiate a plan of postsurgical treatment, stressing patient participation in functional restoration and dispelling unrealistic expectations of complete restoration to normal.

## WEBSITE

http://www.backandbodycare.com

## BIBLIOGRAPHY

1. Bradley WG, Daroff R, Fenichel G, et al: Neurology in Clinical Practice, 5th ed. Philadelphia, Butterworth-Heinemann, 2007.
2. Deyo R, Weinstein J: Low back pain. N Engl J Med 344:363-370, 2001.
3. Frymoyer JW, editor: The Adult and Pediatric Spine, 3rd ed. Philadelphia, Lippincott Williams & Wilkins, 2003.
4. Kaye AH: Essential Neurosurgery, 3rd ed. Philadelphia, Wiley-Blackwell, 2005.
5. Malanga GA, Nadler SF: Nonoperative treatment of low back pain. Mayo Clin Proc 74:1135-1148, 1999.
6. Narayan P, Haid RW: Treatment of degenerative cervical disc disease. Neurol Clin 19:217-229, 2001.

# CHAPTER 8

# MYELOPATHIES

*Randall Wright, MD, and Ericka P. Simpson, MD*

1. **Describe the most important long tracts in the spinal cord, their locations, and their functions.**
   See Table 8-1.

| TABLE 8-1. LONG TRACTS IN THE SPINAL CORD | | |
| --- | --- | --- |
| Tract | Location | Functions |
| Gracile medial | Dorsal column | Proprioception from the leg |
| Cuneate | Lateral dorsal column | Proprioception from the arm |
| Spinocerebellar | Superficial lateral column | Muscular position and tone |
| Pyramidal | Deep lateral column | Motor control |
| Lateral spinothalamic | Ventrolateral column | Pain and thermal sensation |

2. **Draw the anatomic locations of the anterior horn cells, cortical spinal tracts, dorsal column, and spinothalamic tracts.**
   See Figure 8-1.

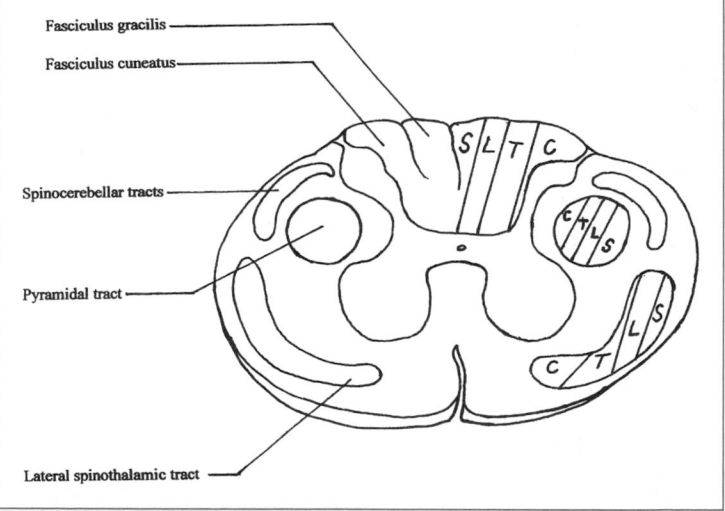

**Figure 8-1.** Relative location of each tract. The cortical spinal and spinothalamic tracts are laminated so that the most lateral fibers are the sacral fibers and the most medial are the cervical. The opposite is true in the dorsal columns; the most lateral fibers are the cervical and most medial fibers are the sacral. This becomes important when distinguishing intramedullary from extramedullary lesions. *C,* cervical; *T,* thoracic; *L,* lumbar; *S,* sacral.

3. **Where do the cortical spinal, dorsal column, lateral spinothalamic, and spinocerebellar tracts decussate (cross)?**
The descending cortical spinal tract decussates in the lower medulla, travels down the spinal cord, and innervates muscles contralateral to its motor strip of origin. The dorsal column tracts enter the spinal cord and ascend ipsilateral to their entry point. They then decussate in the lower medulla. The lateral spinothalamic tract enters the spinal cord and immediately decussates one to two levels above their entry points and then ascends in the spinal cord contralateral to their points of entry. The spinocerebellar tracts do not decussate.

4. **What are the dermatomes at the umbilicus and the nipple line?**
The umbilicus is at T10. The nipple line is at T5.

5. **What is the relationship of the cord segment and its spinal nerves to the vertebral body?**
The spinal cord extends from the medullary cervical junction at the foramen magnum to the level of the body of the first or second lumbar vertebra. The spinal roots exit in relation to their corresponding vertebral body. The first seven cervical nerves exit above the vertebral body, and the eighth exits below C7. The remainder of the spinal roots exit below their corresponding vertebral body.

6. **What are signs of the anterior spinal artery syndrome?**
Anterior spinal artery syndrome occurs when the anterior spinal artery is occluded. This artery supplies blood to the anterior two-thirds of the spinal cord. Occlusion results in bilateral loss of pain and temperature below the lesion, accompanied by weakness and bladder dysfunction. The reflexes may be hyperactive below the level of the lesion. Dorsal column functions (position and vibration sense) are spared.

7. **What is the artery of Adamkiewicz?**
The artery of Adamkiewicz is a major lumbar radicular artery that arises from the aorta and enters the cord between T10 and L3. It supplies the lumbar and lower thoracic segments. It forms anastomoses with the anterior spinal artery in the lower thoracic region, where the watershed area of the spinal cord is located.

8. **What areas of the spinal cord are supplied by the posterior spinal artery?**
The posterior spinal arteries are paired arteries that run dorsolateral to the spinal cord. They extend the length of the cord and supply the posterior third of the cord through circumflex and penetrating vessels. Occlusion of one of these arteries results in ipsilateral deficits in vibratory and proprioceptive sensation below the site of occlusion.

9. **What is a myelopathy?**
A myelopathy is any pathologic process that affects primarily the spinal cord and causes neurologic dysfunction. The most common causes of myelopathies are as follows:
1. Congenital and developmental defects
   - Syringomyelia
   - Neural tube formation defects
2. Trauma
3. Compromise of the spinal cord
   - Cervical spondylosis
   - Inflammatory arthritis
   - Acute disc herniation
4. Spinal neoplasms
5. Physical agents
   - Decompression sickness

- Electrical injury
- Radiation
6. Toxins
    - Nitrous oxide
    - Triorthocresyl phosphate
7. Metabolic and nutritional disorders
    - Pernicious anemia
    - Chronic liver disease
8. Remote effect of cancer
9. Arachnoiditis
10. Postinfectious autoimmune disorders
    - Acute transverse myelitis
    - Connective tissue disease
11. Multiple sclerosis
12. Epidural infections
13. Primary infections (human immunodeficiency virus [HIV])
14. Vascular causes
    - Epidural hematoma
    - Atherosclerotic, abdominal aneurysm
    - Malformation

## KEY POINTS: CLINICAL FINDINGS SUGGESTIVE OF A MYELOPATHY

1. Bilateral upper motor neuron weakness of the legs (paraparesis, paraplegia) or legs and arms (quadriparesis, quadriplegia)

2. Bilateral impairment of sensation with a "sensory level" that separates a region of normal sensation from a region of impaired sensation

3. Bowel or bladder sphincter dysfunction

10. **What is Lhermitte's sign?**
    Lhermitte's sign is present when the patient reports an electric shock–like sensation down the spine with neck flexion. The symptom is produced by stretching or irritating damaged fibers in the dorsal columns of the cervical cord. It may occur in cervical spondylogenic myelopathy, intramedullary lesions such as a demyelinating plaque, or as part of subacute combined degeneration from B12 deficiency.
    Goldblatt D, Levy J: The electric sign and the incandescent lamp. Semin Neurol 5:191-193, 1985.

11. **What is the anal wink?**
    This is not a new way to express your feelings for someone! It is actually a reflex that tests the integrity of S2 to S5 segments. The anal wink reflex is tested by pricking the skin of the perianal region and watching for the external anal sphincter to contract. The absence of this contraction signifies a lesion in the sacral region.

12. **What is "saddle anesthesia"?**
    It is tempting to believe that saddle anesthesia results from prolonged horseback riding. However, this condition describes the sensory loss in the perianal region (saddle) that results from lesions involving the S1 and S2 segments of the spinal cord. It may be accompanied by

sensory loss in the medial aspects of the calf and posterior thigh. Symmetric saddle anesthesia may result from lesions in the conus medullaris.

13. **What is the superficial abdominal reflex?**
The superficial abdominal reflex is elicited by pricking the skin of the abdomen and watching for contraction of the abdominal wall muscles. This reflex is often diminished or absent below the level of a spinal cord lesion. In individuals with excessive adipose tissue in the abdominal region, this reflex may be difficult to observe.

14. **How does the jaw jerk reflex help in localizing lesions in patients with hyperreflexia?**
The jaw jerk is a reflex that involves the contraction of the masseter and temporalis muscles when the patient's lower jaw is tapped. The afferent limb travels via the mandibular branch of the trigeminal nerve to the mesencephalic nucleus of the trigeminal nerve. The efferent limb arises from the motor nucleus of the trigeminal nerve and also travels via the mandibular branch. The jaw jerk is exaggerated with bilateral lesions above the trigeminal nerve but will not be affected by lesions below it in the spinal cord. This is helpful in patients who have hyperreflexia in all four extremities because an exaggerated jaw jerk reflex suggests that the lesion is above the level of the spinal cord (i.e., high brain stem or brain).
   Brazis P: The localization of lesions affecting cranial nerve V (the trigeminal nerve). In Brazis P, Masdeu J, Biller J (eds): Localization in Clinical Neurology, 3rd ed. New York, Little, Brown, 1996.

15. **What is Brown-Sequard syndrome?**
Brown-Sequard syndrome is caused by a lateral hemisection of the spinal cord that severs the pyramidal tract (which has already crossed in the medulla), the uncrossed dorsal columns, and the crossed spinothalamic tract. The region ipsilateral and below the level of the lesion demonstrates upper motor neuron weakness (paralysis), loss of tactile discrimination, loss of position sense, and loss of vibratory sense. The ipsilateral deep tendon reflexes become hyperactive with subsequent spasticity, and an extensor plantar response develops. Contralateral to the lesion, there is loss of pain and temperature sensation below the lesion.

16. **What is spinal shock?**
If the spinal cord is damaged suddenly by mechanical trauma, ischemia, or compression, spinal shock may occur. This is a condition in which there is temporary loss of all spinal reflexes, motor activity, and sensation below the level of the lesion. Flaccid paralysis, hyporeflexia, sensory loss, and loss of bladder tone are cardinal features. There also may be autonomic dysfunction with diffuse sweating and hypotension. Development of upper motor neuron signs may take several weeks.

17. **What is transverse myelitis?**
Transverse myelitis is an inflammatory process that is localized over several segments of the cord and functionally transects the cord. It may occur as an infectious or parainfectious illness or as a manifestation of multiple sclerosis, vasculitis, or an autoimmune process. In a significant number of cases (40%), no specific etiology is ever identified (Figure 8-2).
   Rolak LA: Transverse myelitis. In Samuels MA, Feske SK (eds): Office Practice of Neurology, 2nd ed. Philadelphia, Churchill Livingstone, 2003, pp 420-423.

18. **What are the clinical features of acute transverse myelitis?**
The sudden onset of weakness and sensory disturbance in the legs and trunk is the usual presenting feature. Ultimately, sphincter dysfunction is common. Pain and temperature are usually affected, but proprioception and vibration are often spared. The tendon jerks below the lesion may be initially depressed and then hyperactive. A sensory level indicates the level of the lesion.

Transverse Myelitis Consortium Working Group. Proposed diagnostic criteria and nosology of acute transverse myelitis. Neurology 59:499-505, 2002.

19. **What is cervical spondylosis?**
Cervical spondylosis is a condition in which osteophyte proliferation in the cervical region results in narrowing of the spinal canal. These changes may result in cord compression if the canal diameter becomes small enough, and spinal cord circulation may also be compromised. Spondylitic changes also may compress the spinal nerves that exit through the foramen. If the spinal cord is compressed, upper motor neuron weakness (paresis, hypertonia, hyperreflexia) may be seen. This may appear before sensory impairment. When sensory loss does develop, dorsal columns tend to be more affected than lateral spinothalamic tracts. Bladder and bowel dysfunction is less common.

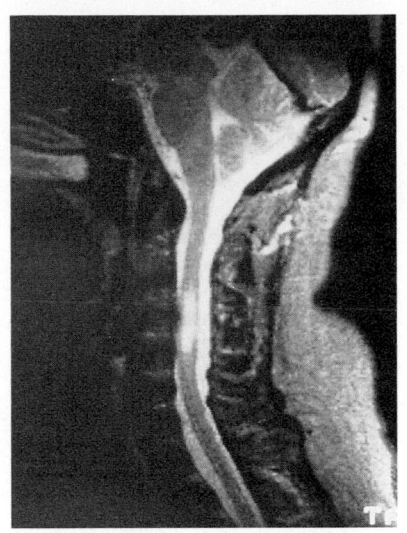

**Figure 8-2.** Sagittal T2-weighted magnetic resonance imaging (MRI) shows increased signal within the cervical cord caused by acute inflammatory transverse myelitis.

20. **Summarize the anatomy of masses that compress the spinal cord.**
    1. **Extramedullary extradural lesions** (outside the spinal cord and outside its dural covering). Such lesions include the following:
       - Epidural metastases from a remote primary neoplasm
       - Epidural abscess
       - Epidural hematoma
       - Herniated disc
    2. **Extramedullary intradural lesions** (outside the spinal cord but inside its dural covering). Such lesions include:
       - Neurofibroma and schwannoma
       - Meningioma
    3. **Intramedullary intradural lesions** (inside the cord itself). Such lesions include the following:
       - Primary cord neoplasms
       - Syringomyelia
       - Metastasis or abscess within the substance of the cord (rare)
       
       See Figure 8-3.

21. **What are the most common neoplasms arising with the spinal cord?**
Most primary spinal cord tumors are astrocytomas, ependymomas, or oligodendrogliomas (Figure 8-4).

22. **What tumors commonly metastasize to the spinal cord?**
Neoplasms typically metastasize to the vertebral bodies and extend into the epidural space, causing extramedullary extradural compression of the spinal cord. The most common metastatic tumors to the spinal cord are: breast, lung, gastrointestinal (GI) tract, lymphoma/myeloma, and prostate.

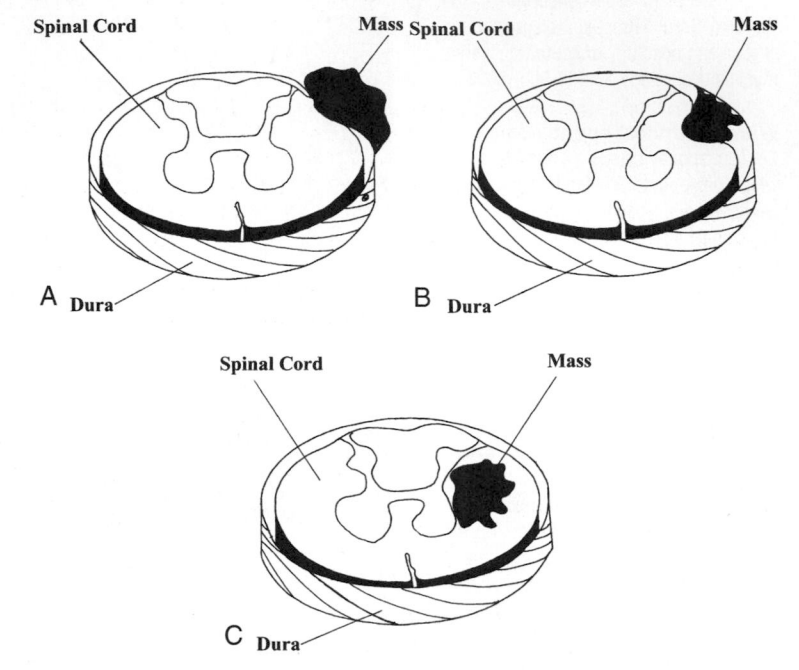

**Figure 8-3.** Location of spinal masses: **A**, extradural extramedullary. **B**, intradural extramedullary. **C**, intradural intramedullary.

23. **Describe the features of extramedullary lesions.**

    Extramedullary lesions are lesions that compress the spinal cord from the outside. They can be extramedullary extradural or extramedullary intradural. Either way, extramedullary lesions cause exterior compression of the spinal cord. Because of the somatotopic organization of the spinal cord, the spinothalamic tracts and the corticospinal tracts are arranged so that the sacral fibers are most lateral and the cervical fibers are the most medial. Because of this, external compression of the spinal cord causes the sacral regions to be affected first, followed by the lumbar, then thoracic, and then cervical. Thus, external

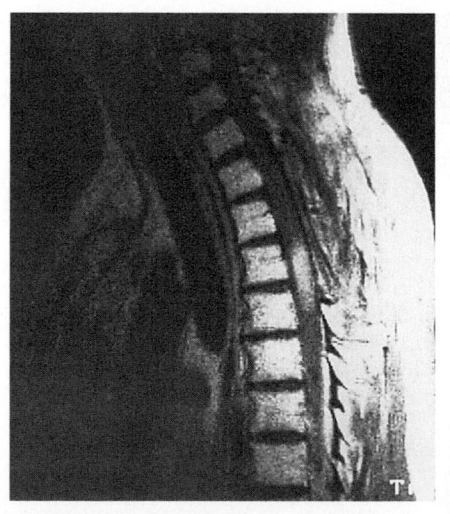

**Figure 8-4.** Sagittal T1-weighted MRI, after gadolinium enhancement, shows an astrocytoma arising within the thoracic spinal cord (an intramedullary, intradural lesion).

compression causes ascending deficits starting in the sacral region and traveling up to one or two levels below the actual level of the lesion.

24. **Describe the features of intramedullary lesions.**
Intramedullary lesions are lesions that originate from within the spinal cord. If the lesion starts within one-half of the cord and grows outward, the innermost fibers are affected first. Once again, the somatotopic organization of the spinal cord is responsible for the clinical presentation. If the lesion is high (i.e., cervical cord), the cervical fibers are affected first, followed by thoracic, then lumbar, and finally sacral. So in this case, **intramedullary lesions cause sacral sparing of sensation.** Because the spinothalamic tracts cross the midline, intramedullary lesions cause sensory loss at one to two levels below their location. As the lesion (tumor) expands outward, the sensory deficits appear to descend as they subsequently affect the cervical, thoracic, lumbar, and finally sacral regions (Figure 8-5).

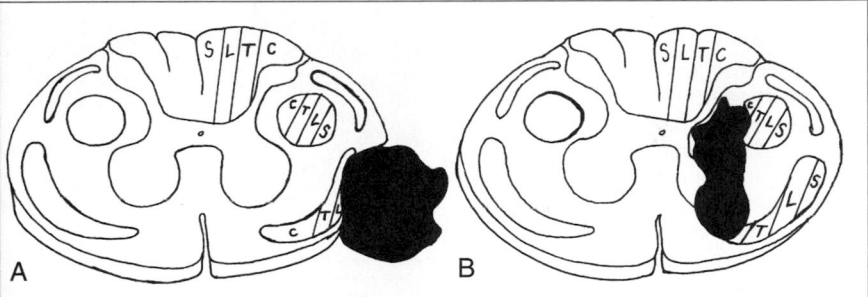

**Figure 8-5.** Extramedullary lesions compress the spinal cord from the outside (**A**), causing the sacral fibers to be affected first. As the lumbar, thoracic, and cervical fibers are compressed, the "level" of injury seems to rise. In intramedullary lesions (**B**), the cervical fibers are affected first, thus causing "sacral sparing."

25. **Describe the features of lesions in the dorsal columns.**
The dorsal columns relay fibers that are involved in proprioception and vibration. These fibers are also arranged somatotopically. However, this time the sacral fibers are medial and the cervical fibers are lateral. Thus lateral lesions within the dorsal column will damage fibers from the cervical region. And conversely, medially located lesions in the dorsal column will damage sacral fibers. Lesions in the dorsal columns may result in deficits in vibration, proprioception, and two-point discrimination. Lhermitte's sign may also be present.

26. **What is syringomyelia?**
Syringomyelia is a longitudinal cystic cavity that develops within the substance of the cord. It may extend over a few or many segments of the cord and even into the medulla (syringobulbia). The cavity is irregular and tends to intrude into the anterior horns of the gray matter and the gray matter dorsal to the central canal. This condition may result from a developmental anomaly, trauma (hyperextension injuries of the neck), or ischemia, or it may be part of an intramedullary tumor.

27. **What are the clinical features of syringomyelia?**
The classic clinical features are dissociated sensory loss (loss of temperature and pain with intact proprioception) and lower motor neuron weakness (flaccid paralysis, atrophy, fasciculations). This occurs because centrally located lesions initially compromise the decussating fibers of the spinothalamic tract, which as you recall, are carrying pain and temperature information. Because of the lamination of the spinal cord, the cervical and thoracic

fibers are affected first (if the lesion is in the cervical region), resulting in a "cape" or "shawl" distribution of sensory loss bilaterally. Dorsal column function is preserved, thus causing the dissociation of sensory loss. With forward extension of the cavity, anterior horn cells are affected, resulting in atrophy, paresis, and areflexia below the lesion. Lateral extension results in an ipsilateral Horner's syndrome. Neurogenic arthropathies may also develop (Figures 8-6 and 8-7).

28. **What part of the spinal cord does Friedreich's ataxia involve?**
    Friedreich's ataxia is an autosomal recessive disorder that arises from triplet expansion of the frataxin gene. It affects the cerebellum, spinal cord, peripheral nerves, and heart. In the spinal cord, the following tracts are affected: the dorsal columns, lateral corticospinal tracts, and the anterior and posterior spinocerebellar tracts. As you can guess by its name, this condition typically presents with ataxia.

29. **What part of the spinal cord is affected in tabes dorsalis?**
    Tabes dorsalis is one of the many manifestations of neurosyphilis, caused by infections of the brain, meninges, or spinal cord by *Treponema pallidum*. When the spinal cord is infected, degeneration of the dorsal columns occurs. This results in profound loss of joint position sense and fine touch.

30. **What is "man-in-a-barrel" syndrome?**
    Man-in-a-barrel syndrome is not to be confused with vacationers to Niagara Falls! Neurologically, this syndrome refers to individuals who suffer from hyperextension injuries to the neck.

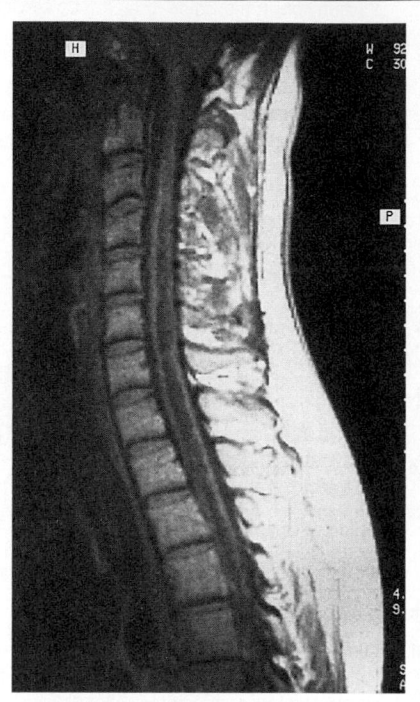

**Figure 8-6.** Sagittal MRI shows an extensive syrinx cavity in the cervical and thoracic spinal cord. This syrinx is associated with a developmental defect—an Arnold-Chiari malformation at the base of the skull (protrusion of the cerebellar tonsils down through the foramen magnum).

This results in quadriplegia in the acute phase, with the arms being much weaker than the legs (like a man with a barrel around his chest). Urinary retention and patchy sensory loss may occur. Recovery of strength may spontaneously occur within minutes to hours, or the deficits may be permanent. Damage to the central gray matter is hypothesized to cause the syndrome.

31. **What is tropical spastic paraparesis?**
    Tropical spastic paraparesis has been recognized clinically for many years in tropical areas and Japan. It is characterized by a chronic course in which mild-to-severe leg weakness develops with increased muscle tone and extensor plantar responses. One-half of patients have posterior column sensory signs, and 15% have optic nerve involvement. The condition is caused by infection with a retrovirus, HTLV-1; thus, it is sometimes called HTLV-1–associated myelopathy (HAM).

Oh LL, Jacobson S: Treatment of HTLV-1 associated myelopathy/tropical spastic paraparesis: Toward rational targeted therapy. Neurol Clin 26:781-797, 2008.

32. **What is subacute combined degeneration of the spinal cord?**
This condition is the result of vitamin B12 deficiency. Most patients with B12 deficiency will present with a peripheral neuropathy that causes a burning, painful sensation in their hands and feet. Examination shows a stocking-glove sensory loss as well as vibratory loss. However, if the spinal cord is affected, it results in demyelination and vacuolar degeneration of the posterior columns and corticospinal tracts. This results in upper motor neuron signs of weakness, increased tone, hyperreflexia, and Babinski's and Hoffmann's signs. Nitrous oxide exposure may produce a similar pathologic picture. Treatment is with intramuscular B12 replacement.
Turner MR, Talbot K: Functional vitamin B12 deficiency. Pract Neurol 9:37-41, 2009.

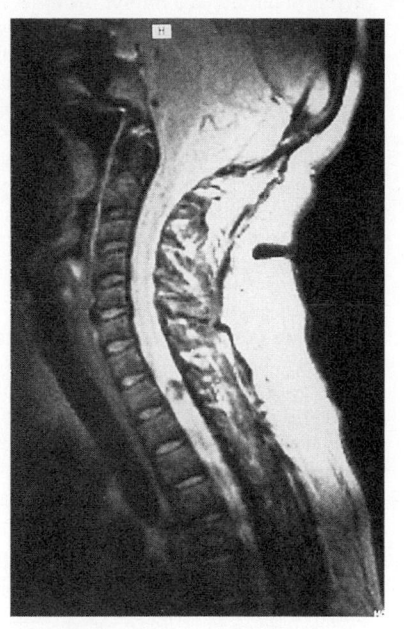

**Figure 8-7.** Sagittal T2-weighted MRI shows a neurofibroma displacing the thoracic spinal cord (an extramedullary, intradural lesion).

33. **What is the micturition reflex?**
Simply stated, the act of voiding is controlled by a delicate balance between reflexive actions and cortical control. Bilateral projections originating from cortical structures descend in the spinal cord just medial to the corticospinal tracts and synapse with preganglionic parasympathetic neurons in the S2, S3, and S4 regions. These fibers then travel out the ventral roots of S2, S3, and S4 to synapse at postganglionic parasympathetic ganglia near the bladder to innervate the detrussor muscle. Muscle spindles located in the detrussor muscle are stretched when the bladder is filled, increasing their firing rate. This signal change increases the firing rate of the preganglionic parasympathetic fibers of S2, S3, and S4, resulting in detrussor muscle contraction, and thus voiding of the bladder. This reflex is normally under the voluntary control of descending inputs from the cortex.

34. **Describe what happens to micturition in spinal cord injury.**
Following bilateral lesions to the spinal cord, the bladder initially becomes flaccid (acute) and eventually becomes spastic (chronic). The reason for this is that the detrusor muscle of the bladder loses its cortical inputs. Like the deep tendon reflexes, it initially becomes flaccid, resulting in urinary retention. As the bladder fills, overflow incontinence may develop because the bladder cannot hold any more urine. As time passes, the detrusor muscle becomes spastic (just as the deep tendon muscles become hyperactive). Small stretches in the detrusor muscle result in voiding. This spastic bladder results in urinary frequency and urgency.

35. **What is cauda equina syndrome?**

The spinal cord ends around the L1/L2 level. If damage occurs at this level or below, the exiting roots (the cauda equina) may be injured. This is typically caused by a herniated disc in the lumbosacral region. This results in weakness and sensory deficits in the lower extremity (which may be asymmetric). Bowel and bladder functions are affected as well. Because the compression is of the nerve roots, a lower motor neuron pattern of deficits is seen. Patellar and ankle reflexes may be absent. Radicular pain is often very prominent and occurs early in the course. It may be worse at night or in the recumbent position. Asymmetric saddle distribution sensory loss may occur, and urinary incontinence may occur late in the course due to a flaccid bladder. Cauda equina syndrome is reversible if intervention is initiated early in the course, so *this syndrome is a neurosurgical emergency!*

36. **What are the clinical signs of conus medullaris lesions?**

Lesions at the base of the spinal cord result in an autonomous neurogenic bladder and paralysis of the muscles of the pelvic floor. There is loss of voluntary control of the bladder because there is no awareness of fullness. This results in urinary retention and secondary overflow incontinence. Constipation, erectile dysfunction, and symmetric saddle anesthesia may also be present. Pain is not a typical part of this condition (which differentiates it from the cauda equina syndrome) but may occur late in the course.

## KEY POINTS: CAUSES OF MYELOPATHY

1. Intramedullary lesions cause sacral sparing sensory loss and symptoms that appear to descend (as the cervical, thoracic, lumbar, and finally sacral regions are affected).

2. Sudden damage to the spinal cord can cause spinal shock, which results in temporary flaccid paralysis, hyporeflexia, sensory loss, and loss of bladder tone.

3. Occlusion of the artery of Adamkiewicz may result in the anterior spinal artery syndrome, causing bilateral weakness, loss of pain and temperature, and hyperreflexia below the lesion with preserved dorsal column functions (position and vibration).

4. Cauda equina syndrome is a neurosurgical emergency that presents with weakness and sensory loss in the lower extremity, prominent radicular pain, saddle anesthesia, and late-occurring urinary incontinence.

## WEBSITE

http://www.spinalinjury.net

## BIBLIOGRAPHY

1. Bradley WG, Daroff R, Fenichel G, et al.: Neurology in Clinical Practice, 5th ed. Philadelphia, Butterworth-Heinemann, 2007.
2. Ropper AH, Samuels M: Adams and Victor's Principles of Neurology, 9th ed. New York, McGraw-Hill, 2009.
3. Rowland L: Merritt's Neurology, 11th ed. Philadelphia, Lippincott Williams & Wilkins, 2005.
4. Simon R, Greenberg D, Aminoff M: Clinical Neurology, 7th ed. New York, McGraw-Hill, 2009.

# CHAPTER 9

# BRAIN STEM DISEASE

*Eugene C. Lai, MD, PhD*

## CLINICAL ANATOMY OF THE BRAIN STEM

1. **What is the functional importance of the brain stem?**
   The brain stem is a small, narrow region connecting the spinal cord with the rest of the brain. It lies ventral to the cerebellum, which it links via the cerebellar peduncles. Its functions are critical to survival. The brain stem is densely packed with many vital structures such as long ascending and descending pathways that carry sensory and motor information to and from higher brain regions. It contains the nuclei of cranial nerves III to XII and their intramedullary fibers. It also possesses groups of neurons that are the major source of noradrenergic, dopaminergic, and serotonergic inputs to most parts of the brain. In addition, other specific nuclear groups, such as the reticular formation, olivary bodies, and red nucleus, lie within the brain stem. In short, it is a complicated but highly organized structure that controls motor and sensory activities, respiration, cardiovascular functions, and mechanisms related to sleep and consciousness. Consequently, a small lesion in the brain stem can affect contiguous structures and cause disastrous neurologic deficits.

## KEY POINTS: MAIN DIVISIONS OF THE BRAIN STEM

1. Medulla

2. Pons

3. Midbrain

2. **Describe the function of the medulla.**
   The medulla (bulb) is the direct rostral extension of the spinal cord. It contains the nuclei of the lower cranial nerves (mainly IX, X, XI, and XII) and the inferior olivary nucleus. The dorsal column pathways decussate in its central region to form the medial lemniscus, whereas the corticospinal tracts cross on the ventral side as they descend caudally. Together with the pons, the medulla also participates in vital autonomic functions such as digestion, respiration, and regulation of heart rate and blood pressure (Figure 9-1).

3. **Describe the function of the pons.**
   The pons (bridge) lies rostral to the medulla and appears as a bulge mounting from the ventral surface of the brain stem. The pons contains nuclei for cranial nerves V, VI, VII, and VIII as well as a large number of neurons that relay information about movement from the frontal cerebral hemispheres to the cerebellum (frontopontocerebellar pathway). Other clinically pertinent pathways in the pons are those for the control of saccadic eye movements (medial longitudinal fasciculus [MLF]) and the auditory connections (Figure 9-2).

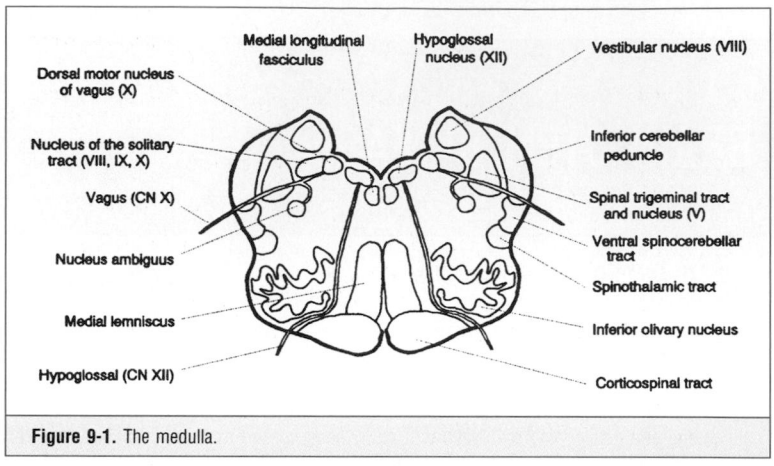

**Figure 9-1.** The medulla.

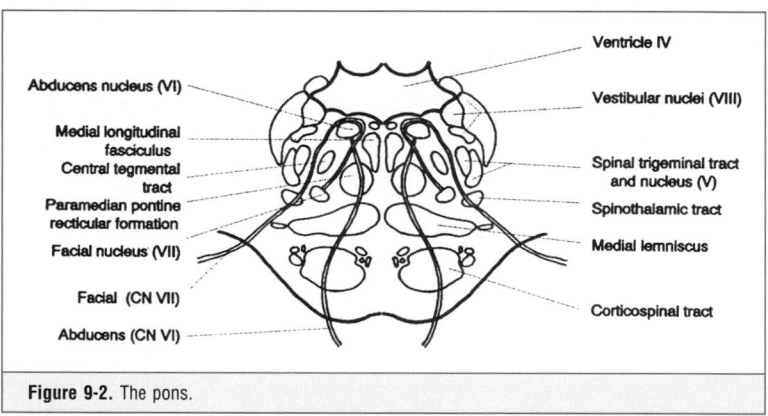

**Figure 9-2.** The pons.

4. **Describe the function of the midbrain.**

The midbrain, the smallest and most rostral component of the brain stem, plays an important role in the control of eye movements and coordination of visual and auditory reflexes. It contains the nuclei for cranial nerves III and IV. Other important structures are the red nuclei and substantia nigra. The periaqueduct area has an important but poorly understood influence on consciousness and pain perception (Figure 9-3).

5. **Which cranial nerves are _not_ found in the brain stem?**

The 12 pairs of cranial nerves are numbered in rostral-caudal sequence. The brain stem contains the nuclei of all cranial nerves except two: the optic (II) nerve, which terminates in the thalamus, and the olfactory (I) nerve, which synapses in the olfactory bulb.

6. **What are the locations and functions of the individual cranial nerves?**

See Table 9-1.

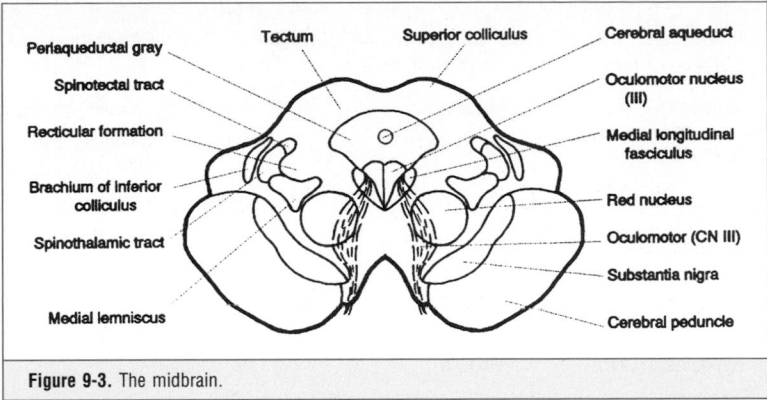

**Figure 9-3.** The midbrain.

## TABLE 9-1. LOCATION AND FUNCTION OF CRANIAL NERVES

| Nerve | Location of Nuclei | Function |
|---|---|---|
| Olfactory (I) | Olfactory bulb | Sensory: smell and olfactory reflex |
| Optic (II) | Thalamus | Sensory: vision and visual reflexes |
| Oculomotor (III) | Midbrain | Motor: eye movement, eyelids, pupillary constriction, accommodation of lens |
| Trochlear (IV) | Midbrain | Motor: eye movement (superior oblique) |
| Trigeminal (V) | Midbrain | Sensory: proprioception for chewing |
| | Pons | Sensory: from face and cornea |
| | | Motor: to masticatory muscles and tensor tympani muscle |
| | Medulla | Sensory: from face and mouth |
| Abducens (VI) | Pons | Motor: eye movement (lateral rectus) |
| Facial (VII) | Pons | Sensory: from skin of external ear, taste from anterior tongue. Motor: facial expression, stapedius muscle movement, salivation, and lacrimation |
| Vestibulocochlear (VIII) | Pons and medulla | Sensory: equilibrium and hearing |
| Glossopharyngeal (IX) | Medulla | Sensory: from middle ear, palate, pharynx, and posterior tongue, taste from posterior tongue. Motor: swallowing, parotid gland salivation |

*(continued)*

**TABLE 9-1. LOCATION AND FUNCTION OF CRANIAL NERVES** *(continued)*

| Nerve | Location of Nuclei | Function |
|-------|-------------------|----------|
| Vagus (X) | Medulla | Sensory: from pharynx, larynx, thorax, and abdomen, taste from epiglottis. Motor: swallowing and phonation. Autonomic: parasympathetics to thoracic and abdominal viscera |
| Spinal accessory (XI) | Medulla | Motor: sternocleidomastoid and upper trapezius muscles |
| Hypoglossal (XII) | Medulla | Motor: tongue |

From Wilson-Pauwels L, Akesson EJ, Stewart PA: Cranial Nerves: Anatomy and Clinical Comments. Toronto, B.C. Decker, 1988.

## KEY POINTS: MAIN FUNCTIONS OF THE CRANIAL NERVES

1. To provide motor or general sensory functions

2. To mediate special senses such as vision, hearing, olfaction, and taste

3. To carry the parasympathetic innervation that controls visceral functions

7. **What is the approach to localizing a brain stem lesion?**
   As a consequence of the unique anatomic arrangements in the brain stem, a unilateral lesion within this structure often causes "crossed syndromes," in which ipsilateral dysfunction of one or more cranial nerves is accompanied by hemiplegia and/or hemisensory loss on the contralateral body. Exquisite localization of a brain stem lesion depends on signs of long-tract (corticospinal and spinothalamic pathways) dysfunction to identify the lesion in the longitudinal (or sagittal) plane and on signs of cranial nerve dysfunction to establish its position in the cross-sectional (or axial) plane. Localization of disorders of the brain stem can be simplified by summarizing the patient's neurologic deficits to answer the following questions: Is the lesion affecting unilateral or bilateral structures of the brain stem? What is the level of the lesion? If the lesion is unilateral, is it medial or lateral in the brain stem?

8. **What are the common symptoms and signs of brain stem lesions?**
   Symptoms
   1. Double vision
   2. Vertigo
   3. Nausea
   4. Incoordination
   5. Gait imbalance
   6. Numbness of the face
   7. Hoarseness
   8. Difficulties with swallowing and speaking

Signs
1. Multiple cranial nerve dysfunctions
2. Gaze palsies
3. Nystagmus
4. Sympathetic dysfunction (Horner's syndrome)
5. Hearing loss
6. Dysphagia
7. Dysarthria
8. Dysphonia
9. Tongue deviation or atrophy
10. Paresis or dysesthesia of the face with contralateral motor or sensory deficits in the body (crossed symptoms)
11. Unilateral hemiparesis with ataxia
12. Significant bilateral brain stem lesions produce altered mental status or coma

9. **What is the approach to localizing an isolated cranial nerve deficit?**
An isolated cranial nerve defect, especially of VI and VII, is most often due to a peripheral and not a brain stem lesion.

10. **How do the presentations of intra-axial and extra-axial lesions of the brain stem differ?**
A lesion that directly affects the tissues of the brain stem is called *intra-axial* or *intramedullary*. It usually presents with simultaneous cranial nerve and long-tract symptoms and signs.
A lesion outside the brain stem is called *extra-axial*. It affects the brain stem by initially compressing and interfering with the functions of individual cranial nerves. Later, as it enlarges, neighboring structures within the brain stem may be affected, causing additional long-tract signs.

11. **What is the differential diagnosis for a brain stem lesion?**

| Intra-axial lesions | Extra-axial lesions |
|---|---|
| Neoplasm | Acoustic neuroma |
| Ischemia/infarct | Meningioma |
| Hemorrhage | Chordoma |
| Vascular malformation | Aneurysms |
| Demyelinating disease | Epidermoid |
| Inflammatory lesion | Arachnoid cyst |

12. **What is the radiographic examination of choice for brain stem lesions?**
Magnetic resonance imaging (MRI) is the examination of choice for suspected brain stem lesions. It provides a highly sensitive and noninvasive method of evaluating the posterior fossa, unhampered by skull base artifact. Enhancement with gadolinium may be useful to characterize breakdown of the blood-brain barrier. MR angiography also may be helpful to investigate further the major branches of the vertebrobasilar system in brain stem ischemia or infarction.

## BRAIN STEM VASCULAR DISEASES

13. **Describe the vascular supply of the medulla.**
The medulla is supplied by the vertebral arteries and their branches. Its blood supply may be further subdivided into two groups, the **paramedian bulbar** and the **lateral bulbar arteries**. The paramedian bulbar arteries are penetrating branches, mainly from the vertebral artery, that

supply the midline structures of the medulla. At the lower medulla, branches from the anterior spinal artery also contribute to this paramedian zone. The lateral portion of the medulla is supplied by the lateral bulbar branches of the vertebral artery or the posterior inferior cerebellar artery.

14. **Describe the vascular supply of the pons.**
    The basilar artery is the principal supplier of the pons. It gives off three types of branches. The **paramedian arteries** supply the medial basal pons, including the pontine nuclei, corticospinal fibers, and medial lemniscus. The **short circumferential arteries** supply the lateral aspect of the pons and the middle and superior cerebellar peduncles. The **long circumferential arteries** together with branches from the anterior inferior cerebellar and superior cerebellar arteries supply the pontine tegmentum and the dorsolateral quadrant of the pons.

15. **Describe the vascular supply of the midbrain.**
    Arteries supplying the midbrain include branches of the superior cerebellar artery, posterior cerebral artery, posterior communicating artery, and anterior choroidal artery. Branches of these arteries, like those of the pons, can be grouped into **paramedian arteries**, which supply the midline structures, and the **long and short circumferential arteries**, which supply the dorsal and lateral midbrain.

16. **What is medial medullary syndrome?**
    Medial medullary (Dejerine's) syndrome is caused by occlusion of the anterior spinal artery or its parent vertebral artery, resulting in the following signs:
    1. Ipsilateral paresis of the tongue (damage to cranial nerve XII), which deviates toward the lesion
    2. Contralateral hemiplegia (damage to corticospinal tract), with sparing of the face
    3. Contralateral loss of position and vibratory sensation (damage to medial lemniscus)

17. **What is the consequence of occlusion of a dominant anterior spinal artery?**
    The central medullary area may be supplied by a single dominant anterior spinal artery. Occlusion of this vessel then leads to bilateral infarction of the medial medulla, resulting in quadriplegia (with face sparing), complete paralysis of the tongue, and complete loss of position and vibratory sensation. The patient will be mute, although fully conscious.

18. **What is lateral medullary syndrome?**
    Lateral medullary (Wallenberg's) syndrome is often due to vertebral artery or posterior inferior cerebellar artery occlusion. Vertebral artery dissection can also be a cause. Damage to the dorsolateral medulla and the inferior cerebellar peduncle results in the following signs:
    1. Ipsilateral loss of pain and temperature sensation of the face (damage to descending spinal tract and nucleus of cranial nerve V)
    2. Ipsilateral paralysis of palate, pharynx, and vocal cord (damage to nuclei or fibers of IX and X) with dysphagia and dysarthria
    3. Ipsilateral Horner's syndrome (damage to descending sympathetic fibers)
    4. Ipsilateral ataxia and dysmetria (damage to inferior cerebellar peduncle and cerebellum)
    5. Contralateral loss of pain and temperature on the body (damage to spinothalamic tract)
    6. Vertigo, nausea, vomiting, and nystagmus (damage to vestibular nuclei)
    7. Other signs and symptoms may include hiccups, diplopia, or unilateral posterior headache. See Figure 9-4.

19. **What is ventral pontine syndrome?**
    Ventral pontine (Millard-Gubler) syndrome is caused by paramedian infarction of the pons and results in the following signs:

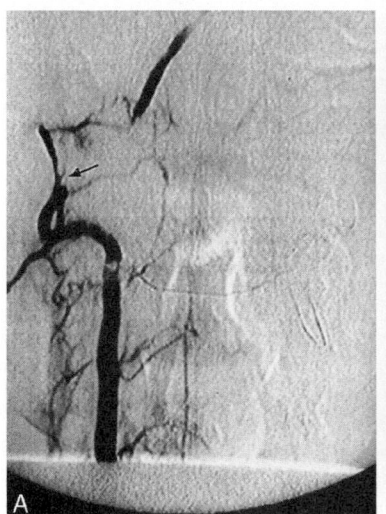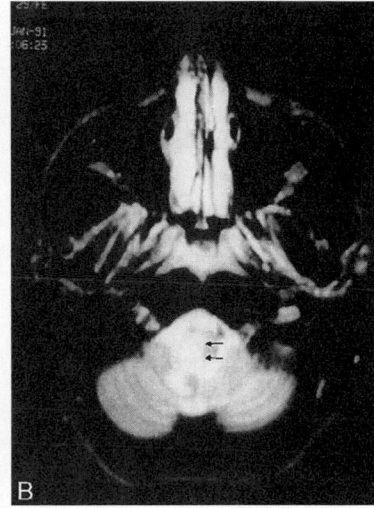

**Figure 9-4.** Dissection of the right vertebral artery (A, arrow) causing a lateral medullary infarct (Wallenberg's syndrome), seen as an area of increased signal (B, arrows) on a T2-weighted MRI of the brain stem.

1. Ipsilateral paresis of the lateral rectus (damage to cranial nerve VI) with diplopia
2. Ipsilateral paresis of the upper and lower face (damage to cranial nerve VII)
3. Contralateral hemiplegia (damage to corticospinal tract) with sparing of the face

20. **What is lower dorsal pontine syndrome?**
    Lower dorsal pontine (Foville's) syndrome is caused by lesions in the dorsal tegmentum of the lower pons and results in the following signs:
    1. Ipsilateral paresis of the whole face (damage to nucleus and fibers of VII)
    2. Ipsilateral horizontal gaze palsy (damage to paramedian pontine reticular formation and/or VI nucleus)
    3. Contralateral hemiplegia (damage to corticospinal tract) with sparing of the face

21. **What is upper dorsal pontine syndrome?**
    Upper dorsal pontine (Raymond-Cestan) syndrome is caused by obstruction of the long circumferential branches of the basilar artery and results in the following signs:
    1. Ipsilateral ataxia and coarse intention tremor (damage to superior and middle cerebellar peduncles)
    2. Ipsilateral paralysis of muscles of mastication and sensory loss in the face (damage to sensory and motor nuclei and tracts of V)
    3. Contralateral loss of all sensory modalities in the body (damage to medial lemniscus and spinothalamic tract)
    4. Contralateral hemiparesis of the face and body (damage to corticospinal tract) may occur with ventral extension of the lesion.
    5. Horizontal gaze palsy may occur, as in lower dorsal pontine syndrome.

22. **What is ventral midbrain syndrome?**
Ventral midbrain (Weber's) syndrome is caused by occlusion of median and paramedian perforating branches and results in the following signs:
   1. Ipsilateral oculomotor paresis, ptosis, and dilated pupil (damage to fascicle of cranial nerve III, including parasympathetic fibers)
   2. Contralateral hemiplegia, including the lower face (damage to corticospinal and corticobulbar tracts)

23. **What is dorsal midbrain syndrome?**
Dorsal midbrain (Benedikt's) syndrome results from a lesion in the midbrain tegmentum caused by occlusion of paramedian branches of the basilar or posterior cerebral arteries or both. It results in the following signs:
   1. Ipsilateral oculomotor paresis, ptosis, and dilated pupil (damage to fascicle of cranial nerve III, including parasympathetic fibers as in Weber's syndrome)
   2. Contralateral involuntary movements, such as intention tremor, ataxia, and chorea (damage to red nucleus)
   3. Contralateral hemiparesis may be present if the lesion extends ventrally.
   4. Contralateral hemianesthesia may be present if the lesion extends laterally, affecting the spinothalamic tract and medial lemniscus.

24. **What is the dorsolateral midbrain syndrome?**
The dorsolateral midbrain syndrome is caused by infarction of the circumferential arteries and results in the following signs:
   1. Ipsilateral Horner's syndrome (damage to sympathetic tract)
   2. Ipsilateral severe tremor that may be present at rest and grossly worsened by attempted movement (damage to superior cerebellar peduncle prior to crossing to the opposite red nucleus). Tremor and ataxia can be present bilaterally if both the superior and cerebellar peduncle and red nucleus are affected.
   3. Contralateral loss of all sensory modalities (damage to spinothalamic tract and medial lemniscus that now ascend together).

25. **What are the symptoms of brain stem transient ischemic attacks?**
Transient circulatory insufficiency in the vertebrobasilar distribution causes brief episodes of brain stem dysfunction characterized by a more patchy and variable presentation. They are often premonitory symptoms of impending brain stem strokes that may result in devastating consequences.
   Symptoms of brain stem ischemia are usually multiple, and isolated findings (such as vertigo or diplopia) are more often caused by peripheral lesions affecting individual cranial nerves.

26. **What is "top of the basilar" syndrome?**
Occlusion of the rostral basilar artery, usually embolic, often results in "top of the basilar" syndrome caused by infarction of the midbrain, thalamus, and portions of the temporal and occipital lobes. This syndrome should be suspected in a patient with sudden onset of unresponsiveness, confusion, amnesia, abnormal eye movement, and visual defect. The neurologic signs may be variable, but the most common include:
   1. **Impairments of ocular movements**—unilateral or bilateral vertical (upgaze, downgaze, or complete) gaze palsy, skew deviation, hyperconvergence or convergence spasms causing pseudo-VI-nerve palsy, convergence retraction nystagmus, and retraction of the upper eyelids.
   2. **Abnormalities in pupils**—small with incomplete light reactivity (diencephalic dysfunction), large or mid-position and fixed (midbrain dysfunction), ectopic pupils (corectopia), oval pupils.
   3. **Alterations of consciousness and behavior**—stupor, somnolence, apathy, lack of attention, memory deficits, and agitated delirium.

4. **Defects in vision**—homonymous hemianopsia, cortical blindness, Balint's syndrome (impaired visual form discrimination and color dysnomia), and abnormal color vision.

5. **Motor weakness, sensory deficits, and reflex abnormalities** are usually variable and subtle and due to the involvement of long tracts at the infarcted region.

This syndrome may be reversible in patients who are younger and do not have significant risks for cerebrovascular disease.

Caplan LR: "Top of the basilar" syndrome. Neurology 30:72-79, 1980.

27. **What is locked-in syndrome?**

Locked-in syndrome occurs in patients with bilateral ventral pontine lesions. Its most common cause is pontine infarction. Other common causes include pontine hemorrhage, trauma, central pontine myelinolysis, tumor, and encephalitis. The patient is quadriplegic because of bilateral damage of the corticospinal tracts in the ventral pons. He or she is unable to speak and incapable of facial movement because of involvement of the corticobulbar tracts. Horizontal eye movements are also limited by the bilateral involvement of the nuclei and fibers of cranial nerve VI. Consciousness is preserved because the reticular formation is not damaged. The patient has intact vertical eye movements and blinking because the supranuclear ocular motor pathways that run dorsally are spared. The patient is able to communicate by movement of the eyelids but otherwise is completely immobile.

Bauby J-D: The Diving Bell and the Butterfly. New York, Alfred A. Knopf, 1997.

28. **What are the common causes of brain stem hemorrhage?**

Pontine hemorrhage is usually caused by uncontrolled systemic hypertension, resulting in a sudden loss of consciousness, quadriparesis, and pinpoint pupils. Progressive central herniation from supratentorial mass lesions can compress the brain stem and cause hemorrhage in the midline of the midbrain (Duret hemorrhage), producing coma and bilateral large and fixed pupils. Diencephalic bleeding, such as thalamic hemorrhage, can dissect into the cerebral peduncles and midbrain, producing acute severe headache, hemiparesis, and III nerve palsy. Small petechial hemorrhages occur in the brain stem of patients with head injuries, blood dyscrasias, or hemorrhagic disorders. Ruptured aneurysms or arteriovenous malformations of the vertebrobasilar system may result in subarachnoid hemorrhage that injures the brain stem.

## KEY POINTS: COMMON CAUSES OF BRAIN STEM ISCHEMIA

1. Atherosclerotic stenosis of vessels of the vestibulobasilar system

2. Embolization from the heart or ulcerated plaques

3. Recurrent hypotension

4. Vertebral steal syndrome

## OTHER BRAIN STEM SYNDROMES

29. **What is Parinaud syndrome?**

Parinaud syndrome is also known as dorsal midbrain or collicular syndrome. The lesion is in the rostral dorsal midbrain, damaging the superior colliculi and pretectal structures. Patients report difficulty in looking up and blurring of distant vision. The common tetrad of findings is as follows:

1. Paralysis of upgaze and accommodation but sparing of other eye movements
2. Normal-to-large pupils with light-near dissociation (loss of pupillary reflex to light with preservation of pupilloconstriction in response to convergence)
3. Eyelid retraction
4. Convergence-retraction nystagmus (eyes make convergent and retracting oscillations following an upward saccade)

Causes include tumors of the pineal gland, stroke, hemorrhage, trauma, hydrocephalus, or multiple sclerosis. The upgaze palsy can be mimicked by progressive supranuclear palsy, thyroid ophthalmopathy, myasthenia gravis, Guillain-Barré syndrome, or congenital upgaze limitation.

30. **What is internuclear ophthalmoplegia?**
Internuclear ophthalmoplegia (INO) is a disorder of horizontal ocular movement due to a lesion in the brain stem (usually in the pons, specifically along the medial longitudinal fasciculus between the VI and III nuclei). Horizontal gaze requires the coordinated activity of the lateral rectus muscle of the abducting eye (innervated by the VI nerve) and the medial rectus muscle of the adducting eye (innervated by the III nerve). This integrated function is regulated by the paramedian pontine reticular formation (or pontine gaze center), which receives input from the contralateral occipital and frontal eyefields and sends fibers to the ipsilateral abducens (VI) nucleus and the contralateral oculomotor (III) nucleus. Fibers from the pontine gaze center run rostrally together with vestibular and other fibers to make up the medial longitudinal fasciculus (MLF).

The cause is commonly multiple sclerosis in young adults, especially when the syndrome is bilateral. In older adults, the syndrome is often unilateral and caused by occlusion of the basilar artery or its paramedian branches. Occasionally, INO can be caused by lupus erythematosus and drug overdose (e.g., barbiturates, phenytoin, amitriptyline). Pseudo-INO occurs rarely as a feature of myasthenia gravis, Wernicke's encephalopathy, and Guillain-Barré syndrome.

Many patients with INO have no symptoms, but some have diplopia or blurred vision. On lateral gaze, the signs of INO include the following:
1. Impaired or paralyzed adduction of the eye ipsilateral to the lesion. The deficit can range from complete medial rectus paralysis to slight slowing of an adducting saccade.
2. Horizontal nystagmus of the abducting eye contralateral to the lesion.
3. Bilateral INO results in defective adduction to the right and left, and nystagmus of the abducting eye on both directions of gaze.
4. Convergence is usually preserved. Skew deviation and vertical gaze nystagmus are sometimes present.

31. **What is "one-and-a-half" syndrome?**
One-and-a-half syndrome is a disorder of horizontal ocular movement characterized by a lateral gaze palsy on looking toward the side of the lesion and INO on looking in the other direction. The location of the lesion is the paramedian pontine reticular formation or VI nerve nucleus. MLF fibers crossing from the contralateral VI nucleus are also involved, causing INO. The common causes of this syndrome are similar to those of INO (e.g., multiple sclerosis, stroke). Hemorrhage or tumor in the lower pons is also in the differential diagnosis. Pseudo–one-and-a-half syndromes may occur with myasthenia gravis, Wernicke's encephalopathy, or Guillain-Barré syndrome. Clinical signs include the following:
1. Horizontal gaze palsy on looking toward the size of the lesion ("one").
2. INO on looking away from the side of the lesion ("half"). This paralyzes adduction and causes nystagmus on abduction. As a result, the ipsilateral eye has no horizontal movement, and the only lateral ocular movement that remains is abduction and nystagmus of the contralateral eye.
3. Associated signs include skew deviation, gaze-invoked nystagmus on vertical gaze, and exotropia of the eye contralateral to the lesion.
4. Vertical ocular movements and convergence are usually intact.

32. **What is bulbar palsy?**
    The bulb is the medulla, and the term *bulbar palsy* refers to a syndrome of lower motor neuron paralysis, affecting muscles innervated by cranial nerves (mainly IX to XII) that have their nuclei closely approximated in the lower brain stem. Muscles of the face, palate, pharynx, larynx, sternocleidomastoid, upper trapezius, and tongue are usually affected. Patients may present clinically with dysarthria, dysphagia, hoarseness, nasal voice, palatal deviation, diminished gag reflex, or weakness of the sternocleidomastoid, upper trapezius, or tongue. Causes of intra-axial lesions include brain stem infarct, syringobulbia, glioma, poliomyelitis, encephalitis, and motor neuron disease (amyotrophic lateral sclerosis [ALS] or progressive bulbar palsy). Extra-axial causes are neoplasms (meningioma or neurofibroma), chronic meningitis, aneurysms, neck trauma, and congenital abnormalities (Chiari malformation or basilar impression).

33. **What is pseudobulbar palsy?**
    Pseudobulbar palsy is a syndrome of upper motor neuron paralysis that affects the corticobulbar system above the brain stem bilaterally. Although it presents with most of the signs and symptoms of bulbar palsy, the causative lesion is not in the brain stem. This condition causes dysphagia, dysarthria, and paresis of the tongue (without atrophy or fasciculations). In contrast to bulbar palsy, the reflex movements of the soft palate and pharynx are frequently hyperactive. The jaw jerk is brisk. Frontal signs (grasp, snout, suck, and glabellar reflex) may be present. Emotional incontinence with exaggerated crying (or, less often, laughing) is also common and may be due to disruption of frontal efferents subserving emotional expression. Multiple lacunar infarcts or chronic ischemia in the hemispheres affecting bilateral corticobulbar fibers usually cause this syndrome. Other causes are ALS and multiple sclerosis.

## OTHER BRAIN STEM DISEASES

34. **What is a brain stem glioma?**
    Brain stem glioma is the most frequent neoplasm affecting the brain stem. It occurs mostly in children and adolescents and is often associated with neurofibromatosis. The tumor arises in the region of the VI nerve nucleus and gradually enlarges to involve the VI and VII nerves and adjacent vestibular structures. Vestibular, cerebellar, and lower cranial nerve symptoms may be present and slowly progressive over a period of months or years before the diagnosis is made because motor and sensory symptoms in the body are usually absent.

35. **What are the common metabolic causes of brain stem dysfunction?**
    Extraocular movements and cerebellar pathways are vulnerable to damage by metabolic insults because they are highly metabolically active. These dysfunctions are usually acute and reversible. The common presentations are ataxia, vertigo, nausea, vomiting, dysarthria, nystagmus, and gaze palsies such as INO. Common causes are alcohol intoxication and overdose of sedative drugs (e.g., barbiturates) and anticonvulsants (e.g., phenytoin).

36. **How does thiamine deficiency affect the brain stem?**
    Wernicke's encephalopathy is a complication of alcoholism and malnutrition resulting in thiamine deficiency. It usually presents with characteristic mental changes of gross confusion, ataxia, extraocular movement abnormalities, and other signs of brain stem dysfunction. The brain stem signs can be readily reversed by parenteral thiamine therapy, but the confusional state may resolve more slowly.

37. **How does demyelinating disease affect the brain stem?**
    Multiple sclerosis often results in demyelination of the fast-conducting, heavily myelinated nerve fibers traveling along the brain stem. These include the cerebellar-vestibular pathways, medial

longitudinal fasciculus, and pyramidal pathways. Bilateral INO is almost pathognomonic of multiple sclerosis. Another hallmark of brain stem multiple sclerosis is the combination of bilateral cerebellar and pyramidal signs producing ataxia and pathologically brisk reflexes.

38. **What is central pontine myelinolysis?**
Central pontine myelinolysis is another demyelinating disease that affects the brain stem white matter, mostly in the central pons and occasionally the cerebral hemispheres. It occurs primarily in patients suffering from malnutrition or alcoholism complicated by hyponatremia. Rapid correction of the hyponatremia has been implicated as a cause of the demyelination. This disorder develops as a subacute progressive quadriparesis with lower cranial nerve involvement. It is usually fatal, but survival with recovered neurologic function is possible. It can be prevented by correcting the electrolyte disturbance gradually rather than rapidly.

Charness ME: Neurologic complications of alcoholism. In Samuels ME, Feske SE (eds): Office Practice of Neurology. Philadelphia, Churchill-Livingstone, 2003, pp 1268–1277.

## VERTIGO

39. **What is vertigo?**
Vertigo is a false sense of movement, either of oneself or of the environment. The feeling may involve the whole body or be limited to the head. It should be distinguished from dizziness or giddiness resulting from near syncope, postural hypotension, hyperventilation, multiple sensory deficits, ataxia, or other etiologies. The spinning or swirling sensations of vertigo are related to disturbances of the vestibular system.

40. **What are the common causes of vertigo?**
The causes of vertigo are central (due to a brain stem lesion) or peripheral (due to an inner ear or vestibular nerve lesion). Central vertigo is almost always accompanied by other signs of brain stem dysfunction, such as double vision, weakness or numbness of the face, dysarthria, or dysphagia. Peripheral vertigo is usually accompanied by tinnitus or hearing loss but no other neurologic abnormalities (Table 9-2).

### TABLE 9-2. COMMON CAUSES OF VERTIGO

| Central | Peripheral |
|---|---|
| Brain stem stroke or transient ischemic attack | Vestibular neuronitis |
| Multiple sclerosis | Benign positional vertigo |
| Neoplasms | Ménière's disease |
| Syringobulbia | Local trauma or posttraumatic |
| Arnold-Chiari deformity basilar migraine | Physiologic (e.g., motion sickness) |
| Cerebellar hemorrhage | Drugs/toxins (e.g., antibiotics, diuretics, antineoplastics, or anticonvulsants) |
| | Posterior fossa tumors/masses (e.g., acoustic neuroma) |

41. **What signs and symptoms help to distinguish central vertigo from peripheral vertigo?**
See Table 9-3.

| TABLE 9-3. CENTRAL VERSUS PERIPHERAL VERTIGO | | |
|---|---|---|
| Signs and Symptoms | Central Vertigo | Peripheral Vertigo |
| Nystagmus | Often vertical or rotatory; may change with direction of gaze; increases with looking toward side of lesion | Mostly horizontal or sometimes rotatory; unidirectional and conjugate; increases with looking away from side of lesion |
| Latency of onset and duration of nystagmus | No latency after head motion; persistent and lasts >60 seconds | Latency after head motion; fatigable and lasts <60 seconds |
| Caloric test | May be normal | Abnormal on side of lesion |
| Brain stem or cranial nerve signs | Often present | Absent |
| Hearing loss, tinnitus | Absent | Often present |
| Nausea and vomiting | Usually absent | Usually present |
| Vertigo | Usually mild | Severe, often rotational |
| Falling | Often falls toward side of lesion | Often falls to side opposite nystagmus |
| Visual fixation or eye closing | No change or increase of symptoms | Inhibits nystagmus and vertigo |

**42. What is vestibular neuronitis?**

Vestibular neuronitis is a condition affecting primarily young adults, causing a sudden attack of vertigo without tinnitus or hearing loss. This benign disorder usually resolves within several days. The etiology is presumed to be a viral infection.

   Baloh RW: Vestibular neuritis. N Eng J Med 348:1027-1032, 2003.

**43. What is Ménière's disease?**

Ménière's disease causes the symptomatic triad of episodic vertigo, tinnitus, and hearing loss. It is caused by an increased amount of endolymph in the scala media. Pathologically, hair cells degenerate in the macula and vestibule.

**44. What is benign positional vertigo? How is it diagnosed?**

Benign positional vertigo is a disorder characterized by paroxysms of vertigo and nystagmus on assumption of certain positions of the head. Hearing tests are normal. The diagnosis is made by performing head maneuvers that elicit the patient's symptoms and nystagmus. The cause is calcification and dislocation of otoliths, which move freely in the semicircular canal, thus abnormally stimulating the hair cells within the semicircular canals.

   Furman JM, Cass SP: Benign paroxysmal positional vertigo. N Eng J Med 341:1590-1596, 1999.

**45. What are canalith repositioning (Epley) maneuvers?**

Epley maneuvers are performed as a treatment for benign positional vertigo. While lying supine, the patient's head is rotated through a series of positions that rolls the otoliths out of the semicircular canals and thus removes the cause of the positional vertigo.

   Epley JM: The canalith repositioning procedure for treatment of benign paroxysmal positional vertigo. Otolaryngol Head Neck Surg 107:399-406, 1992.

## KEY POINTS: BRAIN STEM DISEASE

1. A unilateral lesion within the brain stem often causes "crossed syndromes," in which ipsilateral dysfunction of one or more cranial nerves is accompanied by hemiparesis and/or hemisensory loss on the contralateral body.

2. Symptoms of brain stem disease are usually multiple, and isolated findings (such as vertigo or diplopia) are more often caused by peripheral lesions affecting individual cranial nerves.

3. Brain stem glioma is the most frequent neoplasm found. Other brain stem neoplasms include ependymomas that occur in the fourth ventricle and metastatic lesions that may originate from malignant melanomas or carcinomas of the lung and breast.

4. Ménière's disease presents with the symptomatic triad of episodic vertigo, tinnitus, and hearing loss. It is caused by an increased amount of endolymph in the scala media. Pathologically, hair cells degenerate in the macula and vestibule.

5. The blood supply of the brain stem is derived from the vertebrobasilar system of the posterior circulation.

6. Central pontine myelinolysis occurs primarily in patients suffering from malnutrition or alcoholism complicated by hyponatremia. Rapid correction of the hyponatremia has been implicated as a cause of the pathologic abnormality.

## CONSCIOUSNESS

**46. What are the functions of the reticular formation in the brain stem?**
The reticular formation is composed of a network of diffuse aggregations of neurons distributed throughout the central parts of the medulla, pons, and midbrain. It fills the spaces between cranial nerve nuclei and olivary bodies and intermixes between ascending and descending fiber tracts. Its neurons receive afferent information from the spinal cord, cranial nerve nuclei, cerebellum, and cerebrum and send efferent impulses to the same structures. Their widespread connections give them extensive influence over many neuronal activities. The main functions of the reticular formation are as follows:

1. Activation of the brain for behavioral arousal and different levels of awareness
2. Modulation of segmental stretch reflexes and muscle tone for control of motor function
3. Coordination of autonomic functions, such as control of breathing and cardiovascular activities
4. Modulation of the perception of pain
   Steriade M: Arousal: Revisiting the reticular activating system. Science 272:225-227, 1996.

**47. How do you examine for brain stem dysfunction in a comatose patient?**
When examining a comatose patient, one should be aware of signs and symptoms indicating that the coma is due to brain stem (reticular formation) dysfunction. This is especially true of impending brain stem failure from increased intracranial pressure causing herniation into the posterior fossa. This dysfunction travels in a rostral-caudad direction, ending in death with medullary involvement. Emergency management to reduce the intracranial pressure should be implemented immediately. The following observations are used to monitor the patient's condition:

- Mental status
- Breathing pattern
- Pupillary size and light response

- Spontaneous eye movement or deviation
- Oculocephalic reflex on head turning (doll's eye movement)
- Oculovestibular test of gaze response to ice-water calorics
- Motor response to supraorbital nerve pressure (noxious stimulus)
- Presence of other brain stem reflexes (corneal, gag, and ciliospinal)

**48. How does the clinical examination localize the level of brain stem dysfunction in a comatose patient?**
See Table 9-4.

### TABLE 9-4.  LOCALIZATION OF LEVEL OF BRAIN STEM DYSFUNCTION

| Signs and Symptoms | Subcortical | Midbrain | Pons | Medulla |
|---|---|---|---|---|
| Consciousness | Lethargy or stupor | Coma | Coma | Coma |
| Breathing | Cheynes-Stokes | Central hyperventilation | Apneustic or cluster | Atactic |
| Pupils | Small and reactive | Midposition and fixed (III nucleus); unilateral dilated and fixed (III nerve); large and fixed (pretectal) | Pinpoint fixed, often | |
| Midposition and irregular in shape | | | | |
| Oculocephalic and oculovestibular responses | Present | Absent or abnormal | Absent or abnormal | Absent |
| Motor response to stimulation | Decortication | Decerebration | Decerebration or no response | No response |

**49. How do you test for irreversible loss of brain stem function?**
Brain death is a clinical diagnosis of irreversible cessation of all cerebral and brain stem function. Complete loss of brain stem function begins with apneic coma. On examination, all brain stem reflexes (corneal, pupillary, gag, ciliospinal) are absent. The pupils are midposition or large and fixed. Oculocephalic and oculovestibular reflexes are absent. Muscle tone is flaccid, with no spontaneous facial movement and no motor response to noxious stimuli. This condition should be present for 6 to 24 hours in adults. Metabolic causes (hypothermia, hypotension) and drug effects (neuromuscular blockers, sedative drugs) need to be ruled out. Many local institutions have developed their own, slightly modified criteria for brain death.

Booth CM, Boone RH, Tomlinson G, et al: Is this patient dead, vegetative, or severely neurologically impaired? JAMA 291:870-879, 2004.

### 50. What is the apnea test?

The apnea test is an essential test for the cessation of brain stem function. It stimulates the respiratory centers in the brain stem by inducing hypercarbia. One technique is ventilation of the patient with 100% oxygen for 10 to 30 minutes (depending on the severity of any underlying lung injury) followed by disconnection from the respirator and administration of 100% oxygen through a catheter in the trachea or via T-piece at a flow rate of 6 L/min. Absence of spontaneous respiratory effort with a $PaCO_2$ above 60 mmHg or $> 20$ mm above baseline confirms clinical apnea. Arterial blood gas should be checked before and after the withdrawal of ventilation. Sometimes the test cannot be completed because of ventricular arrhythmias or hypotension. In this situation, the diagnosis of irreversible brain stem dysfunction is made by clinical judgment.

## WEBSITE

1. http://www.nlm.nih.gov/medlineplus/dizzinessandvertigo.html

## BIBLIOGRAPHY

1. Baloh RW: Dizziness, Hearing Loss, and Tinnitus, Philadelphia, F.A. Davis, 1998.
2. Kandel ER, Schwartz JH, Jessell TM: Principles of Neural Science, 4th ed. New York, McGraw-Hill, 2000.
3. Leigh RJ, Zee DS: The Neurology of Eye Movements, 4th ed. Oxford, Oxford University Press, 2006.
4. Posner JB, Saper CB, Schiff N, et al.: Plum & Posner's Diagnosis of Stupor and Coma, Oxford, Oxford University Press, 2007.

# CEREBELLAR DISEASE

CHAPTER 10

*Eugene C. Lai, MD, PhD*

**1. What is the functional importance of the cerebellum?**

The cerebellum coordinates movement and maintains equilibrium and muscle tone through a complex regulatory and feedback system. It receives somatosensory input from the spinal cord, motor information from the cerebral cortex, and input about balance from the vestibular organs of the inner ears. It integrates all this information and aids in organizing the range, velocity, direction, and force of muscular contractions to produce steady volitional movements and posture. It does so by constantly screening its sensory inputs and modulating its motor outputs. The cerebellum also plays an important role in the coordination of the planning of limb movements. In addition, it participates in learning motor tasks, because its function can be modified by experience.

Damage to the cerebellum alone does not impair sensory perception or muscle strength. Rather, it disrupts coordination of limb and eye movements, impairs balance, and decreases muscle tone.

**2. What is the basic anatomy of the cerebellum?**

The cerebellum can be divided into three major lobes by transverse fissures. The primary fissure, located on the upper surface of the cerebellum, divides the cerebellum into an **anterior lobe** and a **posterior lobe**. The posterolateral fissure on the underside of the cerebellum separates the large posterior lobe from the small **flocculonodular lobe**. The cerebellar cortex consists of three layers based on its microscopic anatomy: the molecular cell layer, the Purkinje cell layer, and the granule cell layer. Three pairs of deep nuclei are present within the cerebellum. From medial to lateral these are the fastigial, interposed (may be separated into globose and emboliform), and dentate nuclei. A more functionally useful method of describing the cerebellum is based on its longitudinal zonal patterns and their different connections. A midline zone, known as the **vermis**, separates the two-cerebellar hemispheres on each side. Each hemisphere in turn is composed of an **intermediate zone** and a **lateral zone**. These three zones, together with the flocculonodular lobe, represent the major functional subdivisions of the cerebellum by virtue of their distinct input and output pathways (Figure 10-1).

## KEY POINTS: MAJOR DIVISIONS OF THE CEREBELLUM

1. Flocculonodular lobe

2. Vermis

3. Intermediate zone

4. Lateral zone

**3. What are the connections and functions of the major divisions of the cerebellum?**

See Table 10-1.

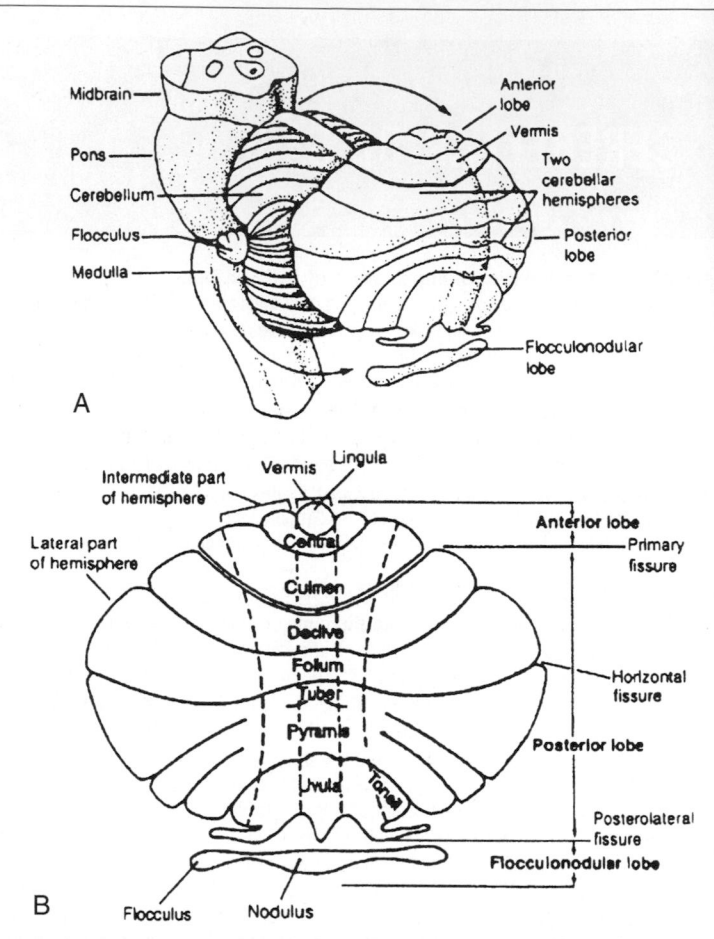

**Figure 10-1.** The cerebellum is divided into anatomically distinct lobes. **A**, The cerebellum is unfolded to reveal the lobes normally hidden from view. **B**, The main body of the cerebellum is divided by the primary fissure into anterior and posterior lobes. The posterolateral fissure separates the flocculonodular lobe. Shallower fissures divide the anterior and posterior lobes into nine lobules. The cerebellum has three functional regions: the central vermis and the lateral and intermediate zones in each hemisphere. From Ghez C: The cerebellum. In Kandel ER, et al. (eds): Principles of Neural Science. New York, Elsevier, 1991.

4. **What are the principal afferent and efferent pathways of the cerebellum?**
   The afferent and efferent pathways to and from the cerebellum course through three pairs of tracts (cerebellar peduncles) that connect the cerebellum to the brain stem:
   1. The **inferior cerebellar peduncle** (restiform body) consists of mainly afferent fibers. A single efferent tract, the fastigiobulbar tract, goes to the vestibular nucleus from the flocculonodular lobe. Afferent fibers enter the inferior cerebellar peduncle from at least five sources, including: (1) the vestibulocerebellar tract, (2) the olivocerebellar tract, (3) the dorsal spinocerebellar tract, (4) the cuneocerebellar tract, and (5) the reticulocerebellar tract.

**TABLE 10-1. CONNECTIONS AND FUNCTIONS OF MAJOR DIVISIONS OF THE CEREBELLUM**

| Functional Division | Major Input | Major Output | Function |
| --- | --- | --- | --- |
| Flocculonodular lobe (vestibulocerebellum) | Vestibular nuclei, labyrinth, visual system | Vestibular nuclei, medial and lateral vestibular tracts | Equilibrium (axial), eye movements, and vestibular reflexes |
| Vermis (spinocerebellum) | Vestibular, visual, and auditory systems, face, proximal body parts | Vestibular nucleus, reticular formation, contralateral motor cortex, and medial descending system via the **fastigial** nucleus | Axial and proximal muscle control and execution, progressive movement |
| Intermediate zone (spinocerebellum) | Spinal cord (distal body parts) | Contralateral red nucleus, motor cortex, and lateral descending system via the **interposed** nucleus | Distal muscle control and execution, progressive movement |
| Lateral zone (cerebrocerebellum) | Contralateral cerebral cortex via pontine nuclei | Contralateral red nucleus, thalamus, motor and premotor cortex via **dentate** nucleus | Motor planning initiation and timing |

2. The **middle cerebellar peduncle** (brachium pontis) consists almost entirely of crossed afferent fibers from the pontine nuclei that transmit impulses from the cerebral cortex to the intermediate and lateral zones of the cerebellum (corticopontocerebellar tract).
3. The **superior cerebellar peduncle** (brachium conjunctivum) consists principally of efferent projections from the cerebellum. Rubral, thalamic, and reticular projections arise from the dentate and interposed nuclei. The fastigiobulbar tracts run with this peduncle for a short distance before it enters the inferior cerebellar peduncle. Afferent fibers include the ventral spinocerebellar tract and the trigeminocerebellar and tectocerebellar projections.

5. **What are the blood supplies to the cerebellum?**
The vertebral and basilar arteries give off three paired branches to the cerebellum: the superior, the anterior inferior, and the posterior inferior cerebellar arteries, which are interconnected by anastomoses. The superior cerebellar artery runs over the superior surface of the cerebellum, while the other arteries supply the inferior surface.

## KEY POINTS: BLOOD SUPPLY TO THE CEREBELLUM

1. The superior cerebellar arteries
2. The anterior inferior cerebellar arteries
3. The posterior inferior cerebellar arteries

6. **What are the clinical tests for cerebellar dysfunction?**
   See Table 10-2. Because most of the tests of cerebellar functions require the cooperation and volitional movement of the patient, clinical features of cerebellar dysfunction cannot be elicited from a paralyzed or comatose patient.

| TABLE 10-2. TESTS FOR CEREBELLAR DYSFUNCTION | |
| --- | --- |
| **Abnormality** | **Methods of Examination** |
| Hypotonia | Passive movement of extremities to check muscle tone; pendular patellar reflexes; rebound phenomenon; inspect for rag doll (flaccid) posture |
| Asynergy | Finger-nose-finger, heel-to-shin, and rapid-alternating supernation-pronation tests to evaluate rate, range, force, and accuracy of voluntary movement |
| Nystagmus | Ocular oscillations through the fields of gaze |
| Dysarthria | Abnormalities in articulation and prosody (scanning or explosive speech, altered accent) |
| Stance and gait | Broad-based stance and gait, difficulty with tandem walk, and postural instability |
| Tremor | Limb tremor at rest, with sustained posture, and during action |

## KEY POINTS: MNEMONIC FOR CEREBELLAR DYSFUNCTION

**H** = **H**ypotonia (loss of muscle tone)
**A** = **A**synergy (lack of coordination)
**N** = **N**ystagmus (ocular oscillation)
**D** = **D**ysarthria (speech abnormalities)
**S** = **S**tation and gait (imbalance, gait ataxia)
**Tremor** = Tremor (coarse intention tremor)

7. **How do you differentiate cerebellar and sensory ataxia?**
   The cerebellum can coordinate and equilibrate movement only if it receives the proper proprioceptive information. Therefore, if the proprioceptive system is defective, the patient has imbalance and ataxia. The proprioceptive defect can be compensated by visual guidance; therefore, the patient with sensory loss exhibits worsening of movement with the eyes closed (Table 10-3).

**TABLE 10-3.  CEREBELLAR VERSUS SENSORY ATAXIA**

|  | Cerebellar Ataxia | Sensory Ataxia |
|---|---|---|
| Hypotonia | Present | Absent |
| Asynergy, dysmetria | Present | Absent |
| Nystagmus | Present | Absent |
| Dysarthria | Present | Absent |
| Tremor | Present | Absent |
| Loss of vibration and position sense | Absent | Present |
| Areflexia | Absent | Present |
| Dystaxia much worse with eyes closed (Romberg test) | Absent | Present |

8. **What are the general principles in localizing a cerebellar lesion?**
   Specific cerebellar regions possess distinct functions. There is also a topical representation of individual body parts in the cerebellum. Thus, signs of cerebellar dysfunction may have localizing significance. Some general principles include the following:
   1. Lesions of the midline impair coordination involving stance and gait.
   2. Lateral lesions impair the limbs ipsilateral to the cerebellar lesion.
   3. Lesions of the cerebellar hemisphere ultimately impair movement on the ipsilateral side of the body because of a double-crossing of the pathways. The ascending cerebellocortical fibers cross in the midbrain and project to the contralateral cortex, and then the descending corticospinal fibers cross back in the medulla to project to the contralateral body.
   4. Lesions of the afferent or efferent pathways to the cerebellum may cause signs similar to lesions of the cerebellum itself.
   5. Lesions of the superior cerebellar peduncle and the deep nuclei usually produce the most severe disturbance of cerebellar dysfunction.

9. **What are the major cerebellar syndromes?**
   There are four major cerebellar syndromes: rostral vermis syndrome, caudal vermis syndrome, hemispheric syndrome, and pancerebellar syndrome. They are distinguished by their presentations and the anatomic regions affected. Recognition of these syndromes may help to narrow the differential diagnosis of cerebellar lesions (Table 10-4).

10. **What are the common acquired diseases of the cerebellum?**
    Acquired cerebellar diseases frequently present as acute ataxia with or without other cerebellar signs. They are often treatable if recognized early. Therefore, one should be astute with the differential diagnosis of acute ataxia so that the disorder can be identified and management plans initiated as early as possible. Cerebellar diseases have a broad differential diagnosis. Initially, they may be divided by etiology into acquired or inherited disorders. Some common acquired cerebellar diseases are as follows:
    1. Vascular diseases
       Infarction (mostly thrombotic, sometimes embolic)
       Hemorrhage (from hypertension, vascular malformation, or tumor)
       Transient ischemic attacks
       Basilar migraine (usually in children)
       Vascular malformation
       Systemic vasculitides (systemic lupus erythematosus)

**TABLE 10-4.   CEREBELLAR SYNDROMES**

| Clinical Syndromes | Region(s) Involved | Distribution of Deficits | Common Causes | Hypotonia | Incoordination of Arms | Incoordination of Legs | Incoordination of Gait and Trunk | Nystagmus | Dysarthria |
|---|---|---|---|---|---|---|---|---|---|
| Cerebellar hemisphere syndrome | Unilateral intermediate and lateral zones | Ipsilateral head and body | Infarct, neoplasm, abscess, demyelination | + | + | + | + | + (bidirectional, coarser, slower on gaze to side of lesion; faster, finer on gaze to other side) | + |
| Rostral vermis syndrome | Anterior and superior vermis | Gait and trunk | Alcoholism Thiamine deficiency | + | + − | + | + | − | − |
| Caudal vermis syndrome | Flocculonodular and posterior vermis | Axial disequilibrium | Midline Neoplasm | + − | − − | + | + | + (variable) | − |
| Pancerebellar syndrome | All regions | Bilateral signs of cerebellar dysfunction | Toxic/metabolic, infectious/ postinfectious, paraneoplastic, degenerative disorders | + | + | + | + | + (variable type) | + |

2. Neoplasms
   Primitive neuroectodermal tumor (PNET or medulloblastoma; in children)
   Astrocytoma (often cystic; midline in children and hemispheric in adults)
   Hemangioblastoma (may be associated with von Hippel-Lindau disease)
   Metastatic tumor (may be multiple)
3. Infections
   Acute cerebellar ataxia of childhood (possible viral etiology)
   Tuberculosis or tuberculoma
   Cysticercosis
   Bacterial infection and abscess (through direct extension of mastoid infection)
   Chronic panencephalitis of congenital rubella infection
   Viral encephalitis (involving cerebellum or brain stem)
4. Inflammatory or autoimmune disorders
   Multiple sclerosis
   Acute postinfectious cerebellitis
   Postinfectious disseminated encephalomyelitis
   Miller-Fisher variant of acute inflammatory polyneuropathy
5. Paraneoplastic syndromes
   Paraneoplastic cerebellar degeneration (PCD, commonly associated with lung, ovarian,
     or breast carcinomas)
   Opsoclonus-myoclonus (secondary to neuroblastoma)
6. Metabolic disorders
   Hypothyroidism
   Hyperthermia
   Hypoxia
   Deficiencies of thiamine (in alcoholics), niacin (pellagra), vitamin E, essential amino
     acids, and zinc
7. Drugs and toxins
   Anticonvulsants: phenytoin, carbamazepine, barbiturates
   Chemotherapeutic agents: 5-fluorouracil, cytosine arabinoside
   Heavy metals: thallium, lead, organic mercury
   Alcohol (may be indirectly due to malnutrition)
   Toluene
8. Developmental abnormalities
   Chiari malformations
   Dandy-Walker syndrome
   Cerebellar aplasia
   Basilar impression
9. Trauma
   Postconcussion
   Hematoma or contusion

11. **What are the major inherited cerebellar diseases?**
    The classification of inherited cerebellar diseases is confusing and nonuniform. These
    diseases usually cause progressive degeneration and atrophy of the cerebellum. They are also
    known as *hereditary ataxias* because their common major neurologic sign is ataxia, or
    clumsiness and incoordination of movement. Inherited diseases can be classified according
    to time of onset, inheritance pattern, known or unknown etiology, and clinical features.
    The more common ones are listed as follows:
    1. **Friedreich's ataxia.** This autosomal recessive disorder is listed separately because it is
       relatively common, with a prevalence of about 1 in 100,000.

2. **Syndromes associated with defective DNA repair** (autosomal recessive)
Ataxia-telangiectasia (low IgA and IgE levels)
Xeroderma pigmentosum
3. **Mitochondrial encephalopathies**
Leigh's disease
Kearns-Sayre syndrome
4. **Syndromes of known metabolic etiology**
Abetalipoproteinemia or hypobetalipoproteinemia (deficient apolipoprotein B)
Wilson's disease (low or absent copper ceruloplasmin)
Refsum's disease (deficient phytanic acid hydroxylase)
Aminoacidurias (Hartnup disease)
Disorders of pyruvate and lactate metabolism (metabolic acidosis)
Urea cycle enzyme defects (hyperammonemia)
Biotinase deficiency (metabolic acidosis)
Hexosaminidase deficiency
Leukodystrophies (metachromatic, Krabbe's)
Ceroid-lipofuscinosis
Niemann-Pick disease
5. **Other inherited syndromes**
Autosomal dominant diseases
Olivopontocerebellar atrophy (ataxia, ophthalmoplegia, optic atrophy)
Spinocerebellar ataxia (ataxia, dysarthria, sensory loss)
Machado-Joseph disease (variable cerebellar, extrapyramidal, and pyramidal involvement)
Autosomal recessive diseases
Ramsay-Hunt syndrome (ataxia and myoclonus)
Behr's syndrome (ataxia, optic atrophy, mental retardation)
X-linked spinocerebellar ataxia (rare)

12. **Summarize the current classification of autosomal dominant spinocerebellar ataxias (SCAs).**
The SCAs are progressive disorders involving a slow degeneration of the cerebellum, often also affecting the brainstem and other regions. Currently, there are at least 28 known genetic loci for SCAs. New genes for SCAs are still being discovered every year. SCAs can be categorized into three major subclasses. The first subclass includes SCAs caused by CAG repeat expansions that encode a repeat of the amino acid glutamine in the disease protein. These "polyglutamine" diseases include SCA 1, 2, 3, 6, 7, and 17. The second subclass comprises the SCAs that are due to repeat expansions situated outside of the protein-coding region of the respective disease genes. They are SCA 8, 10, and 12. A third subclass contains SCAs that are not due to repeat expansions, but are caused by mutations in specific genes. They are SCAs 5, 13, 14, and 27. The molecular mechanisms causing cerebellar degeneration in these disorders are diverse and complex. Much research still needs to be done to understand the pathogenesis and potential treatment of the SCAs.
Soong B-W, Paulson HL: Spinocerebellar ataxias: An update. Curr Opin Neurol 20:438-446, 2007.

13. **What are the common clinical features of autosomal dominant SCAs?**
Dominant SCA syndromes have many overlapping signs that are often difficult to distinguish on clinical grounds. Most of the disorders affect the cerebellum and its pathways, resulting in progressive deterioration of cerebellar function manifested by increasing unsteadiness of gait, incoordination of limb movements, and dysarthria.

14. **What are the clinical features of Friedreich's ataxia?**

Friedreich's ataxia is an autosomal recessive disease that affects the cerebellum, spinal cord, peripheral nerve, and heart. Carbohydrate metabolism is also altered. It has an early onset (before age 20) and a rapidly progressive course. The initial presentation is frequently gait ataxia, but arm ataxia also may be significant. Scoliosis and dysarthria are common. Loss of all tendon reflexes, loss of vibration and position sense, and extensor plantar responses are typical. Other associated features include muscle weakness and atrophy, hypertrophic cardiomyopathy, pes cavus, abnormal ocular motility, diabetes, and deafness. Most patients are confined to a wheelchair by early adulthood. The etiology of Friedreich's ataxia is unknown, but recently the genetic defect was localized to an expanded GAA triplet repeat on chromosome 9. There is presently no effective treatment. Symptomatic treatment of scoliosis by orthopedic intervention and cardiac abnormalities by appropriate medication may prolong survival.

Campuzano V, Montermini L, Molto MD, et al.: Friedreich's ataxia: Autosomal recessive disease caused by an intronic GAA triplet repeat expansion. Science 271:1423-1425, 1996.

15. **What is the difference in the diagnosis of posterior fossa neoplasm in children versus adults?**

Posterior fossa neoplasms account for approximately 50% of the total number of neoplasms in children. The four major types are cerebellar astrocytoma, medulloblastoma (primitive neuroectodermal tumor), ependymoma of the fourth ventricle, and brain stem glioma. In adults, posterior fossa neoplasms are much rarer. They consist mainly of hemangioblastoma, metastatic tumor, acoustic neuroma (schwannoma), and meningioma.

McAllister LD, Ward JH, Schulman SF, et al.: Practical Neuro-oncology. Boston, Butterworth-Heinemann, 2002.

16. **Describe the presentations of cerebellar infarction or hemorrhage. What are the management concerns?**

The presentations of cerebellar infarction and hemorrhage may be indistinguishable. Abrupt onset of headache, vomiting, vertigo, and ataxia, especially in a hypertensive patient, should be considered a neurologic emergency, and vascular etiology should be ruled out. A high index of suspicion may lead to the proper diagnosis with CT or MRI scanning. Expanding hematoma or edema may rapidly lead to brain stem compression and cerebellar herniation accompanied by signs such as hemiparesis, pontine gaze abnormalities, depressed consciousness, irregular breathing, or coma. Prompt surgical evacuation of the hematoma or removal of necrotic cerebellar tissue may be lifesaving.

Amarenco P: The spectrum of cerebellar infarctions. Neurology 41:973-979, 1991.

17. **What are the clinical features and causes of the cerebellopontine angle syndrome?**

Lesions at the space between the cerebellum and the pons often present by compressing and interfering with the functions of the nearby cranial nerves, namely V, VII, and VIII. Involvement of cranial nerve V is often detected by depression or absence of the ipsilateral corneal reflex. Later other sensory and motor functions may be affected, as manifested by numbness of the face and weakness of the mastication muscles. Involvement of cranial nerve VII may produce facial myokymia (involuntary contraction of the facial musculature) or a lower motor neuron paralysis of the ipsilateral face. Hearing loss, tinnitus, and vertigo are features of damage to cranial nerve VIII. As the lesion enlarges, distortion of the brain stem may occur, producing bilateral long-tract signs or obstruction of the aqueduct to cause hydrocephalus and symptoms of increased intracranial pressure. Compression of the cerebellar hemisphere adjacent to the cerebellopontine angle presents with ipsilateral limb ataxia and intention tremor or nystagmus.

Kondziozka D, Lunsford LD, Flickinger JC: Acoustic Neuromas. Curr Treat Options Neurol 4:157-165, 2002.

18. **What is an acoustic neuroma?**
The acoustic neuroma (or schwannoma) is the most common extra-axial lesion that causes cerebellopontine angle syndrome. It originates from Schwann cells in the sheath of cranial nerve VIII, close to the attachment of the nerve to the brain stem. It can be distinguished from other lesions of the cerebellopontine angle by the fact that it involves cranial nerve VIII early; the functions of cranial nerve VII are usually resistant to this tumor and are not affected until much later. The early involvement of cranial nerve VII is sufficient cause to consider the possibility of other lesions, such as meningioma, epidermoidoma, craniopharyngioma, glomus jugulare tumor, and aneurysm of the basilar artery. Intra-axial masses of the brain stem and cerebellum also may cause the syndrome if they are sufficiently large and extend into the cerebellopontine space (Figure 10-2).

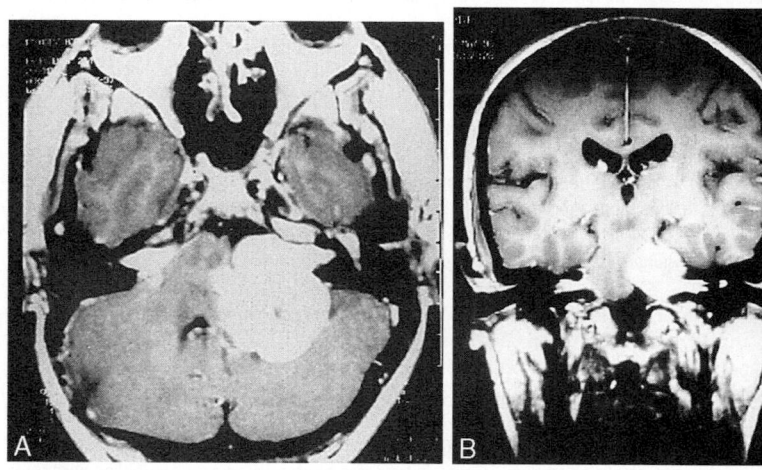

**Figure 10-2.** Gadolinium-enhanced T1-weighted MRIs show bilateral acoustic neuromas (especially large on the left) in a patient with neurofibromatosis. **A**, Axial view. **B**, Coronal view.

19. **What are the clinical features of the cerebellar herniation syndromes?**
Mass lesions in the cerebellum, particularly neoplasms and hematomas, often initially present as nonspecific symptoms such as headache. As the lesions enlarge, the increased pressure causes the cerebellum to herniate in one of two directions—downward or upward.

**Downward herniation** of the cerebellum is most common. Increased pressure in the posterior fossa pushes the cerebellar tonsils downward through the foramen magnum to compress the medulla. It is characterized by progressive vomiting, stiff neck, skew deviation of the eyes, coma, ataxic breathing, apnea, and death. There are no pupillary changes until the patient is terminal. This condition is fatal if not anticipated and prevented early.

**Upward herniation** occurs when the cerebellar mass pushes the cerebellum and upper brain stem through the tentorial opening. The clinical features are caused by progressive compression of the pons and midbrain. The patient is usually obtunded or comatose with small pupils (reactive at first) or anisocoria. Oculocephalic and oculovestibular responses are abnormal. Hemiparesis may progress to quadriparesis and decorticate posturing. Abnormal breathing (central hyperventilation or apneustic breathing) can be observed.

20. **What is the treatment for cerebellar herniation?**
Osmotic agents and hyperventilation may provide temporary relief, but definitive treatment for cerebellar herniations consists of surgical decompression and removal of the mass, if possible.

21. **What is paraneoplastic cerebellar degeneration?**
Paraneoplastic cerebellar degeneration (PCD) is the most common remote effect of neoplasm affecting the brain. It is associated with lung (especially small cell), ovarian, and breast neoplasms and Hodgkin's disease. Cerebellar signs usually begin with gait ataxia, developing over a few weeks to months. The symptoms may progress rapidly to severe and symmetric truncal and limb ataxia with dysarthria and nystagmus. Thus, when an adult develops a rapidly progressing and symmetric cerebellar syndrome, PCD should be promptly considered. Pathologically, severe loss of Purkinje cells affects all parts of the cerebellum. Early neuroimaging studies are typically normal, but later studies show signs of progressive cerebellar atrophy. Cerebellar symptoms may improve in some patients when the causative neoplasms are removed, but they are not improved by plasmapheresis.

22. **What is the cause of PCD?**
An autoimmune process may be the cause of PCD, and antibodies to cerebellar Purkinje cells are observed in patients' sera and spinal fluid. The two main antibodies may be used as markers for patients with PCD. The Yo antibodies (or anti-Purkinje cell cytoplasmic antibodies) are found in gynecologic cancer patients with PCD, whereas the Hu antibodies (antineuronal nuclear antibodies) are present in some patients with small-cell lung cancer with PCD. The pathogenic basis of these antibodies is still uncertain.

Darnell RB: Paraneoplastic neurologic disorders. Arch Neurol 61:30-32, 2004.

Lai EC: Paraneoplastic syndromes. In Rolak LA, Harati Y (eds): Neuroimmunology for the Clinician. Boston, Butterworth-Heinemann, 1997.

# WEBSITES

1. http://www.anatomy.wisc.edu

2. http://www.ataxia.org

# BIBLIOGRAPHY

1. Adams RD, Victor M, Ropper AH: Principles of Neurology, 6th ed. New York, McGraw-Hill, 1997.

2. Kandel ER, Schwartz JH, Jessell TM: Principles of Neural Science, 4th ed. New York, McGraw-Hill, 2000.

3. Lechtenberg R: Handbook of Cerebellar Diseases. New York, Marcel Dekker, 1993.

4. Rolak LA, Harati Y: Neuroimmunology for the Clinician. Boston, Butterworth-Heinemann, 1997.

# CHAPTER 11

# BASAL GANGLIA AND MOVEMENT DISORDERS

*Philip A. Hanna, MD, and Joseph Jankovic, MD*

## ANATOMY AND PHYSIOLOGY

1. **What are the components of the basal ganglia?**

   The basal ganglia are a group of nuclei situated in the deep part of the cerebrum and upper part of the brain stem. Included among these nuclei are the striatum, which is composed of the caudate, putamen, and ventral striatum; the pallidum, which is composed of the internal (medial) and external (lateral) parts of the globus pallidus (GP); the subthalamic nucleus (STN); and the substantia nigra (SN), with the pars compacta (SNc) and pars reticulata (SNr). The putamen and GP are combined to form the lenticular (or lentiform) nucleus because of their lenslike appearance. These interrelated structures are primarily responsible for control of motor functions (Figure 11-1).

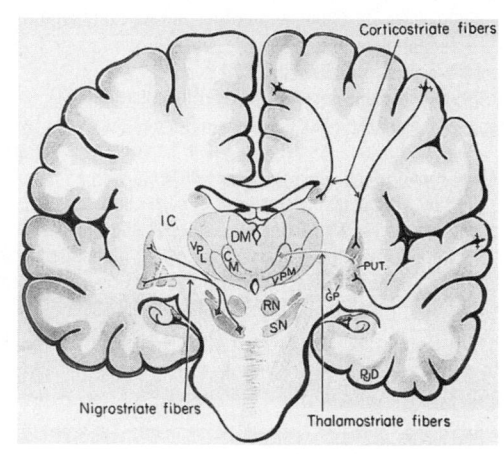

**Figure 11-1.** The basal ganglia and thalamus. *PUT*, putamen; *GP*, globus pallidus; *SN*, substantia nigra; *RN*, red nucleus; *IC*, internal capsule; *VPL*, ventral posterior lateral nucleus; *VPM*, ventral posterior medial nucleus; *CM*, centromedian nucleus; *DM*, dorsomedian nucleus

2. **How are the basal ganglia organized?**

   There are three levels of organization within the basal ganglia. The first level consists of the two major striatal outputs: (1) the indirect pathway to the external segment of the GP (GPe) and (2) the direct pathway to the SNr and internal segment of the GP (GPi). The second level of organization consists of pathways from the cerebral cortex (sublaminae of layer V) to the patch (striosome) and matrix compartments of the striatum (which are organized in a mosaic pattern). The third level of organization is related to the topography of cortical projections to other regions of the striatum.

   DeLong MR, Wichman T: Circuits and circuit disorders of the basal ganglia. Arch Neurol 64:20-24, 2007.

3. **What are the neurotransmitters of the two major striatal output pathways?**
   The majority of the neurons in the striatum are GABAergic medium spiny cells that project to the GPe and SNr. Approximately 50% of these cells also contain substance P and dynorphin and project to the SNr and GPi. The other half of the neurons express enkephalin and project their axons to the GPe. These pathways are, respectively, called striatonigral or direct and striatopallidal or indirect pathways.
   Chase TN, Oh JD: Striatal dopamine- and glutamate-mediated dysregulation in experimental parkinsonism. Trends Neurosci 12(10 Suppl):S86-S91, 2000.

4. **What is the source of the major output of the basal ganglia?**
   The GABAergic neurons of the SNr and the GPi, which may be considered as a single neuronal complex, innervate the mediodorsal and ventral tier thalamic nuclei (which provide feedback to the frontal cortex), the intralaminar thalamic nuclei (which provide feedback to the striatum), the superior colliculus (important in the control of ocular movements), and the pedunculopontine nucleus (seemingly involved in the maintenance of posture).

5. **How many types of dopamine receptors have been identified?**
   Five dopamine receptors, D1 to D5, have now been pharmacologically characterized and cloned.
   The functional significance of this multitude of receptors is not clearly understood. The role of the D1 and D2 receptors in the motor systems has been studied more extensively; activation of the D1 receptors appears to be important in mediating dystonic movements, whereas activation of the D2 receptors may result in chorea. Clozapine, a specific blocker for the D4 receptor, is an effective dibenzodiazepine antipsychotic agent.

6. **How are the D1 and D2 dopamine receptors expressed in the striatum?**
   The D1 dopamine receptor is predominantly expressed on the striatonigral neurons, whereas the D2 receptors are primarily found on the striatopallidal neurons. Evidence suggests that in the striatum the D1 and D2 receptors have an excitatory and inhibitory action, respectively.

## PARKINSONISM

7. **What are the neurophysiologic changes in the basal ganglia in Parkinson's disease (PD)?**
   Neuronal loss in the SNc with consequent dopamine depletion in the striatum is the neurochemical-pathologic hallmark of PD. This dopaminergic deafferentation produces an imbalance in the striatal activity, with hypoactivity of the striatonigral pathway and hyperactivity of striatopallidal pathways. This imbalance results in decreased inhibition (disinhibition) of the STN and increased activity of the GPi/SNr neurons, causing increased inhibition of the thalamic ventral tier nuclei. Because these thalamic nuclei are responsible for the activation of the cortical areas involved in the generation of movements, the final effect of dopamine deficiency is poverty or slowness of movements (hypokinesia).
   Bergman H, Deuschl G: Pathophysiology of Parkinson's disease: From clinical neurology to basic neuroscience and back. Mov Disord 17(Suppl 3):S28-S40, 2002.

8. **What are the cardinal symptoms and signs of parkinsonism?**
   Tremor at rest is one of the most typical signs of parkinsonism. It is characterized by an oscillatory pronation-supination at a 3 to 5 Hz frequency. In addition to the hands, where it assumes an appearance of pill rolling, this type of tremor is commonly observed in the facial musculature (lips and chin) as well as in the legs. Head tremor, however, is rare in parkinsonism, and its presence should suggest the diagnosis of essential tremor (ET).

The term **bradykinesia** is used to describe slowness of movements that often causes the patient difficulty with getting dressed, feeding, and maintaining personal hygiene. Bradykinesia is evident when a patient performs rapid alternating movements, such as pronation and supination of the forearms.

**Rigidity**, often associated with the cogwheel phenomenon, is another hallmark of parkinsonism. Impairment of the postural reflexes is responsible for the falls that are frequently experienced by parkinsonian patients. Parkinsonian gait often reflects a combination of bradykinesia, rigidity, and postural instability.

Jankovic J: Parkinson's disease: Clinical features and diagnosis. J Neurol Neurosurg Psychiatry 79:368-376, 2008.

9. **What are the most common causes of parkinsonism?**
In a highly selected population, such as that attending a movement disorders clinic, PD is responsible for 77.7% of the cases of parkinsonism. The other most frequent causes are parkinsonism-plus syndrome (12.2%), secondary parkinsonism (8.2%), and heredodegenerative parkinsonism (0.6%) (Table 11-1).

---

### TABLE 11-1. CAUSES OF PARKINSONISM

**I. Idiopathic parkinsonism**
PD
    Sporadic form
    Familial form
**II. Secondary parkinsonism**
Drug-induced
    Dopamine receptor blockers (neuroleptics, including antiemetics such as
        metoclopramide)
    Dopamine depleters (reserpine, tetrabenazine)
    Calcium channel blockers (flunarizine, cinnarizine, diltiazem)
    Lithium
    Methyldopa
Hemiatrophy-hemiparkinsonism
Hydrocephalus
    Normal pressure hydrocephalus
    Noncommunicating hydrocephalus
Hypoxia
Infectious diseases
    AIDS
    Intracytoplasmic hyaline inclusion disease
    Creutzfeldt-Jakob disease
    Postencephalitic parkinsonism
    Fungus
    Subacute sclerosing panencephalitis

---

*(continued)*

## TABLE 11-1. CAUSES OF PARKINSONISM *(continued)*

Metabolic
   Acquired hepatocerebral degeneration (chronic liver insufficiency)
   Hypocalcemic parkinsonism
Paraneoplastic parkinsonism
Syringomesencephalia
Toxin
   Carbon disulfide
   Ethanol
   Carbon monoxide
   Manganese
   Cyanide
   Methanol
   Disulfiram
   MPTP
Trauma
Tumor
Vascular
   Multi-infarcts
   Binswanger's disease
   Lower body parkinsonism
**III. Parkinsonism-plus syndromes**
Alzheimer's disease-parkinsonism
Cortical basal ganglionic degeneration (CBGD)
Diffuse Lewy body disease
Multiple system atrophy (MSA)
   Shy-Drager syndrome (SDS)
   Sporadic olivopontocerebellar atrophy (OPCA)
   Striatonigral degeneration
Parkinsonism-dementia-amyotrophic lateral sclerosis
Progressive pallidal atrophy
Progressive supranuclear palsy (PSP)
**IV. Heredodegenerative diseases**

| | |
|---|---|
| Ceroid-lipofuscinosis | X-linked dystonia-parkinsonism |
| Gerstmann-Straussler-Scheinker disease | Disinhibition-dementia-parkinsonism- |
| Familial OPCA | amyotrophy complex |
| Hallervorden-Spatz disease | (chromosome 17) |
| Huntington's disease | Autosomal dominant Lewy body |
| Levodopa-responsiveness | disease |
| (fluctuating) dystonia | Hereditary ceruloplasmin deficiency |
| Machado-Joseph disease | Familial progressive subcortical gliosis |
| (Azorean heredoataxia) | Familial basal ganglia calcification |

*(continued)*

---

**TABLE 11-1.   CAUSES OF PARKINSONISM** *(continued)*

| | |
|---|---|
| Mitochondrial cytopathies with striatal necrosis | Familial parkinsonism with peripheral neuropathy |
| Neuroacanthocytosis | Parkinsonian-pyramidal syndrome |
| Thalamic dementia syndrome | |
| Wilson's disease | |

*PD*, Parkinson's disease; *AIDS*, Acquired immunodeficiency syndrome; *MPTP*, 1-Methyl-4-phenyl-1,2,3,6-tetrahydropyridine; *CBGD*, Cortical basal ganglionic degeneration; *MSA*, Multiple system atrophy; *SDS*, Shy-Drager syndrome; *OPCA*, olivopontocerebellar atrophy; *PSP*, Progressive supranuclear palsy.

---

Azher SN, Jankovic J: Clinical aspects of progressive supranuclear palsy. In Duyckaerts C, Litvan I (eds): Handbook of Clinical Neurology, 3rd Series. Amsterdam, Elsevier. Handb Clin Neurol 89:461-473, 2008.

10. **What causes PD?**
Although PD was first described in 1817, its cause is still unknown. The recognition that 1-methyl-4-phenyl-1,2,3,6-tetrahydropyridine (MPTP) can produce in humans and nonhuman primates a parkinsonian syndrome very similar to PD led to the hypothesis that an MPTP-like substance in the environment could cause PD.

One of the theories about the cause of PD is that, as a result of a defective antioxidant system and increased formation of highly reactive and toxic-free oxygen radicals (oxidative stress), abnormally folded proteins accumulate in the affected neurons and overwhelm the ubiquitin-protease system. When the compensatory autophagic mechanisms fail, this leads to the formation of inclusions in the cytoplasm called *Lewy bodies* and the eventual death of the neuron (see references).

A growing body of evidence supports the notion that genetic factors play an important role in the etiology of PD. Families with an autosomal dominant and recessive transmission of otherwise typical PD have been described, as have monozygotic twins concordant for the disease.

The etiology of PD is still speculative, but a combination of environmental factors may be associated with a genetic predisposition.

Greenamyre JT, Hastings TG: Parkinson's divergent causes, convergent mechanisms. Science 304:1120-1122, 2004.

Klein C, Schlossmacher MG: Parkinson disease, 10 years after its genetic revolution: Multiple clues to a complex disorder. Neurology 69:2093-2104, 2007.

Klein C, Ziegler A: How to predict the risk of Parkinson disease in relatives of parkin mutation carriers: A complex puzzle of age, penetrance, and number of mutated alleles. Arch Neurol 65:443-444, 2008.

Pan T, Kondo S, Le W, Jankovic J: The role of autophagy-lysosome pathway in neurodegeneration associated with Parkinson's disease. Brain 131:1969-1978, 2008.

Tan EK, Jankovic J: Genetic testing in Parkinson's disease: Promises and pitfalls. Arch Neurol 63:1232-1237, 2006.

11. **What are the clinical and pathologic hallmarks of PD?**
Patients with PD may have several combinations of parkinsonian symptoms. Typically, the onset is insidious in the sixth decade of life, and the symptoms usually begin unilaterally or predominate on one side of the body. It is possible to recognize two clinical types of PD:

a tremor-dominant form with earlier age of onset, slower progression, and relatively preserved cognition, and a postural instability and gait difficulty (PIGD) form with more bradykinesia, more rapid progression, and dementia. Furthermore, ET is more likely to coexist in the tremor-dominant form. Pathologically, there is loss of dopaminergic neurons in the SNc, and the surviving neurons contain Lewy bodies (LB). Although to a lesser degree than the SNc, other pigmented nuclei of the brain stem, such as the locus ceruleus and tegmental ventral area, are also involved by a similar process. A recent clinicopathologic study showed that the presence of a resting tremor is more likely to be associated with LB at autopsy. LB has also been demonstrated in nondopaminergic nuclei of the brainstem, olfactory system, and spinal cord. It appears to correlate with the nonmotor "preclinical" manifestations of PD.

Shahed J, Jankovic J: Exploring the relationship between essential tremor and Parkinson's disease. Parkinsonism Relat Disord 13:67-76, 2007.

12. **How specific is the clinical diagnosis of PD?**
Approximately 24% of patients with the clinical diagnosis of PD are found to have another diagnosis at necropsy. Patients with typical symptoms may have variable pathologic findings; conversely, typical pathologic findings can be expressed by dissimilar signs. Findings of asymmetric onset, no evidence for other causes of parkinsonism, and no atypical features of PD increase the specificity of the clinical diagnosis.

Hughes AJ, Daniel SE, Lees AJ: Improved accuracy of clinical diagnosis of lewy body Parkinson's disease. Neurology 57:1497-1499, 2001.

Jankovic J, Rajput AH, McDermott MP, et al.: The evolution of diagnosis in early Parkinson's disease. Parkinson Study Group. Arch Neurol 57:369-372, 2000.

13. **What is the role of anticholinergic drugs and amantadine in the treatment of PD?**
In the early stages of PD, anticholinergic drugs, combined with rasagiline or deprenyl (selegiline), may be used as the primary treatment. With progression of disease, patients require the addition of levodopa. Even in this circumstance, some patients still benefit from using anticholinergics and amantadine. Tremor is occasionally resistant to dopaminergic therapy and may be better controlled with the use of levodopa in association with ancillary medications. In contrast to the anticholinergics, amantadine, a drug that has mild anticholinergic effects and increases the release of dopamine, also improves rigidity and bradykinesia. Furthermore, recent studies have revealed the utility of amantadine in reducing levodopa-induced dyskinesias (LID).

The anticholinergic medications must be used cautiously because, in addition to causing dryness of the mouth and bladder retention, they may produce disorientation, confusion, and memory loss, particularly in the elderly. Amantadine in some patients also may cause cognitive side effects as well as livedo reticularis, ankle swelling, and worsening of CHF.

Jankovic J: Therapeutic strategies in Parkinson's disease. Geriatrics 61:1-11, 2006.

Jankovic J, Stacy M: Medical management of levodopa-associated motor complications in patients with Parkinson's disease. CNS Drugs 21:677-692, 2007.

Pahwa R, Factor SA, Lyons KE, et al: Quality Standards Subcommittee of the American Academy of Neurology. Practice parameter: Treatment of Parkinson disease with motor fluctuations and dyskinesia (an evidence-based review): Report of the Quality Standards Subcommittee of the American Academy of Neurology. Neurology 66:983-995, 2006.

14. **When should levodopa therapy be started in the treatment of PD?**
The mainstay in the treatment of PD is the replacement of dopamine. This therapy was introduced in the 1960s. Instead of using dopamine, which does not cross the blood-brain barrier, the current approach consists of combining levodopa and carbidopa. Levodopa is transformed into dopamine, and carbidopa is a peripheral inhibitor of the enzyme dopa-decarboxylase. The inhibition of this enzyme in the periphery, but not in the brain,

decreases substantially the required levodopa dosage and the occurrence of gastrointestinal side effects (nausea and vomiting). In Europe and other countries, benserazide is available as an inhibitor of dopa-decarboxylase.

The effectiveness of levodopa may be limited by early motor fluctuations and dyskinesia attributed to nonphysiologic stimulation of dopamine receptors by multiple and higher cumulative levodopa doses. This effect is believed to occur more in younger PD patients.

A rational strategy is to start levodopa when the parkinsonian symptoms begin to impair activities of daily living or to interfere with social and occupational functioning. Although Sinemet CR (a continuous-release preparation) may be the preferred starting formulation because constant activation of receptors provides a more predictable and longer response than the intermittent dopaminergic input of regular Sinemet, a 5-year prospective study failed to show any advantage of this preparation over the standard preparation of levodopa/carbidopa. A typical starting dose is Sinemet 25/100, 2 or 3 times/day. Maintenance doses of 200 to 600 mg/day of levodopa may be needed in patients with moderately advanced Parkinson's disease. Other formulations include Sinemet 10/100, Sinemet 25/250, Sinemet CR 50/200, and orally dispersable levodopa/carbidopa, called Parcopa. The dosage of carbidopa should be kept at less than 150 mg/day because it may penetrate the blood-brain barrier and inhibit central dopa-decarboxylase at higher levels. Although some parkinsonologists believe that delaying levodopa therapy is a prudent approach, longitudinal studies show no difference between patients who started on levodopa versus those who started on a dopamine agonists. The approach to early therapy must be individualized. Generally those patients who require symptomatic therapy in order to maintain a satisfactory level of functioning at home and at work are started on levodopa early, whereas those whose symptoms are not troublesome may be started on dopamine agonists.

Hauser RA, McDermott MP, Messing S: Parkinson Study Group: Factors associated with the development of motor fluctuations and dyskinesias in Parkinson's disease. Arch Neurol 63:1756-1760, 2006.

Katzenschlager R, Head J, Schrag A, et al: Parkinson's Disease Research Group of the United Kingdom. Fourteen-year final report of the randomized PDRG-UK trial comparing three initial treatments in PD. Neurology 71:474-480, 2008.

Roach ES: Initial Parkinson's disease therapy: Levodopa, dopamine agonists or both? Arch Neurol 61:1972-1973, 2004.

15. **What are the most common peripheral side effects of levodopa therapy? How are they managed?**
Nausea and vomiting are common side effects in the beginning of the use of levodopa. Most patients overcome this difficulty by taking the medication after meals. In some patients, extra amounts of carbidopa (typically, one 25-mg tablet with each dose of Sinemet) may be necessary. A small proportion of patients have nausea and vomiting despite these measures. Treatment of gastrointestinal (GI) side effects should not include dopamine blockers, such as metoclopramide, because they may cause worsening of PD. Hydroxyzine, trimethobenzamide, diphenidol, cyclizine, or domeperidone are useful alternatives.

The most common cardiovascular side effect is orthostatic hypotension. The management of this complication involves adding salt to the diet; wearing elastic stockings; and using medications such as fludrocortisone, indomethacin, or midodrine.

Jankovic J: Levodopa strengths and weaknesses. Neurology 58(4 Suppl 1):S19-S32, 2002.

16. **What clinical fluctuations are recognized in PD?**
Although the most dramatic fluctuations in patients with PD are related to levodopa therapy, some who have not been previously treated with dopaminergic drugs exhibit fluctuations in severity of their symptoms and signs. Fluctuations are not exclusively motor phenomena. The nonmotor fluctuations (NMF) are classified into three categories: dysautonomic, psychiatric, and sensory. Anxiety, drenching sweat, mental slowing, fatigue, akathisia, and dyspnea are

some common NMFs described in PD. They may occur during "on" or "off" periods and are associated with higher doses of levodopa. Significant improvement in such fluctuations have been reported following chronic subthalamic stimulation. Mood and autonomic functions also fluctuate. For example, some patients display depression when they are "off" and euphoria when they are "on." Fatigue and stress usually make these symptoms more prominent. The most dramatic example of spontaneous fluctuations is paradoxical dyskinesia: under extreme stress, patients completely immobilized by parkinsonism are suddenly able to stand up and run (Table 11-2).

## TABLE 11-2.  CLINICAL FLUCTUATIONS IN PARKINSON'S DISEASE

| Fluctuation | Management |
| --- | --- |
| End-of-dose deterioration ("wearing off") | COMT inhibitors |
| | Increase frequency of levodopa doses |
| | Sinemet CR |
| | Dopamine agonists |
| | Deprenyl |
| | Amantadine |
| | Infusions of levodopa or dopamine agonists |
| Delayed onset of response | Give before meals |
| | Reduce protein |
| | Antacids |
| | Infusions of levodopa or dopamine agonists |
| Drug-resistant "offs" | Increase levodopa dose and frequency |
| | Give before meals |
| | Infusions of levodopa or dopamine agonists |
| Random oscillation ("on-off") | Dopamine agonists |
| | Deprenyl |
| | Infusions of levodopa or dopamine agonists |
| | Levodopa withdrawal |
| Freezing* | Increase dose |
| | Dopamine agonists |
| | Desipramine |
| | Inverted L-shaped cane |

*May not be related to levodopa therapy. *COMT,* catechol-*O*-methyltransferase.

Chaudhuri KR, Healy DG, Schapira AH: National Institute for Clinical Excellence: Non-motor symptoms of Parkinson's disease: Diagnosis and management. Lancet Neurol 5:235-245, 2006.

Olanow CW, Obeso JA: Preventing levodopa-induced dyskinesias. Ann Neurol 47: S167-S176, 2000.

Schrag A, Quinn N: Dyskinesias and motor fluctuations in Parkinson's disease: A community-based study. Brain 123(Pt 11):2297-2305, 2000.

Witjas J, Kaphan E, Regis J, et al.: Effects of chronic subthalamic stimulation on nonmotor fluctuations in parkinson's disease. Mov Disord 22:1729-1734, 2007.

17. **What are some useful strategies in the management of fluctuations in PD?**
    The concept of continuous dopaminergic stimulation has been used as a guiding principle in the prevention and treatment of motor fluctuations. Strategies designed to achieve this goal include the use of MAO inhibitors such as selegiline and rasagiline, COMT inhibitors such as entacapone and tolcapone, dopamine agonists, and subthalamic nucleus (STN) deep brain stimulation (DBS).

    Diamond A, Jankovic J: Treatment of advanced Parkinson's disease. Expert Review of Neurotherapeutics 6:1181-1197, 2006.

18. **What are the most common types of levodopa-induced dyskinesias (LID)? How are they treated?**
    After 3 years of treatment, approximately 50% of patients with PD display some degree of involuntary movements related to levodopa. Phenomenologically, LID may be classified into three main categories:
    1. **Peak-dose dyskinesias** (improvement-dyskinesia-improvement or I-D-I) coincide with the time of maximal clinical improvement and usually consist of choreatic movements. Such dyskinesias may improve with levodopa dose reduction.
    2. **Diphasic dyskinesias** (dyskinesia-improvement-dyskinesia or D-I-D) occur at the onset and/or the end of the "on" period during rising and falling levodopa blood levels and usually consist of dystonia and repetitive stereotypic movements of the legs. Some patients display a combination of the two types and have dyskinesia during the entire "on" period (square-wave dyskinesias). Such dyskinesias may improve with dose increments.
    3. **"Off" dyskinesias**, typically painful dystonias, coincide with the period of decreased mobility. The most common example is early morning dystonia. Dopaminergic stimulation increases "on" dyskinesias and decreases the other two types. Conversely, antidopaminergic drugs improve all forms of LID, although they worsen the PD. Dystonia induced by levodopa may improve significantly with the use of baclofen, an agonist of gamma-aminobutyric acid (GABA) receptors, or local intramuscular injection of botulinum toxin (Table 11-3). Amantadine may reduce dyskinesia without worsening PD symptoms, possibly via NMDA-receptor inhibition. Finally, STN or globus pallidus internus (GPi) DBS may be used to smooth out motor fluctuations and reduce dyskinesias.

    Thanvi B, Lo N, Robinson T: Levodopa-induced dyskinesia in Parkinson's disease: Clinical features, pathogenesis, prevention and treatment. Postgrad Med J 83:384-388, 2007.

    Jankovic J, Stacy M: Medical management of levodopa-associated motor complications in patients with Parkinson's disease. CNS Drugs 21:677-692, 2007.

19. **What is the role of dopamine agonists in the treatment of PD?**
    Dopamine agonists directly stimulate dopamine receptors and, in contrast to levodopa, do not require enzymatic transformation into metabolites. Because dopamine agonists bypass the presynaptic elements of the nigrostriatal system, they have some advantages in relation to levodopa. For example, they cause dyskinesias and clinical fluctuations less frequently and usually have a levodopa-sparing effect. The most established use of dopamine agonists is as an adjunct to levodopa, especially in patients with clinical fluctuations and dyskinesias. Evidence indicates that early introduction of dopamine agonists delays the development of complications of long-term levodopa therapy, such as motor fluctuations and dyskinesias, although this benefit may not be sustained. After 10 years, there is no observable difference between patients initially treated with levodopa or a dopamine agonist with respect to levodopa-induced motor complications.

    Hely MA, Morris JG, Reid WG, et al.: Sydney multicenter study of Parkinson's disease: Non-L-dopa-responsive problems dominate at 15 years. Mov Disord 20:190-199, 2005.

**TABLE 11-3.  LEVODOPA-INDUCED DYSKINESIAS**

| Pattern | Phenomenon | Management |
|---|---|---|
| Peak-dose (I-D-I) | Chorea | Reduce each dose of levodopa |
| | | Add dopamine agonists |
| | Dystonia | Reduce each dose of levodopa |
| | | Clonazepam |
| | | Baclofen |
| | | Anticholinergics |
| | Pharyngeal dystonia | Reduce each dose of levodopa |
| | | Add anticholinergics |
| | Respiratory dyskinesia | Reduce each dose of levodopa |
| | | Add dopamine agonists |
| | Myoclonus | Clonazepam |
| | | Valproate |
| | | Methysergide |
| | Akathisia* | Anxiolytics |
| | | Propranolol |
| | | Opioids |
| Diphasic (D-I-D) | Dystonia | Increase each dose of levodopa |
| | | Baclofen |
| | | Sinemet CR |
| | Stereotypies | Increase each dose of levodopa |
| | | Baclofen |
| Off dyskinesia | Dystonia | Baclofen |
| | | Dopamine agonists |
| | | Anticholinergics |
| | | Sinemet CR |
| | | Tricyclics |
| | | Lithium |
| | | Botulinum toxin |
| | Akathisia* | Anxiolytics |
| | | Propranolol |
| | | Opioids |
| Striatal posture* | Dystonia | Increase levodopa |
| | | Anticholinergics |
| | | Thalamotomy |
| | | Botulinum toxin |

*I-D-I*, improvement-dyskinesia-improvement; *D-I-D*, dyskinesia-improvement-dyskinesia.
*May be unrelated to levodopa therapy.

20. **What dopamine agonists (DA) are available to treat PD? What are their most common side effects?**

Until 1997, only two dopamine agonists (bromocriptine and pergolide) were clinically used in PD. Since then, pramipexole, ropinirole, apomorphine, and rotigotine have become commercially available.

Both bromocriptine and pergolide are ergot derivatives and have the risk of complications such as vasoconstriction (with acroparesthesias and angina); exacerbation of peptic ulcer disease; erythromelalgia; and valvular, pulmonary, and retroperitoneal fibrosis. Pramipexole, ropinirole, and rotigotine are nonergoline agonists and have a lower risk of such complications. The transdermal rotigotine patch was recently taken off the market in the United States due to crystallization of the medication.

Although dopamine agonists display fewer motor complications than levodopa, they may exacerbate peak-dose dyskinesias and cause other undesired dopaminergic effects, such as nausea, vomiting, anorexia, malaise, orthostatic hypotension, confusion, and hallucinations. Furthermore, dopamine agonists have been linked to dopamine dysregulation syndrome, including impulse control disorders as well as hypersexuality, pathologic gambling, compulsive shopping, and other impulsive and compulsive behaviors.

Pan T, Xie W, Jankovic J, et al.: Biological effects of pramipexole on dopaminergic neuron-associated genes: Relevance to neuroprotection. Neurosci Lett 377:106-109, 2005.

Rascol O, Brooks DJ, Korczyn AD, et al.: A five-year study of the incidence of dyskinesia in patients with early Parkinson's disease who were treated with ropinirole or levodopa. 056 Study Group. N Engl J Med 342:1484-1491, 2000.

Stamey W, Jankovic J: Impulse control disorders and pathological gambling in patients with Parkinson's disease. Neurologist 14:89-99, 2008.

Tintner R, Jankovic J: Dopamine agonists in Parkinson's disease. Expert Opin Investig Drugs 12:1803-1820, 2003.

21. **What is the role of surgery in the treatment of PD?**

Deep brain stimulation (DBS) of the ventralis intermedius (VIM) has been shown to be of marked benefit, primarily for tremor, and is able to suppress dyskinesias. DBS involves implanting an electrode in the VIM and delivering high-frequency chronic stimulation via an implantable pulse generator located subcutaneously in the subclavicular area. Patients can turn the device on and off via an external magnet. DBS can be done bilaterally with a lower risk of dysarthria than thalamotomy.

The recognition that PD is associated with hyperactivity of the STN led to the successful treatment of MPTP monkeys by subthalamotomy. Some human patients, inadvertently treated with subthalamotomy instead of thalamotomy, noted improvement not only in tremor but also in bradykinesia. Recent use of STN DBS has demonstrated benefit for contralateral bradykinesia, dyskinesia, and other parkinsonian signs. This was demonstrated by the improvement in off-period motor symptoms and activities of daily living in a recent metanalysis. Patients most likely to benefit had severe off-period symptoms, long disease duration, and a history of good resurgical response to levodopa.

The pallidum, particularly the posteroventral part of the internal segment of the GP (GPi), is also a surgical target in PD. The main benefit of pallidotomy is the marked reduction of contralateral LIDs, with some ipsilateral benefit. Tremor, bradykinesia, and rigidity are also reduced but more variably. After pallidotomy, patients typically have a lower levodopa requirement. DBS into the GPi is receiving increased attention as a treatment for LID as well as other hyperkinesias, including dystonia and tics.

Benarroch EE: Subthalamic nucleus and its connections: Anatomic substrate for the network effects of deep brain stimulation. Neurology 70:1991-1995, 2008.

Diamond A, Jankovic J: Quality of life and cost effectiveness of deep brain stimulation in movement disorders. In Tarsy D, Vitek J L, Starr P, Okun M (eds): Deep Brain Stimulation in

Neurological and Psychiatric Disorders. Current Clinical Neurology Series, Humana Press, Totowa, NJ, 2008.

Hariz MI, Rehncrona S, Quinn NP, et al: Multicentre Advanced Parkinson's Disease Deep Brain Stimulation Group. Multicenter study on deep brain stimulation in Parkinson's disease: An independent assessment of reported adverse events at 4 years. Mov Disord 23:416-421, 2008.

Johnson MD, Miocinovic S, McIntyre CC, et al.: Mechanisms and targets of deep brain stimulation in movement disorders. Neurotherapeutics 5:294-308, 2008.

Tan EK, Jankovic J: Patient selection for surgery for Parkinson's disease. In Lozano AM, Gildenberg PL, Tasker RR (eds): Textbook of Stereotactic and Functional Neurosurgery, 2nd ed. Heidelberg, Germany, Springer-Verlag, 2008.

22. **What is the role of transplant surgery in the treatment of PD?**
Interest in the transplantation of adrenal medulla into the basal ganglia was sparked by the hypothesis that the adrenal chromaffin cells produce dopamine when implanted into parkinsonian striatum. After initial encouraging reports, this procedure has been virtually abandoned in the United States because of its modest benefits and high risk of morbidity. Human fetal mesencephalic transplantation has undergone a great deal of scrutiny. Two double-blind, placebo-controlled trials (real and sham surgery) demonstrated some improvement in clinical measures of PD, particularly in younger patients, but the studies are considered negative with respect to primary efficacy measures. Furthermore, up to half of the patients developed "off" dyskinesias, even without levodopa, and many required GPi DBS to control the troublesome involuntary movements. Finally, some, but not all, patients whose brains were examined many years after the fetal transplant demonstrate synuclein and Lewy body pathology in the grafted tissue. The interpretation of these observations is not clear.

Freed CR, Greene PE, Breeze RE, et al.: Transplantation of embryonic dopamine neurons for severe Parkinson's disease. N Engl J Med 344:710-719, 2001.

Kordower JH, Chu Y, Hauser RA, et al.: Lewy body-like pathology in long-term embryonic nigral transplants in Parkinson's disease. Nat Med 14:504-506, 2008.

Olanow CW, Goetz CG, Kordower JH, et al.: A double-blind controlled trial of bilateral fetal nigral transplantation in Parkinson's disease. Ann Neurol 54:403-414, 2003.

23. **Is there any relationship between Alzheimer's disease (AD) and PD?**
Currently available data do not support the existence of a common etiology for AD and PD. However, approximately 20% of patients with PD have troublesome dementia. AD accounts for an unknown proportion of these cases. Unlike AD, the pattern of dementia in PD is characterized by lack of cortical signs, such as aphasia and apraxia, and the presence of forgetfulness, bradyphrenia, and depression. In a longitudinal study, clinical features that differentiated dementia in PD were cognitive fluctuations, auditory/visual hallucinations, sleep disturbance, and depression. The different patterns suggest that different mechanisms are responsible for cognitive dysfunction in the two diseases, and pathologic studies support this distinction. PD is characterized by relative sparing of the cortex and by neuronal loss in the SN and other subcortical structures, such as the locus ceruleus. LBs are found in the remaining cells. On the other hand, the cerebral cortex is primarily involved in AD; neurofibrillary tangles and deposits of amyloid are the most important lesions. However, a recent study shows that over 50% of patients with AD display parkinsonism and myoclonus during the course of the disease.

Galvin JE, Pollack J, Morris JC: Clinical phenotype of parkinson's disease dementia. Neurology 67:1605-1611, 2006.

Wilson RS, Bennett DA, Gilley DW, et al.: Progression of parkinsonism and loss of cognitive function in Alzheimer's disease. Arch Neurol 57:855-860, 2000.

24. **What are the main clinical features of progressive supranuclear palsy (PSP)?**
Progressive supranuclear palsy is the second most common cause of idiopathic parkinsonism. Typically, the onset is in the seventh decade, with no family history. Patients have

ophthalmoparesis of downgaze, parkinsonism, pseudobulbar palsy, and frontal lobe signs. Eyelid abnormalities are common. For example, patients with eyelid freezing have difficulty with either opening or closing the eyes due to inhibition of levator palpebrae or orbicularis oculi muscles, respectively. The presence of dementia in PSP is controversial. The prevalence of dystonia in patients with pathologically proven PSP is about 13%.

Azher SN, Jankovic J: Clinical aspects of progressive supranuclear palsy. In Duyckaerts C, Litvan I (eds): Handbook of Clinical Neurology, 3rd Series. Amsterdam, Elsevier. Handb Clin Neurol 89:461-473, 2008.

## 25. What is the cause of PSP?

The cause of PSP is unknown. Radiologic and pathologic evidence indicates that a multi-infarct state can cause a picture identical to PSP. Idiopathic PSP is pathologically characterized by marked neuronal cell loss in subcortical structures, such as the nucleus basalis of Meynert, pallidum, STN, substantia nigra, locus ceruleus, and superior colliculi. Other pathologic features include neurofibrillary tangles, granulovacuolar degeneration, and gliosis. Atrophy, generalized or focal (midbrain or cerebellum), is the most common neuroradiologic finding in idiopathic PSP. However, up to 25% of the patients with PSP have no abnormality on computed tomography (CT) and/or magnetic resonance imaging (MRI) of the brain. Growing evidence suggests linkage disequilibrium between a PSP gene and allelic variants of the tau gene.

Litvan I: Update on progressive supranuclear palsy. Curr Neurol Neurosci Rep 4:296-302, 2004.

Rademakers R, Melquist S, Cruts M, et al.: High-density SNP haplotyping suggests altered regulation of tau gene expression in progressive supranuclear palsy. Hum Mol Gen 14:3281-3292, 2005.

## 26. How can PSP be distinguished from PD?

The most distinctive feature of PSP is the supranuclear downgaze palsy, which is not found in PD, the most common misdiagnosis of PSP. The differentiation is particularly difficult when the characteristic supranuclear ophthalmoparesis is not evident, as may be the case in early stages of PSP. Some patients who never develop this finding are found at autopsy to have PSP. The difficulty in establishing the diagnosis of PSP is suggested by an average delay in making the diagnosis of 3.6 years after onset of symptoms. The measurement of midbrain atrophy ratio on MRI and abnormal computerized posturography are useful tools in reliably differentiating early PSP from PD and age-matched controls (Table 11-4).

Oba H, Yagishita A, Terada H, et al.: New and reliable MRI diagnosis for progressive supranuclear palsy. Neurology 64:2050-2055, 2005.

Ondo W, Warrior D, Overby A, et al.: Computerized posturography analysis of progressive supranuclear palsy: A case-control comparison with Parkinson's disease and healthy controls. Arch Neurol 57:1464-1469, 2000.

Osaki Y, Ben-Shlomo Y, Lees AJ, et al.: Accuracy of clinical diagnosis of progressive supranuclear palsy. Mov Disord 19:181-189, 2004.

## 27. What is the treatment for PSP?

Levodopa and dopamine agonists are the most frequently used agents in the treatment of PSP. However, even with high doses, they usually provide only a transient and slight improvement of parkinsonian symptoms. The loss of dopamine receptors in the striatum and the presence of extensive lesions involving other neurotransmitters, such as acetylcholine, probably account for the failure of pharmacologic therapy. Currently, no drug provides sustained relief in patients with PSP. With progression of the disease, patients usually become bedridden and unable to swallow or talk. Gastrostomy is necessary in advanced stages. Death, usually related to respiratory complications, occurs after a mean disease duration of 7 to 8 years.

Lang AE: Treatment of progressive supranuclear palsy and corticobasal degeneration. Mov Disord 20:S83-S91, 2005.

TABLE 11-4. DIFFERENTIAL DIAGNOSIS OF PROGRESSIVE SUPRANUCLEAR (PSP) PALSY AND PARKINSON'S DISEASE

| Clinical Features | PSP | PD |
|---|---|---|
| Age at onset (decade) | 7th | 6th |
| Initial symptoms | Postural and gait disorder | Tremor and bradykinesia |
| Family history | – | ± |
| Multi-infarct state | ± | – |
| Dementia | ± (visual/motor) | ± |
| Downgaze ophthalmoparesis | + | – |
| Eyelid abnormalities | + | ± |
| Pseudobulbar palsy | + | ± |
| Gait | Wide, stiff, unsteady | Slow, shuffling, narrow, festinating |
| Rigidity | Axial (neck) | Generalized |
| Facial expression | Astonished, worried | Hypomimia |
| Tremor at rest | – | + |
| Dystonia | + | ± |
| Corticobulbospinal signs | ± | – |
| Symmetry of findings | + | – |
| Weight loss | – | + |
| Improvement with DA drugs | – | + |
| Levodopa-induced dyskinesias | – | + |

+, yes or present; –, no or absent; *PSP*, progressive supranuclear palsy; *DA*, dopamine; ±, may be present or absent.

28. **What are the most important characteristics of vascular parkinsonism?**
Multiple vascular lesions in the basal ganglia may be associated with parkinsonism. Tremor at rest is not a common finding, and bradykinesia and rigidity tend to be more significant in the legs. In some patients, the findings are virtually limited to the lower extremities; hence the designation lower body parkinsonism. Unlike PD, the gait in patients with vascular parkinsonism is characterized by a broad base. Some patients show stepwise progression. Associated findings, such as dementia, spasticity, weakness, and Babinski's sign, are commonly observed. Neuroradiologic studies, especially MRI, show a multi-infarct state. The response to dopaminergic therapy is usually poor.
    Sibon I, Fenelon G, Quinn NP, et al.: Vascular parkinsonism. J Neurol 251:513-524, 2004.

29. **Is it possible to distinguish drug-induced parkinsonism from PD on clinical grounds?**
Drugs are one of the most common causes of parkinsonism in the general population. Drugs that block postsynaptic dopamine receptors and/or deplete presynaptic dopamine may cause parkinsonism. Clinical studies indicate that drug-induced parkinsonism is indistinguishable from PD. Discontinuation of the offending drug promotes remission of the syndrome in most cases, although sometimes the parkinsonism persists. Such patients may have subclinical PD and require dopaminergic therapy.

30. **What is multiple system atrophy (MSA)?**
Multiple system atrophy is a neuropathologic term that includes Shy-Drager syndrome (SDS), sporadic forms of olivopontocerebellar atrophy (OPCA), and striatonigral degeneration (SND). SDS is characterized by parkinsonism, which occasionally responds to dopaminergic therapy, and dysautonomia. Although cerebellar findings dominate in OPCA, mild parkinsonism and pyramidal signs are also usually recognized. Patients with SND typically have parkinsonism and pyramidal signs with laryngeal stridor, although in some cases, SND is indistinguishable from PD. The division of MSA into SDS, OPCA, and SND is controversial, with some authorities grouping the spectrum into the prominence of either cerebellar or parkinsonisms designated as MSA-A, MSA-C, or MSA-P, respectively. Although usually clinically distinct at onset, with progression symptoms overlap substantially. The three syndromes have a common pathologic substratum consisting of cell loss and gliosis in the striatum, substantia nigra, locus ceruleus, inferior olive, pontine nuclei, dorsal vagal nuclei, cerebellar Purkinje cells, and intermediolateral cell columns of the spinal cord. The characteristic histologic marker—glial cytoplasmic inclusions, which are seen particularly in oligodendrocytes—has helped to distinguish MSA as a clinicopathologic entity. The presence of autonomic dysfunction early on is thought to predict a poor prognosis.
    Hanna PA, Jankovic J, Kirkpatrick JB: Multiple system atrophy: The putative causative role of environmental toxins. Arch Neurol 56:90-94, 1999.
    Wenning GK, Ben-Shlomo Y, Hughes A, et al: What clinical features are most useful to distinguish definite multiple system atrophy from Parkinson's disease? J Neurol Neurosurg Psychiatry 68:434-440, 2000.

31. **What is the treatment for MSA?**
Dopaminergic drugs are the mainstay of the treatment of MSA. However, despite the use of high doses of levodopa, no significant improvement is usually observed. The loss of cells in the striatum and widespread lesions of other neurotransmitters probably accounts for the failure of treatment. The use of midodrine and pyridostigmine may assist in the symptomatic management and control of orthostatic hypotension from autonomic dysfunction.
    Singer W, Sandroni P, Opfer-Gehrking TL, et al.: Pyridostigmine treatment trial in neurogenic orthostatic hypotension. Arch Neurol 63:513-518, 2006.
    Wenning GK, Geser F, Stampfer-Kountchev M, et al.: Multiple system atrophy: an update. Mov Disord 18(Suppl 6):S34-S42, 2003.

32. **What is cortical-basal ganglionic degeneration (CBGD)?**
Patients with CBGD display a combination of cortical (pyramidal signs, myoclonus, progressive aphasia, and apraxia) and subcortical findings (rigidity and dystonia) as well as a distinctive alien limb sign. CBGD is virtually the only disease that causes this constellation of symptoms and signs. CBGD is virtually the only disease that causes this constellation of symptoms and signs, though there appears to be an overlap of CBGD, progressive aphasia, and frontotemporal dementia. Until late stages of the disease, patients do not experience cognitive decline or dysautonomia. Convergence disturbances and oculomotor apraxia are common neuro-ophthalmic signs. The neuropathologic hallmarks are swollen achromatic neurons, neuronal loss, and gliosis in the cerebral cortex, SN, lateral nuclei of the thalamus, striatum, locus ceruleus, and Purkinje layer of the cerebellum. The cause is entirely obscure. No familial forms have been reported. The disease progresses relentlessly until death, usually within 10 years after onset. Response to dopaminergic therapy is usually poor.
    Hanna PA, Doody RS: Alien limb sign. In Litvan J, Goetz CG, Lang AE (eds): Corticobasal Degeneration and Related Disorders. Advances in Neurology Series, Vol. 82. Philadelphia, Lippincott Williams & Wilkins, 2000.
    Kumar R, Bergeron C, Lang AE: Corticobasal degeneration. In Jankovic J, Tolosa E (eds.): Parkinson's Disease and Movement Disorders. 5th ed. Baltimore, William & Wilkins, 2006.

## TREMORS

33. **What is essential tremor (ET)?**

Essential tremor is a neurologic disease characterized by action tremor of the hands in the absence of any identifiable causes, such as drugs or toxins. Other types of tremor, such as isolated head and voice tremor, are also expressions of ET. It is estimated that at least 5 million Americans are affected by ET. Characterized by action-postural tremor of the hands and arms, ET may be asymmetric at onset and have a kinetic component. Patients with severe forms of ET may display tremor at rest. ET is presumably transmitted by an autosomal dominant gene with variable expression. Recently, a familial ET gene (in Icelandic families) was mapped to chromosome 3. In the recent past, three genes (ETM1, ETM2, and a locus on 6p23) have been identified in patients and family members. Supportive criteria for diagnosis of ET include improvement with alcohol, propranolol, and primidone.

Deng H, Le W, Jankovic J: Genetics of essential tremor. Brain 130(Pt 6):1456-1464, 2007.

Lou JS, Jankovic J: Essential tremor: Clinical correlates in 350 patients. Neurology 41:234, 1991.

34. **How can enhanced physiologic tremor be differentiated from ET?**

Physiologic tremor is a rhythmic oscillation with a frequency of 8 to 12 Hz, determined largely by the mechanical properties of the oscillating limb. Under several circumstances, the tremor may be enhanced and appears identical to ET. Enhanced physiologic tremor is the most common cause of postural tremor. However, unlike ET, its frequency can be reduced by mass loading (Table 11-5).

Jankovic J: Essential tremor: Clinical characteristics. Neurology 54(11 Suppl 4):S21-S23, 2000.

### TABLE 11-5. CAUSES OF ENHANCED PHYSIOLOGIC TREMOR

| Stress-induced | Drugs |
| --- | --- |
| Anxiety | Beta agonists (e.g., theophylline, terbutaline, epinephrine) |
| Emotion | Cyclosporine |
| Exercise | Dopaminergic drugs (levodopa, dopamine agonists) |
| Fatigue | Methylxanthines (coffee, tea) |
| Fever | Psychiatric drugs (lithium, neuroleptics, tricyclics) |
| **Endocrine** | Stimulants (amphetamines, cocaine) |
| Adrenocorticosteroids | Valproic acid |
| Hypoglycemia | **Toxins** (arsenic, bismuth, bromine, ethanol withdrawal, |
| Pheochromocytoma | mercury, lead) |
| Thyrotoxicosis | |

35. **What physiopathologic mechanisms underlie ET?**

The pathologic findings in several series have suggested a heterogeneous pathology in ET with the majority showing cerebellar Purkinje cell loss and gliosis. The abnormal pathology appears to be supported by functional imaging studies. Only 14 patients with ET have had a thorough pathologic examination, and no specific abnormality was found. It has been suggested that the postural tremor of ET arises from spontaneous firing of the inferior olivary nucleus, which drives the cerebellum and its outflow pathways via the thalamus to the cerebral cortex and then to the spinal cord. Functional MRI (fMRI) studies have demonstrated increased activation of the cerebellum and red nucleus in ET. Most positron emission tomography (PET) and fMRI evidence indicates that the inferior olive is not likely to be the tremor generator in ET; instead, the generator is probably in the cerebellum. This theory is supported by bilateral overactivity of cerebellar connections by PET in patients with primary writing and primary orthostatic tremor. Clinical data also support a cerebellar role in the pathogenesis of ET: over 50% of patients with ET have difficulty in performing tandem gait, which is considered an indicator of cerebellar function, and hemispheric cerebellar stroke may abolish ipsilateral ET.

Louis ED, Faust PL, Vonsattel JP, et al.: Neuropathological changes in essential tremor: 33 cases compared with 21 controls. Brain 130(Pt 12):3297-3307, 2007.

Shill HA, Adler CH, Sabbagh MN, et al.: Pathological findings in prospectively ascertained essential tremor subjects. Neurology 70(16 Pt 2):1452-1455, 2008.

36. **Is there an association between ET and PD?**
According to different sources, the prevalence of ET in patients with PD ranges from 3% to 8.5%. The prevalence of PD in ET is debated (4.5% to 21.8%). The relatively high frequency of familial tremor (15% to 23%) among patients with PD supports the existence of an etiologic link between PD and ET. An additional ET marker was mapped to chromosome 4p14-16.3 in an autosomal dominant PD family. Furthermore, an allele (263_bp) of the nonamyloid component of plaques (NACP)-Rep1 polymorphism has been associated with sporadic PD in a German and more recently in an American population of patients with PD. The authors conclude that the association of this allele with PD and ET "suggests a possible etiologic link between these two conditions." In addition, Lewy body pathology has been demonstrated in several pathologic series in brains of patients with ET. Further epidemiologic and genetic studies are needed before the controversy about the relationship between PD and ET can be resolved.

Benamer TS, Patterson J, Grosset DG, et al.: Accurate differentiation of parkinsonism and essential tremor using visual assessment of [123I]-FP-CIT SPECT imaging: The [123I]-FP-CIT Study Group. Mov Disord 15:503-510, 2000.

Louis ED, Vonsattel JP, Hong LS, et al.: Essential tremor pathology: A case control study from the essential tremor centralized brain repository. Mov Disord 20:1241, 2005.

Shahed J, Jankovic J: Exploring the relationship between essential tremor and Parkinson's disease. Parkinsonism Relat Disord 13:67-76, 2007.

Tan EK, Matsuura T, Nagamitsu S, et al.: Polymorphism of NACP-Rep1 in Parkinson's disease: An etiologic link with essential tremor? Neurology 54:1195-1198, 2000.

37. **What is the relationship between ET and dystonia?**
Although tremor is frequently found in patients with dystonia, it is not always clear whether the oscillatory movement is a form of dystonia (hence a dystonic tremor) or whether it represents coexistent ET. Postural hand tremor, phenomenologically identical to ET, may precede or be the initial manifestation of dystonia. The lack of demographic and other differences between patients with ET and ET-dystonia supports the notion that ET is a single disease entity with a clinical spectrum that often includes dystonia. Some investigators argue, however, that the postural tremor in patients with dystonia has different clinical characteristics—such as irregularity and a broader range of frequencies, asymmetry of contractions, and associated myoclonus—that distinguish it from ET.

Pal PK: Head tremor in cervical dystonia. Can J Neurol Sci 27:137-142, 2000.

Shaikh AG, Jinnah HA, Tripp RM, et al.: Irregularity distinguishes limb tremor in cervical dystonia from essential tremor. J Neurol Neurosurg Psychiatry 79:187-189, 2008.

38. **What is orthostatic tremor?**
Orthostatic tremor (OT) is a relatively rare but frequently misdiagnosed disorder. It is more common in women, and the onset is typically in the sixth decade. It consists of a rapid (13 to 14 Hz) tremor of the legs triggered by standing. Postural tremor of the hands and a family history of ET are frequent features, suggesting that OT is a variant of ET. Transcranial magnetic

stimulation of the cortex motor area has suggested a supraspinal generator of OT. Clonazepam is the treatment of choice; other less effective options are propranolol, primidone, gabapentin, and phenobarbital.

Gerschlager W, Munchau A, Katzenschlager R, et al.: Natural history and syndromic associations of orthostatic tremor: a review of 41 patients. Mov Disord 19:788-795, 2004.

39. **What other tremors are variants of ET?**

Besides OT, other types of tremor are also considered to be variants of ET. However, some authors argue that the pharmacologic differences between these tremors and ET support the notion that they represent distinct entities. There is evidence, for example, that some isolated site (head tremor) and task-specific tremors, such as primary handwriting tremor, actually represent forms of dystonic tremor. This controversy will not be settled until biologic markers for ET and for dystonia are available (Table 11-6).

Louis ED, Ford B, Barnes LF: Subtypes of essential tremor. Arch Neurol 57:1194-1198, 2000.

### TABLE 11-6. VARIANTS OF ESSENTIAL TREMOR

| Variant | Treatment |
| --- | --- |
| Chin tremor | Propranolol, primidone |
| Facial tremor | Clonazepam, propranolol, primidone |
| Head tremor | Clonazepam, primidone, propranolol, trihexyphenidyl |
| Orthostatic tremor | Clonazepam, propranolol, primidone, phenobarbital |
| Shuddering attacks (childhood) | Propranolol |
| Task-specific tremor (writing) | Propranolol, primidone, trihexyphenidyl, botulinum toxin |
| Tongue tremor | Propranolol, primidone |
| Truncal tremor | Clonazepam, propranolol, primidone |
| Voice tremor | Propranolol, ethanol, botulinum toxin |

40. **Discuss the treatment of ET.**

Propranolol remains the most effective medication for ET, although other beta-blockers also have an antitremor activity. Daily doses of up to 360 mg may be necessary to control tremor.

**Primidone**, an anticonvulsant medication, also has been shown to be highly effective for the treatment of ET in both open and controlled studies. It should be started at low doses (25 mg at bedtime) to avoid the occasional, acute, idiosyncratic toxic reaction characterized by severe nausea, vomiting, sedation, confusion, and ataxia.

Less effective but occasionally useful medications are lorazepam, clonazepam, alprazolam, neurontin, topiramate, and diazepam. A double-blind, placebo-controlled trial revealed mild to moderate benefit of botulinum toxin injections in the treatment of severe hand tremor. Alcohol, although effective in approximately two-thirds of patients with ET, is not recommended because of the possibility of addiction, although ET does not appear to increase the risk of alcoholism.

For intractable ET, contralateral thalamotomy is efficient and well tolerated. The current main surgical treatment for ET is high-frequency thalamic stimulation (DBS), and gamma knife thalamotomy has been shown to suppress completely disabling ET.

Kondziolka D, Onq JG, Lee LY, et al.: Gamma knife thalamotomy for essential tremor. J Neurosurg 108:111-117, 2008.

Ondo W, Hunter C, Vuong KD, et al.: Gabapentin for essential tremor: A multiple-dose, double-blind, placebo-controlled trial. Mov Disord 15:678-682, 2000.

Ondo WG, Jankovic J, Connor GS, et al.: Topiramate in essential tremor: A double blind, placebo controlled trial. Topiramate essential tremor study investigators. Neurology 66:672-677, 2006.

Pilitsis JG, Metman LV, Toleikis JR, et al.: Factors involved in long-term efficacy of deep brain stimulation of the thalamus for essential tremor. J Neurosurg 109:640-646, 2008.

41. **What are the characteristics and most common causes of kinetic tremor?**
Kinetic tremors result from lesions of the cerebellar outflow pathways. The tremor has a 3- to 4-Hz frequency and is typically observed on the finger-to-nose test. In patients with cerebellar lesions, titubation (anterior/posterior oscillation of the trunk and head) and postural tremor of the hands are often seen in addition to the kinetic tremor. Patients who have lesions in the midbrain, involving the superior cerebellar peduncle and nigrostriatal system, also display tremor at rest (midbrain tremor).

Multiple sclerosis, trauma, stroke, Wilson's disease, phenytoin intoxication, acute alcoholic intoxication, cerebellar parenchymatous alcoholic degeneration, and tumor are the most important causes of kinetic tremor.

The treatment of kinetic tremors remains unsatisfactory. Drugs used in the treatment of ET, such as propranolol and primidone, are ineffective in the treatment of kinetic tremors. Isoniazid, carbamazepine, and glutethimide may control kinetic tremor in some patients. Attaching weights to the wrist also may be modestly helpful. Injections of botulinum toxin or thalamotomy may benefit selected patients. Buspirone has been reported to help some patients with mild cerebellar tremor.

Wishart HA, Roberts DW, Roth RM, et al.: Chronic deep brain stimulation for the treatment of tremor in multiple sclerosis: review and case reports. J Neurol Neurosurg Psychiatry 74:1392-1397, 2003.

Yap L, Kouyialis A, Varma TR: Stereotactic neurosurgery for disabling tremor in multiple sclerosis: Thalamotomy or deep brain stimulation? Br J Neurosurg 21:349-354, 2007.

42. **What is the relationship between tremor and peripheral trauma?**
The occurrence of tremor and other movement disorders, especially dystonia and myoclonus, after peripheral trauma is well established. Typically, peripherally induced tremors have rest and action components. Some patients develop a typical picture of parkinsonism, with rest tremor, bradykinesia, hypomimia, and response to levodopa. The physiopathology of this movement disorder is unknown. Although conventional neurophysiologic studies show abnormalities of the peripheral nerves in less than one-half of patients, it is reasonable to speculate that damage to the peripheral nervous system causes sustained changes in the central nervous system connectivity and motor unit sensory reflex feedbacks, which account for the movement disorders. The common association with reflex sympathetic dystrophy suggests that dysautonomia plays a role in the generation of posttraumatic movement disorders. About 60% of patients have predisposing factors such as personal and family history of ET and exposure to neuroleptics.

Treatment is difficult. Anticholinergic agents and antitremor medications, such as propranolol and primidone, are usually ineffective. Clonazepam may provide moderate relief in some patients. Some authors have successfully used injections of botulinum toxin into the affected musculature to control posttraumatic movement disorders. Surgical treatment is another consideration when pharmacologic treatment fails.

Cardoso FC, Jankovic J: Post-traumatic peripherally-induced tremor and parkinsonism. Arch Neurol 52:263-270, 1995.

Costa J, Henriques R, Barroso C, et al.: Upper limb tremor induced by peripheral nerve injury. Neurology 67:1884-1886, 2006.

## DYSTONIA

43. **How is dystonia classified?**

    Dystonia may be classified according to age of onset, genetics, topographic distribution, or etiology (Table 11-7). One aspect of the importance of classification is the recognition of the temporal progression of focal to generalized dystonia in early-onset primary dystonia as compared to late-onset dystonia, which will usually remain localized or segmental. The advancement in identifying several dystonia loci of genes with various modes of inheritance and penetrance has aided genetic counseling in families with dystonia.

    Bressman SB: Dystonia genotypes, phenotypes and classification. Adv Neurol 94:101-107, 2004.

    de Carvalho Aguiar PM, Ozelius LJ: Classification and genetics of dystonia. Lancet Neurol 1:316-325, 2002.

### TABLE 11-7. CLASSIFICATION OF DYSTONIA

| | |
|---|---|
| **Etiology** | |
| Idiopathic | |
|   Familial | |
|   Sporadic | |
| Symptomatic | |
| **Age at onset** | |
| Childhood-onset | 0-12 years |
| Adolescent-onset | 13-20 years |
| Adult-onset | >20 years |
| **Distribution** | |
| Focal | Single body part |
| Segmental | One or more contiguous body parts |
| Multifocal | Two or more noncontiguous body parts |
| Generalized | Segmental crural dystonia and dystonia in at least one additional body part |
| Hemidystonia | One-half of the body |

44. **What is torsion dystonia?**

    Torsion dystonia is a neurologic condition characterized by sustained contractions of both agonist and antagonist muscles, frequently causing twisting and repetitive movements or abnormal postures. Because there is no biochemical, pathologic, or radiologic marker for dystonia, the diagnosis is based on the recognition of clinical features. A characteristic feature of dystonia that helps to differentiate it from other hyperkinetic movement disorders is that dystonic movements are repetitive and patterned. For reasons that are poorly understood, patients with dystonia have the ability to suppress or decrease the involuntary movements by gently touching the affected area (sensory trick or geste antagonistique). Stress and fatigue make dystonia worse, whereas sleep and relaxation improve it.

45. **What features suggest the diagnosis of secondary dystonia?**

    Secondary forms of dystonia, which account for 25% of cases, are suspected in patients with a history of head trauma, peripheral trauma, encephalitis, toxin exposure, drug exposure, perinatal anoxia, kernicterus, and seizures. Abnormal findings such as dementia, ocular motility abnormalities, ataxia, spasticity, weakness, or amyotrophy are often present in patients with secondary dystonia. Furthermore, onset of dystonia at rest instead of with action, early onset of speech involvement, hemidystonia, abnormal laboratory tests, and abnormal brain imaging suggest the diagnosis of secondary dystonia. The list of causes of secondary dystonia is long, but it is important to try to identify those that are potentially treatable, especially Wilson's disease and tardive dystonia (Table 11-8).

### TABLE 11-8. CAUSES OF SECONDARY DYSTONIA

**Metabolic Disorders**
Amino acid disorders
  Glutaric aciduria
  Hartnup's disease
  Homocystinuria
  Methylmalonic acidemia
  Tyrosinosis
Lipid disorders
  Ceroid lipofuscinosis
  GM1-gangliosidose
  GM2-gangliosidose
  Metachromatic leukodystrophy
Miscellaneous metabolic disorders
  Leber's disease
  Leigh's disease
  Lesch-Nyhan syndrome
  Mitochondrial encephalopathies
  Triosephosphate isomerase deficiency
  Vitamin E deficiency
**Neurodegenerative disorders**
Ataxia telangiectasia
Azorean heredoataxia (Machado-Joseph disease)
Familial basal ganglia calcifications
Hallervorden-Spatz disease
Huntington's disease
Infantile bilateral striatal necrosis
Intraneuronal inclusion disease
Multiple sclerosis
Neuroacanthocytosis
Parkinson's disease
Progressive pallidal degeneration
Progressive supranuclear palsy
Rett syndrome
Wilson's disease

**Miscellaneous**
Arteriovenous malformation
Atlantoaxial dislocation or subluxation
Brain tumor
Cerebellar ectopia and syringomyelia
Central pontine myelinolysis
Cerebral vascular or ischemic injury
Drugs
  Anticonvulsants
  Antipsychotics
  Bromocriptine
  Ergot
  Fenfluramine
  Levodopa
  Metoclopramide
Head trauma
Infection
  Acute infectious torticollis
  AIDS
  Creutzfeldt-Jakob disease
  Encephalitis lethargica
  Reye's syndrome
  Subacute sclerosing panencephalitis
  Syphilis
  Tuberculosis
Paraneoplastic brain stem encephalitis
Perinatal cerebral injury and kernicterus
Peripheral trauma
Plagiocephaly
Psychogenic dystonia
Toxins
  Carbon monoxide
  Carbon disulfide
  Methane
  Wasp sting

**46. What are the most common types of idiopathic dystonia?**

The classic idiopathic dystonia, much more common among Ashkenazi Jews, is transmitted by an autosomal dominant gene whose expression is extremely variable. Phenocopies (sporadic cases) account for at least 20% of cases of idiopathic dystonia.

Paroxysmal dystonia encompasses a heterogenous and relatively rare group of conditions. Although psychogenic dystonia accounts for some cases, the majority are thought to be of neurologic origin, possibly representing a form of subcortical epilepsy, arising from the basal ganglia. The organic forms, sporadic or autosomal dominant, can be categorized as either kinesiogenic or nonkinesiogenic. Recently, mutation of the Myofibrillogenesis regulator 1 (MR-1) gene has been identified in 8 of 14 patients with the nonkinesiogenic variant. In the kinesiogenic variety, the attacks are precipitated by sudden movements, lasting less than 5 minutes and recurring up to 100 times per day. Anticonvulsants, such as carbamazepine and phenytoin, are usually effective in preventing the episodes. In the nonkinesiogenic paroxysmal dystonia, the attacks are less frequent (three per day), last longer (minutes to hours), and often are triggered by alcohol, coffee, and fatigue. Clonazepam is partially effective in most patients. Secondary paroxysmal dystonias may be caused by strokes, multiple sclerosis, and trauma to the peripheral and central nervous system (Figure 11-2).

Bruno MK, Lee HY, Aurburger GW, et al: Genotype-phenotype correlation of paroxysmal nonkinesiogenic dyskinesia. Neurology 68:1782-1789, 2007.

Segawa M: Hereditary progressive dystonia with marked diurnal fluctuation. Brain Dev 22 (Suppl 1):65-80, 2000.

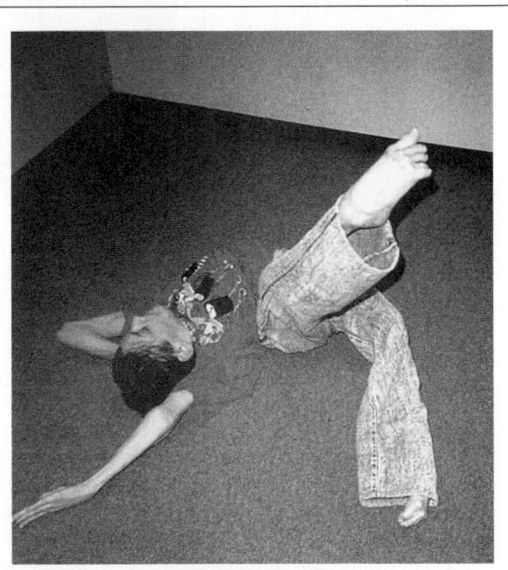

**Figure 11-2.** A patient with childhood-onset generalized dystonia.

**47. Where is the gene for classical dystonia located?**

Molecular genetic techniques link the dystonia (DYT1) gene to chromosome 9 (9q34). The mutation in the DYT1 gene has been characterized as a GAG deletion in the carboxy terminal of the gene that codes for an adenosine triphosphate-binding protein called *torsin A*. Evidence that adult-onset forms of focal dystonia are also related to the same gene awaits confirmation.

Brassat D, Camuzat A, Vidailhet M, et al.: Frequency of the DYT1 mutation in primary torsion dystonia without family history. Arch Neurol 57:333-335, 2000.

Saunders-Pullman R, Shriberg J, et al.: Penetrance and expression of dystonia genes. Adv Neurol 94:121-125, 2004.

**48. What is the most common form of focal dystonia?**

The cervical region is the area most frequently affected by dystonia. Among 1000 patients with dystonia at the Baylor College of Medicine Parkinson's Disease Center and Movement

Disorders Clinic, 76% have cervical dystonia, alone (33% patients) or associated with involvement of other areas. It is slightly more common in women (61%). Depending on the muscles involved, different types of postures are observed. Most patients with cervical dystonia have a combination of abnormal postures, such as torticollis, laterocollis, and anterocollis. Pain is a feature in about 70% of the patients with neck dystonia, whereas tremor, either dystonic or essential-type, is observed in 60% (Figure 11-3).

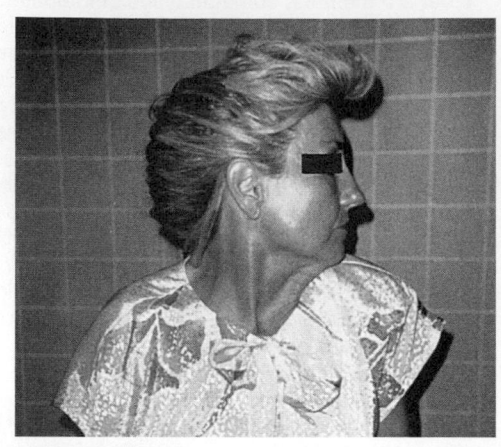

**Figure 11-3.** A patient with cervical dystonia manifested chiefly by torticollis to the left and marked contraction and hypertrophy of the right sternocleidomastoid muscle.

49. **What are the other forms of focal dystonia?**
Blepharospasm, either isolated (11%) or combined with oromandibular dystonia (23%), is the second most common form of focal dystonia. It is defined as an involuntary, bilateral eye closure produced by dystonic contractions of the orbicularis oculi muscles. Blepharospasm is three times more common in women than in men. Onset is usually gradual; often, before the onset of sustained eyelid closure, patients experience excessive blinking triggered by bright light, wind, and stress. With progression, most patients develop dystonia involving other facial muscles as well as the masticatory and cervical musculature. Sensory tricks that help to maintain the eyes open include pulling on the upper eyelids, talking, and yawning. Up to 15% of patients with blepharospasm become legally blind because of inability to keep their eyes open.

Dystonic writer's cramp is a form of task-specific dystonia associated with handwriting. Although able to use their hands for performing daily chores, after a few seconds or minutes of writing patients develop dystonic, usually painful, spasms of the forearm musculature, which prevent them from writing further. With progression of disease, the dystonia becomes less task-specific, occurs during other activities, and may spread to involve more proximal muscles. Approximately 50% of patients develop similar symptoms contralaterally. Other task-specific dystonias occur among musicians (piano player's cramp, guitar player's cramp) and others whose recreational or occupational activities require fine-motor coordination. The actual prevalence of these task-specific dystonias is unknown because only a few patients seek medical attention.

Frucht SJ: Focal task-specific dystonia in musicians. In Fahn S, Hallett M, DeLong M (eds): Dystonia 4: Advances in Neurology, vol 94. Philadelphia, Lippincott Williams & Wilkins 2004, pp 225-230.

50. **What are the most effective medications for the treatment of generalized or segmental dystonias?**
Levodopa, effective in about 10% of children with dystonia, should be tried in all childhood-onset dystonias. If there is no significant improvement in 2 months, levodopa is replaced by anticholinergics. The initial dose of trihexyphenidyl (Artane) is 2 mg twice daily. High doses, sometimes up to 100 mg/day, may be necessary. The benefits may not be

appreciated for 3 to 4 months after initiation of therapy. Moderate-to-dramatic improvement is observed in up to 70% of patients, but the efficacy may decrease with chronic use. The usefulness of these medications, especially in adults, is limited by the occurrence of peripheral (dry mouth and blurred vision) and central (forgetfulness, confusion, hallucinations) side effects. Other drugs that should be tried are baclofen, carbamazepine, benzodiazepines, and antidopaminergics. Extreme caution should be used with dopamine receptor–blocking drugs because of their potential to cause tardive dyskinesia (TD).

Levodopa (in children) and anticholinergics (in adults) are the first options among the systemic drugs. Clonazepam is occasionally highly effective in blepharospasm, whereas baclofen may be particularly useful in cranial dystonia. Systemic treatment of focal dystonias is disappointing, however. If oral medications are ineffective, local injections of botulinum toxin should be considered in patients with focal dystonia. Injections of botulinum toxin into the affected musculature are now considered the first choice of treatment.

51. **What surgical procedure is available for the treatment of dystonia?**
Patients with severe unilateral dystonia (hemidystonia) who are not responsive to medical therapy may benefit from pallidotomy or thalamotomy. More recently, deep brain stimulation (DBS) of the globus pallidus has been an effective treatment option for generalized dystonia in particular.

Coubes P, Cif L, El Fertit H, et al.: Electrical stimulation of the globus pallidus internus in patients with primary generalized dystonia: long-term results. J Neurosurg 101:189-194, 2004.

Vidailhet M, Vercueil L, Houeto JL, et al.: Bilateral deep-brain stimulation of the globus pallidus in primary generalized dystonia. N Engl J Med 352:459-467, 2005.

52. **What is the role of botulinum toxin in the treatment of dystonia?**
Botulinum toxin, one of the most lethal biologic toxins, is produced by the bacteria *Clostridium botulinum*. It acts at the neuromuscular junction, where it binds to the presynaptic cholinergic terminal and inhibits the release of acetylcholine. This functional denervation causes weakness and atrophy. After 3 to 4 months, sprouting and regrowth of the nerve terminals occur.

Botulinum toxin has been found to be effective in 95% of patients with blepharospasm, 90% of patients with spasmodic dysphonia, 85% of patients with cervical dystonia, and a majority of patients with oromandibular and hand dystonia. Patients with generalized dystonia displaying prominent disability in a single region may benefit from application of botulinum toxin to the involved area. The complications of botulinum toxin treatment are limited to local weakness; different consequences depend on the area. For example, patients with blepharospasm may have ptosis, whereas dysphagia is a potential complication of treatment for cervical dystonia. Most complications, however, resolve spontaneously after 2 to 4 weeks. A small percentage of patients (3% to 5% in some series) develop antibodies directed against botulinum toxin.

Anyanwu B, Hanna PA, Jankovic J: Botulinum toxin: Primary and secondary resistance. In Ward A, Barnes MP (eds): Clinical Uses of Botulinum Toxins. Cambridge, Mass: Cambridge University Press, 2007.

Jankovic J: Botulinum toxin in clinical practice. J Neurol Neurosurg Psychiatry 75:951-957, 2004.

Jankovic J, Vuong KD, Ahsan J: Comparison of efficacy and immunogenicity of original versus current botulinum toxin in cervical dystonia. Neurology 60:1186-1188, 2003.

53. **What other conditions may be treated with botulinum toxin?**
Conditions other than dystonia also have been successfully treated with botulinum toxin. Strabismus was the first disease to be treated with botulinum toxin. Ninety percent of patients with hemifacial spasm, a form of segmental myoclonus, improve with injections of the toxin. Over 50% of patients with tremor of the hand and/or head improve with botulinum

toxin. Reports also describe efficacy of this treatment in patients with various disorders associated with abnormal or inappropriate muscle contractions, including tics.

Kwak CH, Hanna PA, Jankovic J: Botulinum toxin in the treatment of tics. Arch Neurol 57:1190-1193, 2000.

## TIC DISORDERS

54. **What are tics?**

Tics are relatively brief, sudden, rapid, and intermittent movements (motor tics) or sounds (vocal tics). They may be repetitive and stereotypic. Tics are usually abrupt in onset and brief (clonic tics) but may be slow and sustained (dystonic tics). Examples of even more prolonged tics (tonic tics) include abdominal or limb tensing. Simple tics are caused by contractions of only one group of muscles and result in a brief, jerk-like movement or single, meaningless sound. Motor tics may also be complex, consisting of coordinated sequenced movements that resemble normal motor acts but are inappropriately intense and timed. Complex vocal tics include linguistically meaningful utterances and verbalizations. Tics, especially if dystonic, are associated with premonitory feelings that are relieved by performing the tics. Unlike other hyperkinetic dyskinesias, tics may be temporarily suppressed, leading some authors to suggest that in many patients they are purposefully, albeit irresistibly, performed (Table 11-9).

### TABLE 11-9. PHENOMENOLOGIC CLASSIFICATION OF TICS

| Motor Tics | Vocal Tics |
|---|---|
| **Simple tics** | **Simple tics** |
| Clonic tics | Blowing |
| Blinking | Coughing |
| Head jerking | Grunting |
| Nose twitching | Screaming |
| **Dystonic tics** | Sneezing |
| Abdominal tensing | Squeaking |
| Blepharospasm | Sucking |
| Bruxism | Throat clearing |
| Oculogyric movements | **Complex tics** |
| Shoulder rotation | Coprolalia (shouting of obscenities) |
| Sustained mouth opening | Echolalia (repetition of someone else's |
| Torticollis | phrases) |
| **Complex tics** | Palilalia (repetition of one's own |
| Copropraxia (obscene gestures) | utterances or phrases) |
| Echopraxia (imitating gestures) | |
| Head shaking | |
| Hitting | |
| Jumping | |
| Kicking | |
| Throwing | |
| Touching | |

**55. What are the most common causes of tic disorders?**
Tourette's syndrome and related disorders are the most important and common causes of tics. However, these dyskinesias may accompany other hereditary disorders or follow acquired diseases (Table 11-10).

---

**TABLE 11-10.  ETIOLOGIC CLASSIFICATION OF TICS**

**Physiologic tics**

| | |
|---|---|
| Mannerisms | Gestures |

**Pathologic tics**

*Primary*

| | |
|---|---|
| Transient tic disorder | Torsion dystonia |
| Chronic tic disorder | Huntington's disease |
|   Chronic motor tic disorder | Neuroacanthocytosis |
|   Chronic phonic tic disorder | |
|   Tourette's syndrome | |

*Secondary (Tourette's)*

| | |
|---|---|
| Chromosomal abnormalities | Infections |
|   Down syndrome |   Creutzfeldt-Jakob disease |
|   Fragile X syndrome |   Encephalitis |
|   XYY syndrome |   Postencephalitic parkinsonism |
|   XXX + 9p mosaicism | Sydenham's chorea |
| Drugs | Mental retardation |
|   Anticonvulsants |   Autism |
|   Dopamine receptor–blocking drugs |   Pervasive developmental disorders |
|   Levodopa |   Rett's syndrome |
|   Stimulants |   Rubella syndrome |
|     Amphetamine |   Static encephalopathy |
|     Cocaine | Others |
|     Methylphenidate |   Carbon monoxide poisoning |
|     Pemoline |   Schizophrenia |
| Head trauma |   Stroke |

---

**56. What features are necessary to make the diagnosis of Tourette's syndrome (TS)?**
According to currently established criteria, the diagnosis of TS requires all of the following features: onset before age 21, multiple motor tics, one or more vocal tics, fluctuating course, and presence of tics for more than 1 year. Tics that last less than 1 year are categorized as transient tic disorder (TTD). TTD is estimated to occur in 5% to 24% of schoolchildren; there is no accurate way to predict whether TTD will evolve into TS. Chronic motor tic disorder (CMTD) or chronic phonic tic disorder (CPTD) have the same criteria as TS, but patients display only either motor or phonic (vocal) tics.

TS, defined by the motor manifestations, is three times more frequent in males, but when obsessive compulsive disorder (OCD) is included, the male preponderance becomes much less significant. The onset is around age 7 years for facial tics with gradual progression in a rostrocaudal fashion. The diagnosis is often delayed because of a tendency to misinterpret or not recognize the tics or behavioral problems as abnormal. Behavioral problems usually precede the onset of tics by 2 to 3 years.

57. **What is the clinical spectrum of tic disorders and Tourette's syndrome?**
A growing body of evidence supports the notion that primary tic disorders represent a clinical spectrum, ranging from the mild TTD to TS. Several studies show that TTD, CMTD, CPTD, and TS are transmitted as inherited traits in the same families, suggesting that they may represent an expression of the same genetic defect. One problem with the current criteria of TS is that they do not take into account the extensive range of psychopathology and academic problems. For example, OCD is encountered in at least 50% of patients and is related to the same gene responsible for the expression of tics. Attention-deficit/hyperactivity disorder (ADHD) is also quite frequent (50% to 60%) among patients with TS, but the genetic association between the two conditions is less well understood. Other behavioral disturbances frequently observed in TS are aggressiveness, anxiety, conduct disorders, depression, learning difficulties, panic attacks, and sleep abnormalities.

58. **How is TS genetically transmitted?**
Tourette's syndrome displays a sex-influenced, autosomal dominant mode of inheritance with variable expressivity as TS, CMTD, or OCD. A recent advance has been the finding of a frameshift mutation in the slit and Trk-like1 (SLITRK1) gene located on chromosome 13q1.1.
Abelson JF, Kwan KY, O'Roak BJ, et al.: Sequence variants in SLITRK1 are associated with Tourette's syndrome. Science 310:317-320, 2005.

59. **How is Tourette's syndrome treated?**
Tics require treatment when they are socially embarrassing, painful (dystonic tics often cause pain), and severe enough to interfere with functioning. Their management relies on the use of dopamine blockers such as fluphenazine, which is more effective and associated with less sedation than other antidopaminergic drugs. Typically, a daily dose of 3 to 6 mg is sufficient to provide adequate relief. These drugs should be used cautiously because of the potential for causing tardive dyskinesia (TD).
The behavioral problems present in TS usually cause more disabilities than tics. Clonidine is considered the first option in the management of ADHD. A significant number of patients experience drowsiness at the beginning of treatment. Once they are stabilized on the medication, they are switched to a clonidine patch. Deprenyl, a specific inhibitor of the enzyme monoamine oxidase type B, the metabolites of which share some properties with amphetamines, has been shown in an open study to represent an effective alternative for treatment of ADHD without causing tics. Clomipramine is the first option to treat OCD, but imipramine, fluoxetine, and sertraline also may be useful. Carbamazepine and lithium are sometimes used in patients with impulse control problems (Table 11-11).
In recent reports, deep brain stimulation has been suggested for treatment of medically refractory patients. It appears promising as both motor and neuropsychiatric improvements have been suggested in these reports.
Maciunas RJ, Maddux BN, Riley DE, et al.: Prospective randomised double blind trial of bilateral thalamic deep brain stimulation in adults with Tourette syndrome. J Neurosurg 107:1004-1014, 2007.
Shahed J, Poysky J, Kenny C, et al.: GPi deep brain stimulation for Tourette syndrome improves tics and psychiatric comorbidities. Neurology 68:159-160, 2007.

| TABLE 11-11. GUIDELINES FOR THE TREATMENT OF TOURETTE'S SYNDROME ||
| Feature | Treatment |
| --- | --- |
| Tics | Fluphenazine |
| | Pimozide |
| | Haloperidol |
| | Trifluoperazine |
| | Molindone |
| | Tetrabenazine |
| | Botox |
| ADHD | Clonidine |
| | Deprenyl |
| | Methylphenidate |
| | Dextroamphetamine |
| OCD | Clomipramine |
| | Fluoxetine |
| | Imipramine |
| | Sertraline |
| Low impulse control | Carbamazepine |
| | Lithium |

*ADHD*, attention-deficit/hyperactivity disorder; *OCD*, obsessive compulsive disorder.

## CHOREA

60. **What is Huntington's disease (HD)?**
Huntington's disease is clinically characterized by the presence of a triad composed of chorea, cognitive decline, and a positive family history. Chorea consists of involuntary, continuous, abrupt, rapid, brief, unsustained, irregular movements that flow randomly from one body part to another. Patients can suppress chorea partially and temporarily and frequently incorporate movements into semipurposeful activities (parakinesia). Affected patients have a peculiar, irregular gait. Besides chorea, other motor symptoms include dysarthria, dysphagia, postural instability, ataxia, myoclonus, and dystonia. Motor impersistence is the inability to maintain constant voluntary muscle contraction such as in the characteristic milkmaid's grip during a handshake. The tone is decreased, and the deep reflexes are often hung up and pendular. All patients eventually develop dementia, mainly characterized by loss of recent memory and impairment of judgment, concentration, and acquisition. Neurobehavioral disturbances occasionally precede motor symptoms and consist of personality changes, apathy, social withdrawal, agitation, impulsiveness, depression, mania, paranoia, delusions, hostility, hallucinations, and psychosis.

Virtually all patients have a family history of a similar condition transmitted in an autosomal dominant fashion. Caudate and putamen atrophy on neuroimaging studies is another feature supportive of the diagnosis of HD.

Jankovic J, Ashizawa T: Huntington's disease. In Noseworthy J (ed): Neurological Therapeutics: Principles and Practice, London, Martin Dunitz, 2003.

61. **What is the Westphal variant?**
    In 10% of cases of HD, the onset is before age 20 (Westphal variant). The disease is then characterized by the combination of progressive parkinsonism, dementia, ataxia, and seizures.

62. **What are other common causes of chorea?**
    It is probable that levodopa-induced chorea in parkinsonism is the most common cause of chorea. Usually this diagnosis is not difficult once the history is available.
    The combination of chorea and psychiatric symptoms can be found in Wilson's disease. However, the diagnosis is easily made by finding a Kayser-Fleischer ring, low-plasma ceruloplasmin, and evidence of hepatic dysfunction. Sydenham's chorea is a form of autoimmune chorea, preceded by a group A streptococcal infection. Rarely encountered in the United States, this condition is one of the most common causes of chorea in underdeveloped areas. Systemic lupus erythematosus and primary antiphospholipid antibody syndrome are other causes of autoimmune chorea. Senile chorea is a condition in which chorea is the only feature; no family history of HD is present.
    Ala A, Walker AP, Ashkan K, et al.: Wilson's disease. Lancet 369:397-408, 2007.

63. **Is it possible to make a diagnosis of HD in asymptomatic individuals?**
    The HD gene (designated IT15) has been identified near the tip of the short arm of chromosome 4 (4p16.3). An unstable expansion of the CAG repeat sequence is present at the 5' end of this large (210 kb) gene. The HD gene encodes a 348-kDa protein called *huntingtin*. Recent studies suggest that the aggregation of mutant huntingtin may be part of the pathogenesis of HD. All patients with HD studied to date have had >36 CAG repeats, but repeat length as short as 29 has been reported with pathologically proven HD. HD families also display "anticipation," or progressively earlier onset of disease in successive generations, typically with increasing CAG repeat size. Such findings allow genetic testing of at-risk individuals before the onset of symptoms. However, until effective treatment is available for HD, many ethical and legal dilemmas associated with genetic testing remain to be solved.
    Ravina B, Romer M, Constantinescu R, et al.: The relationship between CAG repeat length and clinical progression in Huntington's disease. Mov Disord 23:1223-1227, 2008.
    Rosenblatt A, Liang KY, Zhou H, et al.: The association of CAG repeat with clinical progression in Huntington disease. Neurology 66:1016-1020, 2006.

64. **What are the neuropathologic findings in HD?**
    The most important pathologic findings in HD are neuronal loss and gliosis in the cortex and striatum, particularly the caudate nucleus. Chorea seems to be primarily related to loss of medium spiny striatal neurons projecting to the lateral pallidum. This results in functional hypoactivity of the STN with consequent hyperactivity of the thalamic tier. Cortical thinning in various parts such as sensorimotor, parietal, occipital, and inferior temporal lobes is now being recognized in HD and has been associated with earlier cognitive symptoms.
    Rosas HD, Salat DH, Lee SY, et al.: Cerebral cortex and the clinical expression of Huntington's disease: Complexity and heterogeneity. Brain 131(Pt 4):1057-1068, 2008.

65. **Is there any protective treatment for HD?**
    Unfortunately, to date no therapeutic intervention has been capable of halting the relentless progression of HD. In the adult form, death occurs after a mean duration of 15 years, whereas in the juvenile variant the mean survival is 9 years. Tetrabenazine in observational and randomized controlled trials has significantly reduced chorea in HD. Other treatments include neuroleptics, which temporarily relieve chorea and psychosis by interfering with dopaminergic transmission. However, these drugs cause several side effects, including tardive dyskinesia (TD). An alternative approach is to use medications that deplete presynaptic dopamine (e.g., reserpine), which have not been reported to cause TD. Benzodiazepines and antidepressants

are also commonly used for anxiety and depression associated with HD. Fetal transplantation has shown no beneficial results.

Huntington Study Group: Tetrabenazine as antichorea therapy in Huntington disease. Neurology 66:366-372, 2006.

Kenney C, Hunter C, Davidson A, et al.: Short term effects of tetrabenazine on chorea associated with Huntington's disease. Mov Disord 22:10-13, 2007.

## DRUG-INDUCED MOVEMENT DISORDERS

66. **What is an acute dystonic reaction?**
Acute dystonic reaction is an abrupt, drug-induced dystonia, especially of the head and neck. About 2.5% of patients treated with neuroleptics develop ADR within the first 48 hours of treatment. Cocaine use increases the likelihood of ADR. Although it is one of the first described neuroleptic-induced movement disorders, the pathophysiology of ADR remains unknown. Because it follows the use of dopamine receptor–blocking drugs and improves with anticholinergics, it is presumed that changes in the striatal dopamine and acetylcholine are important in the genesis of ADR.

67. **What is tardive dyskinesia?**
Tardive dyskinesia is a hyperkinetic movement disorder caused by dopamine receptor–blocking drugs. According to current criteria, it is possible to make the diagnosis of TD when the hyperkinesia develops during treatment with neuroleptics or within 6 months of their discontinuation and persists for at least 1 month after stopping all neuroleptic agents. It is estimated that 20% of patients exposed to neuroleptics develop TD, but the values range from 13% to 49%. Severe TD seems to be more common in young males and elderly females.

## KEY POINTS: BASAL GANGLIA AND MOVEMENT DISORDERS

1. Loss of pigmented dopaminergic neurons in the substantia nigra is the pathologic hallmark of PD.

2. Sinemet (levodopa) remains the most valuable therapy for PD.

3. Essential tremor is the most common cause of non-parkinsonian tremor.

4. Cervical dystonia (torticollis) is the most common form of focal dystonia.

5. Botulinum toxin is the treatment of choice for most focal dystonias.

6. Tardive dyskinesia is a serious side effect of many neuroleptic drugs.

68. **What is the importance of recognizing stereotypy in an adult patient?**
Stereotypy is defined as a seemingly purposeful, coordinated, but involuntary, repetitive, ritualistic gesture, mannerism, posture, or utterance. Examples of stereotypies include repetitive grimacing, lip smacking, tongue protruding, and chewing movements. The tongue also may move laterally in the mouth ("bon-bon sign"). In addition, patients with tardive dyskinesias, the most common form of adult-onset stereotypy, often exhibit head bobbing, body rocking, leg crossing and uncrossing, picking at clothing, shifting weight, and marching in place.

Stereotypy is the most common form of TD (78% of cases). The second most common form of TD is dystonia (75% of patients). The presence of stereotypies in an adult without mental retardation or untreated schizophrenia strongly suggests the diagnosis of TD, especially in association with other movement disorders commonly present in TD (akathisia, tremor, myoclonus, chorea, and tics) (Figure 11-4).

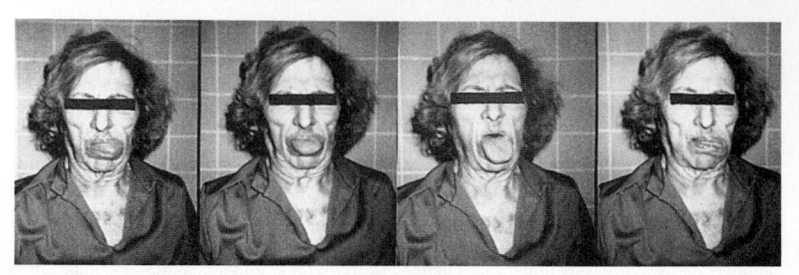

**Figure 11-4.** A patient with tardive dyskinesias manifesting stereotypic orolingual movements.

### 69. What is the pathogenesis of TD?

Because medications that cause TD block the dopamine receptors, dysfunction of striatal dopaminergic systems has been implicated in the pathogenesis. However, the mechanism of production of TD is still not understood. Clinical and experimental evidence suggests that TD and LID share a common pathogenetic mechanism. These studies suggest that TD ultimately results from disruption of the lateral pallidal-subthalamic GABAergic projection, leading to inhibition of the STN. Recent evidence supports the notion that dopamine receptor–blocking drugs exert a neurotoxic effect, resulting in neuronal damage. There is no explanation, however, for the diversity of movement

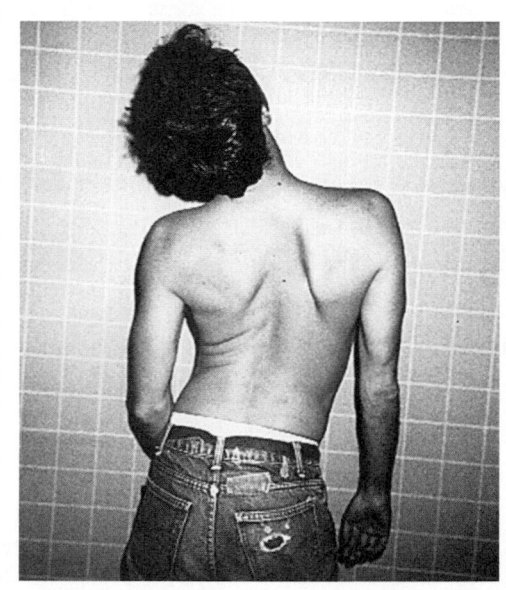

**Figure 11-5.** A patient with axial tardive dystonia.

disorders in TD. The relatively specific pharmacologic profile of each of these dyskinesias suggests that different mechanisms are involved in their generation (Figure 11-5).

**70. How is TD treated?**
The first step in the treatment of TD is to stop the offending drug, which results in spontaneous remission in approximately 60% of cases. Drugs that deplete dopamine, such as reserpine, are the most effective agents for treatment of TD. Tardive dystonia has a less satisfactory response to systemic treatment than other forms of TD. TD may improve with anticholinergic agents, whereas the other types, including stereotypy, may worsen. In patients with focal forms of dystonia, such as cranial and cervical dystonia, injection of botulinum toxin into the affected musculature is a useful and safe alternative. In a small trial, levetiracetam was found to be useful in reducing TD.

Konitsiotis S, Pappa S, Mantas C, et al.: Levetiracetam in tardive dyskinesia: An open label study. Mov Disord 21:1219-1221, 2006.

Ondo WG, Hanna PA, Jankovic J: Tetrabenazine treatment for tardive dyskinesia: Assessment by randomized videotape protocol. Am J Psychiatry 156:1279-1281, 1999.

## OTHER MOVEMENT DISORDERS

**71. How can myoclonus be distinguished from chorea and tics?**
Myoclonus is defined as a brief, sudden, shocklike jerk that may be caused not only by active muscle contractions (positive myoclonus) but also by lapses of muscle contraction (negative myoclonus). Many of the individual movements of chorea are myoclonic, but, unlike myoclonus, they are continuous, occurring in a constant flow. Tics may resemble myoclonus, but they are usually preceded by premonitory feelings, and patients usually have some degree of control over them.

**72. How is myoclonus classified?**
Myoclonus may be classified by etiology, pathophysiology, and distribution (Table 11-12).

| TABLE 11-12. CLASSIFICATION OF MYOCLONUS |
|---|

### Etiology

| | |
|---|---|
| *Physiologic myoclonus* | *Epileptic myoclonus (continued)* |
|   Anxiety |   Fragments of epilepsy |
|   Benign infantile myoclonus with feeding |     Epilepsia partialis continua |
|   Exercise |     Isolated myoclonic epileptic |
|   Hiccup |       myoclonic jerks |
|   Nocturnal myoclonus |     Myoclonic absences in petit mal |
| *Essential myoclonus* |     Photosensitive myoclonus |
|   Autosomal dominant |     Progressive myoclonus epilepsy |
|   Sporadic | *Symptomatic myoclonus* |
| *Epileptic myoclonus* |   Basal ganglia degenerations |
|   Benign familial myoclonic epilepsy |     Cortical basal ganglionic degeneration |
|   Childhood myoclonic epilepsies |     Hallervorden-Spatz disease |
|     Cryptogenic myoclonus epilepsy |     Huntington's disease |
|     Infantile spasms |     Myoclonic dystonia |
|     Juvenile myoclonus epilepsy |     Parkinson's disease |
|     Myoclonic astatic epilepsy |     Progressive supranuclear palsy |

*(continued)*

## TABLE 11–12. CLASSIFICATION OF MYOCLONUS *(continued)*

### Etiology *(continued)*

**Symptomatic myoclonus** *(continued)*

Dementias
  Alzheimer's disease
  Creutzfeldt-Jakob disease
  Gerstmann-Sträussler-Scheinker
    syndrome
Focal lesions
  Dentato-olivary lesions
  Stroke
  Thalamotomy
  Trauma (CNS or peripheral
    nervous system)
  Tumor
Metabolic and toxic encephalopathies
  Biotin deficiency
  Bismuth
  DDT
  Drugs, including levodopa
  Dialysis syndrome
  Heavy metal poisoning
  Hepatic failure
  Hypoglycemia
  Hyponatremia
  Infantile myoclonic encephalopathy
  Methyl bromide

Metabolic/toxic encephalopathies
  (continued)
  Mitochondrial encephalopathy
  Multiple carboxylase deficiency
  Nonketotic hyperglycemia
Physical encephalopathies
  Decompression injury
  Electric shock
  Heat stroke
  Posthypoxia
Spinocerebellar degeneration
Storage disease
  Ceroid lipofuscinosis
  Lafora body disease
  Lipidoses
    GM1-gangliosidosis
    GM2-gangliosidosis
    Krabbe's disease
    Tay-Sachs disease
Viral encephalopathies
  Arbor virus encephalitis
  Encephalitis lethargica
  Herpes simplex encephalitis
  Postinfectious encephalitis
  Subacute sclerosing panencephalitis

### Pathophysiology

| *Cortical* | *Brain stem* | *Spinal* |
|---|---|---|
| Epilepsia partialis continua | Palatal | Propriospinal |
| Focal | Essential | Segmental |
| Generalized | Symptomatic | *Peripheral* |
| Multifocal | Reticular | |
| *Thalamic* | Startle | |

### Distribution

| | | |
|---|---|---|
| Axial | Generalized | Segmental |
| Focal | Multifocal | |

Adapted from Marsden CD: Myoclonus: Classification and treatment. Syllabus for the Movement Disorders Course, AAN, 1992, p. 93.

73. **How is myoclonus treated?**
Recognition of the different types of myoclonus has practical implications because each of the categories has a unique pathophysiologic mechanism and specific treatment. Myoclonus related to metabolic encephalopathies improves with treatment of the metabolic disturbance. Epileptic myoclonus is initially treated with sodium valproate. If toxic reactions occur or the patient is still symptomatic, either clonazepam or primidone may be added. Clonazepam is the first choice in myoclonus arising from the brain stem, but 5-hydroxy-tryptophan, clomipramine, and fluoxetine are useful alternatives. Spinal and other segmental myoclonus also may respond to clonazepam or drugs that enhance serotoninergic transmission, but injections of botulinum toxin in the affected musculature have been the most useful treatment. Recent studies with levetiracetam for the treatment of cortical myoclonus have shown some promising results as an antimyoclonic agent.
   Striano P, Manganelli F, Boccella P, et al.: Levetiracetam in patients with cortical myoclonus: A clinical and electrophysiological study. Mov Disord 20:1610-1614, 2005.

74. **What is asterixis?**
Asterixis is a form of negative myoclonus mainly associated with metabolic encephalopathies; electrophysiologically, it is characterized by the presence of brief silences of electric muscular activity. Although originally described in patients with hepatic encephalopathy, asterixis may be caused by many other conditions. The early stages of metabolic dysfunction assume a rhythmic aspect, resembling tremor. With progression of the underlying cause, when patients hold their arms outstretched, the wrists display a characteristic flexion (caused by electric silence in the antigravity muscles) (Table 11-13).

### TABLE 11-13. CAUSES OF ASTERIXIS

| Hepatic Failure | Drugs | Lesions in the CNS |
|---|---|---|
| Respiratory failure | Anticonvulsants | Medial frontal cortex |
| Renal failure | Salicylates | Parietal lobe |
| Cardiac failure | Levodopa | Internal capsule |
| Chronic hemodialysis | | Thalamus |
| Polycythemia | | Rostral midbrain |

75. **What is stiff person syndrome (SPS)?**
Patients with this rare disorder have progressive, usually symmetric, rigidity of the axial muscles that may fluctuate in intensity. Motion, tactile stimulation, emotion, and startle are common triggering factors of the spasms. EMG shows continuous normal motor unit potentials in the affected muscles despite the patient's attempts to relax. The diagnosis is supported by relief of the rigidity with general and spinal anesthesia, peripheral nerve blocks, and diazepam, which is still the first-line treatment of SPS. In refractory cases, propofol, rituximab, and IVIG have been reported to be of benefit. It should be noted that use of general anesthesia in patients with SPS carries a risk of postoperative hypotonia, especially with concomitant use with muscle relaxants.
   An insight into the pathophysiology of SPS was provided by the finding that 20 of 33 patients had autoantibodies against glutamic acid dehydoxylase (GAD). The hypothesis of an autoimmune etiology of SPS is further supported by the presence of other autoantibodies (e.g., to islet cells and gastric parietal cells), coexistent autoimmune diseases such as

insulin-dependent diabetes mellitus, vitiligo, thyroid disease, family history of presumed autoimmune conditions, and improvement with plasmapheresis and corticosteroid drugs.

Dalakas MG: The role of IVIg in the treatment of patients with stiff person syndrome and other neurological diseases associated with antiGAD antibodies. J Neurol 252(Suppl 1):I19-I25, 2005.

Koerner C, Wieland B, Richter W, et al.: Stiff-person syndromes: motor cortex hyperexcitability correlates with anti-GAD autoimmunity. Neurology 62:1357-1362, 2004.

## 76. What is Wilson's disease?

Wilson's disease is an autosomal recessive disease; the gene is linked to markers located in the q14-21 region on chromosome 13. The prevalence of the disease is estimated to be 1 in 30,000. It is associated with impaired incorporation of copper into ceruloplasmin as well as impaired biliary excretion of copper. The result is copper overloading in the liver, cornea, and brain, particularly in the basal ganglia. Virtually all patients display laboratory and/or clinical evidence of liver insufficiency. The most useful laboratory screening test is plasma ceruloplasmin, which usually is less than 20 mg/dL (normal: 24 to 45 mg/dL).

The most common neurologic findings are parkinsonism, bulbar signs (e.g., dysarthria and dysphagia), dystonia, postural tremor, and ataxia. Psychiatric symptoms, such as depression and psychosis, are particularly common among adults.

MRI of the head may display either decreased or increased signal intensity in the striatum on T2-weighted images. MRI of the midbrain may show a specific "face of a giant panda" appearance, which is produced by reversal of the normal hypointensity of the substantia nigra, midbrain tegmentum, and hypointensity in the superior colliculi.

Ala A, Walker AP, Ashkan K, et al.: Wilson's disease. Lancet 369:397-408, 2007.

## 77. What is the treatment for Wilson's disease?

Early diagnosis is essential because treatment with copper-chelating agents often completely reverses the neurologic and hepatic symptoms. All siblings and cousins should be screened because presymptomatic patients require treatment to prevent development of symptoms. Penicillamine is the drug of choice for Wilson's disease; the typical dose is 250 mg 4 times a day in combination with pyridoxine (25 mg/day). Side effects are initial exacerbation of symptoms, rash, optic neuritis, thrombocytopenia, leukopenia, and nephrotoxicity. Other options to decrease copper overload are triethylene tetramine dihydrochloride, zinc sulphate, and tetrathiomolybdate. Symptomatic treatment of neurologic symptoms includes levodopa, anticholinergics, and injections of botulinum toxin. Liver transplant may be necessary in terminal cases of hepatic insufficiency.

## 78. What are the paraneoplastic movement disorders?

Opsoclonus-myoclonus designates a combination of rapid, erratic, involuntary movements of the eyes, with multifocal myoclonus (dancing eyes–dancing feet syndrome). Most cases occur between ages 6 and 18 months. Fifty percent of cases are related to an underlying neoplasm, especially neuroblastoma. This syndrome also occurs in adults with brain stem encephalitis, either paraneoplastic or infectious (Whipple's disease). Steroids dramatically improve this form of myoclonus. A few cases have been reported in patients with SPS, breast cancer, and autoantibodies against amphiphysin.

Ataxia is another well-established paraneoplastic movement disorder. The mechanism is cerebellar degeneration related to anti-Purkinje cell antibodies. There are also reports of parkinsonism, chorea, dystonia, segmental rigidity, and action and segmental myoclonus as remote effects of neoplasm.

Samii A, Dahlen DD, Spence AM, et al.: Paraneoplastic movement disorder in a patient with non-Hodgkin's lymphoma and CRMP-5 autoantibody. Mov Disord 18:1556-1558, 2003.

## WEBSITES

1. http://www.apdaparkinson.org

2. http://www.psp.org

3. http://www.tsa-usa.org

## BIBLIOGRAPHY

1. Fahn S, Jankovic J: Principles and Practice of Movement Disorders. Philadelphia, Churchill Livingstone, 2007.

2. Jankovic J: The extrapyramidal disorders. In Goldman L, Ausiello D, eds. Cecil Textbook of Medicine, 22nd ed. Philadelphia, WB Saunders, 2004.

3. Jankovic J, Lang AE: Movement disorders: diagnosis and assessment. In Bradley WG, Daroff RB, Fenichel GM, et al (eds): Neurology in Clinical Practice, 4th ed. Philadelphia, Butterworth-Heinemann, 2004.

4. Jankovic J, Tolosa E, eds. Parkinson's Disease and Movement Disorders, 5th ed. Baltimore, Williams & Wilkins, 2006.

# CHAPTER 12

# AUTONOMIC NERVOUS SYSTEM

*Yadollah Harati, MD, FACP, and Shahram Izadyar, MD*

1. **What are the physiologic responses to stimulation of the sympathetic and parasympathetic systems?**
   See Figure 12-1.

| Sympathetic stimulation | Parasympathetic stimulation |
|---|---|
| Tachycardia | Bradycardia |
| Increased heart contractility | Decreased heart contractility |
| Bronchodilation | Bronchoconstriction |
| Decreased peristalsis | Increased peristalsis |
| Mydriasis | Miosis |
| Ciliary muscle relaxation (far vision) | Ciliary muscle contraction (near vision) |
| Bladder internal sphincter contraction | Bladder internal sphincter relaxation |
| Detrusor relaxation | Detrusor contraction |
| Ejaculation | Penile erection |
| Decreased kidney output | Increased exocrine gland secretion (salivary, lacrimal) |
| | |
| Vasoconstriction | Vasodilation |
| Piloerection | |
| Increased sweating | |
| Glycogenolysis, gluconeogenesis | |
| Lipolysis | |

2. **What features of the history must be explored in all patients with suspected autonomic dysfunction?**
   Some cardinal symptoms of autonomic dysfunction may be drug-induced or have a psychogenic etiology. With this caveat in mind, special attention to symptoms involving the following systems is essential when obtaining a history:
   1. **Cardiovascular**—Orthostatic lightheadedness, dizziness, blurred vision, syncope or near-syncope, fatigue, weakness (especially in the legs on standing), headache, and neck ache after prolonged standing (coat hanger phenomenon), postprandial or postexercise lightheadedness or angina pectoris, fainting after alcohol ingestion or insulin injection, palpitations, resting tachycardia, orthostatic cerebral transient ischemic attack symptoms, angina pectoris.
   2. **Sudomotor and vasomotor**—Partial or complete loss of sweating, heat intolerance (hot, flush, dizzy, and weak without sweating), excessive sweating (partial or total), facial and upper trunk gustatory sweating (especially when food incites salivation or with ingestion of cheese), nocturnal sweating, skin cracks on distal extremities, dry and shiny skin, unusually cold or warm feet, reduced skin wrinkling, peripheral edema.
   3. **Secretomotor**—Dry mouth and eyes, increased saliva production.
   4. **Genitourinary**—History of urinary tract infections, lengthened interval between micturitions, increased volume of first morning void, need for straining to initiate and maintain voiding, weakness of stream, postvoid dribbling, sensation of incomplete emptying of bladder, overflow incontinence, frequency and urgency with or without dysuria

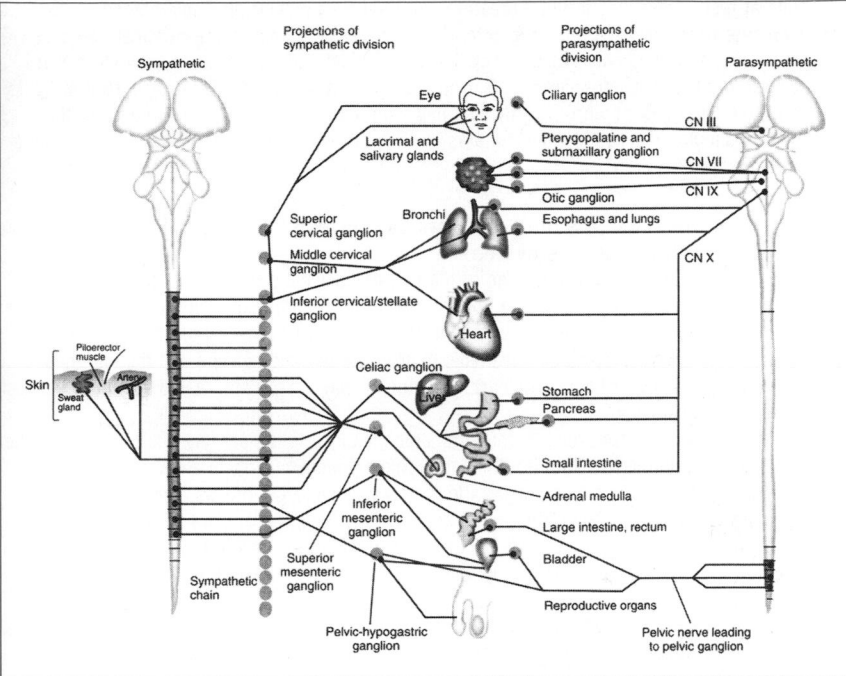

**Figure 12-1.** Sympathetic and parasympathetic nervous systems. From Nadeau SE, Ferguson TS, Valenstein E, et al.: Medical Neuroscience. Philadelphia, Saunders, 2004, p 504.

(with superimposed infection), impotence (difficulty in initiating and/or maintaining erection), reduced or absent waking erection, diminished libido, decreased volume of ejaculation, inability to ejaculate, retrograde ejaculation, reduced vaginal lubrication.

5. **Respiratory**—Irregular breathing or apnea during sleep.
6. **Gastrointestinal**—Dysphagia, retrosternal discomfort, heartburn, anorexia, epigastric fullness during or after meals, recurrent episodes of nausea and vomiting (fasting and/or postprandial) associated with upper abdominal pain, constipation, diarrhea (especially nocturnal), or fecal incontinence (especially at night), weight loss. Note that explosive diarrhea and severe constipation may alternate.
7. **Ocular**—Blurring of vision, trouble focusing, photophobia, difficulty seeing at night, drooping of eyelids.
8. **Factors aggravating symptoms**—Alcohol, continued standing, hot temperature (environmental, hot bath, fever), exercise, bed rest, food ingestion, and hyperventilation.

3. **What physical examination must be performed in all patients with suspected autonomic dysfunction?**
A careful examination of the skin provides valuable clues to the presence of autonomic dysfunction. Particular attention should be given to acral vasomotor and trophic changes of the skin, abnormal sweating patterns, and the presence of allodynia or hyperalgesia. Examination of the eyes (ptosis) and pupillary shape, size, and response to light and accommodation is essential. Cardiovascular examination includes measurement of the heart

rate at rest in response to deep breathing and Valsalva maneuver. Supine blood pressure (BP) and heart rate after 5 to 10 min of rest followed by measurement after active standing for 3 min should be checked in every patient with suspected dysautonomia. If orthostatic hypotension (systolic BP drop >20 mmHg or diastolic BP drop >10 mmHg) is not noted in a patient who nevertheless has symptoms of orthostatic hypotension, the patient should be asked to do 12 squats (orthostatic stress test), after which the standing BP is repeated.

4. **What are the major anatomic differences between the sympathetic and parasympathetic nervous systems?**
   The sympathetic neurons are located in the interomediolateral (IML) and intermediomedial (IMM) columns of the thoracic and upper lumbar spinal cord. Axons of these neurons make synaptic contact with ganglionic neurons in the bilateral paravertebral or largely unpaired prevertebral ganglia. The parasympathetic neurons lie in the brainstem and the intermediate zone of the sacral spinal cord. The parasympathetic relay ganglia are located near or in the wall of the effector organs.

   Because of the close proximity of sympathetic ganglia to the primary efferent sympathetic neurons (IML and IMM columns), the sympathic preganglionic fibers are short, whereas the postganglionic fibers may extend a long way to their target organs. The parasympathetic preganglionic axons, on the other hand, are relatively long myelinated fibers that synapse with parasympathetic relay ganglia located near or within the wall of individual innervated organs. The postganglionic parasympathetic fibers, are, therefore, short (1 mm to several centimeters).

   The number of postganglionic neurons is very close to the number of preganglionic neurons in the parasympathetic system. On the other hand, the high ratio of postganglionic to preganglionic neurons in the sympathetic system explains the massive sympathetic outflow and the wide range of autonomic effects that occur during strenuous and stressful situations. Sympathetic activation can lead to simultaneous and diverse reactions including raised arterial blood pressure, increased blood flow to active muscles, increased muscle glycolysis and blood glucose level, enhanced mental activity and muscular strength, increased sphincter contraction, and decreased gastrointestinal peristalsis. A disorder that predominantly affects the sympathetic nervous system may, therefore, render the body incapable of dealing appropriately with strenuous physical or emotional stimulation. In contrast, the small difference between the number of preganglionic and postganglionic neurons in the parasympathetic system promotes a more localized response and allows a highly specific, controlled output.

5. **Discuss the major neurotransmitters and their receptors in the autonomic nervous system.**
   **Acetylcholine (ACh)** is the neurotransmitter for all preganglionic and for the parasympathetic postganglionic neurons. ACh receptors in the autonomic nervous system are divided into nicotinic and muscarinic types. Nicotinic receptors, of which there are multiple subtypes found mainly in the ganglia, are ligand-gated sodium channels that mediate fast responses. Muscarinic receptors mediate slower responses and are found mostly throughout autonomic effector tissues. Five subtypes of muscarinic receptors ($M_1$ to $M_5$) have been identified and cloned.

   **Norepinephrine (NE)** is the neurotransmitter for most sympathetic postganglionic fibers. Adrenergic receptors are divided into alpha ($\alpha_1$ and $\alpha_2$) and beta ($\beta_1$, $\beta_2$, and $\beta_3$) types and are localized in various autonomic effector tissues. Determining the importance of subtypes $\alpha_1$ ($\alpha_{1A}$, $\alpha_{1B}$, and $\alpha_{1D}$) and $\alpha_2$ ($\alpha_{2A}$, $\alpha_{2B}$, and $\alpha_{2C}$) receptors is a major area of current investigation.

6. **What other neurotransmitters play a role in the autonomic nervous system?**
   Researchers have identified a plethora of neuropeptides that act as neuromodulators or cotransmitters in autonomic signaling. Examples include substance P, calcitonin gene-related peptide (CGRP), somatostatin, vasoactive intestinal peptide, oxytocin, and enkephalins. Less conventional neurotransmitters such as nitric oxide, purines (adenosine triphosphate [ATP]), and carbon monoxide have recently been implicated in autonomic transmission as well. The colocalization of more than one neurotransmitter to a single nerve terminal is well documented.

7. **How useful is measurement of plasma catecholamines in the evaluation of dysautonomia?**
   There are six detectable catecholamines in human plasma: the three main catecholamines of the body (epinephrine, NE, and dopamine), their precursor (L-3,4-dihydroxyphenylalanine [DOPA; levodopa]), and their metabolites (dihydroxyphenylacetic acid [DOPAC] and dihydroxyphenylglycol [DHPG]).
   The main source of plasma NE is the sympathetic network around blood vessels. However, most of the released NE is metabolized before spilling over to the plasma and only a small proportion enters the blood stream unchanged. The plasma level of NE is also affected by its removal rate. Accordingly, an elevated plasma NE level could suggest a high rate of sympathetic activity or a decreased rate of clearance from plasma. Measurement of both NE and DHPG levels can provide further information about the mechanism involved. DHPG is derived from the metabolism of NE following its reuptake in the sympathetic nerve endings. An increased plasma level of NE mediated by increased sympathetic activity is associated with elevated DHPG. On the other hand, if the diminished NE reuptake is the cause of increased NE level, an increase in plasma DHPG would not be observed. Various processes such as emotion, exercise, eating, smoking, caffeine, medications, time of day, blood volume, hypoglycemia, and pathologic states such as cardiac ischemia affect the release, reuptake, metabolism, and removal of this hormone. The plasma NE level, therefore, must be interpreted with caution, taking the influence of the mentioned factors into account.

8. **What is the normal catecholamine response?**
   In normal subjects, the plasma level of NE is 150 to 170 pg/mL after 30 min in the supine position; it increases 50% to 100% above supine values after 5 minutes of standing, and remains constant after 10 minutes of standing.

9. **How does age affect catecholamine measurements?**
   Because plasma NE increases with age, the value must be corrected for age. The mechanism for increase with age is controversial; both reduced clearance and increased release have been suggested. Microneurographic recordings show an increase in muscle sympathetic activity with age, supporting the hypothesis of increased NE release.

10. **Can catecholamine measurements localize the site of autonomic dysfunction?**
    Patients with a neuropathy causing a primarily postganglionic autonomic abnormality (such as pure autonomic failure) have a subnormal plasma level of NE in the supine position that fails to increase during standing. In patients with intact postganglionic neurons (such as multiple system atrophy) the plasma level of NE in the supine position remains within normal limits, but fails to increase upon standing, similar to postganglionic abnormalities. Because of considerable overlap between preganglionic and postganglionic abnormalities in individual patients with autonomic dysfunction, plasma NE values alone are usually not sufficiently diagnostic for the site of the lesion.

11. **What are the central structures that regulate the autonomic functions?**
Telencephalic, diencephalic, and brain stem structures are involved in autonomic control. Insular cortex, anterior cingulate cortex, and amygdala are parts of the telencephalon that are in close contact with the hypothalamus and brain stem and play a central role in integration of bodily sensations and emotions. Hypothalamic and thalamic nuclei, as part of the diencephalic structures, are essential for maintaining the homeostasis of the body and integrating autonomic and endocrine responses. Brain stem structures such as periaqueductal gray, parabrachial nucleus, nucleus tract solitarii (NTS), ventrolateral medullary (LVM), and medullary raphe all play crucial roles in cardiovascular function, respiration, and thermoregulation.

12. **What is the role of the NTS in the central autonomic network?**
This important nucleus, situated at the dorsomedial medulla, receives inputs from neocortical regions and from nuclei of the forebrain, higher brain stem, and diencephalon. The visceral afferents, which convey information important to the reflexive regulation of cardiac rhythm and motility, peripheral vascular tone, respiration, and gastrointestinal motility and secretion, terminate at different parts of this nucleus. Most efferent fibers from the NTS terminate in the parabrachial nucleus, which in turn project to higher brain stem sites, hypothalamus, basal forebrain, and cerebral cortex. Efferent fibers from the NTS also end on the neurons of the reticular formation of the ventrolateral medulla, which in turn project to the IML cell column of the lateral horn of the spinal cord. In addition to autonomic afferent and efferent fibers, the NTS also receives somatic afferents from the spinal cord (dorsolateral horn) and spinal trigeminal lemniscus. This allows the NTS to serve as an integration station for the autonomic and somatic information, playing a vital role in the maintenance of body homeostasis (Figure 12-2). The NTS also plays a major role in gustatory processing within the medulla. There is evidence indicating norepinephrine neurons in the NTS play a role in transmission of signals from the peripheral nervous system to brain structures involved in memory and learning. Recent studies have revealed an actual neuroanatomical pathway between NTS norepinephrine neurons and hippocampus.
   Note: Nucleus tracti solitarii is the correct Latin term for this nucleus. Nucleus tractus solitarious or nucleus tracti solitarious are distorted but commonly used terms.

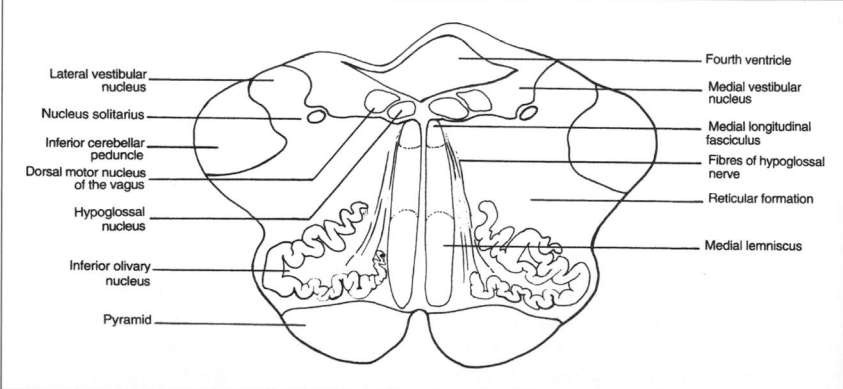

**Figure 12-2.** Transverse section through the rostral medulla, showing the nucleus solitarius or nucleus solitarii. From Crossman AR, Neary D: Neuroanatomy, An Illustrated Colour Text. Edinburgh, Churchill Livingstone, 2000, p 94.

13. **What are the most important peripheral neuropathies associated with autonomic dysfunction?**
See Table 12-1.

### TABLE 12-1. PERIPHERAL NEUROPATHIES ASSOCIATED WITH AUTONOMIC DYSFUNCTION

**Inherited peripheral neuropathies with dysautonomia**

- HSAN I, II, III* (Riley-Day syndrome), IV, and V
- HMSN I and II
- Fabry's disease*
- MEN 2b
- Amyloidosis* (familial amyloid polyneuropathy types I, II, and III)
- Porphyria*
- Some spinocerebellar degenerations

**Infectious, parainfectious, and immune-mediated peripheral neuropathies with dysautonomia**

- Leprosy
- AIDS
- Chagas' disease
- Diphtheria
- Systemic lupus erythematosus
- Systemic sclerosis
- Sjögren syndrome
- Rheumatoid arthritis
- Mixed connective tissue disease
- GBS*
- Inflammatory bowel disease
- Chronic inflammatory neuropathy
- Acute pandysautonomia*
- Pure cholinergic dysautonomia*

**Autonomic neuropathies associated with systemic metabolic disease**

- Diabetes*
- Chronic renal failure
- Alcoholism
- Nonalcoholic liver disease
- Vitamin B12 deficiency
- Paraneoplastic syndrome
- Primary amyloidosis*

**Autonomic neuropathies associated with industrial agents, metals, toxins, and drugs**

- Organic solvents
- Organophosphates
- Acrylamide
- Vacor
- Heavy metals
- Botulism*
- Amiodarone
- Pentamidine
- Doxorubicin
- Vincristine*
- Cisplatinum
- Paclitaxel
- Cisplatinum

AIDS = acquired immunodeficiency syndrome, GBS = Guillain-Barré syndrome, HMSN = hereditary motor-sensory neuropathy, HSAN = hereditary sensory and autonomic neuropathy, MEN 2bn = multiple endocrine neoplasia type 2b.
*Autonomic dysfunction is prominent and clinically important.

14. **What are the salient manifestations of diabetic autonomic neuropathies?**

**Cardiovascular**
Postural hypotension
Resting tachycardia
Painless myocardial infarction
Sudden death

**Gastrointestinal**
Esophageal motor incoordination
Gastric dysrhythmia, hypomotility
(gastroparesis diabeticorum)
Pylorospasm
Uncoordinated intestinal motility ("diabetic diarrhea," spasm)
Intestinal hypomobility (constipation)
Gallbladder hypocontraction (diabetic cholecystopathy)
Anorectal dysfunction (fecal dysfunction)

**Genitourinary**
Diabetic cystopathy (atonic bladder, postmicturition dribbling)
Male impotence
Ejaculatory disorders
Reduced vaginal lubrication, dyspareunia

**Respiratory**
Impaired breathing control
Sleep apnea

**Thermoregulatory**
Sudomotor (diminished, excessive, or gustatory sweating)
Vasomotor (vasoconstriction, vasodilation, neuropathic edema)

**Pupillary abnormalities**
Miosis
Disturbances of dilation
Argyll-Robertson-like pupils

**Neuroendocrine abnormalities**
Reduced pancreatic polypeptide release
Reduced somatostatin release
Reduced motilin and gastric inhibitory peptide release
Enhanced gastrin release
Reduced NE release (orthostatic-, exercise-, and hypoglycemia-induced)
Reduced parathyroid hormone secretion (hypercalcemia-induced)
Elevated atrial natriuretic hormone
Impaired glucose counter-regulation (hypoglycemia unawareness)
Impaired NE release in response to hypoglycemia

15. **What autonomic dysfunction is seen in Guillain-Barré syndrome (GBS)?**
About 65% of patients with GBS have some dysautonomia, and serious disturbances in autonomic function occur in approximately 20% of patients. In fact, dysautonomia is an important cause of death in patients with severe GBS. Afferent baroreflex abnormalities may cause intermittent hypertension and hypotension associated with orthostatic hypotension, which carries a risk of cardiovascular collapse and sudden death. Abrupt fluctuations of blood pressure may precede fatal arrhythmias.

Less frequent and less severe symptoms of autonomic dysfunction include urinary incontinence or retention, constipation, fecal incontinence, gastroparesis, sudomotor dysfunction, and pupillary abnormalities.

16. **Is there a difference in autonomic involvement between different subtypes of GBS?**
There are two major subtypes of GBS: demyelinating, or acute inflammatory demyelinating neuropathy (AIDP), and axonal, or acute motor axonal neuropathy (AMAN). They differ in pathogenesis, clinical course, and response to treatment. They also differ in the extent of autonomic involvement. AIDP patients show the more serious manifestations of cardiosympathetic hyperactivity. Some authors suggest that the long, myelinated, preganglionic neurons of the vagal fibers are vulnerable to demyelinating processes, which eventually leads to the predominance of the sympathetic system involvement in AIDP patients. Others postulate that demyelination of both afferent and efferent limbs of the baroreflex loop are the leading cause of tachycardia in these patients. On the other hand, autonomic manifestations in AMAN patients are limited to hypoactivity sudomotor and skin vasomotor function.

17. **Describe the appropriate management for the blood pressure fluctuations seen in GBS.**

Blood pressure fluctuations in GBS are best monitored in a medical intensive care unit (ICU) setting. Adequate administration of isotonic IV fluids should be started, a bladder catheter should be placed, fluid intake and output should be carefully monitored, and blood pressure should be measured frequently. Most importantly, continuous electrocardiographic (ECG) monitoring is mandatory.

Pressor drugs may be necessary. These must be used with extreme caution because hypersensitivity responses are common. The use of short-acting agents such as dopamine or phenylephrine is recommended. There is often a delay of several minutes in blood pressure responses to pressor drugs. Treatment of paroxysmal hypertension in GBS should be avoided, unless end-organ damage is present. If antihypertensive agents are used, it is best to use short-acting agents (preferably beta-blockers or nitroprusside) that can be titrated to the blood pressure response. Again, hypersensitivity with resultant hypotension is a potential complication. There may be an exaggerated hypotensive response to even small doses of IV drugs (e.g., morphine, furosemide, nitroglycerin, edrophonium chloride, thiopental).

18. **Describe the appropriate management for the arrhythmias seen in GBS.**

Bradycardia of nonsinus origin is probably best treated with a transvenous pacemaker. Sinus tachycardia due to vagal damage occurs in about 50% of patients and usually responds to fluid replacement therapy. Its occurrence in a patient without infection or circulatory cause indicates vagal denervation. Absence of beat-to-beat (R-R) variation of heart rate during normal and deep breathing in a patient with early GBS is an important and reliable index of impending cardiovascular dysautonomia due to vagal nerve dysfunction. Acute atrial fibrillation and ventricular tachycardia are best managed by ICU experts, but if beta-blockers are used, they must have a rapid onset and offset of action.

19. **How long does the cardiovascular instability persist in GBS?**

There is no consistent correlation between the severity of peripheral weakness and the risk of severity of dysautonomia. Cardiovascular instability may be seen in otherwise minimally disabled patients. As a rule, severely affected patients (especially if they require mechanical ventilation) have a higher risk of significant autonomic fluctuations, which resolves when ambulation is regained. The duration of cardiovascular instability ranges from a few days to weeks. It is recommended that the cardiovascular monitoring of the severely affected individuals continue until the ventilatory support is discontinued and they have started to improve clinically.

20. **What is the appropriate management for the other dysautonomias seen in GBS?**

Adynamic ileus and atonic bladder may occur. Adynamic ileus requires upper gastrointestinal (GI) tract decompression via a nasogastric tube and maintenance of nil per os (NPO; Latin, nothing by mouth) status. Urinary retention is treated with an indwelling catheter while the patient is on IV fluids; if present in the rehabilitation phase of GBS, it is treated with sterile intermittent catheterization.

21. **Describe the clinical features of acute autonomic ganglionopathy (AAG).**

AAG (formerly known as acute autonomic neuropathy, acute panautonomic neuropathy, or acute dysautonomia) is an acquired immune-mediated involvement of both sympathetic and parasympathetic components of the autonomic nervous system, with relative or complete sparing of the somatic nerve fibers. Antibodies against ganglionic nicotinic acetylcholine receptors (AchR) are found in about 50% of patients and based on several observations it is suggested that AAG is an antibody-mediated disorder. The typical patient has symptoms related to sympathetic failure (orthostatic hypotension, anhidrosis) or parasympathetic failure (reduced lacrimation and salivation, disturbances of the gastrointestinal motility [such as ileus, diarrhea, and constipation], bladder atony, impotence, fixed heart rate, and fixed pupils). The progression of symptoms is rapid in the majority of cases, while some patients have a more insidious onset of disease, resembling neurodegenerative causes of autonomic failure. There are no controlled trials of effective treatment of AAG and treatment primarily consists of supportive care for orthostatic hypotension and bowel and bladder symptoms. A few case reports suggest that immunomodulatory therapies such as IV gamma-globulin or plasmapheresis may enhance recovery. Recently, a small study demonstrated a substantial clinical improvement in a few patients with combined immunomodulatory therapy.

Wang Z, Low PA, Jordan J, et al.: Autoimmune autonomic ganglionopathy: IgG effects on ganglionic acetylcholine receptor current. Neurology 68:1917-1923, 2007.

22. **What are the autonomic abnormalities seen in primary Sjögren's syndrome (PSS)?**
This autoimmune exocrinopathy, which affects women nine times as frequently as men, is estimated to be second in frequency only to rheumatoid arthritis among collagen vascular diseases. In addition to the clinical presentation, the determination of highly specific autoantibodies, Ro (SS-A) and La (SS-B), directed against low-molecular-weight ribonuclear proteins, aids in the diagnosis of PSS. Signs of all forms of peripheral neuropathy (sensory neuropathy, sensorimotor neuropathy, multiple mononeuropathies, sensory neuronopathy, cranial neuropathy, and entrapment syndromes) may be seen in about 20% of patients with Sjögren's syndrome. Autonomic dysfunction, including Adie's pupil, anhidrosis, urinary retention, orthostatic hypotension, and impaired cardiac parasympathetic function, may be superimposed on a generalized neuropathy. Most studies have shown the presence of autonomic nervous system dysfunction in patients with Sjögren's syndrome; however, autonomic abnormalities have a poor correlation with exocrine dysfunction. Recently, antibodies to M3-receptors in other tissues has led some investigators to assume these antibodies may also be involved in the development of other autonomic nervous system symptoms such as irritable bladder and constipation. Inflammation of the sympathetic ganglia and presence of some cytokines that interfere with neurotransmission have been reported as other possible mechanisms involved in autonomic nervous system dysfunction in PSS.

23. **Name the four most common paraneoplastic autonomic syndromes.**
Lambert-Eaton myasthenic syndrome (LEMS), subacute sensory neuropathy, autonomic neuropathy, and enteric neuropathy.

24. **What is LEMS?**
LEMS is an antibody-mediated autoimmune disease. The target of the aberrant immune response is the presynaptic P/Q voltage-gated calcium channel at the neuromuscular junction. In 90% of patients, antibodies can be detected by radioimmunoassay. The cardinal symptom of LEMS is weakness, usually in the proximal muscles and more prominent in the lower extremities. Extraocular muscles are usually spared. In about 60% of the cases, the syndrome is paraneoplastic, associated almost exclusively with small-cell lung cancer. Onset of symptoms may precede detection of tumor by 1 to 4 years. LEMS is frequently associated with autonomic symptoms, including dry mouth (74%), impotence (41%), constipation (18%), blurred vision (8%), and impaired sweating (4%). Some patients also may have orthostatic lightheadedness, difficulty with micturition, or tonic pupils. About 57% of patients demonstrate cholinergic and adrenergic supersensitivity of pupils when tested with 2.5% methacholine and 0.5% phenylephrine. Tear

production is also reduced. Variations in heart rate and blood pressure may occur with the Valsalva maneuver or deep breathing, and sweat tests also may be abnormal.

Poumand R: Lambert-Eaton myasthenic syndrome. Front Neurol Neurosci 26:120-125, 2009.

### 25. How is LEMS treated?

When an underlying neoplasm is identified, removal or treatment of the tumor usually results in substantial improvement in all symptoms, including those of autonomic dysfunction. In patients who do not have an underlying malignancy, the treatment is directed toward the enhancement of cholinergic function and immunosuppression. Antiacetylcholinesterase agents, guanidine hydrochloride, 4-aminopyridine, and 3,4-diaminopyridine (3,4-DAP) have been used to enhance neuromuscular transmission and improve autonomic dysfunction. Pyridostigmine and prostigmine provide limited symptomatic relief. Immunosuppression with corticosteroids, azathioprine, or cyclosporine as well as immunomodulation with plasma exchange or IV gamma-globulin may prove beneficial in patients with either the non-neoplastic or neoplastic forms of LEMS. A combination of 3,4-DAP and IV gamma-globulin may produce the highest likelihood of improvement. Drugs that adversely affect neuromuscular transmission, particularly those with calcium channel–blocking properties, should be avoided in patients with LEMS. If no malignancy is found, patients with LEMS should undergo screening for small-cell lung cancer every 6 months for a minimum of 2 years, and also be evaluated for other autoimmune disorders.

### 26. What is paraneoplastic subacute sensory neuropathy (SSN)?

Sudden onset and rapid progression of dysesthesia, paresthesia, and lancinating pain and numbness in all limbs and occasionally trunk and face are the characteristics of SSN. Almost 75% of these patients have small-cell lung carcinoma, but other malignancies such as prostate cancer, neuroblastoma, and seminoma have also been associated with SSN. Some patients with this syndrome may have one or several of the following autonomic dysfunctions: orthostatic hypotension, tonic pupils, hypohidrosis, dry mouth, diminished lacrimation, impotence, urinary retention, and constipation. Serum and cerebrospinal fluid (CSF) of patients with this syndrome frequently contain antineuronal nuclear (ANNA-1 or anti-HU) antibody, a polyclonal complement-fixing immunoglobulin G (IgG) that also reacts against a 35 to 40 kDa protein of small-cell lung cancer cells. The neuronal nuclear antigen has the same molecular weight but lacks the 38 kDa band. Treatment of the underlying tumor may result in the partial alleviation of autonomic and somatic symptoms.

### 27. What is paraneoplastic autonomic neuropathy?

Some patients with small-cell lung cancer, pancreatic adenocarcinoma, prostate cancer, or Hodgkin's disease may develop autonomic symptoms (orthostatic dizziness, impotence, dry mouth, urinary retention, or GI symptoms) with no or minimal somatic involvement that may improve with treatment of the tumor. In these patients, the autonomic neuropathy may be part of a generalized paraneoplastic syndrome that variably includes sensory neuronopathy, limbic and brain stem encephalitis, cerebellar degeneration, and a sensorimotor neuropathy. Approximately 40% of patients have antibodies directed against the nicotinic ACh receptors in the autonomic ganglia. The list of antibodies in paraneoplastic autonomic neuropathies has been constantly growing and includes antineuronal nuclear antibodies, Purkinje cell cytoplasmic autoantibody (PCA), and collapsin response-mediated protein 5 (CRMP-5). The presentation of autonomic neuropathy may precede or follow the diagnosis of malignancy.

### 28. What is paraneoplastic enteric neuropathy?

Enteric neuropathy of the GI tract, with or without other symptoms of autonomic dysfunction, may be seen in association with small-cell lung cancer, pulmonary carcinoid, undifferentiated epithelioma, and malignant thymoma. Based on the segment of the GI tract involved, the neuropathy can clinically present as achalasia, gastroparesis, intestinal pseudoobstruction, or megacolon. Patients may subsequently develop other dysautonomic symptoms. The motility disorder may resolve with the treatment of the underlying tumor. The salient GI pathologic features include loss of myenteric plexus neurons, fragmentation and degeneration of axons, and plasma cell and lymphocytic infiltrations. Some patients have elevated titers of antineuronal nuclear antibody (ANNA-1 or anti-Hu), which reacts with antigens shared by the tumor cells and the myenteric plexus neurons.

29. **What is the differential diagnosis of nonpsychogenic causes of male sexual impotence?**
   - Penile arterial insufficiency
   - Excessive venous leakage
   - Spinal cord damage
   - Conus medullaris damage
   - Cauda equina damage
   - Sacral plexus damage
   - Peripheral neuropathies
   - Central and peripheral autonomic disorders
   - Drugs
   - Alcohol
   - Hyperprolactinemia
   - Peyronie's disease

30. **What are the most common cardiovascular disturbances associated with central nervous system (CNS) disease?**
   Cardiac arrhythmias, myocardial injury, and changes in blood pressure.

31. **What cardiac arrhythmias are associated with CNS disease?**
   A number of CNS disorders, including subarachnoid hemorrhage, cerebral infarction and hemorrhage, brain tumors, and head injury, may cause a variety of supraventricular and ventricular arrhythmias unrelated to the any underlying cardiac disease. The incidence of cardiac arrhythmias increases if there is more than one infarction site and is highest in subarachnoid hemorrhage. Some studies suggest that the incidence of cardiac arrhythmias in right hemispheric ischemic lesions is more than left hemispheric lesions. The most common arrhythmia following stroke is atrial fibrillation, whereas in intracranial hemorrhage the incidence of ventriculary tachycardia is high. The occurrence of arrhythmias may further compromise the prognosis of the CNS disease: 4% to 5% of sudden deaths in patients with subarachnoid hemorrhage are attributed to arrhythmias. Arrhythmias occur because of an imbalance between sympathetic and parasympathetic influences on the heart, presumably from an enhanced release of peripheral catecholamines triggered by the central lesion.

32. **What is the nature of the myocardial injury associated with CNS disease?**
   Central nervous system lesions, particularly intracerebral and subarachnoid hemorrhage, may cause a number of ECG abnormalities suggestive of myocardial ischemia. These changes may closely resemble myocardial infarction and include prolongation of the QT interval, ST segment depression, flattening or inversion of T waves, and the appearance of U waves. With the exception of QT interval prolongation and the U waves, these changes usually revert to normal within 2 weeks after the CNS event. Other less frequently observed ECG changes are increased amplitude of the P wave, development of Q waves, ST segment elevation, and T wave elevation, notching, or peaking. Differentiation between a centrally induced ECG abnormality and a true myocardial infarction may be difficult, but the patient must be cared for in a monitored setting until a "true" myocardial infarction is excluded. The ECG changes are thought to be due to a neurogenically mediated excessive release of catecholamines upon cardiac myocytes, resulting in myonecrotic changes. In fact, a higher level of serum catecholamines correlates with a poor outcome in patients with subarachnoid hemorrhage (Figures 12-3 and 12-4).

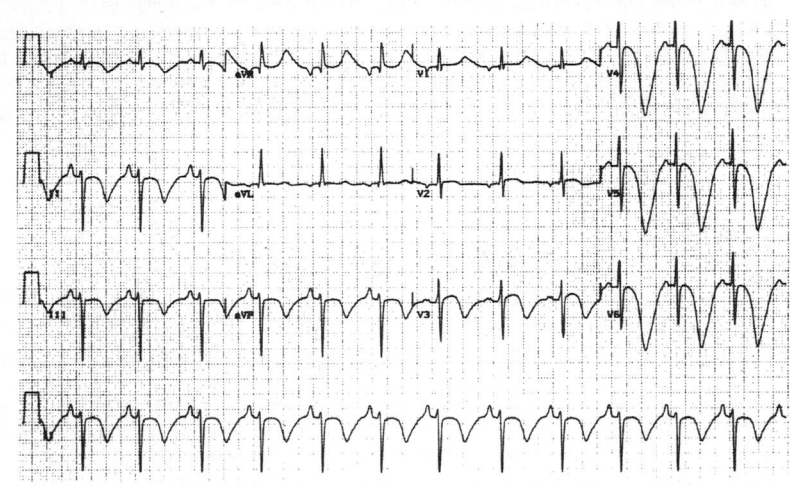

**Figure 12-3.** Electrocardiogram of a 41-year-old woman showing typical central nervous system (CNS) changes of prolonged QT interval and deep, inverted, peaked T waves. These ECG changes were secondary to the traumatic basal ganglion hemorrhage shown on her computed tomography (CT) scan (Figure 12-4).

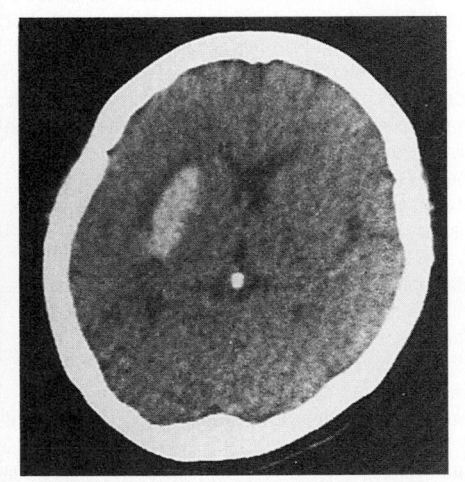

**Figure 12-4.** Computed tomographic (CT) scan showing traumatic basal ganglion hemorrhage.

33. **What is the relationship of changes in blood pressure to CNS disease?**
Lesions of the hypothalamus and medulla oblongata or tumors of the posterior fossa may cause arterial hypertension. Ischemic, degenerative, or destructive lesions of the NTS in the medulla may result in chronic lability of blood pressure. Cushing's response of hypertension, bradycardia, and apnea, an important sign of increased intracranial pressure and potential herniation, also may develop after ischemic lesions of the dorsal medullary reticular formation along the floor of the fourth ventricle. Hypertension caused by posterior fossa tumors is due to the compression of the pressor center at the rostral ventrolateral medulla (RVLM). Such an

increase in blood pressure may present as malignant hypertension and may be indistinguishable from a pheochromocytoma. Patients with normal-pressure hydrocephalus also may have chronic hypertension. Decreased blood pressure is rare with CNS disease, but orthostatic hypotension may accompany brain stem tumors, although the exact mechanism and the specific nuclei involved are not clear.

34. **Which autonomic dysfunctions occur following heart transplantation?**
Heart or heart-lung transplantation result in afferent and efferent denervation (i.e., loss of autonomic control) of the transplanted organ with a relative resting tachycardia, little or no rise in heart rate after standing, and a delayed increase in heart rate in response to exercise. Also, there are no changes in heart rate with the Valsalva maneuver or carotid sinus massage. In general, the heart rate response in such patients depends on the circulating catecholamines. The resting tachycardia seen in severe autonomic neuropathies (e.g., diabetes) resembles that seen in a denervated transplanted heart.

35. **Which neurologic conditions cause hypothermia?**
Experimental studies suggest that lesions of the anterior hypothalamus cause hyperthermia, lesions of the posterior hypothalamus hypothermia, and lesions of the suprachiasmatic nucleus alteration in the circadian rhythm of temperature. Tumors and degenerative or inflammatory processes involving the hypothalamus may produce hypothermia (core body temperature below 35° C).

**Wernicke's encephalopathy**, by damaging the posterolateral hypothalamus and the floor of the fourth ventricle, may present with continuous hypothermia. Prompt treatment with thiamine results in normalization of temperature.

**Paroxysmal hypothermia with hyperhidrosis** (PHH) is a syndrome manifested as episodic hypothermia, lasting between half an hour to 2 hours, associated with excessive sweating. PHH is probably caused by a low core temperature set in hypothalamus and is seen in various conditions including congenital lesions such as Shapiro's syndrome (agenesis of the corpus callosum), hemispheric stroke, hypothalamus lesions, traumatic brain injury, multiple sclerosis, subarachnoid hemorrhage, and human immunodeficiency virus (HIV) infection. The underlying mechanisms of this syndrome are largely unknown, but disturbances in the function of ion channels may play a role in its pathogenesis. PHH may be seen in childhood, sometimes in association with a history of migraine. Oxybutynin, cyproheptadine, clonidine, chlorpromazine, and occasionally antiepileptic medications may control hypothermia and diaphoresis.

**Episodic spontaneous hypothermia** is a rare periodic childhood syndrome with no known systemic cause or underlying brain lesion. Manifestations include episodic hypothermia (<35° C), marked facial pallor, and absent shivering. Some patients may have bradycardia and hypertension. It is believed that this childhood periodic syndrome is related to migraines.

36. **What are the autonomic manifestations that accompany severe brain injury?**
In the initial phase of severe traumatic brain injury, dysautonomic manifestations are frequent. The main features of this syndrome include marked agitation, diaphoresis, hyperthermia, hypertension, tachycardia, tachypnea, and dystonia of limbs. Various names have been given to this complex of symptoms, including paroxysmal sympathetic storm, diencephalic seizures, and hypothalamic-midbrain dysregulation syndrome. Recently, the term paroxysmal autonomic instability with dystonia (PAID) has been proposed, as it captures the cardinal features of this syndrome.

The pathophysiology of PAID seems to be related to the dysfunction of autonomic centers in the diencephalon (thalamus and hypothalamus) or their connections to cortical, subcortical, and brain stem loci that mediate autonomic function. It has been suggested that a disinhibition phenomenon occurs, with loss of cortical and subcortical control of vegetative functions, including blood pressure and temperature. The syndrome is seen in patients with severe head injury (Glasgow coma score ≤ 8) and predicts a worse hospital course as well as a poorer functional outcome in survivors. Treatment options in the acute setting of the syndrome include morphine sulfate, bromocriptine, propranolol, clonidine, gabapentin, benzodiazepines, dantrolene, and, in refractory cases, intrathecal baclofen. In a recent case report, dexmedetomidine, a strong selective α2 agonist, has been used to control the symptoms of this syndrome and the results have been promising.

Srinivasan S, Lim CC, Thrugnanam U: Paroxysmal autonomic instability with dystonia. Clin Auton Res 17:378-381, 2007.

37. **What are the major differences between the syndrome of pure autonomic failure (PAF) and multiple-system atrophy (MSA)?**

MSA, also called Shy-Drager syndrome, is associated with autonomic dysfunction, particularly orthostatic hypotension, and parkinsonian symptoms of akinesia and rigidity, leading to incapacity in a few years. Clinical variants of striatonigral degeneration (predominant symptoms are rigidity and dysarthria) and olivopontocerebellar atrophy (predominant symptoms are ataxia, incoordination, or bradykinesia) have been identified. PAF, also called idiopathic orthostatic hypotension and Bradbury-Eggleston syndrome, is an idiopathic sporadic disorder characterized by orthostatic hypotension, usually accompanied by evidence of more widespread autonomic failure. There are no other neurologic signs, and the natural history is slow progression over 10 to 15 years. Symptoms of autonomic dysfunction in MSA may precede the appearance of neurologic symptoms by up to 5 years. Accordingly, the diagnosis of PAF cannot be made with certainty until prolonged follow-up has been established.

38. **Which autonomic dysfunctions occur in Parkinson's disease (PD)?**

In the classic forms of PD, disturbances in salivation, sweating, bladder and bowel functions, and erection may be seen. Some patients may have orthostatic or postprandial dizziness; however, one should not overlook the possibility that orthostatic symptoms may result from dopaminergic agents used in treatment. The cardiovascular reflexes are generally preserved, although responses may be somewhat reduced. The resting recumbent levels of plasma NE and dihydroxyphenylglycol (DHPG) are lower in patients with orthostatic hypotension (OH) than in patients without OH. These subtle autonomic disturbances in PD are thought to be due to a central rather than a peripheral lesion. Of interest, however, Lewy bodies may be present in the sympathetic ganglia of patients with PD.

39. **What are the most important genetic causes of autonomic failure?**

1. Dopamine/beta-hydroxylase deficiency
2. Familial dysautonomia
3. Fabry's disease
4. Familial amyloidosis
5. Multiple endocrine neoplasia, type 2b
6. Porphyria

40. **What is dopamine beta-hydroxylase (DBH) deficiency? What is the best treatment for this disease?**

Beta-hydroxylase is the last enzyme in the synthesis pathway of norepinephrine (NE) and the encoding gene is located on chromosome 9. Several recessively inherited mutations of this gene have been detected, which result in undetectable levels of NE in the circulation and tissues. Patients with this very rare disorder present with severe orthostatic hypotension, episodic hypoglycemia, and hypothermia. Dihydroxyphenylserine (DOPS), a precursor of NE, has effectively treated these patients.

41. **What is familial dysautonomia?**

Familial dysautonomia (Riley-Day syndrome, hereditary sensory and autonomic neuropathy type III [HSAN-III]) is an autosomal recessive disorder affecting primarily people of Ashkenazi Jewish extraction. It is classified as one of the HSANs, of which at least seven clinically and genetically distinct entities have been identified. It affects the development and survival of sensory, sympathetic, and some parasympathetic neurons. One of every 32 individuals among

Ashkenazi Jews is considered a carrier, and the frequency of occurrence is 1 in 3700 live births among them. The genetic abnormality responsible for the disease has been identified as the splicing mutation in the *IKBKAP* (IKB kinase-associated protein) gene on the distal long arm of chromosome 9. A single noncoding mutation is seen in 99.5% of cases. Two other rare mutations have been identified. Prenatal and preimplantation genetic diagnosis is now available. The cardinal clinical features include: alacrima (absence of tears), absent fungiform papillae of tongue, depressed patellar reflexes, and absent skin response to scratch and histamine injection in a patient from Ashkenazi Jewish or Eastern European Jewish heritage.

Autonomic features result primarily from sympathetic system dysfunction, and include transient and emotionally induced erythematous skin blotching, orthostatic hypotension, hyperhidrosis or erratic sweating, and esophageal and GI transit dysfunction. Dysautonomic crisis is a constellation of symptoms that may occur in response to physiologic or psychologic stress. The main symptoms of dysautonomic crisis include vomiting, tachycardia, excessive sweating, blotching of the skin, piloerection, ileus, and dilation of the pupils.

Rubin BY, Anderson SL: The molecular basis of familial dysautonomia: Overview, new discoveries, and implications for directed therapies. Neuromolecular Med 10:148-156, 2008.

## 42. What is Fabry's disease?

This X-linked recessive metabolic disease, also known as angiokeratoma corporis diffusum, is due to a deficiency of the lysosomal enzyme alpha-galactosidase, with resulting cell storage of the glycolipid ceramide trihexoside in several organs, including the skin (corpora angiokeratomas), kidneys, cardiovascular and pulmonary systems, blood vessels, and central and peripheral nervous systems. Vascular disease develops at a young age, and many patients have a stroke or myocardial infarction before the age of 50 years. The posterior cerebral circulation appears more vulnerable, as suggested by the disproportionately high number of brain stem strokes in this population. The disease displays a remarkable genetic heterogeneity; more than 50 mutations in the alpha-galactosidase A gene have been identified.

Pathologically, there is a prominent lipid deposition in the dorsal root and peripheral autonomic ganglia, which are known to have fenestrated blood vessels and a permeable blood-nerve barrier.

The clinical presentation of autonomic dysfunction includes diminished sweating (which may be due to lipid accumulation in sweat glands rather than neuropathy), absent skin wrinkling after immersion in warm water, reduced cutaneous flare response, reduced tear and saliva production, disturbed intestinal motility, abnormal cardiovascular responses, and abnormal pupillary response to pilocarpine. Peripheral nerve pathology consists of degenerative changes of unmyelinated and small myelinated fibers. Successful renal transplantation corrects many of the abnormalities and increases survival. Regular intravenous infusions of recombinant human alpha-galactosidase A has been used as a hormone replacement therapy (HRT) in patients with Fabry's disease. HRT appears to improve neuropathic pain, renal function, and glomerular pathology and may also improve the overall prognosis of the disease.

## 43. What is familial amyloidosis?

Hereditary amyloidosis is a heterogeneous group of familial diseases that have in common the systemic or localized accumulation of polypeptide amyloid fibrils arranged in beta-pleated sheets. Extracellular amyloid deposits result in disruption of normal tissue structure and function.

The autonomic dysfunction involves both sympathetic and parasympathetic systems. Late onset, predominant sensory symptoms, prominent early autonomic involvement, and frequent association with carpal tunnel syndrome should strongly favor the diagnosis of familial amyloidosis. Genetic testing for detection of Met 30 transthyretin mutation, the most common mutation, is commercially available. The only treatment for familial amyloidosis is liver transplantation. When performed early in the course of the disease, it may stop clinical progression and modestly improve symptoms.

44. **What is multiple endocrine neoplasia type 2b (MEN 2b)?**
    MEN 2b, an autosomal dominant inherited disorder, is characterized by multiple mucosal neuromas (conjunctiva, oral cavity, tongue, pharynx, and larynx), medullary thyroid carcinoma, pheochromocytoma, ganglioneuromatosis, bony deformities, marfanoid appearance, muscle underdevelopment, and hypotonia. Gross and microscopic abnormalities of the peripheral autonomic nervous system affect both sympathetic and parasympathetic systems. Patients have disorganized hypertrophy and proliferation of autonomic nerves and ganglia (ganglioneuromatosis). Neural proliferation of the alimentary tract (Auerbach and Meissner's plexi), upper respiratory tract, bladder, prostate, and skin also may be seen. The clinical autonomic manifestations include impaired lacrimation, orthostatic hypotension, impaired reflex vasodilation of the skin, and parasympathetic denervation supersensitivity of pupils, with intact sweating and salivary gland function. Nerve biopsy shows degeneration and regeneration of unmyelinated fibers. A few point mutations in the *RET* proto-oncogene located on chromosome 10 have been associated with the disease. Genetic testing is critical for detection of young carriers, who can undergo prophylactic thyroidectomy to prevent the development of medullary thyroid carcinoma.

45. **What is porphyria?**
    Acute hepatic porphyrias (acute intermittent porphyria, variegate porphyria, and hereditary coproporphyria) are autosomal dominant hereditary disorders that manifest as acute or subacute, severe, life-threatening neuropathy. The basic genetic defect is a 50% reduction in porphobilinogen deaminase activity (acute intermittent porphyria), protoporphyrinogen-IX oxidase (variegate porphyria), and coproporphyrinogen oxidase (coproporphyria), resulting in abnormalities of heme biosynthesis. In the presence of sufficient endogenous or exogenous stimuli (e.g., drugs, hormones, menstruation, starvation), this partial deficiency may lead to clinical manifestations, including peripheral neuropathy, autonomic dysfunction, skin symptoms, and CNS abnormalities.
    Pathologic involvement of the autonomic nervous system (degeneration of the vagus nerve and sympathetic trunk) may explain certain features of acute attacks, including abdominal pain, severe vomiting, constipation, intestinal dilatation and stasis, persistent sinus tachycardia (100 to 160 min), labile hypertension, postural hypotension, hyperhidrosis, and sphincteric bladder problems.

46. **What are the most important factors in the maintenance of normal blood pressure?**
    1. Blood volume
    2. Vascular reflexes (e.g., reflex arteriolar-venous constriction, baroreflex-induced tachycardia)
    3. Hormonal mechanisms (e.g., increased plasma catecholamines, renin–angiotensin–aldosterone system, arginine, vasopressin, atrial natriuretic factor)

47. **Which age-related physiologic changes predispose to hypotension?**
    Decreased baroreflex sensitivity, impaired neuroendocrine response to changes of intravascular volume (e.g., reduced secretion of renin, angiotensin, and aldosterone), and impaired early cardiac ventricular filling (diastolic dysfunction).

48. **What are the baroreceptors? What is their significance?**
    Baroreceptors are spray-type nerve endings in the walls of blood vessels and the heart that are stimulated by the absolute level of, and changes in, arterial pressure. They are extremely abundant in the wall of the bifurcation of the internal carotid arteries (carotid sinus) and in the wall of the aortic arch. The primary site of termination of baroreceptor afferent fibers is the NTS.
    The function of the baroreceptors is to maintain systemic blood pressure at a relatively constant level, especially during a change in body position. Intact baroreceptors are extremely

effective in preventing rapid changes in blood pressure from moment to moment or hour to hour, but because of their adaptability to prolonged changes of blood pressure (> 2 or 3 days), the system is incapable of long-term regulation of arterial pressure.

Stretching of the baroreceptors as a result of increased blood pressure causes an increase in the activity of the vagal nerve by projection to the nucleus ambiguus. It also causes inhibition of the sympathetic outflow from the RVLM, ultimately leading to decreased heart rate and blood pressure. Conversely, decreased blood pressure results in decreased signal output from the baroreceptors, leading to disinhibition of the central sympathetic control sites and decreased parasympathetic activity. The final effect is an increase in blood pressure.

**49. What are the clinical features of baroreceptor failure?**

Baroreflex failure is a heterogenous entity that can result from abnormalities in vascular baroreceptors, cranial nerve 9 or 10 abnormalities, or brain stem abnormalities that involve the baroreflex control centers such as NTS. As a result of impairment in the baroreflex, these patients have volatile blood pressures and heart rates. The clinical presentation can resemble pheochromocytoma. The ability of clonidine to inhibit neurons of RVLM and therefore to profoundly reduce the blood pressure differentiates these patients from patients with pheochromocytoma.

**50. What are the most common tests to quantitatively evaluate the autonomic nervous system?**

Quantitative sudomotor axon reflex test (QSART) is used to evaluate the sympathetic cholinergic nerves that innervate the sweat glands. Variability of heart rate to deep breathing and Valsalva maneuver are used to assess the cardiovagal component of the autonomic nervous system. Beat-to-beat changes of blood pressure during Valsalva maneuver and tilt-up test screens the adrenergic component of the autonomic nervous system.

**51. Why does skin turn red (flare) after it is scratched?**

The normal skin axon-reflex vasodilation (flare) follows skin stimulation from a simple scratch. The scratch causes activation of unmyelinated sensory nerve terminals (C fibers). The impulse generated by this stimulus travels antidromically, reaches a branch point, and then orthodromically arrives at a skin blood vessel, releasing one or more vasodilating peptides or adenosine triphosphate (ATP). The released substance leads to further histamine release, activating other sensory terminals, creating a cascade of spreading flare response. Released histamine also causes itching. Both the flare response and the itching may be reduced by antihistamines. The absence of a flare response provides evidence of dysfunction of unmyelinated sensory fibers in peripheral neuropathies.

**52. What is a sudomotor axon reflex?**

The sudomotor axon reflex employs the same mechanism as the skin axon-reflex flare, but the neural pathway consists of an axon reflex mediated by the postganglionic sympathetic axon (C fibers) that innervates sweat glands. The axon terminals of these fibers are activated by the local injection of ACh: the generated impulse travels to a branch point where it is deflected and then travels orthodromically to activate a different sweat gland, releasing ACh, which binds to M3 muscarinic receptors. In other words, in the sudomotor axon reflex, the activation of sweat glands results in the reflex activation of another population of nearby glands, the sweat output of which can be quantitatively measured. The quantitative sudomotor axon-reflex test (QSART) is, therefore, a sensitive and reproducible test of the integrity of the postganglionic sympathetic sudomotor axon.

**53. What is the basis for the heart rate variability to deep breathing test?**

Usually, inspiration increases and expiration decreases the heart rate (sinus arrhythmia). This phenomenon is mediated primarily by the vagus nerve. Pulmonary stretch receptors and cardiac mechanoreceptors, as well as baroreceptors, contribute to its generation. The variation of heart rate in inspiration and expiration is age-dependent and is reduced in elderly people (e.g., normal maximal-to-minimal variation in people 10 to 40 years old is >18 beats per minute, but in people 61 to 70 years old, it declines to >8 beats per minute). The test is easy to perform with a commercial ECG machine or appropriately set electromyography (EMG) equipment. While supine with the head elevated to 30 degrees, the patient breathes deeply at 6 respirations per minute (usually for 8 cycles), and minimal and maximal heart rate within each respiratory cycle (5 seconds inspiration followed by 5 seconds expiration) is measured. The simplest index is the heart rate variability (maximum heart rate minus minimum heart rate). Another index, the E/I ratio, is determined by the longest R-R interval on ECG (slow heart rate) divided by the shortest R-R interval (fast heart rate). An abnormal test indicates parasympathetic dysfunction.

**54. What are the confounding factors that influence the heart rate variability to deep breathing?**
Heart rate variability to deep breathing decreases with advancing age (about 3 to 5 beats per minute every 10 years). Rate and depth of breathing, position of the subject, obesity, and medications such as cholinergic agents influence the test results.

**55. What are the four phases of blood pressure variation during a Valsalva maneuver in a person with an intact autonomic nervous system?**
During phase I, increased intra-abdominal and intrathoracic pressure result in compression of the large vessels and aorta and therefore transient increase in the blood pressure, accompanied by a reflex bradycardia. Shortly after, reduction in the venous return to the heart leads to reduced stroke volume and blood pressure (early phase II). This decline in blood pressure triggers the sympathetic nervous system with resultant increase in norepinephrine level, peripheral vascular resistant, and blood pressure (late phase II). When the Valsalva maneuver is released, the sudden decline in intrathoracic pressure causes a concomitant decrease in blood pressure and tachycardia (phase III). Finally, in phase IV in normal subjects, despite the return of the venous return and cardiac output to the baseline values, blood pressure continues to rise as a result of the persistent high peripheral vascular resistant (residual from late phase II). Therefore, blood pressure usually overshoots the baseline in this phase (Figure 12-5).

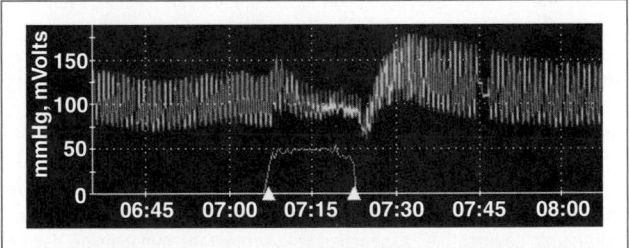

**Figure 12-5.** Blood pressure variation during Valsalva maneuver in a person with intact autonomic nervous system.

**56. What are the changes seen in the blood pressure variation during a Valsalva maneuver in a patient with adrenergic failure?**
In patients with inadequate response of the adrenergic system, the blood pressure fails to increase in late phase II. By the same token, the blood pressure fails to overshoot the baseline level in phase IV (Figure 12-6).

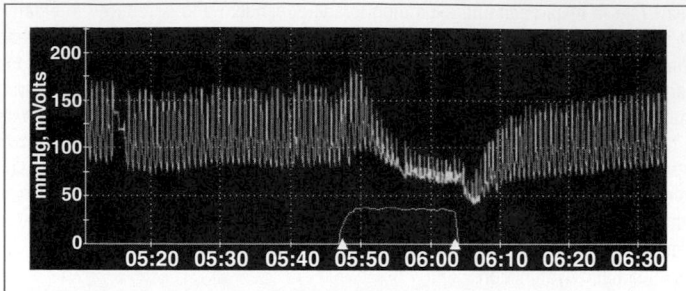

**Figure 12-6.** Blood pressure variation during Valsalva maneuver in a person with adrenergic failure.

57. **What is the Valsalva ratio? What component of the autonomic nervous system is assessed by this ratio?**
    Valsalva ratio is the ratio of maximum heart rate during the Valsalva maneuver divided by the minimum heart rate occurring within 30 seconds of the maximum rate. This ratio is another quantitative value that reflects the integrity of the cardiovagal component of the autonomic nervous system.

58. **How is a tilt table test performed?**
    The patient rests on a tilt table in a supine position for 20 minutes. Then the table is tilted to 70 degrees within 10 to 20 seconds. The blood pressure is measured at 1 and 5 minutes, although different protocols are employed by different labs. In normal individuals, there is a transient reduction in systolic, mean, and diastolic blood pressure following tilt, followed by recovery in 1 minute.

59. **Why do patients with orthostatic hypotension have diurnal variation in blood pressure?**
    Many patients with orthostatic hypotension have supine hypertension, even before they are treated with fludrocortisone or other medications. The reason for supine hypertension remains to be determined, however, it seems that baroreflex dysfunction may play a role. Prolonged supine position at night may lead to natriuresis and diuresis and eventually contracture of intravascular volume. These events cause the orthostatic hypotension to become more severe in the morning.

60. **What is the difference in orthostatic hypotension caused by autonomic dysfunction and that caused by hypovolemia during a tilt table test?**
    In most autonomic neuropathies associated with orthostatic hypotension, failure of vascular reflexes to increase sympathetic outflow to splanchnic and muscular vasculature results in a drop in both systolic and diastolic pressures. However, there is no increase in plasma NE (hypoadrenergic response). Conversely, in orthostatic hypotension secondary to hypovolemia, plasma NE increases excessively in response to standing (hyperadrenergic response).
    In orthostatic hypotension secondary to generalized sympathetic failure, a drop in systolic blood pressure is not associated with reflex tachycardia, whereas in orthostatic hypotension secondary to hypovolemia or deconditioning, with intact sympathetic nerves, reflex tachycardia is prominent. A fall in systolic pressure alone is most likely caused by a non-neurologic disturbance (e.g., hypovolemia).

61. **What are the three main mechanisms of syncope?**
    1. **Orthostatic hypotension** may be due to a reduction in vascular resistance, hypovolemia, drugs, chronic baroreflex failure, or a neurally mediated mechanism (vasovagal syncope triggered by pain or fear). Reflex syncope and vasodepressor syncope are synonymous with vasovagal syncope.
    2. **Fall in cardiac output** may be due to cardiac arrhythmias, obstructions to flow, or myocardial infarction.
    3. **Increased cerebrovascular resistance** may be due to hyperventilation or increased intracranial pressure.
       Molnar SJ, Somberg JC: Neurocardiogenic syncope. Cardiology 114:47-49, 2009.

---

## KEY POINTS: AUTONOMIC NERVOUS SYSTEM

1. Cardinal symptoms of autonomic insufficiency include orthostatic hypotension, bowel and bladder dysfunction, impotence, and sweating abnormalities.

2. ACh is the neurotransmitter for the parasympathetic autonomic system, while the sympathetic system also uses NE (in postganglionic neurons).

3. Diabetic neuropathy is one of the most common causes of autonomic dysfunction.

4. LEMS resembles myasthenia gravis, with autonomic dysfunction, and arises from an autoimmune attack on presynaptic voltage-gated calcium channels.

5. Syncope is seldom a neurologic problem—loss of consciousness is almost always due to cardiovascular disease.

---

62. **What general advice should you give to a patient with orthostatic hypotension secondary to dysautonomia?**
    1. Avoid straining, which results in the Valsalva maneuver, by treating and preventing constipation with a high-fiber diet.
    2. Avoid severe diurnal variation, particularly morning postural hypotension, by head-up tilt or sleeping in a sitting position at night, sitting for several minutes at the edge of the bed before standing, shaving while sitting, or immediately assuming a squatting position, crossing the legs, bending forward and placing the head between the knees, or placing one foot on a chair when presyncopal symptoms occur.
    3. Avoid exposure to a warm environment to prevent uncompensated vasodilation (e.g., travel to warm countries, hot baths).
    4. Avoid postprandial aggravation of orthostatic hypotension by eating smaller and more frequent meals with reduced carbohydrate content.
    5. Avoid a low-sodium diet by increasing the food sodium content to at least 150 mEq.
    6. Avoid dehydration by increasing fluid intake to 2.0 to 2.5 L/day.
    7. Avoid vigorous exercise; moderate isotonic exercises are preferable to isometrics.
    8. Avoid prolonged recumbency.
    9. Avoid vasodilators such as alcohol.
    10. Avoid drugs known to cause vasodilation and/or bradycardia (nitroglycerin or β-blockers).

63. **What are the most common pharmacologic agents used for the treatment of orthostatic hypotension secondary to autonomic failure?**
    Fludrocortisone, a potent mineralocorticoid, is the most common agent in use. Its mechanism of action is increase of the blood volume by retention of sodium from the kidneys. Usually 1 to 2 weeks is required to see the effect. The $\alpha_1$-agonist midodrine stimulates both arterial and

venous systems without directly affecting the CNS or heart. This drug is converted to the active agent desglymidodrine and is best used to elevate the daytime blood pressure. Up to one-fourth of patients may develop supine hypertension, which can best be prevented by taking the last dose at least a few hours before bed time. Recent studies show that a precursor of norepinephrine (L-threo-3,4-dihydroxyphenylserine [L-DOPS]) can be converted to norepinephrine outside of the CNS and improve orthostatic tolerance. $\alpha_2$-Antagonists such as clonidine are sometimes used as an adjunctive therapy, but their use is limited by supine hypertension.

64. **What is postural tachycardia syndrome (POTS)? How is it treated?**
This increasingly recognized condition, often observed in females aged 15 to 50 years, is defined as a syndrome of consistent orthostatic symptoms associated with an excessive heart rate of equal to or greater than 120 beats/min or an increase in the heart rate of 30 beats/min or greater within 5 minutes of standing or tilt up. There is only a minimal or no drop in blood pressure after standing, but the patient feels many of the orthostatic symptoms, including dizziness, fatigue, tremulousness, palpitations, nausea, vasomotor skin changes, hyperhidrosis, or chest wall pain. Some patients with the diagnosis of chronic fatigue syndrome or anxiety or panic disorder may instead have POTS, especially if their symptoms are consistently reproduced after standing and cease after assuming a recumbent position. Patients with orthostatic headaches but no evidence of cerebrospinal fluid leak should also be investigated for POTS.
POTS has heterogeneous etiologies and the exact pathophysiologic mechanisms involved remain elusive, but it is suspected that the symptoms are related to excessive central hypovolemia or excessive pooling of blood due to the sympathetic denervation in the lower extremities. Treatment options include increased intake of fluids and salt (to increase blood volume), fludrocortisone, desmopressin, midodrine ($\alpha_1$-adrenergic agonist that induces vasoconstriction), propranolol, pyridostigmine, and measures to reduce blood pooling in the legs.
Medow A, Stewart JM: The postural tachycardia syndrome. Cardiol Rev 15:67-75, 2007.

65. **What cardiovascular autonomic changes are seen during rapid eye movement (REM) sleep?**
During REM sleep, sympathetic activity of the splanchnic and renal circulation is decreased, but activity by skeletal muscles is increased. Whereas the slow phases of sleep are accompanied by hypotension and bradycardia, which become increasingly more pronounced with the progression of sleep from stage 1 to stage 4, REM sleep is associated with large, transient increases in blood pressure, reversing the hypotension of slow-wave sleep. Direct recording of sympathetic nerve traffic to the skeletal-muscle vascular bed by microneurography shows more than a 50% reduction in sympathetic activity during the slow phases of sleep but a significant increase to the level of wakefulness during REM. This finding may suggest that slow-wave sleep provides a protective effect on the cardiovascular and cerebrovascular systems; during REM sleep or immediately afterward, such protective effects may disappear. This phenomenon may explain why cardiovascular and cerebrovascular events occur more frequently in the early morning hours after awakening.

66. **There is a higher incidence of sudomotor and vasomotor disturbances of the arm with injuries to the lower trunk of the brachial plexus than with injuries to the upper trunk. Why?**
There is a higher density of postganglionic sympathetic fibers in the medial cord of the brachial plexus and the median and ulnar nerves.

67. **During examination of the external ear canal with an otoscope, the patient developed dry cough and became dizzy. Why?**
There is an anatomic explanation. The second branch of the vagus nerve, the auricular nerve, which originates after the vagus nerve has exited from the jugular foramen, is a somatic afferent nerve that provides the sensory fibers for the posterior wall and floor of the external acoustic meatus and the outer surface of the tympanic membrane. Irritation of the external auditory canal and the tympanic membrane by instruments, cerumen, or syringing may, therefore, cause abnormal vagal reflexes, resulting in coughing, vomiting, slow heart rate, or even cardiac inhibition.

68. **What is the syndrome of autonomic dysreflexia observed in tetraplegics? What is the best management?**
Traumatic spinal cord lesions result in markedly abnormal cardiovascular, thermoregulatory, bladder, bowel, and sexual function. In a recently injured tetraplegic in spinal shock, tactile or painful stimuli originating below the level of the lesion induce no change in blood pressure or heart rate. In the chronic stages of spinal cord injury at a level of T6 and above, however, there is an exaggerated rise in the systolic and diastolic blood pressure, accompanied by bradycardia. Transient tachycardia may precede the drop in heart rate. The plasma NE levels are only marginally elevated. The marked hypertension may lead to neurologic complications, including seizures, visual defects, and cerebral hemorrhage. This uncommon but potentially life-threatening phenomenon, called autonomic dysreflexia, is caused by the increased activity of target organs below the lesion supplied by sympathetic and parasympathetic nerves lacking supraspinal modulation. Other clinical manifestations of autonomic dysreflexia include headache, chest tightness and dyspnea, pupillary dilation, cold limbs, flushing of face and neck, excessive sweating of the head, penile erection and discharge of seminal fluid, and contraction of bladder and bowel.
   The prolonged episodes of this syndrome may be prevented if the precipitating cause (e.g., painful tactile or visceral urinary and rectal stimuli) is corrected. It is important that the bladder be emptied before performing any procedure on tetraplegic patients. Blood pressure can often be decreased by elevating the head of the bed.

69. **What are the pathologic causes of hyperhidrosis? How is it treated?**
Spinal cord damage or lesions of the peripheral sympathetic nerves may cause localized hyperhidrosis. Generalized and episodic hyperhidrosis may occur in patients with infectious diseases (night sweats), malignancies, hypoglycemia, thyrotoxicosis, pheochromocytomas, carcinoid syndrome, acromegaly, or diencephalic epilepsy and in patients receiving cholinergic agents.
   Primary or essential hyperhidrosis usually involves limited areas of the body, particularly the axilla, palms, and plantar regions. Axillary hyperhidrosis predominantly affects younger people and may cause social embarrassment. Essential hyperhidrosis is, however, usually self-limiting by the fourth or fifth decade of life. There is no known cause for essential hyperhidrosis, but up to one-half of patients have a family history of a similar condition. Several studies have demonstrated no abnormalities of the sweat glands and have implicated central and preganglionic sympathetic pathway hyperactivity.
   The treatment of essential generalized hyperhidrosis is difficult and requires systemic pharmacotherapy (anticholinergics and diltiazem), topical agents (aluminum chloride), excision of axillary sweat glands, and sympathectomy as the last resort. Recent experience suggests that botulinum toxin injections are a safe and effective treatment for focal or localized hyperhidrosis.

70. **How may mastocytosis be confused with autonomic dysfunction?**
Mastocytosis, or abnormal proliferation of tissue mast cells, may be confused with autonomic dysfunction because of symptoms of flushing, palpitation, dyspnea, chest discomfort, headache, lightheadedness and dizziness, fall in blood pressure, nausea, abdominal cramps, and diarrhea,

which occur episodically. Some patients may have an elevation of blood pressure. Each attack is followed by profound lethargy and fatigue. Episodes may be brief, lasting several minutes, or protracted, lasting 2 to 3 hours. Exposure to heat or emotional or physical stress may precipitate an attack. The presence of flushing and warm sensations are the most important clues differentiating this syndrome from syndromes of orthostatic intolerance.

In adults, there are two main forms of abnormal proliferation of mast cells: cutaneous mastocytosis and systemic mastocytosis. Some patients may experience episodes of systemic mast cell activation but show no evidence of mast cell proliferation in the skin or bone marrow. During an attack, increased serum histamine and prostaglandin $D_2$ may be demonstrated. Pigmented cutaneous lesions (urticaria pigmentosa) that characteristically urticate when stroked (Darier's sign) are frequently observed. Some patients with systemic mast cell activation are hypersensitive to aspirin, and any prostaglandin inhibitor may provoke severe mast cell activation.

71. **When your attending physician pumps you on rounds, why do you get sweaty palms but not sweaty armpits?**

Anxiety and emotional stress primarily aggravate the hyperhidrosis of the palms and soles but not of the axilla. The eccrine sweat glands of the palms and soles, as well as those of the forehead, respond to emotional, mental, or sensory stimuli, whereas the axillary glands respond primarily to thermal stimuli.

## BIBLIOGRAPHY

1. Appenzeller O, Oribe E: The Autonomic Nervous System, Part I, Amsterdam, Elsevier, 1999.

2. Appenzeller O, Oribe E: The Autonomic Nervous System, Part II, Amsterdam, Elsevier, 2000.

3. Freeman R: Autonomic peripheral neuropathy. Neurol Clin 25:277-301, 2007.

4. Goldstein DS: The Autonomic Nervous System in Health and Disease, New York, Marcel Dekker, 2001.

5. Harati Y: Diabetes and the autonomic nervous system. In Appenzeller O (ed): The Autonomic Nervous System, Part II, Revised Series 31, Amsterdam, Elsevier, 2000.

6. Low PA, Benarroch EE: Clinical Autonomic Disorders, 3rd ed. Philadelphia, Lippincott Williams & Wilkins, 2008.

7. Mathias CJ, Bannister R: Autonomic Failure, 4th ed. Oxford, Oxford University Press, 1999.

8. Murali NS, Svatikova A, Somers VK: Cardiovascular physiology and sleep. Front Biosci 8:s636-s652, 2003.

9. Robertson D, Biaggioni I, Burnstock G, Low PA: Primer on the Autonomic Nervous System, 2nd ed. San Diego, Academic Press, 2004.

# CHAPTER 13

# DEMYELINATING DISEASE

*Loren A. Rolak, MD*

## DISEASES OF MYELIN

**1. What is myelin?**

Myelin is the proteolipid membrane that ensheaths and surrounds nerve axons to improve their ability to conduct electrical action potentials. Oligodendrocytes make myelin and wrap it around axons, leaving gaps called nodes of Ranvier, where membrane ionic channels are heavily concentrated and powerful action potentials can thus be generated.

**2. How does demyelination cause symptoms?**

When myelin is stripped away from the axon, the underlying membrane does not contain a high enough concentration of sodium, potassium, and other ionic channels to permit a sufficient flow of ions to cause depolarization. The membrane thus becomes inert. The loss of myelin makes it impossible to depolarize the membrane to conduct an action potential, so the nerve is rendered useless.

**3. What is multiple sclerosis?**

Multiple sclerosis (MS) is the most common condition that destroys myelin in the central nervous system. It affects approximately 250,000 Americans, mostly between the ages of 20 and 40, making it the leading disabling neurologic disease of young people.

**4. How does MS cause demyelination?**

The demyelination is largely an inflammatory process. Lymphocytes, macrophages, and other immunocompetent cells accumulate around venules in the central nervous system and exit into the brain, attacking and destroying the myelin, in what appears to be an autoimmune process. In many patients with MS, a more degenerative (and poorly understood) pathology often appears, with less inflammation and more involvement of axons.

**5. Are there other demyelinating diseases?**

Yes, but they are rare. MS is the only common demyelinating disease in adults. Other rare conditions include:

1. **Central pontine myelinolysis**, a syndrome of myelin destruction in the pons, associated with rapid correction of hyponatremia.
2. **Progressive multifocal leukoencephalopathy**, an opportunistic viral infection of oligodendrocytes, seen most often in patients with acquired immunodeficiency syndrome (AIDS).
3. **Acute disseminated encephalomyelitis**, a postinfectious, acute, autoimmune demyelination.
4. **Inborn errors of myelin metabolism**, usually presenting in childhood:
   - Metachromatic leukodystrophy, a deficiency of the enzyme aryl sulfatase
   - Adrenoleukodystrophy, a defect in metabolism of very long chain fatty acids
   - Krabbe's globoid leukodystrophy, a deficiency of the enzyme galactosylceramidase
5. **Neuromyelitis optica or Devic's disease**, once considered a variant of MS, this is probably a distinct autoimmune disease predominantly affecting the optic nerves and spinal cord.

Patients have relapses, usually every few years, causing primary visual and spinal cord deficits. Severe disability often results. Patients have antibodies to aquaporin-4.

O'Riordan JI: Central nervous system white matter diseases other than multiple sclerosis. Curr Opin Neurol 10:211-214, 1997.

Wingerchuk DM, Lennon VA, Pittock SJ, et al.: Revised diagnostic criteria for neuromyelitis optica. Neurology 66:1485-1489, 2006.

## CLINICAL FEATURES OF MULTIPLE SCLEROSIS

6. **What are the most common symptoms of MS?**
   1. Pyramidal weakness—45%
   2. Visual loss—40%
   3. Sensory loss—35%
   4. Brain stem dysfunction—30%
   5. Cerebellar ataxia and tremor—25%
   6. Sphincter disturbances—20%

7. **Are there any symptoms that MS does not cause?**
   Not many. Virtually every neurologic problem has been described in MS, at least as a case report. However, because MS is predominantly a disease of myelin (white matter), it only rarely causes neuronal (gray matter) symptoms, such as aphasia, seizures, pain, and movement disorders.

8. **What is the clinical course of MS?**
   The clinical course of MS is highly variable and can follow almost any pattern, but many patients have both inflammatory (acute) and degenerative (chronic) symptoms.
   1. **Relapsing-remitting**. Patients have the sudden onset (over hours or days) of neurologic symptoms that usually last several weeks and then resolve, often leaving few or no deficits. The frequency of these relapses is highly variable but averages about one every 2 years.
   2. **Progressive**. Many patients gradually develop chronic progressive disability independent of acute relapses. If this occurs following a series of relapses, patients are labeled "secondary progressive." Approximately 15% of patients have chronic progressive symptoms from the onset, never preceded by any relapsing-remitting phase. Such "primary progressive" patients are often older and have predominantly spinal cord symptoms. Rare patients have both progressive disease and acute relapses simultaneously, and are referred to as "progressive relapsing."

   Confavreux C, Vukusic S, Moreau T, Adeleine P: Relapses and progression of disability in multiple sclerosis. N Engl J Med 343:1430-1438, 2000.

9. **What is the prognosis of MS?**
   MS varies greatly, not only in its symptoms and clinical course but also in its prognosis. Although not a fatal disease, MS is associated with a slight statistical shortening of life span as a result of secondary complications that may afflict severe cases, such as aspiration pneumonia, decubitus ulcers, urinary tract infections, and falls. As a general rule, approximately one third of patients with MS do well throughout their life, without accumulating significant disability. Another one-third accumulate neurologic deficits sufficient to impair activities but not serious enough to prevent them from leading a normal life—holding a job, raising a family. The final third of people with MS become disabled, requiring a walker, wheelchair, or even total care.

10. **What factors help to predict the course of MS?**
    The variability of MS makes accurate prediction fallible, but a few factors may portend a good prognosis:

1. Early age of onset (first symptoms before age 40)
2. Sensory symptoms at onset (as opposed to weakness, ataxia, or other motor abnormalities)
3. A relapsing-remitting course (versus a primary progressive symptom at onset)
4. Female gender: Women do better than men

Rolak LA: Multiple sclerosis. In Evans R (ed): Prognosis of Neurological Disorders. New York, Oxford University Press, 1992, pp 295-300.

11. **What is the EDSS?**
The Expanded Disability Status Score is a number that rates a patient's degree of disability from MS on a scale of 0 to 10. Deficits are determined in various functional systems (motor, sensory, cerebellar, etc.). A patient with a score of 6 requires a cane to walk, and with a score of 8, is confined to a wheelchair. The EDSS is widely used as a standard method of evaluating MS patients.

## DIAGNOSIS

12. **Given the great variability in the signs, symptoms, and clinical course of MS, how can it be accurately diagnosed?**
The diagnosis of MS is one of the most difficult in neurology. Nevertheless, certain clinical criteria can accurately diagnose MS (Table 13-1).

| TABLE 13-1. CLINICAL CRITERIA FOR DEFINITE MULTIPLE SCLEROSIS |
|---|
| Two separate central nervous system symptoms |
| Two separate attacks—onset of symptoms is separated by at least 1 month |
| Symptoms must involve the white matter |
| Age 10 to 50 years (although usually 20 to 40 years) |
| Objective deficits are present on the neurologic examination |
| No other medical problem can be found to explain the patient's condition |

13. **Is there any universally accepted standard for proving the diagnosis of MS?**
Maybe. The "McDonald criteria" incorporate the clinical criteria (discussed above) with features of the magnetic resonance imaging (MRI), spinal fluid, and evoked potentials to confirm a definite diagnosis of MS. The McDonald system can be complex, however, and is not universally embraced.

McDonald WI, Compston A, Edan G, et al.: Recommended diagnostic criteria for multiple sclerosis. Ann Neurol 50:121-127, 2001.

Miller DH, Weinshenker BG, Filippi M, et al.: Differential diagnosis of suspected multiple sclerosis. Mult Scler 14:1157-1174, 2008.

14. **How can the cerebrospinal fluid (CSF) be used to diagnose MS?**
Immunoglobulins are increased in the central nervous system in patients with MS. When the immunoglobulin G (IgG) is examined by electrophoresis, it may concentrate into specific bands. The finding of multiple bands in the IgG region, called oligoclonal bands, is reasonably sensitive and specific for MS. However, it remains unclear how or why oligoclonal bands are produced or exactly what they represent.

Freedman MS, Thompson EJ, Deisenhammer F, et al.: Recommended standard of cerebrospinal fluid analysis in the diagnosis of multiple sclerosis. Arch Neurol 62:865-870, 2005.

15. **Do other diseases have oligoclonal bands?**
Yes, especially inflammatory conditions, such as syphilis, meningoencephalitis, subacute sclerosing panencephalitis (a latent measles infection), and Guillain-Barré syndrome.

16. **How can evoked potentials be used to diagnose MS?**
    1. **Visual evoked potentials** (VEPs) are performed by flashing a checkered pattern in the patient's eyes while recording the electrical response from the visual cortex in the occipital lobe. Usually, a response appears approximately 100 msec after the stimulus is presented to the eye, and a delay implies demyelination in the visual pathways.
    2. **Brain stem auditory evoked potentials** (BAEPs) are performed by giving an auditory stimulus in the ear, such as a clicking sound, while recording from the auditory cortex in the temporal lobe. The sound generates a series of waves as it travels through the brain stem and hemispheres, and a delay in these waves is presumptive evidence of a demyelinating slowing.
    3. **Somatosensory evoked potentials** (SSEPs) are performed by applying an electrical stimulus to the wrist or ankle while recording from the sensory area of the cortex. Slowing can often be detected in the spinal cord, brain stem, or hemispheres if there is demyelination in these areas that delays nerve conduction.

17. **How valuable are evoked potentials for diagnosing MS?**
Evoked potentials can be very helpful by revealing unsuspected areas of demyelination. Studies disagree considerably, but probably about 75% of people with definite MS have an abnormal VEP; about 50% have abnormal SSEPs. Abnormal BAEPs are rare. Most of these patients also have an abnormal magnetic resonance imaging (MRI) scan, however, so evoked potentials usually have only a secondary role in diagnosis.

Gronseth GS, Ashman EJ: Practice parameter: The usefulness of evoked potentials in identifying clinically silent lesions in patients with suspected multiple sclerosis. Neurology 54:1720-1725, 2000.

18. **How can the MRI be used to diagnose MS?**
Because of its sensitivity and noninvasive nature, MRI is the best test to confirm the diagnosis of MS. The inflammatory demyelinated lesions, or plaques, are visualized quite well on MRI. The drawback to MRI is its lack of specificity. The scattered subcortical periventricular white matter abnormalities that characterize MS may occur in various other settings, including cerebrovascular disease, vasculitis, migraine, hypertension, and in some subjects who appear to be normal. For this reason, reliance strictly on MRI may lead to overdiagnosis of MS (Figure 13-1).

Frohman EM, Goodin DS, Calabresi PA, et al.: The utility of MRI in suspected MS. Neurology 61:602-611, 2003.

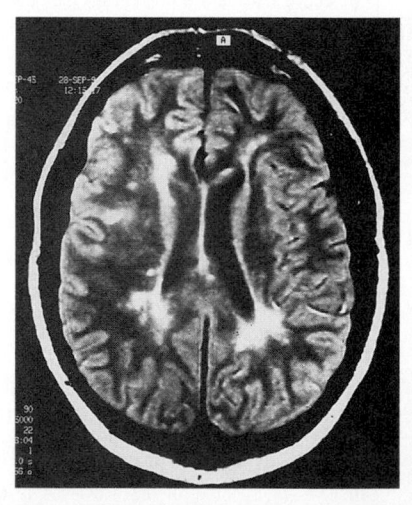

**Figure 13-1.** Axial flair magnetic resonance image (MRI) of the brain shows typical confluent, deep white matter signal intensities characteristic of multiple sclerosis (MS).

19. **Can MS be diagnosed after only one attack of symptoms?**
MS may begin in some patients with a "clinically isolated syndrome" such as a single, monophasic episode of optic neuritis or transverse myelitis. If this patient has an abnormal MRI of the brain (i.e., subclinical disease in another location in the central nervous system), it is virtually certain that he or she has MS. If a repeat brain MRI 1 to 6 months later reveals a new lesion, then the diagnosis of MS can be confirmed, even if a second clinical symptom has not appeared.

## ETIOLOGY

20. **How does the epidemiology of MS provide clues to its cause?**
Some unusual features characterize the epidemiology of MS. MS is more common the farther one moves away from the equator. It most frequently afflicts high socioeconomic classes, such as literate, educated professionals. It is more common in women than men. It primarily strikes people of northern European ancestry and is almost unknown in other racial groups such as Eskimos and Gypsies, a finding that may be related to specific human leukocyte antigen (HLA) type (i.e., immune functions) and genetic predisposition.

The chance of developing MS seems to be set by approximately age 15 years. A person born in a high-risk area (such as Scandinavia) who leaves for a low-risk area (in the tropics) after age 15 years will carry the high risk for developing MS. A person who emigrates before age 15 years acquires the low risk of the new home. In short, the risk of MS is determined before age 15 years, even though the disease itself does not appear, on average, until age 30 years.

Unfortunately, none of these tantalizing epidemiologic findings has yet led to a coherent hypothesis for the etiology of MS. The cause of MS is still unknown.

Compston A, Confavreux C: The cause and course of multiple sclerosis. In Compston A (ed): McAlpines Multiple Sclerosis. Philadelphia, Churchill Livingstone, 2006, pp 69-284.

21. **What evidence suggests that MS is an autoimmune disease?**
1. Pathologically, MS is an inflammatory disease involving lymphocytes and other immunocompetent cells.
2. MS is most common in patients with certain HLA types, implying that genes that control the immune system are related to the development of MS.
3. Oligoclonal bands in the CSF imply an abnormality in the immune system.
4. T-cell subsets are abnormal in MS. Most researchers report decreased numbers of suppressor T-lymphocytes.
5. The animal model of MS, experimental autoimmune encephalomyelitis (EAE), is an immune-mediated disease. Animals injected with myelin basic protein and immune adjuvants can be induced to mount an immune response against the myelin antigens, which damages their own myelin.
Rolak LA: Multiple sclerosis. In Rolak L, Harati Y (eds): Neuro-immunology for the Clinician. Boston, Butterworth-Heinemann, 1997, pp 107-132.

22. **Is MS all one disease?**
That is not clear. Clinically, it is quite heterogeneous, and pathologically this may prove true. New immunopathologic techniques suggest that there may be different patterns of demyelination and immune activation among different patients.
Breij EC, Brink BP, Veerhuis R, et al.: Homogeneity of active demyelinating lesions in established multiple sclerosis. Ann Neurol 63:16-25, 2008.
Luchinetti C, Bruck W, Parisi J, et al.: Heterogeneity of multiple sclerosis lesions: Implications for the pathogenesis of demyelination. Ann Neurol 47:707-717, 2000.

## TREATMENT

23. **What is the role of steroids in MS?**
A number of studies have suggested superiority of steroids over placebo for alleviating relapses of MS. Symptoms resolve more quickly, although it is not clear if treatment of attacks ultimately prevents disability or mitigates the final outcome of the disease. There remains much controversy about the most appropriate steroid preparation, dosage, route of administration, and duration of treatment.

24. **What is the usual steroid regimen in MS?**
The most popular therapy employs intravenous methylprednisolone (Solu-Medrol) in a dose of 500 to 1000 mg daily for 3 to 7 days. This "pulse" of steroids seems effective, at least in the short term, for improving MS symptoms.

25. **What is the role of immunosuppressants in MS?**
Many immune-altering regimens have been used in MS, but prospective, randomized, blinded, controlled, multicentered trials have been few and disappointing. Nevertheless, treatments such as plasmapheresis, cyclophosphamide, azathioprine, methotrexate, and intravenous immunoglobulin still are occasionally used, more for their theoretical benefits than for any proof of efficacy.
   Mitoxantrone (Novantrone), a broad-spectrum immunosuppressant, may slow the accumulation of disability in secondary progressive MS and is the best available treatment for that form of the disease. However, its benefits are modest, and its cardiotoxicity is considerable. There is a slightly increased risk of leukemia as well. Thus, its therapeutic role is limited.
   Noseworthy J, Hartung HP: Multiple sclerosis and related conditions. In Noseworthy J (ed): Neurological Therapeutics, 2nd ed. London, Martin Dunitz, 2006, pp 1224-1254.

26. **What prophylactic drugs are available to decrease attacks of MS?**
There is no cure for MS, but several drugs have been approved in the United States as long-term maintenance therapy to reduce the rate of attacks in relapsing-remitting MS: beta-interferon, glatiramer acetate, and natalizumab. These drugs are indicated for relapsing-remitting disease or clinically isolated syndromes and are probably useless for the progressive, degenerative aspects of MS.

27. **Discuss the role of interferons for the treatment of MS.**
These medications are given by self-injection. Some patients do not tolerate interferons because of their flu-like side effects. From 2% to 20% of patients produce neutralizing antibodies against these drugs as well. Interferons may work by altering T cells so they are less active in the inflammatory process. The approved preparations are as follows:
1. Beta-interferon-1b (Betaseron—subcutaneous QOD)
2. Beta-interferon-1a (Avonex-intramuscular; once weekly)
3. Beta-interferon-1a (Rebif-subcutaneous; three times per week)

28. **Discuss the role of glatiramer acetate (Copaxone) for the treatment of MS.**
Copaxone is a synthetic polypeptide resembling a fragment of the myelin basic protein molecule, and it may work by preventing activation and differentiation of myelin-targeting T-cells. It has few systemic side effects, and the daily injections are usually well tolerated.

29. **Discuss the role of natalizumab (Tysabri) for the treatment of MS.**
Tysabri is a monoclonal antibody given by monthly IV infusions. It is directed against alpha-1-integrin on the blood-brain barrier and prevents T cells from leaving the circulation and entering the central nervous system, thus reducing attacks on the myelin. Because it

also reduces T cell immune surveillance in the brain, the rate of opportunistic infections is increased, especially from progressive multifocal leukoencephalopathy.

Ransohoff FM: Natalizumab for multiple sclerosis. N Engl J Med 356:2622-2629, 2007.

**30. What is the best drug to prevent attacks of MS?**

There is no consensus about which of the drugs is superior or even which patients with MS should be treated at all, or for how long. Studies have shown no superiority of one interferon preparation over any other. Copaxone and the interferons are equally effective. There are not yet any head-to-head trials with Tysabri. Thus, the choice of therapy depends largely on personal preferences of doctors and patients. Although these drugs have all been shown to reduce relapse rates, none have yet been proven to prevent disability, which may depend more on the chronic degeneration process than on relapses.

Mikol DD, Barkhof F, Chang P, et al.: Comparison of subcutaneous interferon beta-1A with glatiramer acetate in patients with relapsing multiple sclerosis. Lancet Neurol 7:903-914, 2008.

## KEY POINTS: DEMYELINATING DISEASE

1. Traditionally, the diagnosis of MS requires two separate symptoms at two separate times, or lesions disseminated in space and in time.

2. The most common symptoms of MS are weakness, numbness, and visual changes.

3. A patient's prognosis and response to treatment depends upon what pattern of MS that he or she has. Relapsing-remitting disease has a better prognosis and response to therapy than progressive MS.

4. No treatment has yet been shown to prevent ultimate disability in MS.

### SYMPTOMATIC TREATMENT

**31. What is the role of symptomatic treatments for MS?**

If MS were cured today, the many sufferers from the disease would still have neurologic deficits. Management of these deficits is an important part of the treatment of MS. The most disabling symptoms reported by patients are fatigue, motor deficits, cerebellar problems, and sphincter disturbance.

**32. What is the best treatment for fatigue in MS?**

Although fatigue seems to be a vague and subjective symptom, it is one of the leading reasons why victims of MS are unable to work. Amantadine has been shown in careful studies to reduce fatigue, usually in doses of 100 mg twice daily, and is the mainstay of treatment. Modafinil and selective serotonin reuptake inhibitors such as fluoxetine also are prescribed. Of course, simple commonsense measures are also useful, such as resting during the day and reorganizing the home and workplace for better efficiency.

Lapierre Y, Hum S: Treating fatigue. International MS Journal 14: 64-71, 2007.

**33. What is the best treatment for motor deficits in MS?**

Unfortunately, little can be done to restore muscle strength. However, spasticity often improves with the use of baclofen (Lioresal) in doses of 60 mg/day or more. Tizanidine (Zanaflex), given up to 8 mg four times/day, produces similarly potent muscle relaxation.

Dantrolene (Dantrium) and diazepam (Valium) are also useful oral antispasticity agents, although their side effects make them less attractive as first-line drugs. Physical therapy can also minimize spasticity.

34. **What is the best treatment for cerebellar tremor and ataxia in MS?**
Therapy for cerebellar deficits is frustrating—these are among the most difficult symptoms to alleviate. Sometimes simple mechanical measures are helpful, such as attaching weights to the ankles or wrists. Drug treatment usually focuses on agents that increase levels of $\gamma$-aminobutyric acid (GABA), which is the primary neurotransmitter of the cerebellum. Benzodiazepines such as clonazepam (Klonopin) may help in a dose of 0.5 mg or more twice daily.

35. **What is the best treatment for urologic problems in MS?**
Urologic consultation is often useful to manage the neurogenic bladder. The most common problem is a hyperreflexic bladder with a small capacity, early detrusor contraction, urinary frequency, and urgency. It can be managed with medications such as oxybutynin (Ditropan), tolterodine (Detrol), or hyoscyamine (Levsinex). A flaccid bladder (more rare) may require self-catheterization. When sphincter-detrusor dyssynergia appears, medications to relax the sphincter, such as the alpha-adrenergic blocking agent prazosin (Minipress), may be useful.

# WEBSITE

http://www.nationalmssociety.org

# BIBLIOGRAPHY

1. Burks JS, Johnson KP: Multiple Sclerosis: Diagnosis, Medical Management, and Rehabilitation, New York, Demos, 2000.
2. Cohen JA, Rudick RA: Multiple Sclerosis Therapeutics, 2nd ed. London, Martin-Dunitz, 2003.
3. Compston A, editor: McAlpine's Multiple Sclerosis, Philadelphia, Churchill Livingstone, 2006.
4. Cook SD, editor: Handbook of Multiple Sclerosis, New York, Marcel Dekker, 2001.
5. Fleming JO: Diagnosis and Management of Multiple Sclerosis, New York, Professional Communications Medical Publishers, 2002.

# CHAPTER 14

# DEMENTIA

*Rachelle Doody, MD, PhD*

## GENERAL CONSIDERATIONS

**1. How is dementia defined? How do definitions vary?**

Dementia is generally regarded as an acquired loss of cognitive function due to an abnormal brain condition. The National Institutes of Health criteria (formerly NINCDS-ADRDA criteria) for the diagnosis of Alzheimer's disease (AD) stress that there must be **progressive** loss of cognitive function, including but not limited to memory loss. The DSM-IV general criteria for dementia include the requirement of **functional decline** that interferes with work or usual social activities in addition to cognitive decline.

American Psychiatric Association: Diagnostic and Statistical Manual of Mental Disorders, 4th ed. Washington, D.C., American Psychiatric Association, 1994.

McKhann G, Drachman D, Folstein M, et al.: Clinical diagnosis of Alzheimer's disease: Report of the NINCDS-ADRDA Work Group under the auspices of Department of Health and Human Services Task Force on Alzheimer's disease. Neurology 34:939-944, 1984.

**2. What is senility? Is it normal?**

Senility is an outdated term. It used to mean cognitive impairment due to aging, which was assumed to be normal. Although memory, learning, and thinking change with age in subtle ways, memory loss and cognitive impairment are not features of normal aging.

**3. What is pseudodementia?**

Pseudodementia has many meanings. It refers to depressed patients who are cognitively impaired and often have psychomotor slowing but do not have one of the well-defined dementia syndromes. The term does not mean that the patient is consciously simulating dementia (malingering) or is cognitively intact but believes himself or herself to be demented (Ganser's syndrome). Some researchers believe that pseudodementia may be a precursor to dementia.

**4. What features are characteristic of pseudodementia associated with depression?**

Patients with pseudodementia may or may not have a history of depressive or vegetative symptoms. They tend to have flat affect, to give up easily when mental status is examined, or to say that they cannot perform a task without even trying it. They often respond surprisingly well when given extra time and encouragement, but they may deny their success. Results of mental status examination are inconsistent; for example, they may fail a simple task but perform a similar, more difficult one correctly. Or they may have variable strengths and weaknesses over repeated testing sessions.

**5. What is Ganser's syndrome?**

It is an involuntary and unconscious simulation of altered mental status (confusion or dementia) in a patient who is not malingering and believes in the validity of his or her symptoms.

6. **What is delirium?**
   Delirium is an acute confusional state.

7. **What features distinguish delirium from dementia?**
   Although this distinction cannot always be made with certainty, several features are helpful. Sudden onset suggests delirium, as do findings of altered consciousness, marked problems with attention and concentration out of proportion to other deficits, cognitive fluctuations (e.g., lucid intervals), psychomotor and/or autonomic overactivity, fragmented speech, and marked hallucinations (especially auditory or tactile). Chronically demented patients may develop delirium in addition to dementia, which will change the clinical picture.

8. **Do all patients with dementia develop psychotic features?**
   No. Psychosis is a variable finding in all types of dementia and is not even clearly related to the stage or severity of dementia.

9. **Which screening instruments are commonly used in diagnosing dementia?**
   The Folstein Mini-Mental Status Examination (MMSE), Short Blessed dementia scale, and Mattis Dementia Rating Scale are commonly used clinically and in experimental studies to screen for dementia and to rate severity of dementia.

10. **What are the limitations of the MMSE in the assessment of dementia?**
    Besides the fact that it has both false-positive (usually depression) and false-negative results (usually early dementia in highly functioning patients), the MMSE also has limitations based on its lack of comprehensiveness.

11. **At what point is a patient too demented to require an evaluation?**
    No patient is too demented to be evaluated. The need to rule out reversible causes and structural lesions always remains. Neurologic and psychometric examinations can be tailored to the level of even the most profoundly demented patients. Further, even severely demented patients may respond to treatments.

12. **What are the most common causes of dementia or conditions resembling dementia?**
    Alzheimer's disease is the most common form of dementia in adults (>80% in most series). Depression with pseudodementia is a frequent cause of cognitive loss and must be ruled out in all patients. Other important causes include multi-infarct or vascular dementia, dementia with Lewy bodies, frontotemporal dementia, and dementia-like syndromes due to alcohol or chronic use of certain prescription drugs.

13. **What uncommon causes of dementia must be considered in the differential diagnosis *of every patient with dementia?***
    1. Toxins (lead, organic mercury)
    2. Vitamin deficiencies ($B_{12}$, $B_1$, and $B_6$, in particular)
    3. Endocrine disturbances (hypothyroidism or hyperthyroidism, hyperparathyroidism, Cushing's disease, and Addison's disease)
    4. Chronic metabolic conditions (hyponatremia, hypercalcemia, chronic hepatic failure, and renal failure)
    5. Vasculopathies affecting the brain
    6. Structural abnormalities (chronic subdural hematomas, normal-pressure hydrocephalus, and slow-growing tumors)
    7. Central nervous system (CNS) infections (including acquired immune deficiency syndrome [AIDS], Creutzfeldt-Jakob disease, and cryptococcal or tuberculous meningitis).

14. **How often is a Wernicke's diagnosis missed and what are the consequences?**
Wernicke's encephalopathy is correctly diagnosed in 1 of 22 patients. The classic features of confusion due to encephalopathy, variable ophthalmoplegia, and ataxia may be complete or only one or two of the features may be present. Untreated, patients can become comatose and death can result.

   Torvik A, et al.: Brain lesions in alcoholics: A neuropathological study with clinical correlations. J Neruol Sci 56:233-248, 1982.

15. **Which dementia syndromes are associated with alcohol?**
The DSM-IV includes alcohol amnestic syndrome (Korsakoff's syndrome), in which the amnestic disorder predominates, as well as a more generalized dementia associated with alcoholism. Both are associated with some degree of visuospatial impairment; neither includes aphasia. Patients with or without dementia may experience an acute, alcohol-related delirium known as Wernicke's encephalopathy (usually with confusion, eye movement abnormalities, and ataxia).

## ALZHEIMER'S DISEASE

16. **How is AD diagnosed?**
First, the presence of dementia must be established clearly by clinical criteria and confirmed by neuropsychological testing. The clinical manifestations must include impairment of memory and at least one other area of cognition. There must be no evidence of other systemic or brain disease sufficient to cause the dementia, and the National Institutes of Health (NIH) criteria suggest basic laboratory studies (which are not all-inclusive) to exclude other disease. The diagnosis is both a diagnosis of exclusion and a diagnosis based on the establishment of certain characteristic features.

   Knopman DS, DeKosky ST, Cummings JL, et al.: Practice parameter: Diagnosis of dementia. Neurology 56:1143-1153, 2001.

   McKhann G, Drachman D, Folstein M, et al.: Clinical diagnosis of Alzheimer's disease: Report of the NINCDS-ADRDA Work Group under the auspices of Department of Health and Human Services Task Force on Alzheimer's disease. Neurology 34:939-944, 1984.

17. **How are the alcohol-related dementias differentiated from AD?**
No absolute features distinguish these conditions. If the patient has a systemic disorder (such as alcoholism) that, in the clinician's opinion, is sufficient to cause dementia, the diagnosis should **not** be probable AD. Possible AD may be used if underlying AD is suspected in an actively drinking patient. The patient should stop drinking with the help of appropriate rehabilitative services. If the dementia improves and the improvement continues or persists for 1 year or more, the diagnosis is not likely to be AD.

18. **Which blood tests are typically ordered in a patient with suspected AD to rule out other causes or contributing factors?**
   1. Chemical analysis (including sodium, blood sugar, calcium, liver enzymes, and renal function)
   2. Complete blood count with differential
   3. Thyroid function tests
   4. Venereal Disease Research Laboratory or equivalent test for syphilis
   5. Vitamin $B_{12}$
   6. Antinuclear antibody (extractable nuclear antigen panel, if positive)
   7. Sedimentation rate

**Additional tests:**

Folate
Serum homocysteine
Serum methylmalonic acid

Serum arterial ammonia
Parathyroid hormone
Serum protein electrophoresis
Cortisol levels
Serum (and urine) drug screens
Hexosaminidase levels
Human immunodeficiency virus (HIV)

**19.  What blood tests can be done to assess the risk for AD?**
Glucose, cholesterol, and homocysteine elevations are risk factors for developing AD, as is an ApoE4 genotype.

**20.  Which ancillary studies (in addition to blood tests) are useful to evaluate patients with suspected AD?**
An imaging study (magnetic resonance imaging [MRI] or computed tomography [CT] with contrast) and neuropsychological testing to confirm dementia are necessary. Electroencephalography (EEG), single-photon emission CT (SPECT), or positron emission tomography (PET) studies and lumbar puncture (LP) may be useful or even necessary. Also consider an electrocardiogram (ECG) (to look for evidence of cardiovascular disease) and chest radiograph.

**21.  When is LP necessary in the diagnostic work-up?**
When symptoms are of short duration (<6 months) or have atypical features, such as rapid progression or severe confusion, an LP should be performed early. It also should be done if clinical or laboratory features suggest a specific etiology that is an indication for LP, such as CNS meningitis or CNS vasculitis.

**22.  What are typical symptoms of early AD?**
Early symptoms of AD include forgetfulness for recent events or newly acquired information, often causing the patient to repeat himself or herself. Other early features are disorientation, especially to time, and difficulty with complex cognitive functions such as mathematical calculations or organization of activities that require several steps.

**23.  What are typical symptoms of moderately advanced AD?**
Advanced AD includes a history of progression of pervasive memory loss sufficient to impair everyday activities, disorientation to place and/or aspects of person (e.g., age), inability to keep track of time, and problems with personal care (such as forgetting to change clothes). Behavioral changes, such as depression, paranoia, or aggressiveness, are more likely in these stages.

**24.  Does progression of AD follow a consistent pattern?**
Definitely not. Salient symptoms and rates of progression vary tremendously.

**25.  What language disturbances do patients with AD experience?**
Early in the disease, most patients have word-finding difficulties that may cause pauses in spontaneous speech or may be detected by asking the patient to name objects (particularly objects with low frequency in the language). As AD progresses, most patients develop problems with comprehension with intact repetition (similar to transcortical sensory aphasia); then repetition becomes affected while speech remains fluent (similar to Wernicke's aphasia). Ultimately, some patients develop expressive speech problems in addition to the above symptoms, or they may just stop talking secondary to inanition and apparent lack of anything to say.

**26.  Does the presence or absence of insight differentiate AD from other dementias?**
Lack of insight into their memory disorder (or anosognosia) occurs in some patients with AD as well as in patients with other dementing disorders. It does not appear to correlate with disease severity and is not useful in differential diagnosis.

Feher E, Doody R, Pirozzolo FJ, Appel SH: Mental status assessment of insight and judgment. Clin Geriatr Med 5:477-498, 1989.

27. **What motor features may be associated with AD? What is their significance?**
Rigidity, bradykinesia, and parkinsonian gait may be associated with more rapid progression of disease (both cognitive decline and activities of daily living). Tremor is rare, differentiating patients with AD from patients with Parkinson's disease to some extent. Myoclonus may occur, and recent evidence suggests its association with a younger age of onset of AD. In very severe AD, patients may have gait apraxia.

28. **What is the genetic defect in early-onset familial AD?**
Some families show a mutation in the gene that encodes amyloid precursor protein on chromosome 21. Other families show mutations on chromosome 14 (in the gene for presenilin 1) or chromosome 1 (in the gene for presenilin 2). It is likely that other genes will be linked to the early-onset familial form of AD. These mutations are rare and account for less than 5% of AD cases.

29. **What is the genetic defect in late-onset familial AD?**
Late-onset familial AD is linked to chromosome 19. It has been demonstrated that the particular inherited form of apolipoprotein E (coded by a gene on chromosome 19) determines the age-dependent risk and age of onset of AD in some patients. Patients who inherit one or more $E_4$ alleles are at greater risk, but only about 50% of AD patients have $E_4$. Other families have been linked to variant forms of TOMM 40, $\alpha$ mitochondrial transport protein on chromosome 19. These gene associations likely represent inherited risk factors rather than genetic forms of AD.

30. **Is there a genetic component to all cases of AD?**
The answer is not clear. Patients with a family history of AD in even one primary relative appear to be at increased risk, and the risk is higher if both parents have AD. Cases that seem to be sporadic are common, although the apolipoprotein E (ApoE) genotype is a clear risk factor for both sporadic and late-onset familial cases. Multiple genetic factors probably account for a predisposition for AD.

31. **What is apolipoprotein E? What is its importance?**
ApoE is a cholesterol-carrying blood protein that comes in three forms: $ApoE_2$, $E_3$, and $E_4$. We inherit one ApoE allele from each parent, and people with one or more $E_4$ alleles have an increased risk for developing AD.

32. **What other disorders have been associated with AD in epidemiologic surveys?**
Patients with Down syndrome are at high risk for AD. Whether families of patients with AD have a higher incidence of Down syndrome remains controversial. Parkinson's disease and a history of head trauma have been associated with AD in some large studies but not in others.

33. **What are the risk factors for AD?**
The presence of $ApoE_4$ and serious head injury in $ApoE_4$-positive people, aging, postmenopausal estrogen deficiency, positive family history (independent of ApoE genotype), elevated serum homocysteine levels, elevated blood glucose and/or cholesterol, and low education level (especially early in development) may be risk factors. Aluminum exposure is frequently cited, but no sound evidence supports the association.

34. **What factors reduce the risk for AD?**
Although definite proof is lacking, perimenopausal/estrogen replacement (but not later in life), anti-inflammatory drugs (including nonsteroidal agents), antioxidants, and the use of statin drugs have been proposed and are under study.

35. **What are the classic neuropathologic changes in AD?**
Senile plaques, neurofibrillary tangles, granulovacuolar degeneration, and amyloid in blood vessels and plaques are classic changes. Plaques and tangles also may be seen in normal brains but are far less numerous; in normal subjects, tangles outside the hippocampus are rare.

36. **Which neuropathologic changes correlate best with the severity of dementia due to AD?**
In most studies, neurofibrillary tangles correlate best with the severity of dementia. Synaptic density has been shown to have an inverse correlation with severity of dementia, at least in some brain regions. Because education seems to increase synaptic density, some have suggested that education may have a protective effect against the manifestation of AD cognitive changes.
Terry RD, Masliah E, Salmon DP, et al.: Physical basis of cognitive alterations in Alzheimer's disease: Synapse loss is the major correlate of cognitive impairment. Ann Neurol 30:572-580, 1991.

37. **Which neuropathologic entities overlap with AD?**
Besides normal aging, dementia with Lewy bodies, Parkinson's dementia, progressive supranuclear palsy, and vascular dementias are sometimes difficult to distinguish from AD because plaques and tangles may occur with other pathologic changes. Clinical correlations are extremely important in such cases.

38. **Which neuropathologically distinct entities may be clinically indistinguishable from AD?**
Vascular dementias (without plaques and tangles), dementia with Lewy bodies, Pick's disease, dementia lacking distinctive histology, and other frontal lobe dementia syndromes may be impossible to distinguish from AD on clinical grounds alone.

39. **What is the clinical picture of frontotemporal dementia?**
This designation includes a group of entities with variable neuropathologic findings and similar clinical features. Patients have early personality changes, particularly impulsivity and Klüver-Bucy type symptoms or withdrawal and depression. Psychiatric symptoms may precede dementia by several years. Memory and frontal executive tasks (e.g., planning, set-shifting, and set maintenance) are much more impaired than attention, language, and visuospatial skills. SPECT or PET studies may show hypofrontality. Neuropathology includes Pick's disease or primary degeneration at multiple brain sites (dementia lacking distinctive histology), usually with gliosis. Many of these cases have been linked to genetic mutations in the tau protein on chromosome 17.
The Lund and Manchester Groups: Clinical and neuropsychological criteria for frontotemporal dementia. J Neurol Neurosurg Psychiatry 57:416-418, 1994.

40. **What is the cholinergic hypothesis?**
The cholinergic hypothesis attempts to explain many of the cognitive deficits in AD (particularly memory disturbance) by a deficiency of cholinergic neurotransmission. Evidence includes the fact that poor memory can be induced in normal people by anticholinergic drugs. Loss of cholinergic projection neurons in the nucleus basalis of Meynert and loss of choline acetyltransferase activity throughout the cortex of patients with AD correlate with the severity of memory loss.

41. **Besides acetylcholine, which transmitters are affected by AD?**
Norepinephrine, somatostatin, dopamine, serotonin, and neuropeptide Y are decreased. Glutamate dysfunction (over production) also may play a role in AD.

42. **What is the role of amyloid in AD?**
Clearly AD is associated with abnormal accumulation of a breakdown product of the amyloid precursor protein known as beta-amyloid or Aß-amyloid, especially in the insoluble form. Amyloid appears to be toxic to cells in vitro, and abnormal accumulation may actually cause cell loss. No one knows why the Aß-amyloid accumulates, but accumulation may be secondary to abnormal processing within neurons.

43. **What is the role of tau protein in AD?**
Tau protein is part of the cytoskeleton of neuronal cells. In damaged cells (e.g., after heat shock), its expression is increased. Tau protein is found in the neurofibrillary tangles of patients with AD. Tau appears to be hyperphosphylated in cells destined to develop neurofibrillary tangles. It may be an early marker of cells with abnormal cytoskeletal function and abnormal metabolism.

44. **What famous people probably had AD?**
    1. Ronald Reagan—U.S. president
    2. Charlton Heston—actor
    3. Rita Hayworth—actress
    4. Immanuel Kant—philosopher
    5. Ralph Waldo Emerson—writer
    6. Maurice Ravel—composer
    7. John James Audubon—painter

45. **What is the treatment for the noncognitive secondary behavioral effects of AD?**
Behavioral symptoms, such as disturbed sleep, depression, anxiety, psychotic features, agitation, and aggressiveness, are amenable to treatment. Behavioral modification, such as entraining sleep-wake cycles and increasing daytime activity, should be tried first for **sleep disorders.**

   **Depression,** particularly early in the disease, may respond to low doses of antidepressants, but drugs with anticholinergic side effects should be avoided. Drugs that act on the serotonergic system may be better tolerated (fluoxetine, paroxetine, citalopram, sertraline), although controlled studies are lacking for patients with AD.

   **Anxiety and agitation** frequently respond to behavioral interventions, such as day center participation, that engage the patient and reduce caregiver stress. Other respite interventions for caregivers may help to reduce patient stress. If symptoms are infrequent, anxiety or agitation may be treated with low doses of anxiolytics as needed, such as chloral hydrate or lorazepam (avoid long-acting drugs). Chronic anxiolytics are not indicated for AD, but short-term therapy with buspirone or lorazepam may be justified during periods of transition or change.

   **Environmental** triggers and pain should always be ruled out as causes of agitation before using drugs. **Severe agitation, aggressiveness, and psychotic features** that disturb the patient should be treated with atypical antipsychotics such as olanzapine, risperidone, and quetiapine, in the lowest doses possible, because these drugs further impair cognition (and sometimes motor performance). Some of these drugs include black box warnings for dementia patients in their labeling. Psychotic features that do not disturb the patient or disrupt the household need not be treated.

   Doody RS, Stevens JC, Beck, C, et al.: Practice parameter: Management of dementia (an evidence-based review). Neurology 56:1154-1166, 2001.

46. **What treatments exist for the primary process of AD?**
The Food and Drug Administration (FDA) has approved five treatments specifically for AD. Tacrine, donepezil, rivastigmine, and galantamine are cholinesterase inhibitors, and Memantine is an N-methyl-d-aspartate (NMDA) receptor antagonist. Studies of estrogen as a treatment for

AD have been negative. Many patients can qualify for experimental studies of potential new AD treatments and should be referred to AD research centers that test medications if they are interested. Available drugs and sites can be identified by calling the National Alzheimer's Disease Association in Chicago.

Doody RS, Stevens JC, Beck, C, et al.: Practice parameter: Management of dementia (an evidence-based review). Neurology 56:1154-1166, 2001.

Doody RS: Prevention and future treatment of Alzheimer's disease. In Doody RS (ed): Alzheimer's Dementia. Delray Beach, Carma Publishing, 2008, pp 115-140.

Reisburg B, Doody R, Stoffler A, et al.: Memantine study group. Memantine in moderate to severe Alzheimers disease. N Engl J Med 348:1333-1341, 2003.

47. **Are there any agents besides prescription drugs that improve cognition or slow functional loss in AD?**
One large-scale double-blind study supports the benefits of vitamin E (1000 IU twice daily) or selegiline, an MAO-B inhibitor (10 mg twice daily) for slowing the time to significant worsening. Vitamin E is better tolerated, and the two should not be used together because combination therapy reduces the benefits.

Sano M, Ernesto C, Thomas RG, et al.: A controlled trial of selegiline, alpha-tocopherol or both as treatment for Alzheimer's disease. N Engl J Med 336:1216-1222, 1997.

48. **What is respite care?**
Respite care is any caretaking arrangement for the patient that temporarily relieves the primary caregiver. It may be as informal as a friend or relative who comes to the home to care for the patient, a part-time in-home aide, or a few days per week at a day center. It also may apply to short-term stays in residential facilities.

49. **What are the responsibilities of physicians and health care workers with respect to respite care?**
The physician or health care worker must introduce the concept of respite care and assure every primary caregiver that he or she will need it sooner or later. Even early in the disease process, activities that are directed toward patients (such as day centers) help promote their autonomy and provide supervision while providing respite to caregivers. Many caregivers feel guilty about not being able to care for the patient alone every day and night. They need to know that all affected families require help in caregiving.

## VASCULAR DEMENTIAS

50. **What entities constitute the vascular dementias?**
1. Multiple large infarctions, which usually involve cortical and subcortical tissue.
2. Single or multiple smaller infarctions that involve critical brain regions.

It is less clear whether diffuse, chronic vascular processes such as Binswanger's disease, leukoaraiosis, or diffuse changes in white matter due to microinfarcts also cause dementia.

51. **Can vascular dementia be diagnosed by CT or MRI alone?**
No. Patients who have changes in white matter on scans or even multiple, definite infarctions may be clinically normal. It is not known how many infarcts or how much change in white matter on a scan translates into dementia for patients who suffer cognitive impairments. Many white-matter signal changes, especially on MRI, do not represent strokes.

Román GC, Tatemichi, TK, Erkinjuntti T, et al.: Vascular dementia: Diagnostic criteria for research studies. Neurology 43:250-260, 1993.

## KEY POINTS: DEMENTIA ✓

1. Dementia must be differentiated from delirium and depression.

2. Dementia is a category, not a diagnosis. The clinician must determine the cause of the dementia.

3. AD is rarely caused by inheriting an abnormal genetic mutation (familial AD). On the other hand, patients may inherit risk factors that predispose them to developing AD, such as APO $E_4$.

4. Both cognitive and behavioral symptoms of dementia can be treated, and long-term therapy may slow decline and help maintain function.

5. Vascular dementia cannot be diagnosed by MRI or CT scan alone.

---

**52. Can dementia occur after a single stroke?**
One prospective study of patients after acute stroke showed that the risk of dementia was 9 to 10 times greater than for matched controls without stroke. A single stroke also can lead to dementia by "unmasking" underlying Alzheimer's disease that has not yet become symptomatic.

    Tatemichi TK, Desmond DW, Mayeux R, et al.: Dementia after stroke: Baseline frequency, risks, and clinical features in a hospitalized cohort. Neurology 42:1185-1193, 1992.

**53. Can neuropsychological testing differentiate vascular dementia from AD?**
Not absolutely. Patchy performances across tests, unilateral motor impairments (e.g., reaction times or finger tapping), and improvements in some but not all areas of cognition over time are typically seen in vascular dementias. Asymmetric finger tapping, however, is also common in AD.

**54. What basic work-up should be done when vascular dementia is suspected?**
The work-up should begin with imaging studies and psychometric testing in addition to the history and physical examination. In most cases, all tests recommended for the diagnosis of AD should be pursued to rule out additional conditions that may cause or contribute to the dementia, including a lipid profile and blood homocysteine levels, which are risk factors for both AD and vascular dementia. Some patients, especially those with clear-cut strokes, may benefit from imaging of the carotid arteries, especially when high-grade stenosis or ulcerated plaques are suspected. An echocardiogram is indicated in patients who have a cardiac history or appear to have had embolic strokes.

**55. What ancillary tests may be useful in diagnosing vascular dementia?**
The EEG may show multiple slow-wave foci, and SPECT or PET scans may show multiple areas of decreased flow or altered metabolism. These tests have not been adequately studied to assess their utility for differentiating the various forms of vascular dementia.

**56. Can vascular dementia be diagnosed in patients with aphasia due to a left hemisphere infarct?**
Patients should not be tested for dementia in the acute phase of stroke, whether aphasic or otherwise. Although most tests for cognitive functioning rely heavily on language abilities, tests of nonverbal memory and reasoning help to support the diagnosis of dementia in an aphasic patient. A history of functional decline not related to language-based tasks is also helpful.

**57. What is the treatment of vascular dementia?**
The FDA has not yet approved any drugs to treat vascular dementia, but research studies suggest that cholinesterase inhibitors and Memantine may be helpful. As for AD, noncognitive

behavioral effects of dementia are amenable to therapy, and respite care should be introduced early. In addition, it is advisable to control vascular risk factors as much as possible (blood pressure, blood glucose, cholesterol, and hypertension). Prophylactic antiplatelet therapy (aspirin, clopidogrel, or ticlopidine), although not of proven benefit for dementia, may be helpful by reducing the risk of future strokes.

## SUBCORTICAL DEMENTIAS

58. **What are the characteristics of subcortical dementias?**
Subcortical dementias lack cortical features, such as aphasia, apraxia, and acalculia. Recall memory is impaired worse than recognition memory. Visuospatial skills are often impaired. Frontal executive deficits, bradyphrenia, anomia, personality changes, and psychomotor slowing are prominent. Dysarthria, abnormal posture and coordination, and adventitious movements may be present.
Cummings JL: Subcortical Dementia. New York, Oxford University Press, 1990.

59. **How do the general features of subcortical dementias differ from cortical dementias?**
The cortical dementias, such as AD, usually involve language and calculations and may involve apraxia and cortical sensory disturbances (e.g., astereognosis, graphesthesia), whereas subcortical dementias do not. Both recall and recognition memory are usually impaired in cortical dementia, whereas recognition memory is relatively preserved in subcortical dementia. Frontal executive functions are lost in proportion to the overall dementia in cortical processes but are prominently affected in subcortical dementia. Bradykinesia and bradyphrenia, as well as other motor features, are usually absent or late findings in cortical dementias but occur early in subcortical dementias. Personality changes are variable in both types but are said to be more prominent early in the course of subcortical dementia.
Cummings JL: Subcortical Dementia. New York, Oxford University Press, 1990.

60. **In what ways do the specific memory disturbances of subcortical dementias differ from those of cortical dementias?**
Problems with short-term spontaneous recall occur in both types, but strategies to enhance encoding and recognition cuing are mainly helpful in subcortical dementias. Incidental memory (details not related to the task at hand, such as what the examiner was wearing) is better in subcortical dementias. Procedural memory (memory involved in learning tasks) is better preserved in cortical dementias. Remote memory usually shows a temporal gradient in cortical dementias but not in subcortical dementias.

61. **Is there a rigid anatomic or functional distinction between cortical and subcortical dementia?**
No. So-called subcortical dementias may give rise to or be associated with cortical changes and vice versa. Huntington's dementia, like most subcortical dementias, causes disturbances of cortical frontal lobe functioning. Patients with (subcortical) Parkinson's disease may show atrophy of cortical cells. Patients with AD have subcortical changes in deep nuclei, such as the nucleus basalis of Meynert and locus ceruleus.

62. **What disorders or clinical syndromes are typically associated with subcortical dementia?**
1. Parkinson's disease
2. Huntington's disease
3. Progressive supranuclear palsy

4. Spinocerebellar degeneration
5. Idiopathic basal ganglia calcification
6. Multiple sclerosis
7. Inflammatory conditions involving the basal ganglia and/or thalamus
8. AIDS
9. Corticobasal degeneration

63. **What are the clinical features of Parkinson's dementia?**
Parkinsonian features sufficient to make a diagnosis of Parkinson's disease usually predate the dementia by at least 1 year. Typically bradyphrenia, dysnomia, and frontal executive dysfunction are present, and depression is common. There may be visuospatial abnormalities, especially on formal testing.

64. **What are the clinical features of Huntington's dementia?**
Psychiatric symptoms or dementia may occur before or after the features of Huntington's disease (e.g., chorea) are well established. Psychiatric features include personality changes, depression, and psychosis. The memory disorder is typical of the subcortical pattern. Language and speech disorders, including dysarthria, reduced spontaneous speech, impaired syntactic complexity, and impaired comprehension, are common, as are visuospatial abnormalities.

65. **What are the clinical features of the dementia associated with progressive supranuclear palsy (PSP)?**
PSP is a syndrome characterized by supranuclear gaze palsy, dystonic rigidity of axial musculature, dysarthria, and pseudobulbar palsy. The dementia is not clearly present in all patients and is difficult to characterize because the associated visual scanning disorder interferes with testing. Memory impairments tend to be mild relative to frontal executive functions.

66. **What is dementia with Lewy bodies?**
A spectrum of disorders probably makes up Lewy body disease, ranging from Parkinson's disease (with Lewy bodies primarily in the subcortical and brain stem regions) to diffuse Lewy body disease, in which Lewy bodies are present throughout the cortex, subcortex, and brain stem. Some authorities describe an intermediate form of Lewy body dementia (senile dementia of the Lewy body type), which is associated with many Lewy bodies in the brain stem and subcortical regions, fewer in the hippocampus, and fewer still in the neocortical region. When Lewy bodies occur in AD brains, the condition may be called Lewy body variant of AD.

67. **What are the clinical characteristics of dementia with Lewy bodies?**
Patients typically exhibit fluctuating confusion and dementia, usually with vivid visual hallucinations and extrapyramidal features. The neuropsychological deficits are not well characterized, and little is known about the natural history of the disorder. A rapid eye movement (REM) sleep disorder is not uncommon.
   McKeith IG, Galasko D, Kosaka K, et al.: Consensus guidelines for the clinical and pathologic diagnosis of dementia with Lewy bodies (DLB). Neurology 47:1113-1124, 1996.

68. **What other disorders are in the differential diagnosis of dementia (not necessarily subcortical) with extrapyramidal features?**
   1. Alzheimer's disease
   2. Parkinson's disease plus dementia
   3. Creutzfeldt-Jakob disease
   4. Binswanger's disease
   5. Multi-infarct or vascular dementia

6. Normal pressure hydrocephalus
7. Dementia lacking distinctive histology
8. Corticobasal ganglionic degeneration
9. AIDS dementia
10. Hallervorden-Spatz disease
11. Neuronal intranuclear inclusion disease
12. GM1 gangliosidosis type III
13. Striatonigral degeneration

69. **How do patients with corticobasal ganglionic degeneration (CBGD) present?**
Patients tend to present either with an alien limb phenomenon and associated motor features (tremor, rigidity, grasp reflex, apraxia, and myoclonus) or with an akinetic-rigid syndrome similar to Parkinson's disease. Dementia frequently develops over time and affects cognitive function pervasively. The neuropsychological deficits are typical of subcortical dementia.

Doody RS, Jankovic JJ: The alien hand and related signs. J Neurol Neurosurg Psychiatry 55:806-810, 1992.

Massman PJ, Kreiter KT, Jankovic J, Doody RS: Neuropsychological functioning in cortical-basal ganglionic degeneration: Differentiation from Alzheimer's disease. Neurology 46:720-726, 1996.

# WEBSITES

1. http://www.alzforum.org

2. http://www.alz.org

3. http://www.nlm.nih.gov/medlineplus/dementia.html

## BIBLIOGRAPHY

1. Behatar M: Analytic Neurology, Boston, Butterworth-Heinemann, 2003.
2. Doody RS, (ed): Alzheimer's Dementia, Delray Beach, Carma Publishing, 2008.
3. Growdon JH, Rossor MN, (eds). The Dementias, Boston, Butterworth-Heinemann, 1998.
4. Noseworthy JH, editor: Neurological Therapeutics, 2nd ed. London, Martin Dunitz, 2006.
5. Trimble MR, Cummings JL: Contemporary Behavioral Neurology. Boston, Butterworth-Heinemann, 1997.
6. Trojanowski J, Clark C, (eds). Neurodegenerative Dementias. New York, McGraw-Hill, 1998.

# CHAPTER 15

# NEUROPSYCHIATRY AND BEHAVIORAL NEUROLOGY

*Heike Schmolck, MD, Salah U. Qureshi, MD, and Paul E. Schulz, MD*

## MEMORY AND AMNESTIC SYNDROMES

1. **What is amnesia, and injury to which areas can cause an amnestic syndrome?**
   Amnesia is a severe, isolated disturbance of memory in the absence of other forms of cognitive dysfunction. Patients are unable to acquire new memories (anterograde amnesia) or recall recent memories (retrograde amnesia). Other memories remain intact, including remote memory (e.g., childhood events), working memory (digit span), and semantic memory (knowledge about things).

   Bilateral lesions of the Papez circuit and related areas can cause an amnestic syndrome while unilateral lesions can produce a milder, but often clinically relevant memory deficit. This includes the medial temporal lobes (hippocampus and entorhinal cortex), the diencephalon (fornix and mamillary bodies; dorsomedial and anterior nuclei of the thalamus), and the basal forebrain cholinergic nuclei (medial septal nuclei and the diagonal band of Broca).

   Isolated, slowly progressive reduced ability to learn new information is referred to as amnestic mild cognitive impairment (aMCI). Many or most patients with aMCI develop Alzheimer's dementia over the next 5 years.

2. **What are the most common etiologies for amnestic syndromes?**
   - Medial temporal lobes—hypoxia, herpes simplex encephalitis, early Alzheimer's disease, Posterior Cerebral Artery (PCA) strokes (thalamic and temporal lobe), surgery
   - Diencephalon-Korsakoff syndrome (thiamine deficiency), thalamic strokes, surgery
   - Basal forebrain—Anterior Cerebral Artery (ACA) aneurysm bleed or clipping (with damage to the small perforating arteries)
   - Substances—alcohol, benzodiazepines (transient, not permanent)

3. **What is declarative memory and how does it differ from nondeclarative memory?**
   Declarative memory (explicit memory) is flexible, requires awareness, allows conscious recollection, and is the type of memory damaged in amnesia. Nondeclarative memory (implicit or procedural memory) does not require the hippocampal circuitry, is not consciously accessible, one is unaware of it and it is inflexible, and it remains intact in amnesia. Examples are conditioning, priming, motor and cognitive skill learning, and habit learning. It requires the cerebellum, basal ganglia, and association cortices. In healthy individuals, both systems work together. In amnesia, implicit learning remains intact; this fact can be utilized for rehabilitation. Even patients with Alzheimer's disease, for example, can learn through this system—the repetition of facts, rather than single presentations, may allow their storage.

4. **What is Ribot's law?**
   Ribot's law states that recent memories are more vulnerable than remote memories and are lost first when memory-relevant structures are damaged. Once memories have become independent of the hippocampal system after consolidation, they are more stable. Most amnestic patients thus have a temporally graded retrograde amnesia.

5. **What are the clinical characteristics of transient global amnesia?**
   Patients develop a sudden, isolated amnestic syndrome without structural brain abnormalities (anterograde and retrograde amnesia), which usually has a duration of 12 to 24 hours. Afterwards, patients will not remember the episode because they were unable to encode new memories during it. Working memory is normal during the episode. On positron emission tomography (PET) or single photon emission computed tomography (SPECT), bilateral temporal hypoperfusion can be demonstrated. The cause of this benign syndrome remains unknown. Because it occurs more often in migraineurs, it could be a migraine equivalent. Risk of recurrence is low, but higher than in the general population.
   Noel A, Quinette P, Guillery-Girard B, et al.: Psychopathological factors, memory disorders, and transient global amnesia. Br J Psychiatry 193:145-151, 2008.

6. **What are the features of psychogenic amnesia?**
   In most cases of psychogenic amnesia, patients exhibit biologically unlikely patterns of impairment. Commonly, autobiographical memory is disproportionately affected, sparing memories of political and entertainment events. It also includes remote memories, which are normally very resistant to damage. New learning (anterograde memory) is often spared. Nevertheless, reversible abnormalities on PET with temporal hypometabolism have been found in some of these patients.

7. **What types of memory difficulties occur with frontal lobe lesions?**
   The dorsolateral prefrontal cortex is important for "metamemory," which has executive control over the memory apparatus. For example, it decides whether a retrieved memory is plausible for a given context, does strategic searching of the memory store, and temporally orders memories.
   An impairment of declarative memory in conjunction with frontal lobe dysfunction may cause confabulation, the inability to distinguish a true memory from a false memory or from a memory inappropriate for the context. Confabulations are a common occurrence in alcoholic Korsakoff syndrome.
   The dorsolateral prefrontal cortex is also important for working memory, which usually holds about 7 to 10 bits of information as long as they are constantly repeated ("phonological loop"). A common test of working memory is the "digit span," in which patients are asked to recall a sequence of up to 7 digits in a row. Working memory is intact in pure amnesia.

8. **What are paramnesias? What are some specific paramnesias and their characteristics?**
   Paramnesias, or misidentifications syndromes, are rare disorders resulting in very specific memory distortions. They are poorly understood and occur most commonly in psychotic disorders but also with medial temporal or prefrontal lesions.
   In *Capgras' syndrome,* a patient has the delusional belief that family members and friends have been replaced by impostors. The patient may also see himself as his own double (Doppelgänger syndrome). As a variant of this syndrome, the patient believes that inanimate objects, such as furniture, a letter, a watch, or spectacles, have been replaced by an exact double. The syndrome has been described with partial limbic lesions superimposed on right hemisphere damage. It is also associated with Lewy body disease. It has been proposed that the Capgras' delusion is the result of intact perception of faces with a loss of the affective response that normally contributes to the recognition of familiar ones. A patient interprets this dissonance in a paranoid, suspicious way, which leads him or her to conclude that the person must be an impostor.
   In *reduplicate paramnesia,* a patient is convinced that a person, a place, or an object exists in duplicate. A disturbed sense of familiarity may produce this phenomenon. A patient may be unable to associate the present situation with a previously experienced and familiar one, and thus give the present situation a different identity.
   In *reduplication of time,* a patient believes that he or she exists in two different, parallel time points.
   In *autoscopy,* a patient believes that his or her body is a duplicate of another body.
   In *Foley's syndrome,* a patient believes that his or her image belongs to someone else.

In *Fregoli's syndrome,* a patient believes that a familiar person has taken on the appearance of another person to persecute him or her.

In *intermetamorphosis,* a patient believes that he or she has switched identities with another individual, or believe that other people or objects have changed physically and psychologically into someone else.

Sinkman A: The syndrome of Capgras. Psychiatry 71:371-378, 2008.

9. **Which areas are responsible for encoding, storage, and retrieval of information?**
   - The hippocampal system is concerned with encoding and consolidating information.
   - Long-term storage generally occurs in the temporo-parietal cortices. The left hemisphere stores primarily verbal or general knowledge (i.e., semantic/lexical information) and the right nonverbal or autobiographical information.
   - Retrieval uses prefrontal and distributed temporo-parietal networks; the role of the hippocampal system in retrieval is time limited.

## APHASIAS

10. **What is the definition of aphasia and how does it differ from dysarthria?**
    Aphasia is an acquired disturbance of language whereas dysarthria is an acquired disorder of speech production.
    Pulvemuller F, Berthier ML: Aphasia therapy on a neuroscience basis. Aphasiology 22:563-599, 2008.

11. **Which are the nonfluent aphasias and which are the fluent aphasias?**
    The anterior aphasias are nonfluent, and include Broca's, global, mixed transcortical, and transcortical motor. The posterior aphasias are fluent, including Wernicke's, transcortical sensory, and usually thalamic.

12. **Which aphasias spare repetition and which have impaired repetition?**
    Repetition is spared in those outside the perisylvian fissure area, including transcortical motor, transcortical sensory, and thalamic aphasias. Repetition is impaired in the perisylvian aphasias, including Broca's, Wernicke's, conduction aphasia, and pure word deafness.

13. **What are the clinical characteristics of nonfluent aphasia?**
    Impaired articulation, impaired melodic production, reduced phrase length (five or less words per phrase), and decreased grammatical complexity. Often a guideline of less than 15 words per minute is used to define nonfluent aphasias.

14. **What are the clinical features of Broca's aphasia and where is the lesion responsible for it?**
    Speech is nonfluent, effortful, agrammatic and telegraphic, with poor ability to name, semantic and phonemic paraphasic errors, impaired repetition, and relatively spared comprehension. The lesion is in Broca's area (the frontal operculum, Brodmann areas 44 and 45), inferior left frontal gyrus, the surrounding frontal areas and the underlying white matter and subjacent basal ganglia.
    Keller SS, Crow T, Foundas A, et al.: Broca's area: Nomenclature, anatomy, typology, and asymmetry. Brain Lang 109:29-48, 2009.

15. **What are the clinical features of aphemia and where is the lesion that underlies it?**
    Aphemia is poor speech output with sparing of comprehension and writing. Their speech output can be slow and halting. Aphemia has been reported with lesions of the lower motor strip (cortical dysarthria), supplementary motor cortex, and several other areas.

16. **What are the clinical features of anomic aphasia and where is the lesion that underlies it?**
A person with anomic aphasia has an isolated deficit in word-finding. Otherwise, his or her speech is fluent with good comprehension and good repetition. Lesions producing this aphasia localize less specifically than other aphasias. They may be in the temporo-parieto-occipital association area. This is also a common chronic residual syndrome for other acute aphasias after rehabilitation.

17. **What are the clinical features of conduction aphasia and where is the lesion that produces it?**
Conduction aphasia is a fluent aphasia, with good comprehension, poor repetition, paragrammatic errors, anomia, paraphasic errors, good recitation, and good reading aloud. While any type of paraphasia may be seen, the vast majority of substitutions involve phonemes resulting in literal (phonemic) paraphasic errors. The lesion usually involves the left inferior parietal lobule, especially the anterior supramarginal gyrus. Often the lesion is in the subcortical white matter, deep to the inferior parietal cortex, involving the arcuate fasciculus or the extreme capsule immediately below it—both structures are connected to the temporal and frontal cortex.

18. **What are the clinical features of Wernicke's aphasia and where is the lesion responsible for it?**
It is characterized by fluent speech, good articulation, good or sometimes exaggerated prosody (the expressivity of language), impaired naming, phonemic and semantic paraphasias, poor auditory and reading comprehension, impaired repetition, and fluent but empty writing. It is usually caused by damage to the posterior sector of the left auditory association cortex, Brodmann area 22. Often there is involvement of Brodmann areas 37, 39, and 40, or all three.

19. **What are the clinical features of transcortical motor aphasia and where are the lesions responsible for it?**
Spontaneous speech is nonfluent, with good repetition and good comprehension, delayed initiation of output, brief utterances, semantic paraphasic errors, and echolalia. Lesions of the supplementary motor area or its connections to Broca's area are responsible.

20. **What are the clinical features of transcortical sensory aphasia and where is the lesion responsible for it?**
Spontaneous speech is fluent, with good repetition, echolalia, impaired auditory and reading comprehension, right visual field deficits, and rare motor and sensory deficits. Lesions outside of Wernicke's area in the surrounding temporal-parietal area are responsible.

21. **What are the clinical features of mixed transcortical aphasia, where is the lesion responsible for it, and what is its vascular territory?**
There is absent spontaneous speech, impaired comprehension, and intact repetition. Stock phrases, such as "you know" and "the thing is," and echolalia are pronounced. The lesion includes the areas that cause transcortical motor and sensory aphasias: the dorsolateral frontal region anterior to the motor cortex and the temporal-parietal-occipital junction. This lesion may be caused by hypoperfusion in the distribution of the left internal carotid artery, which produces a watershed stroke.

22. **What are the clinical features of the anterior subcortical syndrome and where is the lesion associated with it?**
It includes dysarthria, decreased fluency, mildly impaired repetition (less than Broca's aphasia), and mild comprehension deficits. It results from strokes in the vicinity of the left basal ganglia, most commonly including the anterior putamen, caudate nucleus, and the anterior limb of the internal capsule.

23. **What are clinical features of the thalamic subcortical aphasias?**
Lesions involving the anterior nuclei and anterior medial intramedullary region can produce an aphasia that is similar to a transcortical sensory aphasia. Spontaneous speech is grammatically correct but terse with elements of echolalia. Comprehension is impaired and repetition is fairly good. Anomia, agraphia, and impaired reading are usually present. Lesions in the posterior thalamus produce no language impairment.

24. **What are the clinical features of global aphasia and where are the lesions that produce it?**
Spontaneous speech is nonfluent with poor repetition and poor comprehension. The output is restricted to meaningless speech sounds or stereotypes. These lesions involve Broca's and Wernicke's area. They may be combined cortical-subcortical or purely subcortical.

25. **What are the features of expressive, receptive, and transcortical sensory aprosody and where are the lesions that produce them?**
In expressive aprosody, speech is monotonous, does not convey emotions, and is amelodic. The lesion producing this is approximately in the right hemispheric equivalent to Broca's area.
   In receptive aprosody, the patient is unable to comprehend emotional and tonal aspects of communication. The lesion producing this is approximately in the right hemisphere equivalent to Wernicke's area.
   In transcortical sensory aprosody, there is good spontaneous and repetitive affective prosody as well as spontaneous gesturing. There is poor affective comprehension of language and gesture.

26. **What is alexia and how does it differ from dyslexia?**
Alexia is an acquired disorder of written language comprehension, that is, difficulty in reading. Dyslexia refers to developmental difficulties with reading.

27. **What are the different types of dyslexia and where are the lesions responsible for them?**
In deep dyslexia, there are semantic errors, concrete words are easier to read, articles and pronouns are difficult to read, and there is an inability to read nonwords. The responsible lesion is in the perisylvian area and is associated with aphasia.
   In phonologic dyslexia, there is reading without print-to-sound conversation and impaired reading of non-word letter strings. The responsible lesion is localized in dominant perisylvian cortex, superior temporal lobe, and angular gyrus.
   In surface dyslexia, there is the inability to pronounce words of nonphonologic pronunciation. The lesion is poorly localized. This condition can be seen with Alzheimer's disease.

28. **What is alexia without agraphia and where is the lesion responsible for it?**
Alexia without agraphia (pure word blindness or acquired pure alexia) is the inability to read despite preserved ability to write. It is associated with a lesion in the dominant occipital lobe (frequently producing a homonymous hemianopia), and a disconnection of the nondominant occipital lobe from the dominant parietal lobe via a lesion of the inferior splenium of the corpus callosum. Alternately, it can occur with lesions of the dominant lateral geniculate body and splenium of corpus callosum or with a single lesion of the dominant occipito-temporal periventricular white matter behind, beneath, and beside the occipital horn of the lateral ventricle. It is most often associated with infarction in the distribution of the dominant hemispheric posterior cerebral artery.

29. **Where is the lesion responsible for alexia with agraphia?**
The lesion responsible for alexia with agraphia is usually associated with a lesion of the angular gyrus (Table 15-1).

30. **What percentage of people are left-handed?**
Less than 5% of people use their left hands for all skilled tasks, 60% are strongly right-handed, and 35% have a mixed hand preference.

**TABLE 15-1. THE APHASIAS**

| Aphasia | Fluency | Repetition | Naming/Word Finding | Comprehension | Reading | Writing | Paraphasic Errors | Lesion Location |
|---|---|---|---|---|---|---|---|---|
| Transcortical motor | NF | Good | | Good | | | Semantic | Supplementary motor |
| Mixed transcortical | NF | Good | | → | | | | Watershed distribution |
| Aphemia | NF | | | NI | | NI | | Lower motor strip, SMA |
| Anterior subcortical (basal ganglia) | Dysarthria, decreased fluency | Mild → | | Mild → | | | | Basal ganglia – putamen and caudate |
| Global | NF | → | → | → | → | → | | Broca's and Wernicke's |
| Broca's | NF | → | Poor | Relatively NI | → | → | Semantic and phonemic | Frontal operculum/ Brodmann 44 and 45 |
| Conduction | F | → | Anomia | NI | | | Phonemic | Arcuate fasciculus |
| Wernicke's | F | → | → | → | | → | Semantic and phonemic | Posterior temporal/ Brodman 22, 37, 39, or 40 |

| | | | | | | | | |
|---|---|---|---|---|---|---|---|---|
| Transcortical sensory | F | Good | | → | | → | Semantic | Temporo-parietal |
| Anomic | F | Good | | NI | | | | T-P-O association |
| Thalamic | F | Good – fairly | Severe | → | → | → | | Ant, VA, DL, VL, Ant DM nuclei |
| Alexia w/o agraphia | F | Good | | NI | → | NI | | Left occipital plus posterior corpus callosum |
| Alexia with agraphia | F | Good | | NI | → | → | | Angular gyrus |

T-P-O = temporo-parieto-occipital, VA = ventroanterior, DL = dorsolateral, VL = ventrolateral, DM = dorsomedial, F = fluent, NF = non-fluent, NI = not impaired, ↓ = impaired

## APRAXIAS

31. **What is apraxia?**
Apraxia is the loss of the ability to perform a learned, familiar, purposeful motor act despite having the desire and the physical ability to perform the movements. This occurs in the absence of a primary disturbance in attention, comprehension, motivation, coordination, or sensation that would preclude that act.
Gross RG, Grossman M: Update on apraxia. Curr Neurol Neurosci Rep 8:490-496, 2008.

32. **What are the features of ideational apraxia and where is the responsible lesion?**
Ideational apraxia is the inability to perform a sequence of learned acts. They are multistep acts such as making coffee, preparing a meal, or mailing a letter. It is usually seen with diffuse brain injury, delirium and dementia, or with frontal lobe lesions. It is thought to represent a primary disturbance of attention and executive functions that interferes with the coherence of sequenced motor output.

33. **What is ideomotor apraxia and where is the lesion responsible for it?**
It is the inability to perform learned familiar movements to command. The lesion usually includes the dominant inferior parietal area (and/or the arcuate fasciculus), which is believed to contain spatiotemporal representations of learned skilled movements ("praxicons"). These are then translated into motor output through the mediation of the premotor cortex.

34. **What is sympathetic apraxia and where is the lesion underlying it?**
It is an ideomotor apraxia of the left hand, commonly associated with a right hemiparesis and a Broca's aphasia. It is caused by left frontal lesions disconnecting the left inferior parietal lobe from the right premotor cortex so that praxicons for the left hand cannot reach the hand area of the right frontal lobe.

35. **What are the features of anterior callosal apraxia?**
An anterior callosal lesion disconnects the right premotor cortex (left hand) from the left hemisphere (left inferior parietal lobe), yielding an apraxia to verbal commands confined to the left hand (left ideomotor apraxia). Sympathetic and anterior callosal apraxias are essentially the same syndrome due to interruption of the same pathway, but the lesion in sympathetic apraxia is much larger, causing other deficits (e.g., aphasia and hemiparesis).

36. **What is limb-kinetic apraxia and where is the lesion that produces it?**
It is a loss of dexterity and coordination of fine distal limb movements. The lesion producing it usually includes the contralateral supplementary motor cortex.

37. **What is dressing apraxia and where is the lesion that produces it?**
It is not a true apraxia. The difficulty in dressing is a result of the inability to align the body axis with the axis of the garment, a complex visuospatial task. Dressing apraxia is a nondominant parietal lobe symptom that is often associated with left visual field deficits and other deficits of visuospatial integration and construction (drawing).
Lesions in the right parietal-occipital-temporal region cause problems with complex perceptual-spatial actions, such as route-finding and navigating the body with respect to solid objects such as beds and chairs.
Another problem arising from this region is "hemineglect" in which one-half of the body is neither clothed nor groomed, and attention to one-half of the patient's extrapersonal space is severely diminished.

38. **What is constructional apraxia and where is the lesion underlying it?**
It involves difficulty in copying figures and designs (drawing) but is not caused by a true apraxia. It is also associated with right parietal lobe lesions (Table 15-2).

## TABLE 15-2. FORMS OF APRAXIA

| Type of Apraxia | Poor Actions | Lesion Location | Associated Features |
|---|---|---|---|
| Ideational apraxia | Sequence of learned acts | Diffuse | Dementia, delirium |
| Ideomotor apraxia | Learned familiar movements to command | Dominant inferior parietal | |
| Sympathetic apraxia | Left hand ideomotor | Left frontal | Right HP, Broca's aphasia |
| Anterior callosal apraxia | Left hand ideomotor | Corpus callosum | None |
| Limb-kinetic apraxia | Distal limb reduced dexterity and coordination | Contralateral SMA | |

HP = hemiplegia, SMA = supplementary motor area

## PERCEPTUAL DISORDERS AND AGNOSIAS

39. **What is agnosia?**
Agnosia is the inability to recognize objects despite adequate perception in the modality in which the object is presented.

# KEY POINTS: NEUROBEHAVIORAL DEFINITIONS

1. Amnesia: severe, isolated disturbance of memory in the absence of other forms of cognitive dysfunction.

2. In anterograde amnesia, patients are unable to acquire new memories; in retrograde amnesia, patients are unable to recall recent memories.

3. Aphasia is an acquired disturbance of language, whereas dysarthria is an acquired disturbance of speech production.

4. Apraxia: loss of ability to perform a learned, familiar, purposeful motor act despite the desire and physical ability to do so.

5. Agnosia: the inability to recognize an object despite adequate perception in the modality in which the object is presented.

40. **What is topographagnosia and where is the lesion responsible for it?**
Topographagnosia is the inability to navigate complex spatial layouts, such as a city, a building, or even one's home, and to describe verbally or with a map how to get to a specific

place or room. This difficulty is often combined with some degree of unilateral neglect. It can be seen in right occipito-parietal damage or in bilateral temporo-parietal lesions, damaging the "parahippocampal place area" (PPA). Spatial orientation can also be disturbed in memory disorders and bilateral lesions of the visual system.

**41. What is anosognosia and where is the lesion responsible for it?**
Anosognosia is the unawareness of illness or impairment, such as hemiparesis or blindness, and is most commonly observed with right parietal lesions.

**42. What is anosodiaphoria and where is the lesion that produces it?**
Anosodiaphoria is a disorder in which patients recognize a deficit, such as hemiparesis and or hemisensory deficit, but are indifferent to it. It may be seen with right hemisphere lesions.

**43. What is prosopagnosia and where is the lesion responsible for it?**
Prosopagnosia (face-blindness) is the inability to recognize familiar faces. Patients can perform a *generic recognition* ("it is a face") and are able to tell age, gender, and emotional expression but are unable to identify the *specific* person. They rely on voice, posture, clothing, etc., to make the identification. Commonly, patients also are unable to identify other specific members of a general class, for example, car brands or birds. The disorder is commonly associated with unilateral or bilateral visual field defects. It is often associated with achromatopsia because of involvement of the fibers projecting from the inferior lip of the occipital lobe.
Prosopagnosia is associated with bilateral inferior occipito-temporal lesions affecting both fusiform gyri. The posterior fusiform gyri contain an area called the fusiform face area (FFA) that is specialized in facial processing and identification. Adjacent areas are specialized in identifying individual members of other general classes of objects (birds, cars, buildings, etc.).
Gruter T, Gruter M, Carbon CC: Neural and genetic foundations of face recognition and prosopagnosia. J Neuropsychol 2:79-97, 2008.

**44. What is simultanagnosia and where is the lesion underlying it?**
Simultanagnosia is a disorder of visual perception and attention characterized by the inability to interpret complex visual arrays despite preserved recognition of single objects.
Simultanagnosia occurs predominantly in patients with high occipito-parietal lobe disease such as bilateral infarcts in the posterior watershed region, venous infarcts due to sagittal sinus thromboses, and in some patients with Alzheimer's disease.

**45. What is cerebral achromatopsia and where is the lesion that is responsible it?**
Achromatopsia is an acquired lack of color vision. Lesions of the occipital cortex below the calcarine sulcus produce upper quadrantanopia and achromatopsia in the preserved inferior visual field. Hemi-achromatopsia can result from contralateral inferotemporal lesions of the fusiform and lingual gyri.

**46. What is neglect and where are the lesions that produce it?**
Neglect is a lack of attention to events and actions in one-half of personal and extrapersonal space. The inattention to stimuli from that hemi-space can involve all modalities, as well as motor acts and motivation.
The posterior parietal cortex is believed to be critical for spatial attention in that it integrates distributed spatial information across all sensory modalities.
Although neglect is classically attributed to right parietal lesions, it can be seen with damage to many other cortical and subcortical areas. The most profound neglect is seen with right parietal lesions, followed by left frontal and then left parietal lesions (Table 15-3).

**TABLE 15-3. FORMS OF AGNOSIA OR NEGLECT**

| | Definition | Associated Features | Anatomic Localization |
|---|---|---|---|
| Topographagnosia | Inability to navigate complex layouts | Unilateral neglect—often | Right O-P or bilateral T-P |
| Anosognosia | Unawareness of impairment | Often left hemiparesis | Right parietal |
| Anosodiaphoria | Recognize deficits, but indifferent to them | Often a HP or hemisensory deficit | Right hemisphere |
| Prosopagnosia | Inability to recognize familiar faces | Unable to identify other specific member of a class, such as car brands; visual field defects | Bilateral inferior occipito-temporal |
| Simultanagnosia | Inability to interpret complex visual scenes | | High O-P (e.g., posterior watershed) |
| Achromatopsia | Lack of color vision | Quadrantanopia | Occipital cortex below the calcarine sulcus; inferotemporal |
| Neglect | Lack of attention in one-half of space | | Posterior right parietal; then left frontal or left parietal |

HP = hemiplegia, O-P = occipito-parietal, T-P = temporo-parietal

## NEUROBEHAVIORAL SYNDROMES

47. **What are the behavioral alterations observed with lesions of the orbitofrontal cortex?**
Impulsive and antisocial behavior (disinhibition, hypersexuality, excessive eating, breaking of social conventions, compulsions, hoarding, and cluttering), high-risk behavior (inability to foresee or learn from negative consequences), unstable mood (lability, irritability, hypomania, mania), inappropriate jocularity (*witzelsucht*; *moria*), and impaired olfactory recognition. These behaviors may be seen with lesions of the orbitofrontal cortex, ventral caudate, globus pallidus, and mediodorsal thalamus. During the examination, patients are often stimulus bound and show utilization behavior.

48. **What is utilization behavior and what does it mean to be "stimulus bound"?**
Utilization behavior refers to a patient's inability to suppress the urge to manipulate or use an object in a correct way but in an unacceptable context—for example, drinking from the

examiner's cup or writing with the examiner's pen. A patient that is stimulus bound is attracted to each new stimulus, unable to ignore stimuli that are not relevant to the current task. The patient is thus unable to maintain the attention required to pursue one task to full completion.

49. **What are the behavioral alterations associated with lesions of the medial frontal cortex?**
Impoverished speech and apathy, which can be to the extreme of akinetic mutism, lack of motivation and drive, poor initiation, lack of goal formation, loss of planning, paucity of thought, and profound psychomotor (cognitive) slowing. These changes may occur with lesions of the medial frontal cortex, anterior cingulate cortex, nucleus accumbens, globus pallidus, and mediodorsal/ventral anterior thalamus.

50. **What are the behavioral alterations noted with lesions of the dorsolateral prefrontal cortex?**
Depression and apathy, reduced verbal fluency (dominant side), reduced nonverbal fluency (nondominant side), psychomotor slowing, poor set-shifting, impaired abstraction and logical thinking, inability to understand humor, poor judgment, poor response inhibition, impaired free recall and intact recognition memory, poor memory organization, poor temporal sequencing of events, poor visual construction strategies, poor working memory, reduced divided attention, reduced sustained attention, perseveration on sequential motor tasks, and environmental dependency.
Verbal dysdecorum is disinhibited, poorly monitored verbal output that is socially unacceptable and is seen most frequently following damage to the right frontal convexity. These behaviors occur after lesions of the dorsolateral prefrontal cortex, head of the caudate, globus pallidus, and mediodorsal/ventral anterior thalamus.

51. **What is the alien hand syndrome, where is the lesion that produces it, and what is the vascular territory of that lesion?**
With this syndrome, an individual's nonparalyzed hand appears to carry out activities that cannot be controlled by the individual. It can include behaviors like inappropriate grasping, taking off one's glasses, and throwing off one's covers.
It is a disconnection syndrome caused by damage to the corpus callosum that can be seen with occlusion of the anterior cerebral artery. It can also be observed in corticobasal degeneration.
Assal F, Schwartz S, Vuilleumier P: Moving with or without will: Functional neural correlates of alien hand syndrome. Ann Neurol 62:301-306, 2007.

52. **What are the features of Gerstmann's syndrome and where is the responsible lesion?**
It is characterized by four primary symptoms: acalculia, agraphia or dysgraphia, an inability to identify fingers (finger agnosia), and right-left confusion. These occur in the absence of additional language deficits.
The underlying lesion includes the angular gyrus in the dominant hemisphere. A pure Gerstmann's syndrome is rare: more commonly, it is associated with aphasia and/or other parietal lobe symptoms.

53. **What is Geschwind's syndrome and where is the responsible lesion?**
It includes a cluster of personality traits: circumstantiality (excessive verbal output, stickiness, hypergraphia); altered sexuality (loss or alteration of sexual interests and a craving for overly close interpersonal relationships); and intensified mental life (deepening of many emotions, often resulting in religious or philosophical preoccupation; a strong moralistic sense).

These personality traits have been attributed to temporal lobe epilepsy and are hypothesized to result from chronic epileptic activation or "kindling" within the amygdala. The specificity of these features for temporal lobe epilepsy is poor, however.

54.  **What lesions are associated with obsessive-compulsive behavior?**
The majority of structural lesions associated with the development of obsessive-compulsive behavior have involved the frontal lobe and or frontal-basal ganglia network connections.

55.  **What is the Balint's syndrome and where is the responsible lesion?**
It includes misreaching under visual guidance (optic ataxia), failure to scan and integrate an entire visual scene or picture (simultanagnosia), and ocular apraxia.
Patients with these symptoms usually have bilateral lesions of the occipito-parietal junctions.

56.  **What is Anton's syndrome and where are the lesions associated with it?**
Anton's syndrome is the combination of cortical blindness and denial of blindness. It is typically associated with bilateral posterior cerebral artery infarctions producing "cortical" blindness plus memory impairment.

57.  **What are the features of Klüver-Bucy syndrome and where is the lesion associated with it?**
Docility, placidity, hypersexuality, and hyperorality may be seen as part of the Klüver-Bucy syndrome. Hypermetamorphosis (a desire to explore everything) is also associated. This syndrome is seen in monkeys with experimental bilateral temporal lobectomies.
Occasionally, aspects of this syndrome are seen in human patients with bilateral lesions of anterior temporal lobes, including the amygdala. Herpes simplex encephalitis is one cause of this syndrome in humans.

## KEY POINTS: EPONYMOUS SYNDROMES

1. Gerstmann's syndrome: acalculia, agraphia, finger agnosia, right-left confusion.

2. Geschwind's syndrome: circumstantiality, altered sexuality, intensified mental life.

3. Balint's syndrome: optic ataxia, simultanagnosia, ocular apraxia.

4. Anton's syndrome: cortical blindness with denial of blindness.

5. Klüver-Bucy syndrome: docility, placidity, hypersexuality, hyperorality, hypermetamorphosis.

58.  **What is the Charles-Bonnet syndrome and when does it occur?**
Vivid, well-formed visual hallucinations in the setting of poor vision occurring in mentally healthy, most often elderly, individuals. Severe macular degeneration and glaucoma are common etiologies, but optic nerve damage can also predispose to the disorder. Hallucinations are usually of people, animals, or objects, often "Lilliputian," and perceived as pleasurable by many patients.

59.  **What neurodegenerative diseases are associated with depression?**
Major depression is frequent in Parkinson's disease, occurring in 40% to 60% of the patients during the course of their illness. It also occurs in more than 40% of Huntington's disease patients, and suicide occurs in close to 10%.

Major depression and suicide are less common in Alzheimer's dementia, fronto-temporal dementia, Amyotrophic Lateral Sclerosis (ALS), and olivopontocerebellar degeneration, but they do occur.

Structural or functional lesions in the left anterior frontal lobe are more often associated with depression than other focal brain lesions.

## WEBSITE

http://www.searchmedica.com/search.html?Q=neurobehavioural%20disorder

## BIBLIOGRAPHY

1  Apostolova LG, Cummings JL: Psychiatric manifestations in dementia. In continuum: Lifelong learning in neurology. Dementia 13:165-179, 2007.

2  Damasio AR, Damasio H: Aphasia and the neural basis of language. In Mesulam MM (ed): Principles of Behavioral and Cognitive Neurology, 2nd ed. New York, Oxford University Press, 2000.

3  Cappa S, Demonet JF, Fletcher P: Cognitive Neurology: A Clinical Textbook, Oxford University Press, 2008.

4  Heilman KM, Valenstein E, eds. Clinical Neuropsychology, 4th ed. New York, Oxford University Press, 2003.

5  Morgan JE: Textbook of Clinical Neuropsychology, London, Taylor and Francis, 2008.

6  Vallar G: Spatial neglect, Balint-Holmes and Gerstmann's syndrome, and other spatial disorders. CNS Spectr 12:527-536, 2007.

# DYSARTHRIA, DYSFLUENCY, AND DYSPHAGIA

*David B. Rosenfield, MD*

# CHAPTER 16

## DYSARTHRIA

1. **Which parts of the brain are involved in speech motor output?**
   Human speech production involves coordination among respiration, laryngeal activity, and supralaryngeal articulatory movement. The lower motoneurons that control the respiratory movements reside in the anterior portion of the cervical, thoracic, and upper lumbar spinal cord. Motoneurons controlling laryngeal closure reside in the nucleus ambiguous. Neurons directly responsible for the supralaryngeal musculature are the trigeminal motor nucleus, facial nucleus, rostral portion of the nucleus ambiguus, hypoglossal nucleus, and anterior horn cells at the rostral portion of the cervical spinal cord. These lower motor neurons and the bilateral inputs from multiple realms (including motor cortex) of both hemispheres constitute the underlying neural input of speech motor production.

2. **What is dysphonia?**
   Dysphonia is an abnormality in phonation (sound output from the larynx).

3. **What is the difference between speech compromise and language compromise?**
   Speech is motor output. Speech compromise is a deficiency in the way speech sounds. It refers to the underlying motor component. Language compromise involves errors in syntax, word choice, or how sounds are put together. Talking with food in one's mouth causes speech compromise. An aphasic patient has acquired language compromise.

4. **What is the primary difference between communication among animals and humans?**
   Animals have a system of communication, whereas humans have a system of language. Animals do not have a generative grammar, whereas humans do. However, the brain of an animal must learn to control the sound output, just as a human does.

5. **What is dysarthria?**
   Dysarthria, although implying a problem of articulation only, is a defect in phonation as well as resonance. Phonation is sound production (from larynx). Resonance is how the sounds are altered in the cavity between the larynx and vocal fold and the lips/nares (e.g., hyponasal, hypernasal).

6. **What are the causes of dysarthria?**
   Dysarthria may be due to compromise of the brain, brain stem, cerebellum, nerve, neuromuscular junction, or muscle. All diseases that affect these regions, considerable in number, may cause dysarthria, particularly myopathy, myositis, myasthenia gravis, neuropathies, motor neuron disease, cerebellar disease, tumors of the brain and brain stem, Parkinson's disease, and various other movement disorders.

7. **What determines prognosis in dysarthria when it is caused by damage to the cerebral hemispheres?**
   Patients with damage in only one hemisphere have a much better prognosis for dysarthria than patients with damage in both hemispheres.

8. **Where can the brain be stimulated during ongoing speech to cause speech arrest?**
   In right-handed people, just about anywhere in the left hemisphere and in the area of the motor strip on the right. Stimulation of the supplementary motor area, bilaterally, induces speech arrest.

9. **What happens when Broca's area is electrically stimulated?**
   If Broca's area is stimulated while someone is talking, the person stops talking. If it is stimulated while a person is not talking, a grunted sound is elicited.

10. **What happens when Wernicke's area is electrically stimulated?**
    If Wernicke's area is electrically stimulated while someone is talking, the person stops talking. If it is stimulated during silence, a sound may be elicited but not a sentence of word output.

11. **What is the Wada test?**
    The Wada test involves injection of a short-acting barbiturate into the carotid artery of one hemisphere to render the patient plegic, numb, and blind on the side opposite to the injection. If language "resides" on the injected side, the patient also becomes aphasic. The test is named after Dr. Jun Wada.

12. **How does the Wada test relate to handedness?**
    The correlation is excellent. Over 95% of persons who become aphasic when only one particular hemisphere is injected during the Wada test have handedness pertaining to dominance of the injected hemisphere.

13. **List common brain/brain-stem causes of dysarthria.**
    Structural compromise of the corticobulbar tracts (unilaterally or bilaterally) or cranial nerve nuclei V, VII, X, or XII may cause dysarthria. Common diseases that cause such compromise are stroke, tumor, demyelinating disease, motor neuron disease, and collagen disease.

14. **What are the speech signs in Parkinson's disease?**
    Phonation is weak, pitch varies little, volume is low, and the patient is hoarse. Accelerated rate, repetitive dysfluencies, and imprecise consonants may occur. Reduced vocal intensity and abnormal articulation contribute to the impaired intelligibility of many patients with Parkinson's disease. Speech treatment usually focuses on improving articulation and rate but has met with limited success.

15. **What are the speech signs in hyperkinetic dysarthria-chorea?**
    Sudden alterations in pitch and loudness, phonatory arrest, strained hoarseness, and sudden alterations in precision of vowels and consonants.

16. **What are the speech signs in hyperkinetic dysarthria-phonatory tremor?**
    Rhythmic alterations in pitch and loudness, adductor phonatory arrests, and compensatory strain or strangle.

17. **What are the speech signs in Gilles de la Tourette's syndrome?**
    Grunts, barks, squeaks, throat clearing, gurgling, moaning, snorting, sniffing, whistling, clicking, lip smacking, spitting, unintelligible sounds, echolalia, coprolalia, and dysfluencies.

18. **What are the speech signs in cerebellar disease?**
Phonation may be associated with tremor and variations in loudness. Irregular articulatory breakdown, imprecise consonants, and sometimes excessive and equal stress in all syllables of words are present.

19. **List the nerve-damage causes of dysarthria.**
Collagen disease, viral infection, diabetes, and alcohol.

20. **What are the speech signs in motor neuron disease?**
Phonation is strained, harsh, wet, and sometimes fluttering during vowel prolongation. Speech is hypernasal. Articulation is slow, consonants are imprecise, phrases are short, and vowels are distorted.

21. **What is the effect of a fifth cranial nerve (trigeminal) lesion on speech output?**
Phonation and velopharyngeal function are normal, mandibular muscles are weak, and vowels and consonants are imprecise.

22. **How does a lesion of the seventh cranial nerve (facial) affect speech?**
Phonation and velopharyngeal function are normal, the orbicularis oris is weak (causing difficulty in producing "p" sounds), vowels are imprecise, and labial consonants are imprecise.

23. **How does the tenth cranial nerve (vagus) lesion affect speech?**
Phonation is hoarse and breathy, and volume is low. Speech is hypernasal if the lesion is above the pharyngeal branch.

24. **What is the effect of a twelfth cranial nerve (hypoglossal) lesion on speech?**
Phonation and velopharyngeal function are normal. The tongue is weak, demonstrating atrophy and fasciculation. The patient may have drooling, imprecise vowels, and imprecise lingual consonants.

25. **Which muscles adduct the vocal folds?**
Thyroarytenoid, interarytenoid, lateral cricothyroid, and lateral cricoarytenoid.

26. **Which muscles abduct the vocal folds?**
Posterior cricoarytenoid.

27. **Which nerves innervate which muscles in the larynx?**
All of the muscles in the larynx are innervated by branches from the recurrent laryngeal nerve.

28. **What are the causes of recurrent laryngeal nerve paralysis?**
    1. Inflammation (viral disease, collagen disease, pulmonary tuberculosis, coccidioidomycosis)
    2. Polyneuropathy (especially diabetes and alcohol)
    3. Trauma (intubation, neck trauma, head trauma, mediastinoscopy, radical neck dissection, carotid endarterectomy, cardiovascular surgery, thyroidectomy, esophageal resection for carcinoma)
    4. Neoplasm
    5. Syringomyelia
    6. Idiopathic

29. **List the causes of bilateral abductor vocal cord paralysis in adults.**
    1. Thyroidectomy
    2. Neck malignancy
    3. Poliomyelitis

4. Brain stem stroke
5. Guillain-Barré syndrome
6. Demyelinating disease
7. Central nervous system neoplasm
8. Central nervous system infection
9. Charcot-Marie-Tooth disease
   **Rare causes**: foreign bodies near the larynx, bilateral carotid dissection, neck infection, head or neck trauma, substernal thyroid, idiopathic.

30. **How does myasthenia affect speech?**
    Myasthenia's effects are similar to those of a myopathy, but speech improves with rest.

31. **What is the effect of myopathy/myositis on speech output?**
    Phonatory output is hoarse, breathy, and diplophonic and has low volume. The speech is hypernasal, and vowels and consonants may be compromised, depending on the muscles involved.

32. **Name four muscle disturbances that can cause dysarthria.**
    Collagen disease, polymyositis, dermatomyositis, and hypothyroidism.

33. **Define spasmodic dysphonia.**
    Spasmodic dysphonia is effortful, strained speech associated with a sensation of strain and strangle.

34. **What is the most common presentation of spasmodic dysphonia?**
    Strain in the throat, interruption of sound while talking, and difficulty in getting words out but with no evidence of associated aphasia.

35. **What are the neurologic causes of spasmodic dysphonia?**
    Laryngeal tremor, laryngeal dystonia, and other movement disorders involving the laryngeal neuromotor system. It also may be a symptom of psychiatric disease.

36. **What is the prognosis in spasmodic dysphonia?**
    When the condition is associated with tremor, the prognosis is fairly good with therapy. Many experts contend that patients do fairly well with speech therapy; others opt more strongly for various medications, including botulinum toxin injections.

37. **What are the speech characteristics of corticobasal degeneration?**
    Speech characteristics of corticobasal degeneration (CBD) include dysfluency, nonfluent-like aphasia, phonologic errors incorporating what some term "speech apraxia," and elements of oral (buccofacial) apraxia. Be careful about diagnosing CBD as the culprit of speech compromise unless oral apraxia is also present.

## DYSFLUENCY

38. **What are the prevalence and characteristics of developmental stuttering?**
    Developmental stuttering is much more common among males than females (ratio of 4:1). Some argue that everyone stutters, some for just a few minutes or few hours. The prevalence of stuttering in childhood is 4% and in adulthood slightly more than 1%. Developmental stutterers stutter at the beginning of sentences and phrases, are more fluent when their speech is markedly slowed and drawn out, and do not stutter when they sing. Other fluency-evoking maneuvers include repetitive reading, choral reading, and interference by loud, broadband noise with hearing of one's own speech. Development stutterers are emotionally bothered by their dysfluent output.

**39. Can a previously fluent person become a stutterer after brain injury?**

Yes. Acquired stutterers stutter throughout the sentence, whereas developmental stutterers usually stutter at the beginning of sentences and phrases. In addition, fluency-evoking maneuvers, such as singing, do not help acquired stutterers but render developmental stutterers almost totally fluent. As opposed to developmental stutterers, acquired stutterers are only minimally distraught at their compromised output.

**40. What are the causes of acquired stuttering?**

The causes of acquired stuttering include compromise to either hemisphere, anterior or posterior. The damage is usually mild. The damage may be due to stroke, vasculitis, infection, tumor, trauma, or metabolic compromise. Psychogenic causes also exist.

**41. Describe the characteristics of cluttering.**

The clutterer's speech is characterized by excessive speed, repetitions, interjections, disturbed prosody, and sometimes inconsistent articulatory disturbances. Some contend that such patients have errors in grammar, are hyperactive, and have poor concentration. Although his or her rate of speech may not always be markedly increased, the listener usually has the sensation that it is. As opposed to a developmental stutterer, a clutterer frequently is unconcerned about his or her speech deficit.

**42. What are the characteristics of palilalia?**

Palilalics compulsively repeat phrases or words with reiteration at increasing speed and with a decrescendo volume.

**43. Which diseases are associated with palilalia?**

Postencephalitic Parkinson's disease, idiopathic Parkinson's disease, and pseudobulbar palsy.

**44. Dysfluency can be associated with which aphasias?**

Broca's aphasia, transcortical motor aphasia, and primary progressive aphasia.

**45. What is primary progressive aphasia?**

Primary progressive aphasia (PPA) is a focal dementia defined as progressive dissolution in speech and language function, including anomia (inability to retrieve nouns upon demand), agrammatism (inappropriate word order or use of prepositions), or loss of semantic knowledge about words and objects. The degenerative process may later spread to affect not only language but other cognitive functions, ultimately causing a more global dementia.

**46. Where is the lesion in PPA?**

Neuroimaging studies in PPA show metabolic dysfunction and atrophy in the left inferior frontal, perisylvian, and temporal cortices.

## DYSPHAGIA

**47. What is dysphagia?**

Dysphagia (difficulty in swallowing) is a subjective symptom as opposed to an objective sign until delay or disruption in the swallowing mechanism can be documented. If no objective evidence of dysphagia can be documented, globus hystericus should be considered. Dysphagia may be due to mechanical factors that physically narrow the oropharyngeal lumen and obstruct food passage or to neuromotor diseases that cause inadequate food bolus propulsion into the stomach.

48. **List the three stages of swallowing.**
    1. Oropreparatory stage (food passes from mouth into pharynx).
    2. Pharyngeal transfer stage (food passes through the pharynx, over the larynx, and into the esophagus).
    3. Esophageal stage (food is transported from proximal esophagus, the upper one-third of which contains striated muscle, to the lower two-thirds, which consists of smooth muscle, across the lower esophageal sphincter, and into the stomach).

49. **What is the swallow reflex?**
    The swallow reflex mediates the first stage of swallowing into the second. It consists of several movements. The soft palate moves upward (velar elevation), closing the passageway between the oral and nasal cavity; the pharyngeal muscles contract (pharyngeal peristalsis), the larynx elevates, and posterior flexion of the epiglottis closes the airway to the trachea. Vocal cord closure occurs, followed by relaxation of the cricopharyngeus muscle, the upper esophageal sphincter.

50. **What is the role of the vagus nerve in swallowing?**
    The vagus nerve supplies motor fibers to the striated muscle of the esophagus. Thus, a serious consequence of damaging the vagus at the origin of the esophageal branch is dysphagia. A high vagotomy permanently paralyzes the striated muscle at the upper one-third of the esophagus. Peristalsis in the lower two-thirds of the esophagus is an automatic function, mediated by the intrinsic myoenteric plexuses and smooth muscle.

## KEY POINTS: DYSARTHRIA, DYSFLUENCY, DYSPHAGIA

1. Dysarthria is a defect in the way speech sounds, which can arise from many causes, whereas aphasia is a defect in the use of language and arises from the dominant cerebral cortex.

2. Developmental stutterers have problems with the initial, beginning sounds of words, whereas acquired stutterers may stumble anywhere in the sentence.

3. Swallowing is mediated primarily by the vagus nerve.

51. **Are there different types of dysphagia?**
    Dysphagia may be due to mechanical problems or neuromotor problems. Each of these realms has an oropharyngeal and an esophageal component.

52. **What are the symptoms of oropharyngeal dysphagia?**
    The symptoms typically occur immediately upon swallowing and include the sensation of food sticking in the neck, pain while swallowing, nasal regurgitation of food or fluids, and coughing and choking due to aspiration. Discomfort in the midneck area may be present.

53. **List the causes of oropharyngeal neuromotor dysphagia.**
    1. Motor neuron disease
    2. Brain tumor
    3. Stroke
    4. Neuropathy (includes mechanical nerve injury)
    5. Demyelinating disease
    6. Degenerative disease (especially spinocerebellar)
    7. Syringobulbia
    8. Myasthenia gravis

9. Myopathy (including oculopharyngeal muscular dystrophy, hypothyroidism, polymyositis, dermatomyositis)
10. Parkinson's disease
11. Cerebral palsy
12. Tardive dyskinesia
13. Cricopharyngeal achalasia
14. Xerostomia (dry mouth)
15. Sjögren's syndrome

54. **What are the causes of oropharyngeal mechanical dysphagia?**
1. Oropharyngeal tumor
2. Zenker's diverticulum
3. Cervical osteophytes
4. Dislocation of temporomandibular joint
5. Macroglossia
6. Congenital abnormalities
7. Tight circumoral tissue due to scleroderma/burns
8. Neck surgery
9. Retropharyngeal mass
10. Large goiter

55. **What are the symptoms of mechanical dysphagia?**
Symptoms related to mechanical (oropharyngeal, oroesophageal) dysphagia are usually caused by difficulty in swallowing solid foods, progressing to difficulty in swallowing liquids. When the disorder is advanced, patients cannot swallow their own salivary secretions. Symptoms may occur immediately, seconds, or minutes after swallowing, depending on the level and chronicity of the underlying process. More rostral levels of dysfunction cause earlier symptoms.

56. **What causes esophageal neuromotor dysphagia?**
1. Scleroderma
2. Achalasia
3. Diffuse esophageal spasm
4. Polymyositis and dermatomyositis (usually oropharyngeal)
5. Idiopathic autonomic dysfunction
6. Postvagotomy dysphagia
7. Neuropathy (vagal disease, especially diabetes)
8. Amyloidoses (primary or secondary)
9. Symptomatic esophageal peristalsis (nutcracker esophagus)

57. **List the causes of esophageal mechanical dysphagia.**
1. Esophageal carcinoma
2. Metastases to esophagus
3. Benign esophageal tumor
4. Inflammation
5. Strictures of the esophagus
6. Pancreatitis with pseudocysts
7. Pancreatic tumors
8. Postvagotomy hematoma/fibrosis
9. Thoracic aorta aneurysm
10. Posterior mediastinal mass
11. Large hiatal hernia
12. Dysphagia lusoria (abnormal origin of the right subclavian artery)

## WEBSITE

1. http://www.voice-center.com

## BIBLIOGRAPHY

1. Buckingham HW, Christman SS: Aphasia in Stemmer B, Whitaker HA, (eds): Handbook of the Neuroscience of Language, London: Academic Press, 2008, pp 127-146.

2. Damasio AR, Damasio AH: Aphasia and the neural basis of language. In Marsel Mesulam M, (ed): Principles of Behavioral and Cognitive Neurology, 2nd ed., Oxford, Oxford University Press, 2000, pp 294-315.

3. Gorno-Tempini ML, Dronkers NF, Rankin KP, et al.: Cognition and anatomy in three variants of primary progressive aphasia. Ann Neurol 55:335-346, 2004.

4. Hillis AE: Aphasia: Progress in the last quarter of a century. Neurology 69:200-213, 2007.

5. Mega MS, Alexander NP, Cummings JL, Benson DF: The aphasias and related disturbances. In Joint RJ, Griggs RC, (eds): Baker's Clinical Neurology on CD-ROM. Philadelphia, Lippincott William & Wilkins, 2000.

6. Rosenfield DB: Stuttering and dysfluency. In Stemmer B, Whitaker HA, (eds): Handbook of the Neuroscience of Language, London, Academic Press, 2008, pp 309-318.

7. Rosenfield DB, Barroso AO: Difficulties with speech and swallowing. In Bradley WG, et al. (ed): Neurology and Clinical Practice, 3rd ed., Boston, Butterworth-Heinemann, 2000, pp 171-186.

# CHAPTER 17

# VASCULAR DISEASE

*David Chiu, MD, FAHA*

## CLINICAL FEATURES

1.  **What is stroke?**
    Stroke is a clinical syndrome defined by acute neurologic deficits in the setting of focal disruption of cerebral circulation. There are a number of subtypes, including atherothrombotic, cardioembolic, lacunar, and hemorrhagic strokes. Rather than representing diagnostic closure, a stroke should, therefore, prompt a search for an etiologic explanation.

2.  **How common is stroke?**
    Stroke is the most common disabling neurologic disease. It is the third leading cause of death in the industrialized world after heart disease and cancer. In the United States, about 750,000 strokes and 150,000 resulting deaths occur annually. Stroke is the leading cause of serious disability in adults.

3.  **What is the most common presenting symptom of stroke?**
    The most common symptom of stroke is hemiparesis. The second most common disabling symptom is aphasia.

4.  **What is the clinical profile of an atherothrombotic stroke?**
    An atherothrombotic stroke may be sudden, stuttering, or stepwise in onset. The "classic" history is a patient who awakens from sleep with deficits. This stroke subtype results from thrombosis associated with atherosclerotic lesions of the large-size and medium-size arteries in the neck or brain. Strokes caused by carotid disease are included in this category. The mechanism of cerebral infarction in this setting is often artery-to-artery embolism of platelet-fibrin thrombi or atherosclerotic material rather than purely hemodynamic.

5.  **What is the clinical profile of a cardioembolic stroke?**
    The typical cardioembolic stroke has an abrupt temporal profile, with deficits that are maximal at onset. There may be improvement of deficits shortly afterward if the embolus breaks up and travels to more distal branches of the affected artery. The "classic" history is an onset of symptoms during activity or associated with palpitations or a Valsalva maneuver. The heart and aortic arch are sources of such emboli.

6.  **What is the clinical profile of a lacunar stroke?**
    The four classic lacunar stroke syndromes are as follows: (1) pure motor hemiparesis, with face, arm, and leg equally affected; (2) pure hemisensory stroke; (3) clumsy hand-dysarthria; and (4) ataxic hemiparesis, characterized by ipsilateral incoordination out of proportion to the degree of weakness. Other lacunar stroke syndromes have been described, but these four are the most widely recognized. Lacunar strokes are associated with hypertension and/or diabetes mellitus and are related to occlusion of small perforating arterioles by lipohyalinosis or microatheroma.

7.  **What is the clinical profile of a hemorrhagic stroke?**
    Hemorrhagic strokes have a clinical profile that may not be clearly distinguishable from ischemic strokes. A prominent decrease in level of consciousness can be a clue. Headache, nausea, vomiting, severe hypertension, or other signs of raised intracranial pressure also

suggest a hemorrhagic stroke. Common sites for hypertensive intracerebral hemorrhage are the putamen, thalamus, pons, cerebellum, and hemispheric lobes. Hemorrhagic strokes can result from ruptured cerebral aneurysms with subarachnoid hemorrhage (SAH), ruptured arterial venous malformations, or amyloid angiopathy.

8. **What percentage of strokes can be attributed to each type?**
   See Table 17-1.

### TABLE 17-1. TYPES OF STROKES

| Type | Percentage of Strokes | Onset | MRI or CT Scan | Other Features |
|---|---|---|---|---|
| Atherothrombotic | 20 | May be gradual | Infarction | Carotid bruit |
| Cardioembolic | 30 | Sudden | Cortical infarction, may undergo spontaneous hemorrhagic transformation | Underlying heart disease, peripheral emboli, strokes in different vascular territories |
| Lacunar | 20 | May be gradual | Small, deep infarction | Pure motor or sensory stroke |
| Other ischemic/ cryptogenic | 20 | Varied | Varied | Young patient, risk factors absent |
| Hemorrhagic | 10 | Sudden | Hyperdensity on CT | Depressed level of consciousness, nausea and vomiting, headache |

MRI = magnetic resonance imaging, CT = computed tomography

## KEY POINTS: COMMON SUBTYPES OF STROKE

1. Atherothrombotic
2. Cardioembolic
3. Lacunar
4. Hemorrhagic

9. **What are the main anatomic syndromes in cerebrovascular disease?**
The first anatomic challenge is to localize the lesion to the anterior or posterior circulation. The anterior or carotid artery territory encompasses the frontal lobes, parietal lobes, basal ganglia, internal capsule, and a major portion of the temporal lobes. The posterior or vertebrobasilar territory includes the brain stem, cerebellum, thalamus, occipital lobes, and mesial and inferior temporal lobes.

10. **What are the major symptoms of a vascular event affecting the anterior circulation?**
Hemiparesis with or without ipsilateral hemisensory loss is the most common symptom of a stroke in the carotid circulation, although lesions in the brain stem can also produce hemiplegia. A specific pattern of hemiparesis can be a helpful clue. Weakness affecting the face and arm greater than the leg suggests a stroke in the middle cerebral artery territory, whereas a deficit mainly involving the leg is characteristic of an anterior cerebral artery stroke.
Aphasia, neglect, apraxia, and seizures are other signs of involvement of the internal carotid artery territory. Gaze deviation to the side opposite the hemiparesis is highly suggestive as well.
Amaurosis fugax or transient monocular visual loss implies ischemia in the territory of the ophthalmic artery, the first branch of the internal carotid artery. A homonymous hemianopia, if associated with some of the deficits discussed above, usually represents subcortical involvement of the optic radiations.

11. **What signs suggest posterior circulation localization?**
Brain stem findings suggest disease involving the vertebrobasilar system and its branches. Diplopia, dysarthria, dysphagia, dizziness/vertigo, and ataxia are among the classic symptoms of vertebrobasilar disease. Dizziness is the least specific symptom of vertebrobasilar disease but the most common. Crossed findings (an example being loss of pinprick and temperature sensation on one side of the face and the contralateral extremities) show a brain stem pattern, which stems from the decussation of various long tracts at different levels of the brain stem.
Vertebrobasilar insufficiency is in the differential diagnosis of syncope, although other focal findings will typically be present. A major stroke in the territory of the basilar artery can produce coma, quadriparesis, and decerebrate posturing.

12. **What are the most important causes of stroke in the anterior circulation?**
The most important etiologies of stroke in the anterior circulation are internal carotid artery stenosis, cardiac embolism, atherothrombotic disease of the major intracranial branches (especially the middle cerebral artery), and small vessel disease of the penetrating arteries.

13. **What are the most important causes of stroke in the posterior circulation?**
Posterior circulation symptoms often relate to atherosclerosis of the vertebrobasilar arteries or aortic arch, or small vessel disease in the penetrating branches. Cardiac embolism to the vertebrobasilar circulation has a predilection for the distal basilar territory, especially the terminal branches of the basilar artery, the posterior cerebral arteries.

14. **What is the basic evaluation of a suspected stroke?**
The first stage in evaluation is the **history**. The described symptoms suggest the initial localization. The time course of stroke is relatively acute, but some details may be clues to the pathogenesis of the individual event. Onset during sleep or a stuttering progression suggests an atherothrombotic mechanism or a lacunar stroke, whereas sudden onset with maximal deficit at the beginning suggests a cardiac embolism. The **physical examination** includes assessment of the patient's cardiovascular system for the presence of heart murmurs, congestive heart failure, cardiac arrhythmias, carotid bruits, and signs of peripheral vascular disease. The **neurologic examination** focuses on the major deficit and a search for important associated signs that aid in localization.

15. **Which initial laboratory studies should be obtained for patients with a stroke?**
Laboratory studies, which are indicated upon initial evaluation, are a complete blood count (CBC), platelet count, prothrombin time (PT), partial thromboplastin time (PTT), electrolytes, glucose, blood urea nitrogen (BUN), creatinine, chest radiograph, and electrocardiogram (ECG). These provide both general medical assessment and evaluation for some of the complications and underlying risk factors. Subsequent laboratory analysis should include a fasting lipid profile.

In selected cases, antithrombin III, protein C and protein S, activated protein C resistance (factor V Leiden mutation), and prothrombin gene mutation studies may indicate an inherited hypercoagulable state. Anticardiolipin antibody and lupus anticoagulant can point to antiphospholipid antibody syndrome as a stroke etiology. Hyperhomocysteinemia is a risk factor for atherosclerosis and thrombosis. Blood cultures should be obtained in any patient with suspected endocarditis.

If vasculitis is suspected as the underlying cause, screening is done by measurement of erythrocyte sedimentation rate (ESR), rapid plasma reagin (RPR), antinuclear antibody (ANA), rheumatoid factor, serum protein electrophoresis (SPEP), and complement levels C3, C4, and CH50.

16. **What initial imaging should be performed in acute stroke?**
Noncontrast computed tomography (CT) scanning of the brain is often the initial imaging study performed for the acute stroke patient. The distinction between ischemic and hemorrhagic stroke is readily made by CT. Practical advantages of CT over magnetic resonance imaging (MRI) are its more rapid availability, lesser need for patient cooperation, and greater suitability for critically ill or potentially unstable patients.

MRI is often the favored imaging modality for nonacute stroke patients, where its greater sensitivity for ischemic stroke, especially in the posterior fossa, becomes an important advantage. Special MRI sequences add to the range of information provided. Diffusion-weighted imaging, for example, allows the acuity of ischemic lesions to be determined. MR angiography (MRA) or CT angiography (CTA) are valuable screening studies for arterial stenosis or aneurysms (Figures 17-1 and 17-2).

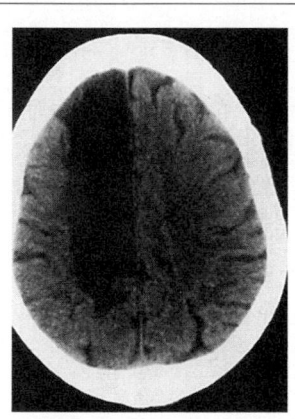

**Figure 17-1.** Noncontrast computed tomography (CT) scan of the brain showing a well-established ischemic stroke in the territory of the anterior cerebral artery.

## KEY POINTS: CAUSES OF STROKE IN THE ANTERIOR CIRCULATION

1. Internal carotid artery stenosis

2. Cardiac embolism

3. Atherothrombotic disease of the major intracranial branches

4. Small vessel disease of the penetrating arteries

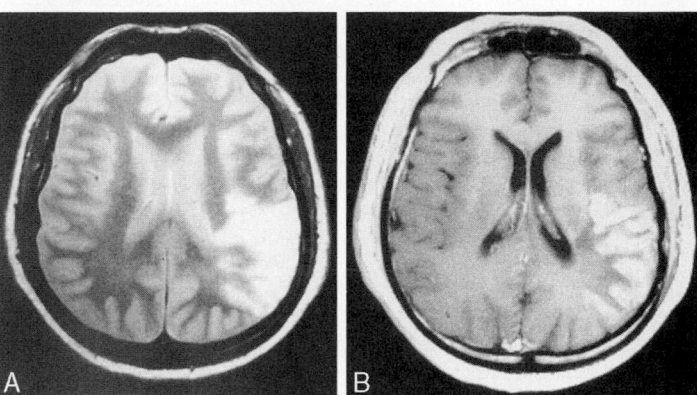

**Figure 17-2.** Magnetic resonance (MR) image of an acute ischemic stroke in the posterior area of the middle cerebral artery territory. The stroke is shown on a proton density technique (A), and a gadolinium-enhanced T1 image (B), which demonstrates the gyral enhancement characteristic of many infarcts.

**17. What cardiac work-up may be useful in stroke?**

A cardiac examination, ECG, and chest radiograph may be all that is necessary in some cases of stroke. Transthoracic echocardiography is frequently performed and is useful in assessing ventricular and valvular function. Transesophageal echocardiography (TEE) is more sensitive than transthoracic echo for the detection of atrial and aortic abnormalities, especially patent foramen ovale, atrial septal aneurysm, left atrial appendage thrombus, and aortic arch atheroma.

Cardiac and/or Holter monitoring is frequently performed and occasionally reveals unsuspected cardiac arrhythmias such as intermittent atrial fibrillation. Myocardial infarction is a common cause of death after stroke, especially in patients with cardiac risk factors. Evaluation for coronary artery disease can be performed with stress thallium cardiac scans. Although this technique may be useful in identifying occult coronary artery disease, its routine use has not yet been established.

**18. What other imaging methods may be useful in evaluating stroke?**

Carotid Doppler ultrasound may be useful in screening the extracranial internal carotid arteries for atherosclerotic disease. Its accuracy depends on the experience of the laboratory performing the test. MRA or CTA also may be used to evaluate the carotid circulation, the vertebrobasilar system, the circle of Willis, and the anterior, middle, and posterior cerebral arteries and their major branches. Because of flow disturbance at a site of stenosis, MRA tends to overestimate the degree of stenosis compared with contrast angiography.

Contrast cerebral angiography provides the most detailed and reliable information about the presence of carotid and intracranial disease. In experienced hands, the complication rate should be less than 1% (Figure 17-3).

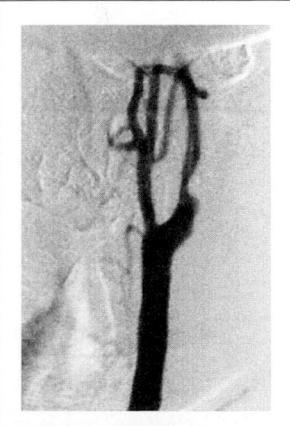

**Figure 17-3.** Contrast angiography showing atherosclerotic stenosis of the left internal carotid artery.

19. **What is the role of transcranial Doppler (TCD) imaging in assessment of strokes?**
Transcranial Doppler can provide information about blood flow in intracranial arteries. Blood flow velocities can be measured in the middle cerebral, anterior cerebral, posterior cerebral, vertebral, and basilar arteries by using different ultrasound "windows" in the skull. Decreased flow in the middle cerebral artery may be evidence of stenosis more proximally in the internal carotid; increased flow velocity may be evidence of stenosis or vasospasm in the middle cerebral artery. The technique also may be used to confirm cross filling of the middle cerebral artery on one side from the contralateral internal carotid artery via the circle of Willis.

## RISK FACTORS

20. **What are the major risk factors for stroke?**
The most important established risk factor for stroke is age, and the second is hypertension. Additional well-established risk factors are:

| | |
|---|---|
| 1. Gender (male) | 8. Smoking |
| 2. Family history | 9. Increased hematocrit |
| 3. Diabetes mellitus | 10. Elevated fibrinogen level |
| 4. Cardiac disease | 11. Hemoglobinopathy |
| 5. Prior stroke | 12. Drug abuse, such as cocaine |
| 6. Transient ischemic attacks | 13. Hyperlipidemia |
| 7. Carotid bruits | |

Wolf PA: Epidemiology and stroke risk factors. In Samuels MA, Feske S (eds): Office Practice of Neurology. New York, Churchill Livingstone, 1996, pp 224-237.

21. **What other risk factors have been described?**

| | |
|---|---|
| 1. Diet | 7. Infection |
| 2. Oral contraceptives | 8. Hyperhomocysteinemia |
| 3. Sedentary lifestyle | 9. Migraine |
| 4. Obesity | 10. African-American race |
| 5. Peripheral vascular disease | 11. Geography (the "Stroke Belt") |
| 6. Hyperuricemia | 12. Alcohol consumption |

22. **What is the significance of hypertension as a risk factor for stroke?**
From a public health standpoint, hypertension is the most important modifiable risk factor for stroke. The risk of all stroke subtypes is increased threefold to fourfold by hypertension. Treatment significantly lowers both the risk of a first-time stroke and the risk of stroke recurrence. Remaining unresolved questions include the optimal blood pressure range and the relative efficacy of different antihypertensive agents with respect to secondary stroke prevention.

23. **What forms of cardiac disease are risk factors for stroke?**
People with heart disease of almost any type have more than twice the risk of stroke compared with people with normal cardiac function. Coronary artery disease is a major association, both as an indicator of the presence of systemic atherosclerosis and as a potential source of emboli from mural thrombi due to myocardial infarction. Congestive heart failure of any etiology is associated with increased stroke. Hypertensive heart disease, whether detected clinically, by left ventricular hypertrophy (LVH) on ECG, or by echocardiogram, is associated with an increased risk of both thromboembolic and hemorrhagic strokes.

Another major stroke risk factor is atrial fibrillation, which is strongly associated with cerebral embolism. Atrial fibrillation due to rheumatic valvular disease has the strongest association, increasing stroke risk by 17 times. Nonvalvular atrial fibrillation has also been shown to increase stroke risk, especially with advancing age.

Various other cardiac lesions have been associated with stroke, such as patent foramen ovale, atrial septal aneurysm, aortic arch atheroma, left atrial appendage thrombus, spontaneous echo contrast, and mitral valve prolapse. Many of these are poorly seen with transthoracic echo but readily detected on transesophageal echo. The appropriate therapy of many of these lesions with respect to stroke remain to be clarified.

### 24. Is smoking an established risk factor for stroke?
Meta-analysis of epidemiologic studies has shown that cigarette smoking confers an increased risk for stroke, that the degree of risk correlates with the number of cigarettes smoked, and that smoking cessation decreases risk, with the incidence reverting to that of nonsmokers by 5 years after smoking cessation. Smoking confers increased risk in all age groups and both sexes. The association exists not only for ischemic stroke but also SAH due to cerebral aneurysms.

### 25. What is the single strongest risk factor for stroke?
Age is the strongest single stroke risk factor. About 30% of strokes occur before the age of 65; 70% occur in those 65 and over. Stroke risk roughly doubles for every decade of age after 55 years.

### 26. What is the role of abnormal lipids in stroke? What is the role of drug abuse?
Elevated cholesterol is associated with atherosclerosis and ischemic stroke. Lipid-lowering therapy with statins in ischemic stroke patients with low-density lipoprotein (LDL) cholesterol greater than 100 moderately reduces the risk of stroke recurrence. Very low cholesterol, on the other hand, may be a risk factor for hemorrhagic stroke.

Drugs of abuse also increase stroke risk. Cocaine and amphetamines are associated with intracerebral and SAH. Intravenous drug use increases the risk of endocarditis and ischemic stroke.

## KEY POINTS: CAUSES OF STROKE IN THE POSTERIOR CIRCULATION

1. Atherosclerosis of vertebrobasilar arteries or aortic arch

2. Small vessel disease in penetrating arteries

3. Cardiac embolism

### 27. Do oral contraceptives increase stroke risk in women?
The early, high-estrogen oral contraceptives were reported to increase the risk of stroke in young women. Lowering the estrogen content has decreased this problem but not eliminated it altogether. The risk factor is strongest in women over 35 years who are also smokers. The presumed mechanism is an increased coagulation tendency mediated by estrogen stimulation of liver protein production, including clotting factors. An autoimmune mechanism has also been suggested in rare cases.

Recent randomized clinical trials showed that hormone replacement therapy also moderately increases the risk of stroke and other thromboembolic complications.

### 28. Which clotting system abnormalities are associated with stroke?
Rare inherited abnormalities of the blood clotting system include antithrombin III deficiency, protein C and protein S deficiency, activated protein C resistance (factor V Leiden mutation), and prothrombin gene mutation. Antiphospholipid antibodies and hyperhomocysteinemia also promote thrombosis.

29. **Summarize the most important treatable stroke risk factors.**
The most important modifiable risk factors for stroke are hypertension, smoking, heart disease, and hyperlipidemia. The presence of prior stroke or transient ischemic attack (TIA) is also an important treatable risk factor. Other modifiable risks include diabetes, hyperhomocysteinemia, alcohol consumption, drugs of abuse, oral contraceptives, and obesity.

Rokey R, Rolak LA: Epidemiology and risk factors for stroke and myocardial infarction. In Rolak LA, Rokey R (eds): Coronary and Cerebral Vascular Disease. Mt. Kisco, NY, Futura, 1990, pp 83-117.

## THERAPY

30. **What are the most common causes of death in patients admitted to the hospital with a stroke?**
The leading causes of death in the first month after a stroke are the following: (1) the neurologic sequelae of the stroke; (2) pneumonia; (3) pulmonary embolism; and (4) cardiac disease. An essential part of stroke treatment is therefore the treatment and prevention of medical complications.

31. **What is the treatment for a completed stroke?**
Intravenous tissue plasminogen activator (tPA) given within the first 3 hours of an acute ischemic stroke significantly improves the likelihood of a good neurologic outcome. Candidates for thrombolytic treatment should have a potentially disabling deficit that is not rapidly resolving. Important contraindications include the presence of hemorrhage or extensive acute hypodensity on the CT scan, a stroke or severe head injury in the previous 3 months, history of intracranial hemorrhage, major surgery in the previous 2 seeks, active or recent bleeding, severe uncontrolled hypertension (systolic blood pressure [SBP] > 185 mmHg or diastolic blood pressure [DBP] > 110 mmHg), thrombocytopenia, abnormal prothrombin or partial thromboplastin time, pregnancy, and myocardial infarction-related pericarditis.

A 0.9 mg/kg dose of tPA is given as an intravenous infusion, 10% as a bolus and the remainder over 1 hour to a maximal dose of 90 mg. Other antithrombotic drugs, such as aspirin and heparin, should be withheld in the first 24 hours, and blood pressure maintained under 185/110 mmHg.

32. **What are the risks of thrombolytic therapy?**
Under strict adherence to these treatment guidelines, the risk of symptomatic intracerebral hemorrhage is 6%. Half are fatal. The risk of intracranial hemorrhage increases significantly if the guidelines are violated. Thrombolysis may be associated with a higher risk of hemorrhage if treatment is administered after 3 hours, a higher dose or different thrombolytic agent is used, aspirin or heparin is given in the first 24 hours, or blood pressure is not maintained under 185/110 mmHg. Despite the recognized risks of thrombolysis, treatment increases by 50% the likelihood of an excellent recovery and reduces the number of patients who die or are left severely disabled.

33. **What is the role of intra-arterial thrombolysis?**
Intra-arterial thrombolytic therapy has been demonstrated to be beneficial in patients with strokes due to middle cerebral artery occlusion up to 6 hours after onset of symptoms. The potential advantages of intra-arterial over intravenous administration (confirmation of arterial occlusion, lower doses of thrombolytic agent, higher patency rates) need to be balanced against the disadvantages (time delay to treatment, less readily available resources).

**34. What advances in acute stroke treatment may be anticipated?**
Mechanical clot retrieval devices are currently undergoing clinical evaluation. Several putative neuroprotective drugs are also currently in clinical trial testing. By targeting one or more steps of the ischemic cascade, these drugs reduce neuronal injury and neurologic disability in experimental models of stroke.

**35. What is the role of Coumadin therapy in cerebrovascular disease?**
Coumadin is the stroke-preventive treatment of choice in patients at high risk for cardiogenic emboli. Coumadin is effective in long-term use for the reduction of stroke risk in nonvalvular atrial fibrillation as well as in rheumatic valvular-related atrial fibrillation and intracardiac thrombus. The benefit of Coumadin depends on the risk of stroke versus the risk of a major bleeding event while on Coumadin. Although the target international normalized ratio (INR) is 2 to 3 in most cases, it is higher for patients with mechanical cardiac valves and may be lower for very elderly patients or those at higher risk for hemorrhagic complications. The bleeding risk is related to the intensity of anticoagulation. The risk of embolic stroke with different cardiac lesions can be stratified as shown in Table 17-2.

**TABLE 17-2. RISK STRATIFICATION FOR PATIENTS IN ATRIAL FIBRILLATION**

**High risk (≥5% per year)**

Valvular heart disease (e.g., mitral stenosis, prosthetic mechanical valve)
Recent-onset congestive heart failure (within 3 months)
Prior thromboembolism
Thyrotoxicosis
Systolic hypertension
Severe left ventricular dysfunction by ECG
Demonstration of intracardiac thrombus

**Moderate risk (3% to 5% per year)**

Age ≥60 years
Mitral annulus calcification
Diuretic therapy
Silent cerebral infarction by CT

**Low risk (<3% per year)**

Lone atrial fibrillation, chronic or paroxysmal, age <60 years

**Uncertain risk**

Diabetes mellitus
Left atrial enlargement
Coexistent carotid artery disease
Recent-onset versus chronic atrial fibrillation
Reduced cerebral blood flow

ECG = echocardiogram, CT = computed tomography
(From Halperin JL, Hart RG: Atrial fibrillation and stroke: New ideas, persisting dilemmas. Stroke 19:937, 1988.)

36. **What is the approach to primary stroke prevention?**
    The mainstay of primary stroke prevention is risk factor management. Although aspirin is often used for primary prevention of myocardial infarction, it has not consistently demonstrated benefit in preventing first-time stroke.

37. **What treatment is used to prevent a stroke in patients with TIA or prior stroke?**
    Aspirin remains the most popular drug used for secondary stroke prevention. The standard dose is 31 to 325 mg per day. Higher doses are not more effective and are associated with greater hemorrhagic and gastrointestinal side effects.

38. **Which antiplatelet agents other than aspirin are used for the prevention of stroke?**
    Clopidogrel 75 mg per day is more effective than aspirin at preventing recurrent ischemic events (stroke, myocardial infarction, and vascular death). The relative risk reduction is 8% to 9%. Clopidogrel is indicated in patients who are aspirin-intolerant and should be considered in patients at high risk of recurrent stroke.
    Aspirin combined with extended-release dipyridamole is another effective secondary stroke prevention regimen. The benefit of the two agents is additive in this combination. Headache is the most common side effect attributable to the dipyridamole component.
    Ticlopidine is a platelet adenosine diphosphate (ADP) receptor antagonist chemically related to clopidogrel. It has a superior efficacy compared to aspirin, but side effects include rash, diarrhea, and neutropenia necessitating CBC monitoring. For these reasons, ticlopidine is rarely used as a first-line agent.
    Sacco RL, Diener HC, Yusuf S, et al.: Aspirin and extended-release dipyridamole versus clopidogrel for recurrent stroke. N Engl J Med 359:1238-1251, 2008.

39. **What is the role of carotid endarterectomy in cerebrovascular disease?**
    Carotid endarterectomy has been proven to prevent recurrent ischemic stroke in patients with high-grade carotid stenosis. In symptomatic patients with an internal carotid artery stenosis of 70% or greater, surgery significantly reduces the risk of subsequent stroke. There is a smaller benefit in symptomatic patients with 50% to 70% stenosis. Lesions less than 50% are better treated medically. An advantage for carotid endarterectomy has also been demonstrated for asymptomatic lesions of 60% or greater, but the absolute reduction in stroke risk is much smaller.

40. **Which factors affect the benefit of carotid endarterectomy?**
    Surgical morbidity and mortality are the key factors determining benefit in carotid surgery. The efficacy of endarterectomy assumes a surgical morbidity and mortality rate of 6% or less for symptomatic carotid disease and 3% or less for asymptomatic disease. The benefit of surgery may be lost when surgical morbidity and mortality exceeds these rates.

41. **What other interventions are available for cerebrovascular disease?**
    Endovascular interventions such as angioplasty, stenting, or both, are an established alternative to carotid endarterectomy in patients who are poor surgical candidates. Angioplasty/stenting procedures may emerge as options for patients with intracranial carotid, vertebral, basilar, or middle cerebral artery lesions not amenable to surgical treatment.
    Extracranial-intracranial bypass surgery may be considered in selected patients with ischemic symptoms secondary to carotid occlusion and demonstrated hemodynamic insufficiency.
    Hemicraniectomy is a life-saving decompressive procedure proven to be of benefit in appropriate patients with malignant hemispheric brain infarction resulting in cerebral edema and incipient brain herniation.
    Surgical evacuation of intracerebral hematomas is also sometimes performed as a lifesaving procedure. As a routine treatment for intracerebral hemorrhages, surgery has not been demonstrated to improve neurologic outcome.

## SUBARACHNOID HEMORRHAGE

42. **What percentage of strokes result due to hemorrhage?**
About 15% to 20% of strokes are due to hemorrhage; roughly one-half of these are due to SAH. SAH is a relatively more common stroke subtype in the young. Although the actual incidence of SAH increases with age, SAH accounts for a smaller proportion of strokes as the incidence of atherothrombotic stroke rises.

43. **What predisposes to SAH?**
SAH is common after trauma. SAH due to ruptured saccular or berry aneurysm is the most serious type with the greatest morbidity and mortality. SAH also may be a consequence of rupture of an arteriovenous malformation (AVM). Ingestion of cocaine or amphetamines may be associated with SAH. Hypertension, cigarette smoking, and alcohol consumption are also risk factors (Figure 17-4).

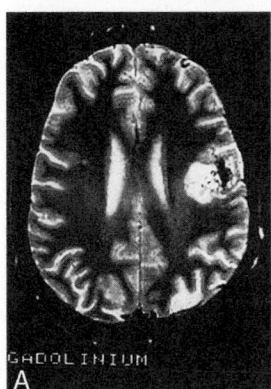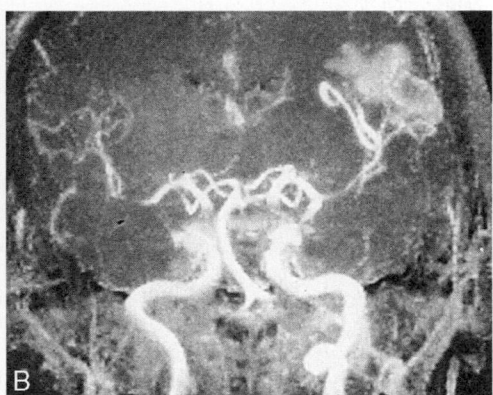

**Figure 17-4.** (A) MR appearance of a left frontoparietal arteriovenous malformation. (B) The characteristic appearance on an MR angiogram.

44. **Where are most intracerebral aneurysms located?**
Eighty percent of aneurysms occur in the anterior circulation and 20% in the posterior circulation. The most common locations are the following: (1) the anterior communicating artery (30%); (2) the junction of the posterior communicating artery with the internal carotid artery (25%); and (3) the bifurcation of the internal carotid and middle cerebral artery (20% to 25%). Aneurysms are multiple in about 25% of the patients. About 3% of intracerebral aneurysms are associated with polycystic kidney disease. Fibromuscular dysplasia is accompanied by intracranial aneurysms in about 25% of the cases.

45. **What is the clinical profile of SAH?**
SAH is characterized by sudden severe headache, often described as "the worst headache of my life," with or without focal neurologic deficit, and often with altered mental status. Aneurysmal SAH may be preceded by a moderately severe headache caused by an initial "sentinel bleed." Clinical deterioration can result from rebleeding from untreated aneurysms. SAH may not be suspected from the initial headache, causing delay in diagnosis and treatment.

46. **What is the work-up of SAH?**
The initial test in suspected SAH is a noncontrast CT scan of the brain, which may reveal blood in the cisterns, sylvian fissure, or sulci around the convexities. There also may be intraparenchymal blood, suggesting the location of the ruptured aneurysm responsible for the hemorrhage. The aneurysm itself may be visible. The amount of subarachnoid blood visible on the CT scan correlates with extent of bleeding and prognosis. The CT scan may be negative in 10% of SAHs. When SAH is strongly suspected clinically and the initial CT scan is negative, a lumbar puncture is necessary.

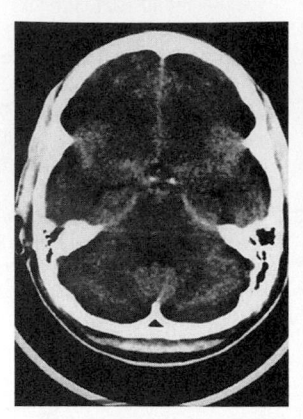

Once SAH is confirmed, neurosurgical consultation should be obtained to plan possible surgical management. Cerebral angiography is necessary for identification of the site of bleeding. Angiography should be obtained emergently if early surgical management is a consideration. Angiography may fail to identify the underlying lesion because of vasospasm or thrombosis preventing visualization of the responsible aneurysm. Repeat angiography may be necessary if initial angiography fails to identify the bleeding source (Figure 17-5).

**Figure 17-5.** Noncontrast CT scan showing an acute subarachnoid hemorrhage, with blood diffusely filling cerebrospinal fluid (CSF) spaces.

47. **What are the treatment options for SAH due to ruptured aneurysm?**
Early surgical repair of a ruptured aneurysm is indicated in patients with a favorable clinical grade to prevent rebleeding. The definitive treatments are surgical clipping of the aneurysm or endovascular obliteration by catheter-directed placement of thrombogenic coils. In patients undergoing aneurysm clipping, surgery should be performed within the first 48 hours of onset of symptoms or be postponed 10 to 14 days because of the risk of vasospasm. Careful blood pressure control is necessary to prevent rebleeding in patients with unclipped aneurysms, and blood pressure must be monitored continuously during this phase.

48. **What is the basic medical management of SAH?**
The general nonsurgical management centers on treatment and prevention of vasospasm and medical complications. Hypertensive hypovolemic therapy is often used to ameliorate the ischemic complications of vasospasm. Nimodipine is administered at a dosage of 60 mg every 4 hours for 3 weeks. If the patient cannot take the medication by mouth, it is administered by nasogastric tube. Because nimodipine lowers blood pressure and may cause bradycardia or atrioventricular (AV) block, the patient's blood pressure and ECG must be monitored during initial therapy.

49. **What clinical grading system is used to characterize patients with SAH?**
Patients with SAH are graded on a clinical scale of I to V, based primarily on level of consciousness and presence of focal neurologic signs.
- Grade I: Awake, with no symptoms or mild headache and/or nuchal rigidity
- Grade II: Awake, with moderate-to-severe headache and nuchal rigidity
- Grade III: Drowsy or confused, with or without focal deficits
- Grade IV: Stuporous, with moderate-to-severe hemiparesis and signs of increased intracranial pressure
- Grade V: Comatose with signs of severe increased intracranial pressure

This clinical grading scale has prognostic significance. Grade I or II patients have the best prognosis and should undergo early cerebral angiography and definitive intervention, particularly if evaluation is within the first 48 hours of onset. Grade IV and V patients have a poor prognosis and warrant medical management until their clinical state improves. Angiography may be performed later if patients improve sufficiently to warrant more definitive care.

50. **Which focal neurologic signs commonly accompany SAH? What is their mechanism?**
Focal neurologic signs associated with an aneurysm of the posterior communicating artery are ptosis, pupillary dilatation, and impaired extraocular movements due to compression of the third nerve. Pupillary dilatation suggests external compression of the third nerve because the fibers for pupillary constriction are superficial, whereas those for the extraocular muscles are deeper in the nerve. Development of focal neurologic signs may be a consequence of intraparenchymal extension of blood or ischemia due to vasospasm.

## KEY POINTS: COMPLICATIONS OF SUBARACHNOID HEMORRHAGE

1. Intraparenchymal extension

2. Seizures

3. Vasospasm

4. Acute hydrocephalus

5. Rebleeding

51. **What systemic complications are common in SAH?**
Fever may occur in SAH due to infection, especially pneumonia or urinary tract infection. An inflammatory response to the blood in the cerebrospinal fluid (CSF) also may lead to fever, and the clinical picture may mimic acute meningitis. Hyponatremia may occur due to cerebral salt wasting syndrome or syndrome of inappropriate antidiuretic hormone (SIADH); the proper treatment (fluid and electrolyte resuscitation versus free water restriction) requires an assessment of the patient's volume status. SAH may cause acute ECG changes, especially prolongation of the QT interval, T-wave inversion, and cardiac arrhythmias. An ECG should be obtained during the initial evaluation, and the cardiac rhythm monitored continuously in the intensive care unit (ICU) with treatment of rhythm disturbances as necessary. A rare complication of SAH is neurogenic pulmonary edema. Development of congestive heart failure due to underlying heart disease or respiratory failure due to acute respiratory distress syndrome also may occur.

52. **What central nervous system (CNS) complications occur in SAH?**
**Rebleeding** can cause worsening headache or a decline in the level of consciousness. **Intraparenchymal extension** can cause focal deficits due to mass effect, including development of cerebral edema and herniation. **Seizures** are another complication of SAH related to the irritant effect of blood.
**Vasospasm** occurs with aneurysmal SAH but usually not with other causes of SAH. It can lead to focal ischemic injury and infarction. TCD can be used to monitor the flow velocity of the middle cerebral artery; vasospasm leads to a characteristic increase in the measured flow velocity.
**Acute hydrocephalus** may develop, usually communicating hydrocephalus due to obstruction of the pacchionian granulations in the venous sinuses by blood. It may be treated in the short term by ventriculostomy or permanently by ventriculoperitoneal shunting if necessary. Patients in higher clinical grades are more likely to experience clinical deterioration.

53. **What is the prognosis in patients with SAH?**
The prognosis of SAH correlates with the clinical grade. Prognosis is best in grade I or II (Table 17-3).

| TABLE 17-3. PROGNOSIS IN PATIENTS WITH SUBARACHNOID HEMORRHAGE | | | |
|---|---|---|---|
| Grade | Deterioration (%) | Rebleed (%) | Death (%) |
| I | 5 | 10-15 | 3-5 |
| II | 20 | 10-15 | 6-10 |
| III | 25 | 10-20 | 10-15 |
| IV | 50 | 20-25 | 40-50 |
| V | 80 | 25-30 | 50-70 |

## BIBLIOGRAPHY

1. Caplan LR: Brain Ischemia: Basic Concepts and Clinical Relevance. London, Springer, 1995.
2. Daniel WG, Kronzon I, Mugge A (eds): Cardiogenic Embolism. Baltimore, Williams & Wilkins, 1996.
3. Kase CS, Caplan LR: Intracerebral Hemorrhage. Boston, Butterworth-Heinemann, 1994.
4. NASCET Collaborators: Beneficial effect of carotid endarterectomy in symptomatic patients with high-grade carotid stenosis. N Engl J Med 325:445-453, 1991.
5. National Institute of Neurological Disorders and Stroke rtPA Study Group: Tissue plasminogen activator for acute ischemic stroke. N Engl J Med 333:1581-1587, 1995.
6. Vermuelen M, Lindsay KW, Van Gihn J: Subarachnoid Hemorrhage. London, W.B. Saunders, 1992.

# CHAPTER 18

# NEURO-ONCOLOGY AND CANCER PAIN

*Yvonne Kew, MD, PhD, and Everton A. Edmondson, MD*

## PRIMARY BRAIN TUMORS

1. **How many different types of primary brain tumors are classified by the World Health Organization (WHO)?**
There are more than 100 different types, with heterogeneous biologies and divergent clinical outcomes.

   Louis DN, Ohgaki H, Wiestler OD, Cavenee WK (eds): WHO Classification of Tumours of the Central Nervous System. Lyon, France, IARC, 2007.

2. **What is the incidence of all primary central nervous system (CNS) tumors in the United States?**
The incidence is 14.8 cases per 100,000, with an estimated 43,800 primary tumors diagnosed in the United States in 2005. About 18,500 of these tumors were malignant. Malignant primary brain tumors cause a disproportionate morbidity and mortality. Morbidity is from the tumor location, progression, and pressure effects. Approximately 12,700 deaths are attributed to malignant primary CNS tumors in the United States each year. Malignant brain tumor is the most common cause of cancer death in children up to age 19, the second most common cause of cancer death in young men 20 to 39 years of age, and the fifth most common cause of cancer death in young women 20 to 39 years of age.

3. **Are supratentorial brain tumors more common in adults or children?**
Two-thirds of the brain tumors in adults present supratentorially; in children, the reverse is true.

4. **What is the most common category of brain tumors?**
Gliomas account for 68% of all primary brain tumors, with glioblastoma multiforme (GBM) accounting for 50% of all the gliomas. Extension of the tumor across the corpus callosum, with central necrosis, is unique to GBM (Figure 18-1).

   Ohgaki H, Dessen P, Jourde B, et al.: Genetic pathways to glioblastoma: A population-based study. Cancer Res 64:6892-6899, 2004.

5. **What features guide the WHO classification for gliomas?**
The WHO classification categorizes gliomas into four grades based upon their histology. Tumors are assessed for key histologic characteristics, including cellularity, atypical cells, mitoses, microvascular proliferate, and necrosis. Grade I includes

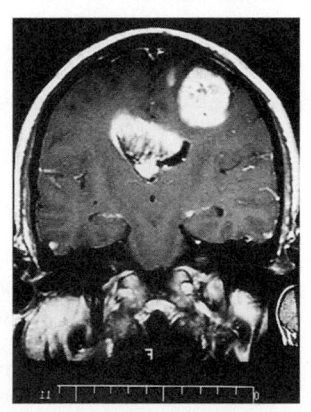

**Figure 18-1.** Gadolinium-enhanced T1-weighted magnetic resonance imaging (MRI) of the brain showing a malignant glioblastoma multiforme, with characteristic extension across the corpus callosum.

well-circumscribed gliomas such as pilocytic astrocytomas, subependymal giant
cell astrocytomas, and dysembryoplastic neuroepithelial tumors (DNET), which can be cured by
complete tumor resection. Grades II through IV are all infiltrative and cannot be completely resected
surgically. WHO grade II or low-grade gliomas include fibrillary astrocytoma, oligodendroglioma,
and mixed oligoastrocytoma. These usually present between the second and fourth decades of life.
The median survival is 5 years for astrocytomas and 10 years for oligodendrogliomas. WHO
grade III comprises anaplastic astrocytoma (AA) and anaplastic oligodendrogliomas (AO), which
tend to occur at ages between 35 and 55 years. Median survival is about 3 years for AA and 5 years
for AO. WHO grade IV glioma or GBM is most frequent at ages 45 to 65, with a median survival of 1
year. The higher grades have high cellularity with poor differentiation, pleomorphic nuclei, and
frequent mitoses. GBM tumors also have neovascularization and necrosis.

   Louis DN, Ohgaki H, Wiestler OD, Cavenee WK (eds): WHO Classification of Tumours of the
Central Nervous System. Lyon, France, IARC, 2007.

6. **What is the customary total radiation dose administered to the brain for primary
   tumors such as gliomas?**
   Radiation therapy of 5400 to 6000 rads delivered in fractions over 6 weeks is commonly
   recommended as the first-line therapy following surgery for malignant gliomas (WHO grades
   III and IV gliomas) with or without adjuvant chemotherapy with temozolomide at 75 mg/m$^2$.
   Intensity-modulated radiation therapy (IMRT) allows for the radiation doses to conform
   precisely to the 3D shape of the tumor, maximizing the dose to the tumor bed and minimizing
   radiation to adjacent normal tissue.

7. **List some of the standard chemotherapy for glioma treatment.**
   Temozolomide (150 to 200 mg/m$^2$ days 1 to 5 for 4 weeks) is an oral alkylating drug
   commonly used as first-line chemotherapy after radiation for malignant glioma. Nitrosoureas
   are commonly used drugs in chemotherapy regimens, such as carmustine (BCNU) as a single
   agent (200 mg/m$^2$ IV for 8 weeks) or in combination with procarbazine (60 mg/m$^2$ days
   8 to 21), CCNU (110 mg/m$^2$ PO day 1), and vincristine (1.4 mg/m$^2$ days 8 to 29) for 6 weeks.
   Currently, various clinical trials are underway to study the effectiveness of molecular targeted
   therapy either used alone or in combination with cytotoxic drugs like temozolomide. Avastin or
   bevacizumab (a monoclonal antibody that blocks vascular endothelial growth factor)
   presumably decreases blood supply to the tumor and probably will be approved by the U.S.
   Food and Drug Administration (FDA) for treating patients with recurrent GBM.

8. **What genetic alterations are frequently seen in oligodendrogliomas?**
   Loss of heterozygosity (LOH) for chromosomes 1p and 19q are often (67% to 80%) observed
   in oligodendrogliomas and confers upon these tumors an increased chemosensitivity and
   improved patient survival. In some institutions, these genetic analyses are done routinely for
   any glioma tissue that has features of oligodendroglioma.

9. **Which primary brain tumors have a higher propensity to bleed?**
   Oligodendrogliomas, but because of the much higher incidence of GBM, brain tumors that
   present with hemorrhage are most likely to be GBM.

10. **What are the two most common brain tumors in children?**
    Medulloblastoma and pilocytic astrocytoma, both of which often present infratentorially and
    together represent about a quarter of all pediatric brain tumors.

11. **What prognostic indices determine a poor chance for survival with a diagnosis
    of medulloblastoma?**
    Poor prognostic features include the following: (1) subtotal resection; (2) malignant cells in
    cerebrospinal fluid (CSF); (3) documented spinal cord metastasis on neuroimaging; and (4)
    age younger than 4 years.

12. **What is the 5-year survival rate for good-risk patients with medulloblastoma?**
Survival for good-risk patients (normal CSF, >75% resection, older than 4 years of age, no metastases) is 70% with maximal treatment. The 5-year survival rate for poor-risk patients is only 25%.

13. **Which CNS tumors are more likely to metastasize?**
Medulloblastoma has a high propensity to metastasize within the CSF pathway and may metastasize outside the CNS (e.g., bone marrow invasion).

14. **What population is most at risk for ependymoma?**
These tumors are most common in the first decade, and the frequency drops significantly after age 30 years. Ependymoma is the most common intraventricular tumor in children. In adults, it is virtually confined to the spinal cord.

15. **The incidence of meningioma increases with age. True or false?**
True. Meningioma is rare in the first two decades and increases progressively thereafter.

16. **What are the sites of predilection for meningiomas?**
The parasagittal and convexity region has the highest incidence, followed by sphenoid ridge, olfactory groove, suprasellar region, posterior fossa, spine, periorbital region, temporal fossa, and falx—in that order.

17. **What is the treatment of choice for meningioma?**
If the tumor is resectable, surgery is the treatment of choice. Radiation and chemotherapy are of limited value. Unresectable, large meningiomas can be irradiated, and shrinkage may occur, but transformation to a sarcoma or higher malignant grade is a risk. Chemotherapy is limited to the treatment of meningeal sarcoma.

18. **Which tumors have a high incidence of calcification on neuroimaging?**
Calcifications are seen in more than 50% of oligodendrogliomas and with high frequency in craniopharyngiomas and meningiomas. Metastatic melanoma and renal cell carcinoma are hemorrhagic tumors that may exhibit exuberant calcific changes on neuroimaging.

19. **Neurofibromatosis is associated with what types of CNS tumors?**
Optic glioma associated with neurofibromatosis type 1 (NF-1) and bilateral vestibular schwannoma (acoustic neurinoma) associated with neurofibromatosis type 2 (NF-2).

20. **Which tumors occur in the pineal area?**
Tumors in the pineal region include germinoma (most common), germ cell tumors (teratoma, choriocarcinoma, yolk sac tumor, embryonal carcinoma), pineocytoma, pineoblastoma, astrocytoma, and meningioma.

21. **Alpha-fetoprotein (AFP) and human chorionic gonadotropin (HCG) are markers for tumors in what area of the brain?**
Germ cell tumors usually present in the pineal region or around the third ventricle and may secrete HCG if they are of trophoblastic origin (e.g., choriocarcinoma) and high levels of AFP if they are of yolk sac origin.

22. **What is primary CNS lymphoma?**
Primary CNS lymphoma (PCNSL) involves the brain without evidence of systemic lymphoma. Much controversy surrounds its site of origin. More than half of these tumors present in the hemispheres, with a periventricular predilection. In immunocompetent patients the peak age of onset is 60 to 70 years. Twenty-five percent to 50% are multiple in immunocompetent

patients, and 60% to 85% are multiple in acquired immune deficiency syndrome (AIDS) and post-transplantation individuals. The incidence of primary CNS lymphoma has decreased in patients with AIDS with the introduction of highly active antiretroviral therapy (HAART) therapy. CNS lymphoma has a high predilection to affect the leptomeninges. Most CNS lymphomas have a large B-cell histology; few are T-cell types (Figure 18-2).

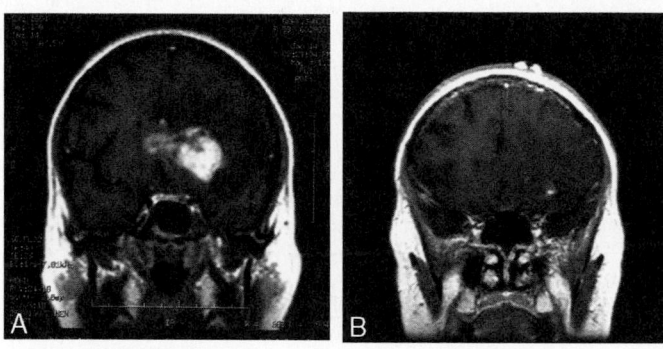

**Figure 18-2.** Before (A) and after (B) 1 week of steroid treatment intended for the vasogenic edema but note that the enhancing butterfly lesion is disappearing. This is pathognomonic for lymphoma due to the sensitivity of the clonal B-cells to steroid therapy. The first image was mistaken for GBM, the most common and lethal primary brain tumor.

23. **What staging tests help to exclude systemic lymphoma in patients with CNS lymphoma?**
   Computed tomography (CT) scans of the chest, abdomen, and pelvis and gallium scans (a nuclear medicine test) can be helpful. Currently body positron emission tomography (PET) scans are more widely used in place of gallium scans.

## KEY POINTS: PRIMARY BRAIN TUMORS ✔

1. About 65% of primary brain tumors are gliomas.

2. Glioblastoma multiforme accounts for 45% to 50% of all gliomas.

3. The two most common brain tumors in children are medulloblastoma and juvenile pilocytic astrocytoma.

4. Medulloblastoma has a high propensity to metastasize.

5. Primary CNS lymphoma is histiocytic lymphoma in the CNS without evidence of systemic lymphoma.

24. **Are pituitary tumors more likely to produce hormone when they are intrasellar or extrasellar in extent?**
   Intrasellar microadenomas are more likely to be hormone-producing, whereas chromophobe adenoma, the more common pituitary tumor, is large, extends outside the sella frequently, and seldom produces hormone (Figure 18-3).

25. **What oral medication is commonly used to treat prolactinoma?**
Bromocriptine and cabergoline reduce prolactin secretion by acting like dopamine and are used in many instances to shrink an intrasellar pituitary prolactinoma.

26. **What are the most common tumors of the foramen magnum and skull base?**
Meningioma, schwannoma, glomus jugulare, and metastatic tumors (Figure 18-4).

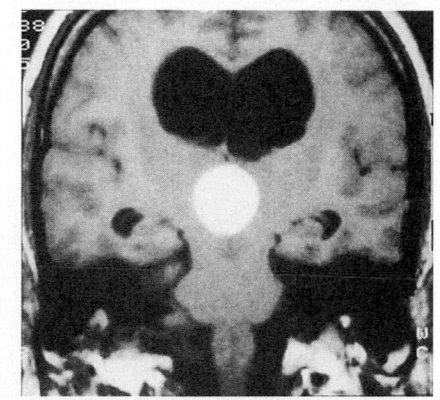

**Figure 18-3.** T1-weighted MRI showing a cystic craniopharyngioma, resulting in the noncommunicating hydrocephalus with round-appearing lateral ventricles.

27. **Which tumor is likely to present in the region of the clivus with evidence of bony erosion?**
Chordoma arising from the clivus is the second most common site for this tumor, following the sacrum. Bony erosion results from direct tumor invasion and enzymatic digestion.

28. **What are the most common tumors arising from the cerebellopontine angle?**
The most common tumors in this area include schwannoma and meningioma; others seen in this region include cholesteatoma and metastatic diseases.

29. **What is von Hippel-Lindau syndrome?**
Hippel-Lindau syndrome is an autosomal-dominantly inherited condition that commonly presents with CNS and retinal hemangioblastoma and renal cysts. Other findings may include pheochromocytoma, pancreatic cysts, and other systemic tumors. It is associated with *VHL* gene mutations, which is a tumor suppressor gene located on chromosome 3.

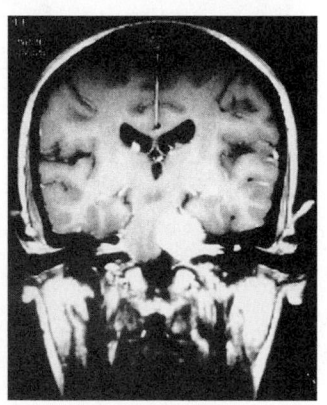

**Figure 18-4.** T1-weighted MRI shows a gadolinium-enhancing tumor of the left glomus jugulare, arising at the skull base and compressing the brain stem.

30. **What types of tumors are found in the intradural, extramedullary region of the spinal cord?**
Schwannoma, neurofibromas, and meningioma.

31. **Which tumors arise in the intradural intramedullary region of the spinal cord?**
By far, the most common tumors occurring within the substance of the spinal cord parenchyma are astrocytomas and ependymomas.

## BRAIN AND SPINE METASTATIC DISEASE

32. **Metastatic disease accounts for what percentage of CNS tumors?**
Most CNS cancers are metastatic, with an incidence of 170,000/year in the United States. About half of CNS metastases are multiple (Figure 18-5).

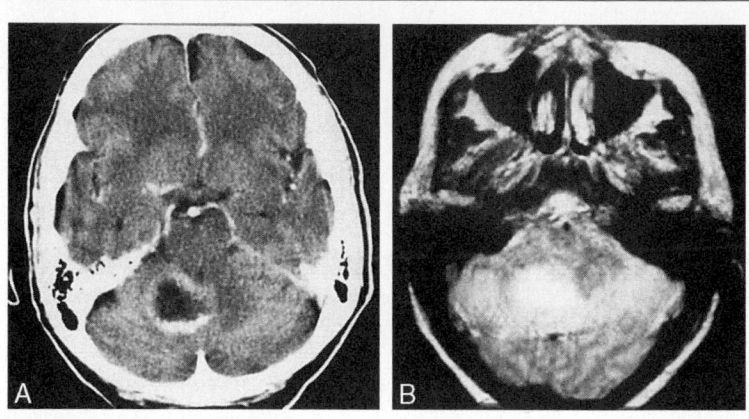

**Figure 18-5.** Small-cell carcinoma of the lung metastatic to the cerebellum shown on contrast-enhanced CT scan (A) and proton-density MRI (B).

33. **Does gross total resection of a solitary metastasis improve survival?**
Surgical resection followed by radiotherapy improves survival in a selected subpopulation. Reasonable candidates are patients who have no evidence of disease elsewhere, who are ambulatory, and in whom gross total resection can be achieved without significant risk of inducing major neurologic deficits.

34. **Without radiation therapy, what is the usual life expectancy of a patient with brain metastasis?**
The mean life expectancy with steroids alone is 1 month. Radiation therapy extends the mean survival time to 4 to 6 months.
    Biswas G, Bhagwat R, Khurana R, et al.: Brain metastases - evidence based management. J Cancer Res Ther 2:5-13, 2006.

35. **What is the role of stereotactic radiosurgery (SRS) in the treatment of brain metastases?**
Patients with four or fewer metastases may be candidates for noninvasive SRS if the lesions are smaller than 3 cm. SRS is more effective against "radioresistant tumors." Patients treated with SRS and whole brain radiation (WBRT) require less salvage therapy. The combined approach of surgery, SRS, and WBRT when appropriate appears to improve survival in 25% to 35% of patients where extracranial disease is well controlled.
    Lindvall P, Berg-Strom P, Lofroth PO, Bergenheim TA: A comparison between surgical resection in combination with WBRT or hypofractionated stereotactic irradiation in the treatment of solitary brain metastases. Acta Neurochir 151:1053-1059, 2009.

36. **Is gamma knife better than SRS for the treatment of brain metastases?**
    Gamma knife uses a cobalt source placed in a circular array to aim gamma radiation to the
    target lesion(s). Both gamma knife and SRS achieve similar good clinical results.

37. **Which solid tumors most commonly metastasize to the brain?**
    The lung is the most common, followed by breast, melanoma, renal, and colorectal cancers.

38. **Which CNS metastases most commonly bleed?**
    Melanoma, renal cell cancer, and choriocarcinoma. Lung cancer is also included in the
    differential diagnosis because of its high frequency of brain metastasis.

39. **What are the clinical features of epidural spinal cord compression? How is it
    diagnosed and treated?**
    The most common presentation is acute or subacute back pain, which occurs in more than
    90% of cases. The pain may even be radicular, such as a shooting dermatomal pain or a
    band-like aching in the trunk. A sensory level is a strong indicator of a myelopathy. Paraparesis
    and bowel/bladder dysfunction usually indicate a more serious cord compression (with a
    worse prognosis).
       Plain films should be obtained in patients with cancer who present with any of the
    above signs or symptoms. Magnetic resonance imaging (MRI) of the spine or myelogram/CT
    is indicated in any patient whose presenting symptoms include back pain with corresponding
    x-ray or bone scan lesions or neurologic deficits consistent with radiculopathy or myelopathy.
       Patients whose deficits are minimal and who are ambulatory at the time of diagnosis of epidural
    cord compression have the best prognosis following institution of treatment. In contrast, only 13%
    of patients who were paraplegic at the time of diagnosis demonstrated significant neurologic
    improvement with radiation therapy or surgery. Most studies indicate that surgery is no better than
    radiotherapy for epidural cord compression; therefore, oncologists regard radiation therapy as the
    treatment of choice with two exceptions: patients with radioresistant tumors and patients who have
    previously received radiation at the involved site are candidates for surgery.
       When the diagnosis of acute epidural cord compression is entertained as a significant
    possibility, IV dexamethasone, 100 mg, should be given immediately over one-half to 1 hour
    and subsequently 4 mg every 6 hours if the diagnosis is confirmed by neuroimaging.
       Hessler C, Burkhardt T, Raimund F, et al.: Dynamics of neurological deficit after surgical
    decompression of symptomatic vertebral metastases. Spine 34:566-571, 2009.

40. **Most tumors that result in epidural spinal cord compression do so by direct
    extension from bone metastasis. How does lymphoma gain access to the
    epidural space?**
    In contrast to lung, breast, and other solid tumors, lymphoma may extend via the foramina into
    the epidural space. Normal plain radiographs of the spine in the face of epidural lymphoma
    are not uncommon.

## KEY POINTS: METASTATIC DISEASE

1. The annual incidence of metastatic CNS disease is almost 10 times that of primary CNS tumors.

2. Lung cancer most commonly metastasizes to the brain, followed by breast cancer,
   melanoma, renal cancer, and colorectal cancer.

3. The most common presentation of epidural spinal cord compression is acute or subacute
   back pain.

41. **How can the clinician distinguish between radiation-induced plexopathy and cancerous invasion of the plexus?**
Radiation-induced plexopathy is far less likely to present with pain, whereas weakness occurs early. Also, more than half of the reported cases of radiation plexopathy have myokymic discharges on electromyogram (EMG) in contrast to none of the cancerous cases.

## LEPTOMENINGEAL CARCINOMATOSIS

42. **What is the clinical presentation of leptomeningeal carcinomatosis?**
Leptomeningeal carcinomatosis (also known as carcinomatous or neoplastic meningitis) may present in myriad ways. Altered mental status is common, as are seizures, multiple cranial and root signs, and headache. The onset may be fulminant, as in lymphoblastic leukemia, or subacute, with stuttering multifocal deficits and deterioration of cognitive function, as in some patients with breast cancer and leptomeningeal carcinomatosis. The prognosis is poor, especially in metastasis from solid tumors.

43. **Which cancer is the most common cause of leptomeningeal disease in children?**
Leukemia.

44. **Which solid tumor has the greatest prevalence of leptomeningeal carcinomatosis?**
Breast cancer is the most common source in adults, followed by lung cancer and melanoma.

45. **What is the diagnostic yield of CSF examination to establish the diagnosis of leptomeningeal disease?**
The first tap has a 50% yield, but by the third tap the yield increases to 85%. The CSF may show elevated protein, increased cells, or positive cytology.

46. **What ancillary testing may help to determine the presence of leptomeningeal disease other than CSF examination?**
Enhanced CT scan of the brain or MRI may reveal leptomeningeal deposits, meningeal enhancement, or hydrocephalus.

47. **Name two chemotherapeutic agents used for the treatment of leptomeningeal disease.**
Methotrexate and cytosine arabinoside are used intrathecally to treat leptomeningeal carcinomatosis. Systemic chemotherapy is also often effective.

## NEUROLOGIC COMPLICATIONS RELATED TO CANCER AND THERAPY

48. **How often are neurologic problems encountered in patients with cancer? Name several common and uncommon examples.**
Neurologic complications are seen in approximately 30% of cancer patients during some point of their course. Excluding metastasis, common problems include metabolic effects, infection, vascular disease, and paraneoplastic syndromes. Others include complications related to cancer therapy (e.g., radiation encephalopathy, radionecrosis, chemotherapy-induced neuropathies, psychosis, cerebellar dysfunction, leukoencephalopathy). It is not uncommon to find multiple neurologic problems in the same patient. Multifocal structural disease may coexist with metabolic or infectious complications, creating a major diagnostic challenge.

49. **Stroke and other cerebrovascular complications are the third most common problem in cancer patients. Which complications are relatively unique to patients with cancer?**
Stroke may occur as a result of **disseminated intravascular coagulation with or without accompanying sepsis. Venous occlusion** may arise from dehydration, direct tumor invasion, or side effects of treatment such as L-asparaginase. **Embolic complications** include nonbacterial thrombotic endocarditis (NBTE), a disorder characterized by sterile platelet-fibrin debris on endocardium and valves. **Septic emboli** are due to pathogens such as fungi, staphylococci, and gram-negative agents and occur most frequently in patients who have indwelling lines and are neutropenic, or in bone marrow recipients. **Tumor emboli** most commonly result from atrial myxoma but may occur with lung tumors. Serial neuroimaging is often required to confirm that a tumor embolus is present. **Sludging due to leukostasis** may result in altered mental status, seizures, and waxing and waning focal/multifocal signs secondary to leukemic crisis. **Multifocal cerebral hemorrhage** may be seen with acute promyelocytic leukemia. Necrotizing infections such as *Mucor* may cause a stroke by **direct invasion of the artery**. Whole brain radiation may induce direct injury to brain tissue as well as blood vessels, which are sometimes treated with anti-platelet or anti-coagulation therapy.

50. **What is progressive multifocal leukoencephalopathy (PML)?**
Progressive multifocal leukoencephalopathy is a multifocal demyelinating disease caused by JC virus infection. It is a progressive disorder most commonly found in immunocompromised hosts such as patients with cancer or AIDS and transplant recipients. Stroke-like events are common.
Epker JL, van Biezen P, van Daele PL, et al.: Progressive multifocal leukoencephalopathy. Eur J Intern Med 20:261-267, 2009.

51. **What are the three most common neurologic complications related to cytomegalovirus (CMV) infection?**
CMV may cause Guillain-Barré syndrome, retinitis, and encephalitis.

52. **Is cryptococcal meningitis restricted to patients with AIDS or cancer or other immunocompromised patients?**
No. Although it is more common in such patients, it may occur in immunocompetent people.

53. **How common is varicella zoster infection in patients with lymphoma?**
The incidence is estimated to be about 15%. Dissemination is relatively common in patients with cancer. Rarely, stroke or a necrotizing CNS lesion may result from varicella zoster infection.

54. **What situations that are relatively unique to patients with cancer may result in acute altered mental status?**
Altered mental status may occur as a complication of chemotherapy with agents such as ifosfamide, procarbazine, 5-fluorouracil, methotrexate, cytosine arabinoside, and methylmelamine. Leptomeningeal disease may result in chronic, subacute, or abrupt changes in mental status. A common cause of abrupt mental obtundation in a patient with leptomeningeal disease is hydrocephalus. Subclinical seizures or status epilepticus also may occur.

55. **What are the potential neurologic complications of chemotherapy and biologic response modifiers?**
See Table 18-1.

## TABLE 18-1. SIDE EFFECTS OF CHEMOTHERAPY AND IMMUNOTHERAPY

| Side Effects | Comments |
| --- | --- |
| **Drugs causing encephalopathy** | |
| Alpha-interferon | |
| Cytosine arabinoside | |
| Cisplatin | Commonly from electrolyte imbalance |
| 5-Fluorouracil | |
| Hexamethylmelamine | |
| Ifosfamide | |
| Interleukin-2 | |
| L-Asparaginase | Can cause hemorrhage or thrombotic insults as well as reversible encephalopathy without parenchymal insult |
| Methotrexate | |
| Nitrogen mustard | |
| Procarbazine | |
| VP-16 (high dose) | |
| **Drugs causing neuropathy** | |
| Adriamycin | Rare |
| Cytosine arabinoside | Rare |
| Cisplatin | Ototoxicity and sensory neuropathy |
| Procarbazine | |
| Taxol | |
| Vincristine | |
| **Drugs causing myelopathy** | |
| Cytosine arabinoside | Administered intrathecally |
| Methotrexate | Administered intrathecally |
| Thiotepa | Administered intrathecally |
| **Drugs causing cerebellar dysfunction** | |
| Cytosine arabinoside | |
| 5-Fluorouracil | |
| Ifosfamide | |
| Procarbazine | |

Adapted from Paleologos NA: Complications of chemotherapy. In Biller J (ed): Iatrogenic Neurology. Boston, Butterworth-Heinemann, 1998, pp 439-461.

56. **Name two chemotherapeutic agents that may cause parkinsonism.**
The interleukins (alpha-interferon and IL-2) and hexamethylmelamine.

57. **Which hormonal drug may cause retinopathy?**
Tamoxifen may result in retinopathy after prolonged use.

58. **Name three chemotherapeutic agents that may induce thrombotic thrombocytopenic purpura (TTP).**
    Bleomycin, cisplatin, and mitomycin-C have been reported to trigger TTP. Seizures and encephalopathy are commonly seen in TTP, which is accompanied by renal failure, hemolysis, schistocytes, fever, and thrombocytopenia.

59. **Name two drugs that enhance leukoencephalopathic changes induced by radiation therapy.**
    Methotrexate and cytosine arabinoside may enhance leukoencephalopathy. Both drugs may induce this problem without prior radiation therapy.

60. **What is the peak time course to note radiation myelopathy?**
    Delayed progressive myelopathy peaks at 9 to 18 months after radiation therapy, although a transient myelopathy may occur within the first month to first 2 years. Progressive myelopathy increases in incidence as the radiation dose increases and is much more common with doses greater than 4400 rads.

61. **What are early side effects of cranial radiation therapy?**
    Within the first few days of radiation treatment, cerebral edema occurs and may result in headache, lethargy, nausea, vomiting, and exacerbation of preexisting neurologic deficits. Dexamethasone ameliorates these symptoms and should be started prophylactically to minimize early ill effects from radiation.

62. **How soon may delayed symptoms of cranial radiation occur?**
    Delayed signs may appear as soon as 1 to 4 months after completing radiation therapy and resemble early symptoms—somnolence, worsening of preexisting deficits, headache.

63. **When is the peak incidence for focal cerebral radionecrosis?**
    Radionecrosis peaks at 18 months after radiotherapy but may occur many years later.

64. **Name two CNS tumors induced by radiation therapy.**
    The peripheral nerves and plexus within the radiation port can develop painful nerve sheath tumors years after radiation therapy. Children treated with whole-brain radiation for lymphoblastic leukemia are at risk for developing gliomas if they are long survivors.

## PARANEOPLASTIC SYNDROMES

65. **Define paraneoplastic syndromes and the most important known syndromes involving the neuromuscular systems.**
    Signs or symptoms resulting from damage to organs or tissues that are remote from the site of malignant neoplasm or its metastases are probably caused by immune-mediated mechanisms and usually precede the diagnosis of cancer. CSF study may reveal mild pleocytosis (30 to 40 white cells/mm$^3$), a slightly elevated protein level (50 to 100 mg/dL), and an elevated IgG level during early course of the disease; these changes disappear within several weeks to months. In CSF of paraneoplastic cerebellar degeneration, fluorescent-activated cell sorting has revealed that more than 75% of white cells are of T-cell origin, with small component of B cell and natural killer cells.
    Most symptomatic paraneoplastic syndromes are rare, affecting about 0.01% of patients. Exceptions include Lambert-Eaton myasthenic syndrome, which affects 3% of patients with small-cell lung cancer; myasthenia gravis, which affects about 15% of patients with thymoma;

and demyelinating peripheral neuropathy, which affects about 50% of patients with rare osteosclerotic form of plasmacytoma (the polyneuropathy, organomegaly, endocrinopathy, M protein, and skin changes [POEMS] syndrome). Categories of paraneoplastic syndromes include:
1. Brain and cranial nerves: limbic encephalitis, brain stem encephalitis, cerebellar degeneration, opsoclonus-myoclonus, optic neuritis, cancer-associated retinopathy, chorea, and parkinsonism.
2. Spinal cord: necrotizing myelopathy, inflammatory myelitis, motor neuron disease (amyotrophic lateral sclerosis [ALS]), subacute motor neuronopathy, and stiff-person syndrome.
3. Dorsal-root ganglia: sensory neuronopathy.
4. Peripheral nerves: autonomic neuropathy, acute sensorimotor neuropathy (Guillain-Barré syndrome and brachial neuritis), chronic sensorimotor neuropathy, vasculitic neuropathy, and neuromyotonia.
5. Neuromuscular junction: Lambert-Eaton myasthenic syndrome, myasthenia gravis.
6. Muscle: dermatomyositis, necrotizing myopathy, and myotonia.
   Darnell RB, Posner JB: Paraneoplastic syndromes involving the nervous system. N Engl J Med 349:1543-1554, 2003.

66. **What is the most important diagnostic testing for paraneoplastic syndromes?**
    Identification of antibodies in patient serum (and CSF) has substantially advanced our ability to make an early diagnosis (Table 18-2).

TABLE 18-2. ANTIBODY TESTING FOR PARANEOPLASTIC SYNDROME

| Antibody | Tumor | Paraneoplastic Symptoms |
| --- | --- | --- |
| Anti-Hu (ANNA-1) | Small-cell lung cancer, neuroblastoma, prostate cancer | Paraneoplastic encephalomyelitis, paraneoplastic sensory neuronopathy, paraneoplastic cerebellar degeneration, autonomic dysfunction |
| Anti-Yo (PCA-1) | Ovarian, breast, and lung cancers | Paraneoplastic cerebellar degeneration |
| Anti-Ri | Breast, gynecologic, lung, and bladder cancers | Ataxia with or without opsoclonus-myoclonus |
| Anti-Tr | Hodgkin's lymphoma | Paraneoplastic cerebellar degeneration |
| Anti-VGCC | Small-cell lung cancer | Lambert-Eaton myasthenic syndrome |
| Anti-retinal (anti-recoverin protein) | Small-cell lung cancer, melanoma, gynecologic cancers | Cancer-associated retinopathy, melanoma-associated retinopathy |
| Anti-amphiphysin | Breast and small-cell lung cancers | Stiff-person syndrome, paraneoplastic encephalomyelitis |
| Anti-CRMP5 (anti-CV2) | Small-cell lung cancer, thymoma | Paraneoplastic encephalomyelitis, cerebellar degeneration, chorea, sensory neuropathy |

*(continued)*

**TABLE 18-2. ANTIBODY TESTING FOR PARANEOPLASTIC SYNDROME** *(continued)*

| Antibody | Tumor | Paraneoplastic Symptoms |
|----------|-------|-------------------------|
| Anti-PCA-2 | Small-cell lung cancer | Paraneoplastic encephalomyelitis, cerebellar degeneration; Lambert-Eaton myasthenic syndrome |
| Anti-Ma1 | Lung and other cancers | Brain stem encephalitis, cerebellar degeneration |
| Anti-Ma2 (-Ta) | Testicular cancer | Limbic brain stem encephalitis |
| ANNA-3 | Lung cancer | Sensory neuronopathy, encephalomyelitis |
| Anti-mGluR1 | Hodgkin's lymphoma | Paraneoplastic cerebellar degeneration |
| Anti-VGKC | Thymoma, small-cell lung cancer | Neuromyotonia |
| Anti-MAG | Waldenstrom's macroglobulinemia | Peripheral neuropathy |

From Darnell RB, Posner JB: Paraneoplastic syndromes involving the nervous system. N Engl J Med 349:1543-1554, 2003.

---

# KEY POINTS: NEUROLOGIC COMPLICATIONS AND PARANEOPLASTIC SYNDROMES

1. Neurologic complications are seen in about 30% of patients with cancer.

2. Common problems include metabolic effects, infection, vascular disease, and paraneoplastic syndromes.

3. The most important test for paraneoplastic syndrome is identification of antibodies in patient serum and cerebrospinal fluid.

---

67. **What are the characteristic features of Lambert-Eaton syndrome?**
    This disorder of the neuromuscular junction is characterized by fatigability, limb-girdle weakness (usually more in the legs than arms but not invariably), marked incremental response to 20 to 50 Hz of repetitive electrical stimulation, and, in roughly half of cases, dryness of the mouth and impotence due to cholinergic interference. **Ptosis and extraocular dysmotility are not features of this syndrome**.

68. **How frequently is dermatomyositis seen as a paraneoplastic problem in adults?**
    Roughly 10% of cases are associated with underlying malignancy. The most common sources are lung, breast, ovaries, and gastrointestinal (GI) tract. The index of suspicion should be higher in patients older than 40 years of age.

69. **What is carcinomatous neuromyopathy?**
This is not a discrete entity. Commonly weakness and reduced reflexes are accompanied by muscle atrophy, but the problem could be primarily a neuropathy or neuronopathy or a combination of myopathy and neuropathy. Findings on neurodiagnostic studies vary significantly.

70. **Opsoclonus-myoclonus is associated with which neoplasm?**
This syndrome of myoclonic jerks and abnormal eye movements is seen with neuroblastoma in children, but in adults, lung cancer is the usual underlying neoplasm.

## CANCER PAIN

71. **What percentage of patients with cancer die unrelieved of pain?**
It is estimated that 25% of patients with cancer die without adequate pain relief.
Nersesyan H. Slavin KV: Current approach to cancer pain management: Availability and implications of different treatment options. Ther Clin Risk Manag 3:381-400, 2007.

72. **What factors preclude adequate treatment of cancer pain?**
Ironically, it is not lack of treatment options or technology that hampers pain treatment, but factors such as opiophobia (fear to use narcotics), inadequate understanding of the origin of the pain (is it nociceptive or neuropathic?), and failure to prioritize pain and suffering as an urgent symptom requiring treatment. Recently, the Joint Commission has mandated that pain should be documented as the fifth vital sign in history and physical examination and subsequent progress noted of hospital pains. This mandate has stimulated a greater focus on addressing pain in recent years. It is to be hoped that future studies will reveal whether this mandate has made a positive impact on the management of pain in general.

73. **What is the difference between nociceptive pain and neuropathic pain?**
Nociceptive pain arises from injury or disease in soft-tissue or other somatic structures. Neural structures are not affected. Pain emanating from neural injury or dysfunction is neuropathic pain. Neuropathic pain usually has bizarre or unfamiliar qualities, such as intense burning provoked by light innocuous touch (allodynia). The pain may extend beyond the confines of injury (spatial summation or extension). Paroxysmal, lancinating pain may occur. Itchy, creepy, crawly, intense tingling, or icy hot sensations may be experienced (dysesthesia).

74. **How is nociceptive pain treated?**
Nonsteroidal anti-inflammatory drugs (NSAIDs) and acetaminophen can adequately relieve mild nociceptive pain. Opiates work well for severe pain. Nonpharmacologic measures such as transcutaneous electrical nerve stimulation (TENS) and local heat or cooling may also be useful.

75. **How may neuropathic pain develop in patients with cancer?**
Patients may experience neuropathic pain from invasion of neural structures by tumor (brachial and lumbosacral plexus, epidural space), as a byproduct of treatment such as surgical severance (e.g., thoracotomy, mastectomy, and amputation), or as a side effect of chemotherapy such as cisplatin.

76. **What types of treatment are available for neuropathic pain?**
There are a plethora of treatments available to combat neuropathic pain:
- Anticonvulsants—pregabalin (Lyrica), gabapentin (Neurontin), oxcarbazepine (Trileptal), zonisamide (Zonegran), etc.

- Antidepressants—tricyclics such as amitriptyline, doxepin, nortriptyline, and imipramine; serotonin and norepinephrine reuptake inhibitors (SNRIs) such as duloxetine (Cymbalta).
- Anesthetics—mexiletine orally; ketamine IV/IM, intranasal, and PO (PO is unpredictable); lidocaine infusion for hyperacute neuropathic pain; and regional nerve blocks with bupivicaine or lidocaine, among others.
- Atypical antipsychotics—drugs such as quetiapine (Seroquel) can be used in patients who are agitated due to severe pain or who have great difficulty with self-soothing (manifested as emotional irritability, negativity, and excessive demands for physical presence and care from others).
- Topical agents—compounded gels such as bupivicaine/ketamine combinations or lidocaine/ ketoprofen combinations are just a small sample of various compounded gels that can be employed for regional pain often associated with an area of hyperpathia.
- Opiates—opiate analgesics can be used for neuropathic pain, although patients are relatively resistant or partially responsive to this category of medications.
- Physical measures—TENS, epidural spinal cord stimulation, local cooling or warmth (hot or cold packs).

77. **For a patient who is taking morphine, 30 mg every 4 hours, what would be the equivalent effective dose (equianalgesic dose) of hydromorphone?**
The correct dose is 7.5 mg every 4 hours. Because hydromorphone is available in 4 mg tablets, a dose of 8 mg every 4 hours is appropriate. Equianalgesic dose conversion charts are a useful guide, but bear in mind that bioavailability and psychophysiologic responses do vary from one patient to another. Thus, most clinicians would start with less than the full dose recommended via the dose conversion chart, for example, 75% of the full dose (Table 18-3).

### TABLE 18-3. OPIATE DOSE CONVERSION

| Drug | Route | Equianalgesic Dose (mg) | Conversion from IV to PO | Conversion to Morphine |
|---|---|---|---|---|
| Morphine | IV/IM | 10 | 3 | = |
| | PO | 30 | | = |
| Levorphanol | IV/IM | 2 | 2 | 5 |
| | PO | 4 | | 7.5 |
| Methadone | IV/IM | 10 | 2 | = |
| | PO | 20 | | 1.5 |
| Fentanyl | IV | 0.1 (100 µg) | — | 100 |
| Hydromorphone | IV/IM | 1.5 | 5 | 6.7 |
| | PO | 7.5 | | 4 |
| Meperidine | IV/IM | 75 | 4 | 0.13 |
| | PO | 300 | | 0.1 |
| Oxycodone | IV/IM | 15 | 2 | 0.67 |
| | PO | 30 | | = |
| Codeine | IM | 130 | 1.5 | 0.8 |
| | PO | 200 | | 0.15 |
| Pentazocine | IM | 60 | 2.5 | 6 |

*(continued)*

| TABLE 18-3. | OPIATE DOSE CONVERSION *(continued)* | | | |
|---|---|---|---|---|
| Drug | Route | Equianalgesic Dose (mg) | Conversion from IV to PO | Conversion to Morphine |
| | PO | 150 | | |
| Butorphanol | IM | 2 | = | 0.2 |
| Nalbuphine | IM | 10 | = | 1 |

IM, intramuscularly; IV, intravenously; PO, orally; =, no conversion needed

78. **Patient-controlled analgesia (PCA) is an effective parenteral method of delivering analgesics. How does PCA work?**
Patients with cancer who cannot tolerate oral medication because of nausea and vomiting, bowel obstruction, postoperative status, or marked moment-to-moment fluctuation in pain are candidates for PCA. A computerized pump delivers opiate analgesics in a variety of permutations: continuous-drip rate (basal rate), intermittent boluses (PCA doses) without a basal drip, or PCA doses superimposed on a basal rate. The physician predetermines the limit of PCA doses allowable per hour and the basal rate (continuous-drip dosage). Patient satisfaction with this modality is high because of self-empowerment, immediate access to medication rather than waiting for medication upon request, and flexible dosing.

## KEY POINTS: CANCER PAIN

1. About 25% of patients with cancer die unrelieved of pain.

2. Nociceptive pain arises from injury or disease in soft-tissue or other somatic structures.

3. Neuropathic pain arises from neural injury or dysfunction.

4. Patient-controlled analgesia is an effective parenteral method of delivering analgesics.

79. **What types of pain syndromes are relatively opiate-resistant?**
Patients with metastatic bone pain and those with neuropathic pain are more apt to experience suboptimal relief from opiates.

80. **What are the alternatives for patients with opiate-resistant cancer pain?**
Metastatic bone pain may respond to combination therapy consisting of NSAIDs or corticosteroids in conjunction with an opiate drug. Radiation therapy frequently alleviates metastatic bone pain. Patients with neuropathic pain may require tricyclic antidepressants, anticonvulsants, or oral anesthetic agents (e.g., mexiletine). In some instances, chronic epidural infusion of anesthetic and opioids is necessary.

81. **Is intravenous administration of opioid medication superior to the oral route?**
Generally, oral medication is just as effective as parenteral injections if the dose is adequately titrated. Intravenous medications work faster, but their duration of action is shorter. Intravenous dosing has an advantage in the patient with intractable nausea and vomiting, obstruction, or hyperacute pain who requires delicate but aggressive dose adjustments.

82. **What types of pharmacologic agents are infused intrathecally for pain control?**
Intraspinal opioid administration is approved by the FDA for the treatment of cancer pain and intractable chronic noncancer pain. The most commonly used drugs are morphine, fentanyl, and sufentanil. Nonopiate regimens for pain control also include intrathecal clonidine, baclofen, and ziconotide.

    Newsome S, Frawley BK, Argoff CE: Intrathecal analgesia for refractory cancer pain. Curr Pain Headache Rep 12:249-256, 2008.

    Williams JA, Day M, Heavner JE: Ziconotide: An update and review. Expert Opin Pharmacother 9:1575-1583, 2008.

83. **What are the therapeutic options for patients who suffer from vertebral fractures— osteoporotic versus pathologic fractures from malignancy?**
Provided that there is a relative lack of retropulsion of bone fragment into the spinal canal, the use of kyphoplasty or vertebroplasty is a reasonable option. Kyphoplasty entails the insertion of a hollow needle through the pedicle of the vertebra to reach the vertebral body, where a balloon inflates to restore vertebral height. Cement is then infused into the marrow space of the vertebral body. Vertebroplasty is similar, with the exception that restoration of vertebral height is not attempted, but cement is injected. These measures are FDA approved for osteoporotic fractures, but they are being employed in selected cases of pathologic vertebral fracture. Generally, radiotherapy is attempted first, and if there is still movement-elicited pain, vertebroplasty or kyphoplasty is a reasonable option provided that the epidural space is not too crowded with bone or epidural metastases. If there is significant retropulsion of bone or epidural metastasis, the procedure could provoke significant cord or thecal sac compression.

84. **What is complex regional pain syndrome (formerly called reflex sympathetic dystrophy [RSD])?**
Complex regional pain syndrome (CRPS) is characterized by pain (usually burning in quality), autonomic instability (demonstrated by swelling or discoloration, warmth, regional coldness, goose bumps, etc.), and no evidence for other explanations for this regional pain (no cellulitis, venous thrombosis, or focal traumatic injury such as fracture). There are two subtypes: CRPS-1 is the aforementioned pain syndrome that occurs in the absence of any somatic nerve injury; the other subtype, CRPS-2, results from a focal nerve or CNS injury. Causalgia is the former term used for burning pain secondary to focal nerve injury, such as median neuropathy, which is a classic example of CRPS-2.

    Albazaz R, Wong YT, Homer-Vanniasinkam S: Complex regional pain syndrome: A review. Ann Vasc Surg 22:297-306, 2008.

85. **List some of the most common treatments for CRPS.**
    - Sympathetic nerve block
    - Topical anesthetic agents such as compounded bupivacaine/ketamine cream or lidocaine gel
    - Anticonvulsants such as gabapentin, pregabalin, oxcarbazepine, and rarely, ethosuximide
    - Anesthetics such as oral mexiletine or IV ketamine infusion
    - Physical therapy, including mobilization, desensitization with fluidotherapy, or hot/cold contrast bath
    - Psychologic therapy, including biofeedback, cognitive restructuring, treatment of depression/anxiety with pharmacotherapy and psychotherapy
    - Epidural spinal stimulation
    - Intrathecal therapy with opioids, Clinidine, or ziconotide

86. **List some examples of treatments available for individuals with neuropathic pain that has been resistant to opioids, anticonvulsants, and antidepressant therapy.**
    - Intravenous lidocaine infusion
    - Intravenous ketamine infusion

■ Intrathecal therapy with a combination of agents such as ziconotide or clonidine with opioids
Edmondson EA, Simpson RK, Stubler DK, and Beric A: Systemic lidocaine therapy for post-stroke pain. Southern Medical Journal 86:1093-1096, 1993.

# WEBSITES

1. http://www.braintumor.org

2. http://www.btfc.org

## BIBLIOGRAPHY

1. Bernstein M, Berger M: Neuro-oncology: The Essentials. New York, Thieme, 2008.

2. Black PM, Loeffler JS: Cancer of the Nervous System, 2nd ed. Philadelphia, Lippincott Williams & Wilkins, 2004.

3. Levin VA (ed): Cancer in the Nervous System, 2nd ed. New York, Oxford University Press, 2002.

4. Schiff D: Principles and Practice of Neuro-oncology. New York, McGraw-Hill, 2005.

# CHAPTER 19

# HEADACHES

*Pankaj Satija, MD, and Howard Derman, MD*

## GENERAL PRINCIPLES

1. **What is the incidence of headaches of all types?**
   About 90% of adults report at least one episode of severe or disabling headache sometime in their life span.

2. **Are headaches more common in males or females?**
   Women outnumber men 3 to 1 in incidence of migraine headaches. This ratio is reversed for cluster headaches, which occur largely in men (70%). Muscle contraction headaches have a slightly increased incidence in female patients, but they are seen almost equally in both genders.

3. **Does the location of head pain help to differentiate headache types?**
   Typically, migraines start on one side of the head, involving the frontal area, usually in and about the eye and cheek, although they may radiate to involve the whole head. Cluster headaches are usually periorbital in location, and patients may report a boring, excruciating pain above and behind the eye. Muscle contraction headaches are classically described as band-like pain in the temporal region, occasionally extending back to the occipital region and forward to the forehead.

4. **Which cranial structures are sensitive to pain?**
   Certain pain-sensitive cranial structures are capable of producing headaches. The brain itself is insensitive to pain (Table 19-1).

| TABLE 19-1.   PAIN-SENSITIVE CRANIAL STRUCTURES |
| --- |
| Skin |
| Fascia |
| Scalp vessels |
| Head and neck muscles |
| Periosteum of the skull and upper cervical vertebrae |
| Orbital structures and the eyeball |
| Salivary glands |
| Teeth and gums |
| External auditory canal and tympanic membrane |
| Mucus membranes of the paranasal sinuses |
| Tempomandibular joints |
| Dura mater within the skull |
| Dural blood vessels |
| Great venous sinuses |
| Pain-sensitive fibers of the fifth, ninth, and tenth cranial nerves |

5. **When is a headache a sign of a serious neurologic problem?**
   Some indications that a headache may be due to a serious underlying illness include:
   1. Sudden onset of severe headache
   2. Headache accompanied with signs of systemic illness (impaired mental status, fever, seizures, or focal neurologic signs)
   3. New headaches beginning after age 50
   4. Headaches increasing in frequency and severity
   5. New onset headache in a patient with risk factors for human immunodeficiency virus (HIV) infection or cancer
   6. Papilledema
   7. Headache subsequent to head trauma

6. **What common, serious diseases may present as a headache?**

   | | |
   |---|---|
   | Primary brain tumor | Meningitis |
   | Metastatic brain tumor | Temporal arteritis |
   | Abscess | Pituitary apoplexy |
   | Hypertension | Stroke |
   | Subdural hematoma | Hydrocephalus |
   | Intracerebral hemorrhage | Glaucoma |
   | Subarachnoid hemorrhage | |

7. **Is there a place for narcotic analgesics in treatment of headaches?**
   Narcotic analgesics at best have a limited role in treatment of headaches. They should routinely be strongly discouraged. The role of opioids is made more complex because of the closely related issues of medication-overuse headache and transformed migraine. If used for intractable headaches unresponsive to other therapies, they should be used by experts in carefully selected patients. A talk with the patient about the issue of narcotic analgesia before starting therapy is often helpful.
   Lipton RB, Bigal ME: Opioid therapy and headache: A cause and a cure. Neurology 62: 1662-1663, 2004.

## MIGRAINE HEADACHES

8. **What is the age of onset for migraine headaches?**
   Migraines typically begin in teenage years and seldom begin after age 40.
   Sabharwal RK: Migraine: A common cause of headache. Indian J Pediatr 70[Suppl]: S39-S44, 2003.

9. **What is the frequency of attack in migraine headaches?**
   Migraines are highly variable but usually occur once or twice per month. Some migraineurs have headaches more sporadically, 3 to 4 times per year. Some women report a strong association with menstruation.

10. **What are the common symptoms of migraine?**
    1. Unilateral headache (60% of cases). The unilateral headaches typically change sides from one attack to the next. The pain may begin as a dull ache but then becomes throbbing and possibly incapacitating.
    2. Visual or sensory loss
    3. Anorexia, nausea, vomiting
    4. Cold hands and feet
    5. Photophobia and phonophobia
    6. Mood changes

11. **What are the five phases of a complete migraine attack?**
    1. **Prodrome**. Premonitory symptoms lasting hours to days may precede 40% to 60% of migraine attacks. The symptoms may include sleepiness, irritability, fatigue, mood changes, yawning, and cravings for sweet or salty foods.
    2. **Aura**. The aura occurs within 1 hour of the headache and is most commonly visual or sensory.
    3. **Headache**. The headache itself is commonly unilateral and may be pulsatile.
    4. **Headache termination**
    5. **Postdrome**. After termination of the headache, the complete migraine attack ends with the postdrome or hangover phase.

12. **How often are migraines accompanied by an aura?**
    An estimated 35% of migraines are accompanied by an aura. This type of headache is known as a classic migraine. Migraine without an aura is known as common migraine.

13. **What are the common auras of migraine?**
    Visual auras are the most common and include photopsias, flashing lights, scintillating scotomata, and fortification (geometric) spectra. Sensory auras are the next most common, especially numbness or paresthesias in a cheiro-oral (face and hand) distribution. Dysphasia may occur. Motor weakness, symptoms of brain stem dysfunction, and changes in level of consciousness are less common and signal particular subtypes (hemiplegia and basilar migraines).

14. **What are the characteristics of migraine with aura?**
    The patient must have two attacks with at least three of the following four characteristics:
    1. One or more fully reversible aura symptoms, indicating focal cerebral, cortical, or brain stem dysfunction.
    2. At least one aura symptom develops gradually over 5 min or more and/or different symptoms occur in succession.
    3. Each symptom lasts 5 min or more but less than 60 min.
    4. The migraine headache must follow the aura within 60 min or less.

15. **What are the characteristics of migraine without aura?**
    The patient must have at least five attacks that fulfill the following criteria:
    1. The duration of the headache must be 4 to 72 hours.
    2. The headache must have at least two of the following characteristics: unilateral location, pulsating quality, moderate-to-severe pain that inhibits or prohibits daily activities, and aggravation by routine physical activity.
    3. During the headache, the patient must suffer at least one of the following: nausea and vomiting, or photophobia and phonophobia.

16. **What is status migrainosus?**
    Status migrainosus refers to an attack of migraine with a headache phase lasting more than 72 hours. The pain is severe (a diagnostic criterion) and debilitating.

17. **What is the pathophysiology of migraine?**
    The underlying mechanism of migraine is complex and, as yet, incompletely understood. The pulsatile pain is thought to be mediated by heightened excitability of the peripheral trigeminovascular neurons of the fifth cranial nerve, which is sensitized in susceptible individuals. Genetics plays a distinct role in this sensitization. Activation of these neurons results in neurogenic inflammation as plasma proteins (substance P, calcitonin gene-related peptide, and neurokinins) extravasate from the blood vessels the trigeminal nerve innervates. Following peripheral activation of trigeminovascular neurons, "central sensitization" occurs in

second-order neurons within the brain stem, resulting in cutaneous allodynia, a heightened sensitivity of the skin during migraine.

New data from functional brain imaging techniques support theories of a cortical spreading depression during migraine aura, which correlates with spreading oligemia, and cortical spreading depression in turn activates the trigeminal system.

Recent MRI studies have shown changes in deep white matter and basal ganglia that occur with increasing frequency and duration of migraine, suggesting that migraine may be a progressive disease.

18. **Does serotonin play a role in migraine?**
Serotonin is widely distributed throughout the body, with 90% concentrated in the gastrointestinal (GI) tract and the remainder in the brain and platelets. During a migraine attack, the blood level of serotonin may decrease, whereas urinary concentration may increase. This shift in serotonin levels may trigger changes in blood vessels and blood flow, and also alter pain perception in the brain. Serotonin thus may play a role (as yet incompletely understood) in the etiology of migraine. Certain medications such as amitriptyline, nortriptyline, and sumatriptan, which have an effect on serotonin metabolism, are useful in treatment of migraine headache.

Hamel E: Serotonin and migraine: Biology and clinical implications. Cephalalgia 27:1293-1300, 2007.

Peroutka SJ: Serotonin receptor subtypes: Their evolution and clinical relevance. CNS Drugs 4(Suppl 1):18-36, 1995.

Schwedt TJ: Serotonin and migraine: The latest developments. Cephalalgia 27:1301-1307, 2007.

19. **Can certain foods bring on migraine?**
Certain foods are known to precipitate a migraine, as some patients note during history taking, but the only food clearly associated with increasing frequency of migraine is red wine. Foods commonly identified as exacerbating migraine include:
- Foods rich in tyramine (cheese, red wine)
- Foods containing monosodium glutamate (Chinese and Mexican food)
- Foods containing nitrates (cold cuts—bologna, salami, smoked meats)
- Pickled, fermented, marinated foods (pasta salads)
- Alcoholic beverages (especially red wine)
- Caffeinated beverages (soft drinks, tea, and coffee)

20. **Is there a genetic component to migraines?**
Both familial clustering and twin studies suggest that significant genetic mechanisms underlie migraine. Several genes (*CACNA1A, ATP1A2*, and *SCN1A*) have been implicated in the genetics of familial hemiplegic migraine (a subtype). However, the identification of genes predisposing to more common forms has been less successful. Five genomewide screens have found several loci (4q24, 14q21.2-22.3, 6p12.2-21.1, 19p13, Xq24-28, and 15q11-13) with significant evidence of linkage to migraine with and without aura. The many linkage peaks detected in these screens support the hypothesis that migraines are heterogeneous and include some relatively strongly penetrant variants at the family level. The effect at the population level is not known and needs further clarification by larger studies.

Russell MB: Genetics in primary headaches. J Headache Pain 8:190-195, 2007.

Wessman J, Terwindt GM, Kaunisto MA, et al.: Migraine: A complex genetic disorder. Lancet Neurol 6:521-532, 2007.

21. **What are the most useful drugs for acute, abortive therapy of migraines?**
The most useful abortive migraine treatments are ergotamines, Midrin, or the triptans.

Silberstein SD, Dodick D, Freitag F, et al.: Pharmacological approaches to managing migraine and associated comorbidities—Clinical considerations for monotherapy versus polytherapy. Headache 47:585-599, 2007.

22. **Is ergotamine helpful therapy for migraines?**
Ergotamine derivatives can be helpful in patients who have migraine with a clear-cut prodrome. Ergotamine is available in oral, sublingual, suppository, injectable, and inhalation forms. Because of the extreme nausea and vomiting seen with some migraines, the suppository and sublingual preparations are the most useful and tolerable. When using sublingual or suppository form, the usual dosage is 2 mg. The patient may take 3 doses per headache, separated by 1½ hours, up to 9 doses per week.

23. **What is Midrin? Is it useful in headaches?**
Midrin is a combination medication that consists of dichloralphenazone (a muscle relaxant), isometheptene (a vasospasm agent), and acetaminophen. It may be used either as a prophylactic medication (1 pill 2 to 3 times/day) or as abortive therapy (2 pills with onset of headache and then 1 pill every hour after that, up to 5 pills total).

24. **What is sumatriptan?**
Sumatriptan (Imitrex) was the first of a new class of medications, the 5-hydroxytriptamine (5-HT) receptor agonists. It may be administered subcutaneously (6 mg), nasally (20 mg), or orally (50 mg), and provides relief in 70% of patients. The chief side effects are chest tightness and flushing. It should not be used concomitantly with ergotamines or in patients with heart disease.

25. **What other 5-HT receptor agonists are beneficial for migraines?**
Since the success of sumatriptan, several similar agents have been marketed, including zolmitriptan, frovatriptan, eletriptan, almotriptan, rizatriptan, and naratriptan. The triptans differ somewhat in pharmacologic profile, but all are roughly comparable in effectiveness. They are generally preferred over ergotamines or Midrin as first-choice therapy for migraine.
Adelman JU, Belsey J: Meta-analysis of oral triptan therapy for migraine: Number needed to treat and relative cost to achieve relief within 2 hours. J Manag Care Pharm 9:45-52, 2003.
Ferrari MD, Roon KI, Lipton RB, Goadsby PJ: Oral triptans in acute migraine treatment: A meta-analysis of 53 trials. Lancet 358:1668-1675, 2001.

26. **Can different triptans be combined in abortive treatment of migraine?**
In general, different drugs should not be combined (e.g., rizatriptan and sumatriptan), but different forms of the same medicine can be used (e.g., nasal sumatriptan followed in 2 hours by oral sumatriptan).

27. **Can more than one class of medications be combined for aborting migraine?**
Few studies have suggested the advantage of combining a triptan plus a nonsteroidal anti-inflammatory drug/cyclo-oxygenase-2 (NSAID/COX-2 selective inhibitor) with regard to efficacy, reduction of recurrence, and improvement of sustained pain-free measures over the treatment with either drug used alone. Treximet (combination of sumatriptan 85 mg and naproxen sodium 500 mg) was granted FDA approval in 2008 for treatment of an acute migraine with or without aura in adults. It may be used as abortive therapy (1 pill at the onset of headache and then 1 pill after 2 hours, up to 2 pills total in 24 hours).
Hill KP, Hope O: Combination of sumatriptan and naproxen for migraine. JAMA 298:1276, 2007.

28. **Are the triptans used only as abortive medications in migraine?**
Because of its longer half-life, naratriptan (Amerge) is useful as a prophylactic agent in menstrual migraine. If a woman has headaches at a predictable time of the month, especially if

she is taking birth control pills, use of naratriptan each morning 1 to 2 days before the period and through day 3 of the period may be helpful.

Pringsheim T, Davenport WJ, Dodick D: Acute treatment and prevention of menstrually related migraine headache. Neurology 70:1555-1563, 2008.

29. **Which group or groups of drugs represent first-line therapy for migraine prophylaxis?**
Tricyclic antidepressants, beta-blockers, calcium channel blockers, and anticonvulsants are the drugs of choice for migraine prophylaxis.

30. **What are the indications for prophylactic treatment of migraine?**
When headaches occur at a frequency of two or more per month or, more importantly, when the headaches affect the patient's day-to-day life (causing absence from work or school), prophylactic therapy is indicated.

Ramadan NM: Current trends in migraine prophylaxis. Headache 47(Suppl 1):S52-S57, 2007.

31. **Which tricyclics are the most helpful prophylactic agents?**
Tricyclic antidepressants work through an action independent of their antidepressant effect. Among the many tricyclic antidepressants, amitriptyline (Elavil) is most useful for migraine therapy. Other drugs that may be successful include doxepin (Sinequan), nortriptyline (Pamelor), and imipramine (Tofranil).

32. **In prescribing a tricyclic antidepressant for migraine, what dosage should be considered?**
In the case of amitriptyline, it is best to start at a dose of 25 mg at bedtime because patients often become lethargic with initial dosing. The level may be increased to a maximal dose of 200 mg by raising the dose slowly (25 mg/week over 3 to 4 weeks). However, doses greater than 100 mg are often associated with significant side effects, such as dry mouth, constipation, and urinary hesitancy. Patients also may become quite sedated. Finally, weight gain is often an intolerable side effect.

33. **Are beta-blockers useful as prophylaxis for migraine?**
Beta-blockers, especially propranolol, have been used effectively for migraine prophylaxis for many years. Propranolol is safe and has few side effects. The usual dose is 80 mg long-acting (LA); it may be increased to 160 mg LA, as indicated. Pulse monitoring is important, and the drug dose may be increased to 160 mg if the pulse stays greater than 60.

34. **Which calcium channel blocker is most effective in migraine?**
Verapamil is the most useful in migraine and is usually started at a dose of 180 mg at night. The dose may be increased as necessary to 240 mg at night over a 4-week period. Verapamil is well tolerated. Another very effective calcium channel blocker, Flunarizine, is not available in the United States.

35. **Are other calcium channel blockers useful in migraine?**
Nifedipine started at 30 mg/day has proved to be useful in migraines; nicardipine, 20 to 60 mg/day, also has been efficacious in migraine prophylaxis. Both nifedipine and nicardipine should be started only after failure of verapamil.

36. **Is sodium valproate effective and well tolerated in migraine prophylaxis?**
Sodium valproate (Depakote) may be helpful in migraine prophylaxis. Its mechanism of action is unclear but may be related to a reduction of excitatory neurotransmission through facilitation

of GABA-ergic activity in the brain or blockade of aspartate release. Depakote ER dosed in the evenings is now available. Most common adverse effects of valproate therapy are nausea, vomiting, gastrointestinal distress, tremor, and alopecia. Valproate is potentially teratogenic and should not be used by pregnant women or women considering pregnancy.

37. **Is there a difference in treating seizures as opposed to migraine with valproate in terms of dosing and drug level?**
Migraine usually responds to lower doses than seizures. Some migraineurs may respond to doses as small as 125 mg twice daily, and an average of 650 mg in divided doses is successful in 70% of patients. It is not necessary to monitor or follow drug levels in treating migraine.

38. **How does topiramate work in migraine prophylaxis? What are the adverse effects?**
Topiramate works for migraine prophylaxis primarily by decreasing neuronal hyperexcitability through antagonism of excitatory glutamatergic neurotransmission and a concomitant enhancement of GABA-ergic inhibition. Several animal studies have shown that systemic administration of topiramate inhibits trigeminovascular activation. It should be started at 25 mg at night and titrated for response slowly over several weeks to the maximum of 100 mg twice a day. The most common adverse events reported are paresthesias, drowsiness, diarrhea, decreased appetite, and weight loss.
   Silberstein SD: Topiramate in migraine prevention. Headache 45(Suppl 1):S57-S65, 2005.
   Silberstein SD, Diener HC, Lipton R, et al.: Epidemiology, risk factors, and treatment of chronic migraine: A focus on topiramate. Headache 48:1087-1095, 2008.

39. **How should you decide among a beta-blocker, tricyclic antidepressant, calcium channel blocker, or anticonvulsant in migraine prophylaxis?**
It is essential to consider a patient's coexisting or comorbid disease, work habits and other factors, such as dosing schedule and exercise programs. The drug used should be the one that has the best risk-to-benefit ratio for the individual patient and takes advantage of the drug's side effect profile. Anecdotal reports seem to favor beta-blockers for patients who have significant visual problems (flashing lights, zigzag lines, fortification spectra) with their headaches. In patients who are underweight, markedly anxious or depressed, or who have a sleep problem, a tricyclic antidepressant may be more appropriate. In contrast, an overweight or epileptic patient may be best treated with Topiramate. The drugs are about equally effective, and studies have not identified any one as clearly superior to the others.
   Afridi S, Kaube H: Prophylactic therapy for migraine. Curr Treat Options Neurol 5:431-440, 2003.
   Silberstein SD, Dodick D, Freitag F, et al.: Pharmacological approaches to managing migraine and associated comorbidities—Clinical considerations for monotherapy versus polytherapy. Headache 47:585-599, 2007.

40. **What is the role of Botox treatment in headaches?**
Botulinum toxin has been studied in patients with primary headaches, namely tension-type headache (TTH), chronic migraine (CM), and chronic daily headache (CDH). The antinociceptive effect appears to be separate from its paralytic properties and may be due to the inhibition of release of neurotransmitters from synaptosomes resulting in decreasing peripheral sensitization of nociceptive sensory nerve fibers. The results of randomized, double-blind, placebo-controlled trials on botulinum toxin have so far been inconsistent in proving its efficacy over placebo injections. Further research is continuing to determine efficacy, specific muscle targets, and subgroups of patients as appropriate candidates.
   Ashkenazi A, Silberstein S: Botulinum toxin type A for the treatment of headache. Arch Neurol 65:146-149, 2008.

41. **How does pregnancy affect treatment of headache?**
    Nonpharmacological approaches, such as rest, exercise, cognitive behavior therapy, hydration, diet, and prenatal vitamins and minerals should be employed first. When pregnant patients must use some medication for their headaches, either acetaminophen or aspirin may be helpful. If these do not work, then and only then is the use of narcotics justified. Codeine is probably the safest medication to use judiciously for headaches during pregnancy. Finally, a tricyclic antidepressant or cyproheptadine (Periactin) may be used.
    Goadsby PJ, Goldberg J, Silberstein SD: Migraine in pregnancy. BMJ 336:1502-1504, 2008.

42. **Are any drugs clearly contraindicated in pregnant patients?**
    Ergotamine derivatives and any drug with a vasospastic component are contraindicated. Valproate should be avoided for its teratogenic properties. Usually, after a heart-to-heart talk, most pregnant patients are willing to proceed during their entire pregnancy without medication if they are convinced that drugs may in some way harm the fetus.

43. **What are other forms of migraine?**
    Familial hemiplegic migraine and basilar-type migraine are forms of migraine where the aura includes motor weakness and posterior fossa symptoms (dysarthria, vertigo, tinnitus, decreased hearing, diplopia, ataxia, and decreased level of consciousness respectively). Accompanying migraine-like headache and the total reversibility of these symptoms help differentiate it from a stroke.
    A number of less well-described disorders including cyclical vomiting, abdominal migraine, benign paroxysmal vertigo and retinal migraine occur more commonly in children and are likely precursors of classic migraine, which presents later in life.

## CLUSTER HEADACHES

44. **What is the age of onset for cluster headaches?**
    The mean age at onset for cluster headaches is 28 years and they may occur as late as age 45.

45. **What symptoms are associated with cluster headaches?**
    Nocturnal predilection is common and patients are often aroused from sleep by an attack. The headache strikes abruptly, without any aura, around and behind one eye. The pain is unilateral, extremely severe and lasts 20 to 60 min. They almost always remain on the same side of the head during cluster periods. Patients report nasal stuffiness, rhinorrhea, forehead sweating, and redness and lacrimation of the eye ipsilateral to the head pain. There also may be partial Horner's syndrome with ptosis and miosis on the side of the head pain. In contrast to migraine, patients are restless during the pain of cluster headache.

46. **What gives cluster headaches their name?**
    The headaches occur during a short time span; this cluster then recurs periodically. A typical cluster of headaches may last 4 to 8 weeks, with 1 to 2 headaches per day during the cluster. Patients may go 6 months to 1 year before another cluster occurs.

47. **Are all cluster headaches associated with this episodic pattern?**
    Sixty-seven percent of patients with cluster headaches report an episodic pattern, but 33% have one to four headaches every month without a quiescent period.

48. **What is the differential diagnosis of cluster headaches?**
    - Trigeminal neuralgia
    - Cyclical migraine

- Sinus infection
- Raeder's paratrigeminal neuralgia

49. **How are acute attacks of cluster headaches managed?**
   - Oxygen inhalation
   - Locally applied anesthetic agents
   - Ergotamine
   - Dihydroergotamine (DHE) injections
   - Sumatriptan
   - Octreotide

50. **How is oxygen used in cluster headaches?**
   The average dose of oxygen is 8 L/min for 10 min, which relieves pain in approximately 80% of patients. Oxygen therapy must be instituted very early in the head pain, and some patients have a rebound headache once the oxygen is stopped.

51. **What prophylactic medications may be considered for patients in the midst of a cluster?**
   Calcium channel blockers, particularly verapamil, have been used in cluster attacks at doses starting at 180 mg at night and increased to 360 mg as tolerated. Steroids, ergotamine, lithium, and topiramate also may provide relief. Minimally invasive procedure of greater occipital nerve blockade has now been shown to be efficacious in cluster headache.

52. **Are steroids helpful in cluster headaches?**
   Steroids can be quite useful in two ways. For acute attacks, a tapering dose of 60 mg, 40 mg, and 20 mg of prednisone over 3 days may be helpful. If the patient is in the midst of a cycle, a tapering course starting at 60 mg, decreasing to 0 mg over a 3-week period, is recommended.

53. **Is lithium useful in cluster headache?**
   Lithium carbonate is an excellent prophylactic treatment of cluster headaches. Patients usually benefit from a dose of 600 to 900 mg/day, maintaining a therapeutic level of 0.4 to 0.8 mEq/L.

54. **What is the treatment for rhinorrhea and lacrimation associated with clusters?**
   Cyproheptadine (Periactin), a drug that works as an antihistamine and also has an effect on serotonin, may be useful. The dose is usually 2 mg by mouth 3 times/day. Side effects include sedation and appetite enhancement; these issues must be discussed with the patient before starting medication.

55. **What is the pathophysiology of cluster headaches?**
   Cluster headache is a form of trigeminal autonomic cephalalgia. An acute attack involves activation of the trigeminovascular system, as shown by the distribution of pain predominantly in the ophthalmic division of the trigeminal nerve and evidence of changes in cranial concentrations of neuropeptides such as calcitonin gene-related peptide (CGRP), substance P, and neurokinin A during the attack.
   The clinical feature of circadian periodicity, changes in hormonal concentration, and functional imaging studies have suggested a role of the hypothalamus. Evidence is available for anatomical and physiological connections between the hypothalamus and the trigeminovascular system, and a defect in these connections is likely the basis of cluster headaches.
   Goadsby PJ: Pathophysiology of cluster headache. Lancet Neurology 1:251-257, 2002.

56. **What are the surgical options for cluster headaches?**
Surgical treatment of cluster headache should only be considered after a patient has exhausted all medical options or when a patient's medical history precludes the use of typical cluster abortive and preventive medications. Various surgical procedures aimed at lesioning or decompressing the trigeminal ganglion or nerve and the cranial parasympathetic system have been evaluated. Radiofrequency rhizotomy, gamma knife radiosurgery, microvascular decompression, nerve root sectioning, and deep brain stimulator in the posterior inferior hypothalamus have all shown some promise but more evidence is required for defining the standard of care. Success of these procedures requires careful selection of patients and surgical expertise.

57. **What are trigeminal autonomic cephalalgias (TACs)?**
TACs are a group of primary headache disorders, which are characterized by strictly unilateral pain, together with ipsilateral cranial parasympathetic autonomic symptoms. TACs include cluster headache (CH), paroxysmal hemicrania (PH), and short-lasting unilateral neuralgiform headache attacks with conjunctival injection and tearing (SUNCT syndrome). TACs differ in the length and frequency of attacks and in their response to drug treatment. It is important to recognize and differentiate between these syndromes because they respond very well, but very selectively, to therapy.

58. **What is hemicrania continua?**
Hemicrania continua is a rare form of primary headache marked by continuous pain on one side of the face that varies in severity. The continuous pain may be superimposed by occasional attacks of more severe pain. Autonomic and migraine-like symptoms may accompany the exacerbations. Most patients experience attacks of increased pain three to five times per 24-hour cycle. Indomethacin, an NSAID, is the treatment of choice and response to therapy is necessary for establishing this diagnosis.

## TENSION HEADACHES

59. **What is a tension headache?**
A tension headache is dull, persistent pain that occurs in the temporal region in a band-like distribution and may radiate forward to the frontal region or posteriorly to the occipital region. It is also referred to as a muscle contraction headache.

60. **What causes tension headache?**
The cause of tension headaches is open to debate. It has not been possible to relate them very well to any particular psychological profile. Some authoritative studies suggest that they are variants of migraine headaches and share the processes of trigeminal activation and central sensitization as common denominators. The underlying stimuli for these processes may arise from tight, tense muscles, but not all studies verify this association.

61. **What are the different types of tension headaches?**
Episodic and chronic.

62. **What are the characteristics of an episodic tension headache?**
The patient must have at least 10 previous headache episodes fulfilling the following diagnostic criteria:
1. The headache must last from 30 minutes to 7 days.
2. A minimum of two of the following pain characteristics: pressing or tightening pain, mild-to-moderate intensity, bilateral location, no aggravation with physical activity.

3. It is not associated with nausea or vomiting, although anorexia may occur. Either photophobia or phonophobia may occur but not both.

**63. What are the characteristics of a chronic tension headache?**
1. Average headache frequency of 15 days per month for 6 months or 180 days per year.
2. Frequently associated with analgesic overuse.
3. Migrainous features may be superimposed intermittently.

**64. What is the treatment for tension headache?**
Treatment of the acute tension headache includes drugs that are primarily analgesics, such as NSAIDs. Chronic suppressive therapy is usually required, and the most effective agents are serotonergic tricyclics such as amitriptyline. Another noradrenergic and specific serotonergic antidepressant, mirtazapine (Remeron), has shown promise as an effective prophylactic agent in several studies.
Couch JR: Chronic daily headache. Curr Treat Options Neurol 5:467-479, 2003.
Tajti J, Almási J: [Effects of mirtazapine in patients with chronic tension-type headache. Literature Review]. Neuropsychopharmacol Hung 8:67-72, 2006.

**65. What is analgesic rebound headache?**
A well-described headache syndrome is associated with analgesic abuse, including over-the-counter medications such as aspirin and acetaminophen (Tylenol). Typically patients take 10 to 20 pills/day and have headaches on a chronic basis, generally daily. A similar syndrome is recognized with overuse/daily use of triptans. Such patients must be switched to suppressive agents such as tricyclics and weaned from analgesics completely.
Katsarava Z, Jensen R: Medication-overuse headache: Where are we now? Curr Opin Neurol 20:326-330, 2007.

**66. Are any nonpharmacologic treatments useful for tension headaches?**
Nonpharmacologic approaches, including physical therapy to the head and neck regions, relaxation techniques, cognitive-behavioral therapy, and biofeedback, either alone or in combination, have been useful in tension headache. However, the benefits are generally short-lived, and long-term results are unknown. Other therapies used are ultrasound, electrical stimulation, spinal manipulation, and acupuncture. More clinical studies are needed to evaluate their role.

**67. What is the role of peripheral nerve blocks in headache management?**
The most widely employed peripheral nerve block for headache is greater occipital nerve (GON) block. The rationale behind this procedure for headache treatment comes from evidence of convergence of sensory input to trigeminal nucleus caudalis neurons from both cervical and trigeminal fibers. Although it is not standardized, typically the nerve is infiltrated with a local anesthetic (lidocaine, bupivacaine, or both). A corticosteroid is added by some physicians. Several studies have suggested efficacy of GON block in the treatment of migraine, tension headache, cluster headache, and chronic daily headache, however, few of these are blinded controlled trials. Despite a favorable clinical experience, more evidence via controlled studies is needed to better assess the role of GON block in the treatment of migraine and other headaches.
Ashkenazi A, Levin M: Greater occipital nerve block for migraine and other headaches: Is it useful? Curr Pain Headache Rep 11:231-235, 2007.
Fredriksen TA: Cervicogenic headache: Invasive procedures. Cephalalgia 28(Suppl 1):39-40, 2008.

## KEY POINTS: HEADACHES

1. Most patients with a headache due to a serious underlying illness will have an abnormal physical examination. The sudden onset of "the worst headache of my life" should raise concern about an intracranial hemorrhage.

2. The use of narcotic analgesics for treatment of headaches should be strongly discouraged.

3. The first-choice drugs for acute migraine therapy are the triptans.

4. The best treatment for tension headache is usually amitriptyline plus an NSAID.

5. Temporal arteritis should be considered in any elderly patient with new headaches.

### SPINAL TAP HEADACHES

**68. Are headaches frequent after lumbar puncture?**
Approximately 20% to 25% of patients have a headache after lumbar puncture. Headaches occur whether or not the tap is traumatic and regardless of the amount of spinal fluid removed.

**69. Do patients with postspinal tap headache have other complaints?**
Patients are often severely disabled by nausea and vomiting along with the headaches. Characteristically, the headache is much worse when the patient is upright and improves dramatically when the patient lies flat in bed.

**70. What is the treatment for postspinal tap headache?**
The first step is to reassure the patient that the headache eventually will go away. The patient must remain flat in bed as much as possible. Simple analgesics are recommended. Finally, if the headache becomes disabling, blood patch therapy with a second spinal tap may be indicated.

### POSTCOITAL HEADACHES

**71. What is coital cephalgia?**
Coital cephalgia refers to headaches that occur before (20%) and after orgasm (75%). They occur with equal frequency in men and women. Preorgasmic headaches are characterized by a bilateral dull ache in the muscles of the head and neck. They begin as sexual excitement builds and can be prevented or reduced by deliberate muscle relaxation. Orgasmic headaches are sudden in onset, pulsatile, and fairly intense; they involve the entire head. These headaches may typically last from a few minute to a few hours.

**72. Are headaches that occur with intercourse a sign of subarachnoid hemorrhage?**
Less than 2% of patients who present with subarachnoid hemorrhage secondary to aneurysm leakage have leakage with intercourse. More often than not, headaches that occur with intercourse are either migraine or muscle contraction in origin.

**73. What is the treatment for postcoital cephalgia?**
The mainstay of treatment of coital headaches is reassurance to both patient and their partner. The headaches are generally self-limiting. For frequent recurrent headaches, an NSAID often prevents headaches. Other options may be to use ergotamine a few hours prior to sexual activity or prophylaxis with a beta-blocker.

## HEADACHES FROM BRAIN TUMORS OR MASS LESIONS

**74. Are headaches associated with a brain tumor different from other types of headaches?**
The headaches associated with a brain tumor may present in much the same fashion as headaches associated with muscle contraction. The headaches may be daily and are seldom severe.

**75. What special features in the history and physical examination should be considered when brain tumor is a concern?**
Patients often awake early in the morning with headaches. Neurologic examination usually reveals focal abnormalities as well as papilledema on funduscopic examination.

## PSEUDOTUMOR CEREBRI

**76. What is pseudotumor cerebri?**
Pseudotumor cerebri, or benign intracranial hypertension, is increased Intracranial pressure (ICP) without evidence of malignancy and is manifested primarily by headaches and visual obscuration. A pulsatile tinnitus in one or both ears that may be exacerbated by the supine or bending position often accompanies the headache.

**77. How can one make the diagnosis of pseudotumor cerebri?**
Patients are generally obese females. The neurologic examination is normal. A magnetic resonance imaging (MRI) or computed tomography (CT) scan is usually normal as well. The pressure is elevated on spinal fluid examination, which confirms the diagnosis.

**78. What etiologic factors are associated with benign intracranial hypertension?**

1. Mastoiditis and lateral sinus thrombosis
2. Head trauma
3. Oral progestational drugs
4. Marantic sinus thrombosis
5. Cryofibrinogenemia
6. Addison's disease
7. Hypoparathyroidism
8. Tetracycline therapy
9. Hypervitaminosis A

**79. What are the visual complaints of patients with benign intracranial hypertension?**
Visual acuity is usually normal, but patients may report transient obscurations of vision. Their visual fields may show enlargement of the blind spot, and examination may show optic disc edema.

**80. What medicines are useful in benign intracranial hypertension?**
Usually, treatment includes the use of acetazolamide at 500 mg 1 or 2 times/day or prednisone at 20 to 40 mg/day. Patients may need to be on treatment for up to 6 months at a time.

**81. Aside from medication, what other treatments are used for benign intracranial hypertension?**
Patients are generally treated with repeat spinal taps to maintain pressures in the normal range. For patients who have progressive visual field loss, surgical approaches such as lumboperitoneal, ventriculoperitoneal, or ventriculoatrial shunts may be employed. Another approach to decrease optic nerve pressure is optic nerve sheath fenestration. All these procedures are fairly successful in carefully selected patients.

**82. Are there headaches associated with low cerebrospinal fluid (CSF) pressure?**
These headaches may be worsened by getting up and improved by lying down. There may be a leak of CSF demonstrated on imaging studies and inflammation of the meninges may be noted.

## TEMPORAL ARTERITIS

**83. What is temporal arteritis?**
Temporal arteritis is a granulomatous arteritis affecting large-size and medium-size arteries of the upper part of the body, including the temporal vessels. Histologic studies reveal intimal thickening and lymphocytic infiltration of the media and adventitia.

**84. What is the clinical setting of temporal arteritis?**
Patients generally present after age 60. Women develop temporal arteritis 2 to 3 times more frequently than men. The headaches are sometimes abrupt in onset, and patients also complain of polymyalgia pain and stiffness in the neck, shoulders, and back and sometimes in the pelvic girdle.

**85. Describe the headache associated with temporal arteritis.**
Severe pain may be experienced in one temple but often occurs in the occipital area, face, or side of the neck. Jaw claudication occurs in about half of the patients. Severe scalp tenderness may occur during simple acts such as resting the head on a pillow, combing hair, or wearing hats and eyeglasses. The pain may have a throbbing character.

**86. Are there any serious complications of temporal arteritis?**
The most severe complication is loss of vision, which may not be reversible.

**87. How does one make a diagnosis of temporal arteritis?**
In addition to clinical findings, ancillary data include an elevated sedimentation rate and positive temporal artery biopsy.

**88. If temporal arteritis is suspected or diagnosed, is there any treatment?**
Treatment involves immediate use of large doses (i.e., 40 to 60 mg) of prednisone daily for the first week, with gradual reduction over the next 4 to 6 weeks to a maintenance dose of 5 to 10 mg/day. Sedimentation rates can be followed, and when the sedimentation rate is normal for 4 months, further tapering of medication is justified.

## WEBSITES

1. http://www.ahsnet.org

2. http://www.migraines.org

## BIBLIOGRAPHY

1. Clinch R: Evaluation of acute headaches in adults. Am Fam Physician 63:2001-2008, 2001.
2. Lipton RB, Bigal ME (eds): Migraine and Other Headache Disorders. New York, Taylor and Francis Group, 2006.
3. Olesen J, Tfelt-Hansen P, Welch KMA: The Headaches. Philadelphia, Lippincott Williams & Wilkins, 2000.
4. Tarvez T: A practical approach to headache treatment. J Pharm Pract 20.2:123-136, 2007.
5. Victor M, Ropper AJ (eds): Neurology, 7th ed. New York, McGraw-Hill, 2001.

# CHAPTER 20

# SEIZURES AND EPILEPSY

*Philip Kurle, MD, and Paul Rutecki, MD*

## DESCRIPTION AND CLASSIFICATION

**1. What is a seizure and what is epilepsy?**

A seizure is a single event characterized by the abnormal excessive synchronized firing of cortical neurons that usually results in altered perception or behavior. Between 7% and 10% of the population will have a seizure at some point in their lives. Epilepsy is the condition of recurrent unprovoked seizures caused by an inherent brain abnormality. Between 0.5% and 1% of the population currently has epilepsy, and the lifetime risk of epilepsy is about 3%.

French JA and Pedley TA: Initial management of epilepsy. NEJM 359:166-176, 2008.

**2. How are seizures classified?**

Seizures are classified according to their clinical and electroencephalographic (EEG) characteristics. A classification scheme proposed in 1981 has been accepted and useful for years but has limitations.

I. Partial seizures
  A. Simple partial seizures (consciousness not impaired)
  B. Complex partial seizures (consciousness impaired)
    1. Impairment of consciousness at onset
    2. Simple partial seizure onset followed by impaired consciousness
  C. Partial seizures evolving to generalized tonic-clonic convulsions (GTC)
    1. Simple partial evolving to GTC
    2. Complex partial evolving to GTC
II. Generalized seizures
  A. Absence seizures
    1. Typical
    2. Atypical, complex
  B. Myoclonic seizures
  C. Clonic seizures
  D. Tonic seizures
  E. Tonic-clonic seizures
  F. Atonic seizures (astatic)

From the Commission on the Classification and Terminology of the International League Against Epilepsy: Proposal for revised clinical and electroencephalographic classification of epileptic seizures. Epilepsia 22:489-501, 1981.

**3. What features distinguish partial from generalized seizures?**

Partial seizures start focally and have clinical and electrographic features that indicate onset from a single unilateral brain region. Primary generalized seizures appear to arise from both cerebral hemispheres at once. The manifestations of focal seizures depend on the area of the brain involved. The more restricted the brain region involved, the more limited the symptoms and the less likely that consciousness will be impaired. Localized seizures may then spread to adjacent areas or to contralateral or other more distant regions through thalamocortical and interhemispheric pathways, eventually resulting in secondarily generalized seizures.

4. **What are the clinical features (semeiology), EEG patterns, and common causes of seizures from different areas of the brain?**
See Table 20-1.

**TABLE 20-1. LOCALIZATION FEATURES AND COMMON CAUSES OF SEIZURES**

| Region | Typical Semiology | EEG | Etiology |
|---|---|---|---|
| Frontal | Often nocturnal, occur in clusters, often brief < 30 sec. Other symptoms relate to subregion of frontal lobes (adversive turning). Complex motor automatisms such as bicycling, pelvic thrusting, or other sexual gestures. Vocalizations common, minimal postictal symptoms. | Frontal or anterior vertex epileptiform discharges. Occasionally frontal bisynchronous discharges. | Trauma, malformations such as cortical dysplasia or cavernous angiomas, strokes, tumors, infections, anoxia. Some genetic syndromes. |
| Mesial temporal | Auras common: olfactory, gustatory, rising epigastric sensation, déjà vu, experiential phenomenon. Behavioral arrest, automatisms of the mouth (oroalimentary) and ipsilateral hand (manual). Semipurposeful or repetitive stereotypical movements. Contralateral dystonic posturing. Significant postictal confusion. | Temporal epileptiform discharges localized to anterior temporal region or sphenoidal electrodes, if used. Rhythmic theta activity. | Mesial temporal sclerosis, postinfectious, trauma. |

*(continued)*

TABLE 20-1. LOCALIZATION FEATURES AND COMMON CAUSES
OF SEIZURES *(continued)*

| Region | Typical Semiology | EEG | Etiology |
|---|---|---|---|
| Lateral temporal | Auras more likely to be auditory, vertiginous, visual distortions, early aphasia symptoms. | Lateral temporal epileptiform discharges and rhythmic theta activity. | Lateral cortical lesions and dysplasias. Cavernous angiomas. Genetic. |
| Parietal | Rare. May reflect activity of association cortex activity and include elementary or unusual formed sensory phenomena, nausea/abdominal, dysphasia or speech arrest. | Parietal epileptiform discharges. | Usually due to cortical lesions such as infarcts, cortical dysplasia, malignancies. |
| Occipital | Usually consist of unformed visual phenomena. May be negative visual symptoms. | Occipital epileptiform discharges, unilateral or bisynchronous. | Cortical lesions such as infarcts, dysplasia, or malignancies, but also as an idiopathic epilepsy syndrome (benign epilepsy with occipital paroxysms). |

5. **What causes primary generalized seizures? At what age do they usually start?**
Primary generalized seizures (i.e., seizures that cannot be localized to one cerebral hemisphere at onset) usually have a genetic predisposition. The seizures usually begin before the age of 20 and are not associated with well-defined auras (an aura is the first subjective symptom of the seizure and represents a focal seizure).

6. **Construct a chart describing the major types of primary generalized seizures.**
See Table 20-2.

## TABLE 20-2. FEATURES OF PRIMARY GENERALIZED SEIZURES

| Seizure Type | Semiology | EEG |
|---|---|---|
| Absence | Sudden behavioral arrest, staring, may have some automatisms. No aura, no postictal confusion. | Generalized 3 Hz spike-and-wave discharges, exacerbated by hyperventilation. Background usually normal. |
| Atypical absence | Sudden behavioral arrest, and staring, but more prolonged with more prominent automatisms than absence. | Generalized 1.5-2.5 Hz spike-and-wave discharges. Often less regular and less symmetrical than absence. Background usually abnormal. |
| Atonic | Sudden loss of tone in postural muscles, resulting in drop attacks. Usually with brief impairment of consciousness. Minimal postictal state. | Low-voltage fast activity, polyspike and wave, or electrodecrement. |
| Tonic | Generalized or occasionally asymmetric hypertonia. May have sudden or gradual onset. Seldom lasts more than 1 min. Respiratory muscle contraction—"ictal cry." | Often associated with generalized 10 Hz or faster activity. |
| Tonic-clonic | Loss of consciousness with initially generalized tonic contractions, followed by rhythmic generalized jerking of all four extremities. | Initially generalized 10 Hz activity in the tonic phase, followed by rhythmic spike-wave, slow-wave, or sharp-slow wave activity. |

7. **How can focal seizures with behavioral arrest (complex partial seizures) and absence seizures be differentiated clinically?**
   Three main features may help to differentiate complex partial from absence seizures:
   1. Complex partial seizures, unlike absence seizures, may be preceded by a well-defined aura.
   2. On average, complex partial seizures last 90 seconds, whereas absence seizures usually last only 10 to 15 seconds.
   3. After a complex partial seizure, the patient is usually confused or has some postictal cognitive problem. Absence seizures are not associated with a postictal state, and patients return to their baseline cognitive state at the end of the seizure.
   **Note**: Automatisms are common with both absence and complex partial seizures.

8. **Define the term *epileptic syndrome*.**
   An epileptic syndrome is a composite of signs and symptoms that may be associated with certain acquired pathologies or etiologies (symptomatic), lack an identifiable pathology or etiology (cryptogenic), or are likely genetic and follow a well-defined and accepted characteristic pattern (idiopathic). Like seizures, epileptic syndromes are classified by

localization or generalization of seizure activity. Syndromes may be associated with focal seizures that begin in one area of the cortex or generalized seizures that appear throughout the cortex at onset. Syndromic classification of patients is useful because some of the syndromes have well-defined prognoses. In addition, more appropriate antiepileptic drug therapy can be guided by syndromic classification. The most recent list of epilepsy syndromes is found at the International League Against Epilepsy website (http://www. ilae-epilepsy.org).

9. **List the four most common inherited epileptic syndromes.**
   1. Febrile convulsions
   2. Benign childhood epilepsy with centrotemporal spikes
   3. Childhood absence epilepsy
   4. Juvenile myoclonic epilepsy
   The first three syndromes usually are associated with seizures that remit spontaneously. Juvenile myoclonic epilepsy persists and usually responds to treatment with antiepileptic drugs.

10. **Describe the Lennox-Gastaut syndrome.**
    This epileptic syndrome usually begins before age 5 and is characterized by tonic-axial, atonic, and atypical absence seizures. Most patients also have myoclonic, partial, and tonic-clonic seizures. The EEG is characterized by a slow ($< 3$ Hz) frontocentral dominant spike and wave pattern, and patients have mental retardation. The seizures are difficult to control, and status epilepticus associated with stupor, jerks, and changes in tone is common. About 60% of patients have a clear underlying cause of encephalopathy (symptomatic). The remaining cases are cryptogenic or idiopathic.
    Arzimanoglou A, French J, Blume WT, et al.: Lennox-Gastaut syndrome: A consensus approach on diagnosis, assessment, management, and trail methodology. Lancet Neurol 8:82-93, 2009.

11. **What are "benign" febrile seizures?**
    Benign febrile seizures (convulsions) are an inherited predisposition to developing a tonic-clonic seizure with a high fever. The description is limited to convulsions associated with high fever in children younger than the age of 5 (usually between 6 and 36 months of age), with no cause for the seizure other than the fever. Benign febrile seizures are common, occurring in 3% to 5% of children younger than the age of 5. Most patients have only one or two seizures. Recent genetic analysis of families with febrile convulsions has defined specific associated gene defects (see Question 21, table 20-4).

12. **Are febrile seizures a risk factor for the development of epilepsy?**
    A single, isolated febrile seizure of short duration probably does not greatly influence the later development of epilepsy. In general, if there are no other reasons to suspect recurrent seizures, such children are not treated. The following features, however, have been identified as risk factors for the development of epilepsy:
    1. Underlying neurologic or developmental abnormality
    2. Family history of nonfebrile seizures
    3. Prolonged febrile convulsions
    4. Multiple febrile convulsions
    5. Atypical or focal features (complex febrile seizures)

13. **Describe the syndrome of benign childhood epilepsy with centrotemporal spikes.**
    This syndrome accounts for about 15% to 20% of epilepsy cases younger than the age of 15 years. The seizures, which are mostly nocturnal, are associated with focal motor activity of

the face and salivation and may generalize secondarily. Sensory symptoms may occur around the mouth in addition to motor components. Speech may not be possible. The EEG is characterized by a prominent centrotemporal sharp wave with otherwise normal background. The sharp waves occur more frequently during sleep. This epilepsy remits spontaneously after the age of 16, regardless of treatment. Treatment for partial epilepsy may be instituted, depending on how disruptive the seizures are.

14. **Characterize juvenile myoclonic epilepsy.**
This syndrome is characterized by myoclonic seizures that often occur shortly after wakening and generalized tonic-clonic seizures that tend to be precipitated by sleep deprivation. Interictally, the EEG shows a 4 to 6 Hz generalized spike-wave pattern. The myoclonic jerks are associated with a spike-wave discharge, and usually consciousness is not lost. Unlike the other common idiopathic epilepsies, juvenile myoclonic epilepsy does not remit with age. Valproate appears to be the most effective therapy, and topiramate, lamotrigine, levetiracetam, and primidone are often successful second-line agents. Some of the other newer antiepileptic drugs (AEDs) also may prove to be beneficial.

15. **Name some famous people who had seizures.**
   1. Julius Caesar–Roman emperor
   2. Lord Byron—poet
   3. Vincent van Gogh—artist
   4. Peter the Great—Russian ruler
   5. Fyodor Dostoyevsky—author
   6. Hector Berlioz—composer

## PHYSIOLOGY

16. **What systemic physiologic changes occur during a seizure?**
For both absence and complex partial seizures, the patient may have a variety of autonomic alterations, including changes in pulse rate, sweating, salivation, pupillary dilatation, and incontinence. The most dramatic systemic changes occur during generalized tonic-clonic seizures with an increase in blood pressure and pulse rate, increased autonomic nervous system activation, a metabolic acidosis, a drop in $P_{O_2}$ and an increase in $P_{CO_2}$ during the apneic tonic phase, and, rarely, hyperkalemia or rhabdomyolysis. Prolonged generalized tonic-clonic seizures may have serious consequences including hyperkalemia or rhabdomyoloysis.

17. **What CNS physiologic changes occur during a seizure?**
During a seizure, blood flow and glucose utilization in the brain are increased. Accompanying the neuronal activity may be an increase in lactate and a decrease in pH, alterations in the concentration of neurotransmitters, an increase in extracellular potassium, and a decrease in extracellular calcium. Generalized tonic-clonic seizures and most complex partial seizures activate the hypothalamus and increase serum prolactin, a finding that may help to differentiate epileptic from nonepileptic (psychogenic) seizures. Prolactin also may be elevated after syncope and hence cannot differentiate seizures from syncope.

## ETIOLOGY

18. **What are the identifiable causes of seizures as a function of age?**
See Table 20-3.

| TABLE 20-3. COMMON CAUSES OF SEIZURES BY AGE | | | |
|---|---|---|---|
| Neonate to 3 Years | 3 to 20 Years | 20 to 60 Years | Older than 60 Years |
| Prenatal injury | Genetic | Brain tumors | Vascular disease |
| Perinatal injury | predisposition | Trauma | Brain tumors |
| Metabolic defects | Infections | Vascular disease | (especially |
| Congenital | Trauma | Infections | metastatic |
| malformations | Congenital | | tumors) |
| CNS infections | malformations | | Trauma |
| Postnatal trauma | Metabolic defects | | Systemic metabolic |
| | | | derangements |
| | | | Infections |

19. **What are the metabolic causes of seizures?**
    1. Hypocalcemia
    2. Hyponatremia
    3. Hypoglycemia
    4. Liver failure
    5. Renal failure
    6. Anoxia
    7. Nonketotic hyperglycemic states
    8. Inherited metabolic diseases

20. **What drugs are common causes of seizures?**
    Seizures may be caused by many drugs, both prescribed and illicit. Cocaine and amphetamines are the two drugs of abuse most commonly associated with seizures. Some drugs produce seizures at toxic levels, including penicillin, lidocaine, aminophylline, and isoniazid. Other drugs, such as bupropion and clozapine, appear to lower seizure threshold and, in susceptible individuals, may produce seizures. Whenever a patient presents initially with a seizure, toxicology studies are indicated. The other setting associated with seizures is withdrawal from drugs, particularly alcohol, barbiturates, or benzodiazepines.

21. **What are channelopathies? Do they cause epilepsy?**
    A channelopathy is a disorder, usually inherited, of ion channels. Although first described in neuromuscular disorders (periodic paralyses), the channelopathies in Table 20-4 may cause or predispose to epilepsy.

22. **Which factors predict the development of epilepsy after head trauma?**
    Open head trauma produced by bullets or shrapnel is associated with a 50% or greater chance of developing epilepsy. Closed head trauma, such as after automobile accidents or blunt injuries, carries a much lower risk (5% or less). Factors that predispose to the development of epilepsy after head trauma include a seizure within 2 weeks of injury, depressed skull fracture, loss of consciousness for longer than 24 hours, cerebral contusion, subdural hematoma, or subarachnoid blood, and age older than 65.
    Temkin NR: Preventing and treating post-traumatic seizures. Epilepsia 50(suppl 2):10-30, 2009.

| TABLE 20-4. CHANNELOPATHIES AND EPILEPSY | | |
|---|---|---|
| Channel Type | Gene | Disorder |
| Potassium (voltage-gated) | KCNQ2 M-type potassium channel subunit (with KCNQ3) | Benign familial neonatal seizures |
| | KCNQ3 M-type potassium channel subunit (with KCNQ2) | Benign familial neonatal seizures |
| Sodium (voltage-gated) | SCN1A α subunit of $Na_v1.1$ (somatic sodium channel) | Generalized epilepsy with febrile seizures plus (GEFS+) and severe myoclonic epilepsy of infancy |
| | SCN2A α subunit of $Na_v1.2$ (axonal sodium channel) | GEFS+ |
| | SCN1B $\beta_1$ subunit of sodium channels | GEFS+ |
| Nicotinic acetylcholine receptor (ligand-gated) | CHRNA4 $\beta_2$ subunit of nicotinic receptors (with $a_4$) | Autosomal dominant nocturnal frontal lobe epilepsy |
| | CHRNB2 $\beta_2$ subunit of nicotinic receptors (with $a_4$) | Autosomal dominant nocturnal frontal lobe epilepsy |
| GABA$_A$ (ligand-gated) | GABRG2 $\gamma_2$ subunit (brain inhibitory synapses) | GEFS+ |

From Kullmann DM, Hanna MG: Neurological disorders caused by inherited ion-channel mutations. Lancet Neurol 2002 1:157-166.

23. **Should antiepileptic drugs be used after head trauma to prevent the development of epilepsy?**
There is no definitive answer to this question. The most recent study assessing phenytoin concluded that therapy was useful only during the first week after head trauma. At later dates, the side effects produced by phenytoin appeared to be detrimental to patients with severe neurologic damage after head trauma. Valproate also has been found to be ineffective as a prophylactic agent after head trauma. At present, no drug clearly has been shown to be effective prophylaxis against post-traumatic epilepsy.
   Chang BS, Lowenstein DH: Practice parameter: Antiepileptic drug prophylaxis in severe traumatic brain injury. Neurology 60:10-16, 2003.

## DIAGNOSTIC TESTING

24. **How many EEGs are needed to establish the diagnosis of epilepsy?**
Epilepsy is a clinical diagnosis and cannot be excluded by normal EEGs. The answer depends on the type of epilepsy and results of studies vary. Overall, from 29% to 69% of patients with the clinical diagnosis of epilepsy had interictal epileptiform activity on a single EEG.

Multiple EEGs, up to four, may enhance the yield up to 92%, but further EEGs have minimal benefit. Untreated patients with absence seizures usually have an abnormal routine EEG. The diagnostic yield of EEG also may be increased by prolonged monitoring, including sleep.

Gilbert DL, Sethuraman G, Kotagal U, Buncher CR: Meta-analysis of EEG test performance shows wide variation among studies. Neurology 60:564-570, 2003.

25. **Which patients with seizures should have magnetic resonance imaging (MRI) scans?**
Patients with partial seizures or focal features on EEG should have MRI scans to look for a brain lesion associated with their seizures (Figure 20-1). Patients with clear-cut primary generalized epilepsy based on EEG and clinical features usually do not require MRI scanning.

26. **What is the value of PET scanning in patients with epilepsy?**
Positron emission tomography (PET) scans have helped us to understand some of the metabolic changes that occur during seizures. PET scans demonstrate hypermetabolism or increased glucose uptake during the seizure. Most patients, however, are studied during the interictal period. In this setting, patients with epilepsy that have focal onset may show an area of hypometabolism in the region of seizure onset and a decrease in glucose

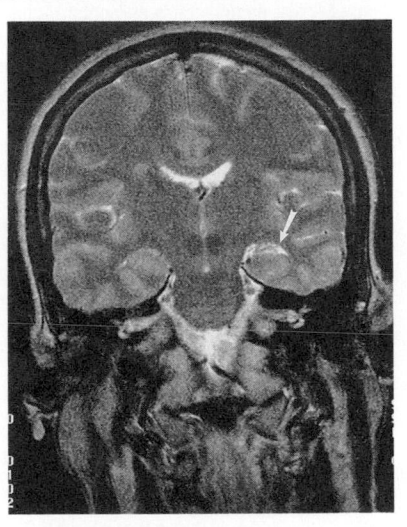

**Figure 20-1.** MRI scan in a patient with partial complex seizures. The arrow shows sclerosis in the hippocampus of the left temporal lobe (mesial temporal sclerosis).

uptake. PET scanning has been useful in helping to localize seizure onset in patients with intractable, complex partial seizures who are being evaluated for surgical therapy.

27. **What is a single-photon emission computed tomography (SPECT) scan? What role does it have in evaluating patients?**
Single-photon emission computed tomography (SPECT) usually uses a radioactive isotope that demonstrates blood flow. SPECT scans may identify areas of decreased blood flow interictally. If given at the start of a seizure or shortly thereafter, an increase in blood flow correlates with the area of seizure onset. SPECT scanning is primarily useful in the presurgical evaluation of patients with intractable epilepsy; it is most useful if an ictal scan can be obtained. Subtraction of the interictal scan from the ictal scan and superimposition on a MRI scan can provide an anatomic and physiologic picture of the epileptogenic zone.

O'Brien TJ, So EL, Mullan BP, et al.: Subtraction peri-ictal SPECT is predictive of extratemporal epilepsy surgery outcome. Neurology 55:1668-1677, 2000.

## THERAPY

28. **When should antiepileptic treatment be initiated?**
People should be treated with antiepileptic medication when the clinician thinks that the person will probably have another seizure without treatment. The seizure type or syndrome may help

with this decision. For example, absence seizures are rarely isolated and so require therapy, whereas febrile seizures are often isolated and therapy is not indicated. Between 20% and 70% of people with an isolated, unprovoked generalized tonic-clonic seizure will never have another seizure. Ideally, it would be best not to treat these patients.

29. **Which patients are at highest risk for recurrent seizures?**
Seizure recurrence is more likely if the patient has focal neurologic deficits, mental retardation, an EEG that demonstrates epileptiform abnormalities, or a structural brain lesion. In these patients, it is reasonable to begin antiepileptic therapy. In patients with a well-defined provocative etiology, it is best to treat the underlying process rather than the seizures themselves, particularly in clear-cut cases of alcohol withdrawal seizures and drug-induced seizures.

30. **When should antiepileptic treatment be stopped?**
Treatment should be stopped when it is the physician's opinion that the patient probably will not have seizures off medications. Certain seizure types and benign epileptic syndromes will remit. Patients with absence seizures usually "outgrow" their seizures, and therapy is no longer needed. Benign childhood epilepsy with centrotemporal spikes also remits. Recent studies suggest that approximately one-third of adult patients and one-fourth of children who are seizure-free for 2 years will relapse after termination of antiepileptic medication.

31. **Which patients are most likely to have further seizures after their medications have been stopped?**
Risk factors for recurrence include:
1. Prolonged period before seizures were controlled
2. High frequency of seizures before control
3. Neurologic abnormalities
4. Mental retardation
5. Complex partial seizures
6. Consistently abnormal EEGs

32. **Which antiepileptic drugs are most appropriate for different seizure types?**
The choice of AED is dictated by the types of seizures that the patient has. If possible, monotherapy should be used.
   The selections in Table 20-5 are based on side effects as well as effectiveness. Phenobarbital and primidone are as efficacious as phenytoin and carbamazepine but are more likely to produce side effects. Tonic and atonic seizures are often resistant to therapy, and valproate seems to be most efficacious. Tonic and clonic seizures may be secondarily generalized, and phenytoin, carbamazepine, lamotrigine, topiramate, levetiracetam and zonisamide can be helpful.
   Curatolo P, Moavero R, LoCastro A, Cerminara C: Pharmacotherapy of idiopathic generalized epilepsies. Expert Opin Pharmacother 10:5-17, 2009.

33. **Construct a table of all major antiepileptic medications to compare their mechanism of action, metabolic profile, common dosages, and significant side effects.**
See Table 20-6.

34. **In general, how often should AEDs be given?**
Antiepileptic drugs should be given at least every half-life. Some medications may need to be given more frequently because of peak-dose side effects. For example, patients tolerate twice-daily or thrice-daily dosing of ethosuximide better than a single daily dose. In some cases, pharmacokinetics (drug metabolism, half-life) may not match pharmacodynamics (drug effect), and medication is given at intervals longer than the half-life. For example, levetiracetam has a half-life of 6 to 8 hours but is given twice daily.

TABLE 20-5.  FIRST-LINE AND SECOND-LINE DRUGS FOR SPECIFIC SEIZURE TYPES*

| Drugs | Partial Seizures and Localization-Related Epilepsy | Epilepsies | | | |
|---|---|---|---|---|---|
| | | Tonic-Clonic | Generalized Seizures and Epilepsies | Myoclonic | Atonic/Tonic |
| First-line | Lamotrigine<br>Carbamazepine<br>Phenytoin<br>Valproate<br>Oxcarbazepine | Lamotrigine<br>Valproate<br>Phenytoin<br>Carbamazepine | Lamotrigine<br>Ethosuximide<br>Valproate | Valproate<br>Levetiracetam<br>Lamotrigine<br>Zonisamide<br>Topiramate | Valproate<br>Lamotrigine<br>Topiramate<br>Rufinamide |
| Second-line | Primidone<br>Phenobarbital<br>Felbamate | Topiramate<br>Primidone<br>Phenobarbital<br>Felbamate | Topiramate<br>Clonazepam | Primidone<br>Phenobarbital<br>Clonazepam<br>Ethosuximide<br>Felbamate | Levetiracetam<br>Phenytoin<br>Phenobarbital<br>Primidone<br>Clonazepam |
| Add-on† | Levetiracetam<br>Topiramate<br>Zonisamide<br>Gabapentin<br>Lacosamide<br>Tiagabine | Levetiracetam<br>Zonisamide | Zonisamide | | Felbamate<br>Zonisamide |

*Listed in order of authors' preference.
†May be effective as monotherapy but approved only as add-on agents.

## TABLE 20-6. MAJOR ANTIEPILEPTIC MEDICATIONS

| AED, Trade Name, Manufacturer, Year Released | Mechanism | Metabolism | Common Dosages | Therapeutic Level, Half-Life | Common or Significant Side Effects |
|---|---|---|---|---|---|
| **Phenobarbital,** generic by various manufacturers, 1912 | Prolongs opening of GABA-ergic $Cl^-$ channels, increases GABA inhibition. | Hepatic > renal. Enzyme inducing. 20%-45% protein bound. | For status epilepticus: 20 mg/kg loading dose. Neonates: 2-5 mg/kg/day divided b.i.d. Adults: 100-300 mg divided b.i.d. Children: 3-7 mg/kg/day divided b.i.d. | Therapeutic range: 15-40 mg/L. Half-life: 24-168 hours. Takes 2-3 weeks to achieve steady state if no loading dose given. | Sedation, depression, cognitive slowing, respiratory depression, hepatic dysfunction, lupus-like syndrome, erythema multiforme, osteomalacia. |
| **Phenytoin,** Dilantin by Parke-Davis, 1938 | Blocks voltage-dependent $Na^+$ and $Ca^{2+}$ channels, reduces high-frequency firing. | Hepatic > renal. Enzyme inducing. 90% protein bound. Nonlinear kinetics. | Loading dose 20 mg/kg. Maintenance 5 mg/kg/day, may divide b.i.d. Adjust dose based on level (nonlinear kinetics). For level 7-10 mg/L, increase dose by 50 mg/day. Level <7 increase dose by 100 mg/day. | Therapeutic range: 10-20 mg/L. Check unbound level (0.5-3 mg/L) if CCr <10, albumin <3.2 mg/dL, on valproate, pregnant, or suspected toxicity. Half-life: average 22 hours (range 7-42 hours, nonlinear kinetics). | Cerebellar atrophy, ataxia, megaloblastic anemia, neuropathy, gingival hyperplasia, nystagmus, osteomalacia. |
| **Primidone,** Mysoline by Athena Neurosciences, 1954 | Enhances GABA inhibition, essentially as phenobarbital, but may also have additional activity. | Renal > hepatic. Enzyme inducing. Protein bound. | Adults: start 100-125 mg qhs, increase by 100-125 mg/day every 3 days to initial target of 250 mg t.i.d. Children: start 50-60 mg/day, increase by 50 mg/day every 3 days to initial target of 10-25 mg/kg/day divided t.i.d. | Therapeutic range: Primidone: 5-12 mg/L. Phenobarbital: 15-40 mg/L. Half-life: Primidone: 8-22 hours. Phenobarbital: 56-140 hours. Phenylethylmalonamide: 10-25 hours. | Sedation, depression, cognitive slowing, respiratory depression, hepatic dysfunction, lupus-like syndrome, erythema multiforme, osteomalacia. |
| **Ethosuximide,** Zarontin by Parke Davis, 1960 | Blocks T-type calcium channels, reduces thalamocortical excitability | Hepatic > renal. | Adults: 1000 mg/day in divided doses t.i.d. Children: 20 mg/kg/day | Therapeutic range: 40-100 mg/L. Half-life: 30-60 hours. | Sedation, nausea/vomiting, headache, personality changes, psychosis. |

| Drug | Mechanism | Metabolism | Dosing | Therapeutic range / Half-life | Side effects |
|---|---|---|---|---|---|
| Tegretol XR by Novartis, Carbatrol by Shire, 1974 | Na$^+$ and Ca$^{2+}$ channels, reduces high-frequency firing | metabolite: carbamazepine 10-11 epoxide. Enzyme inducing. | <12: start 10-20 mg/kg/day div b.i.d. or t.i.d., increase by 5-10 mg/kg/day weekly, target 20-35 mg/kg/day div b.i.d. or t.i.d. Take with food. | 4-12 mg/L. Half-life: initially 25-65 hours with induction, 12-17 hours. | diplopia/blurred vision, nausea, hyponatremia, SIADH, elevated LFTs, osteomalacia, photosensitivity. |
| **Valproic acid**, Depakote, Depakote ER, Depakene by Abbott, 1978 | Blocks voltage-dependent Na$^+$ and Ca$^{2+}$ channels, reduces high-frequency firing. ?Potentiates GABA. | Hepatic N-glucuronidation and beta-oxidation *CYP450*. >90% protein bound. | Adults and children: start 10-15 mg/kg/day b.i.d. or t.i.d. Increase by 5-10 mg/kg/day weekly. Max 60 mg/kg/day. | Therapeutic range: 50-125 mg/L. Half-life: 9-12 hours, children, 5-13 hours, 20 hours with ER preparation. | Tremor, weight gain, elevated LFTs, increased bleeding, thrombocytopenia, hyperammonemia, ? polycystic ovary syndrome, fragile hair, osteomalacia. |
| **Felbamate**, Felbatol by Wallace, 1993 | NMDA blocker (glycine site), enhances GABA inhibition, blocks Na$^+$ channels. | Renal > hepatic. | Adults: start 1200 mg/day t.i.d. or q.i.d. Increase by 1200 mg/ day weekly. Max 3600 mg/day. Children: start 15 mg/kg/day div t.i.d., increase by 15 mg/kg/ day weekly. Max 3600 mg/day. | Therapeutic range: 30-80 mg/L. Half-life: 20-23 hours. | Requires informed consent regarding idiosyncratic reactions - aplastic anemia and hepatic failure. Headache, drowsiness, agitation, weight loss, nausea/ vomiting, tachycardia. |
| **Gabapentin**, Neurontin by Parke-Davis, 1993 | Increases brain GABA levels, may work at Ca$^{2+}$ channels. | Renal >95% unchanged | Adults: start 300 mg qhs, increase by 300 mg/day every 1-3 days. Max 3600 mg/day div t.i.d. Children: start 10-20 mg/kg/ day div t.i.d., increase by 10-20 mg/kg/day. Max 50 mg/kg/day div t.i.d. | Therapeutic range: 2-12 mg/L. Half-life: 4-6 hours. | Somnolence, fatigue, ataxia, weight gain, edema, TTP, leukopenia, tinnitus. |

*(continued)*

## TABLE 20-6. MAJOR ANTIEPILEPTIC MEDICATIONS (continued)

| AED, Trade Name, Manufacturer, Year Released | Mechanism | Metabolism | Common Dosages | Therapeutic Level, Half-Life | Common or Significant Side Effects |
|---|---|---|---|---|---|
| **Lamotrigine.** Lamictal by Glaxo Wellcome, 1994 | Voltage-dependent Na$^+$ channel blocker. Decreases release of excitatory neurotransmitters. | Hepatic > renal. | Starting titration varies if on other drugs. Adults (with valproate): start 25 mg/day, increase by 25 mg b.i.d. every 1-2 weeks, initial target 100 mg b.i.d. Monotherapy or enzyme-inducing AEDs: start 25 mg b.i.d., increase by 50 mg every week, target 200 mg b.i.d. Children (with valproate): 0.15 mg/kg/day for 2 weeks, then 0.3 mg/kg/day for weeks 3-4. On monotherapy or enzyme-inducing AEDS: 0.6 mg/kg/day for first 2 weeks, then 1.2 mg/kg/day for weeks 3-4., target 5-15 mg/kg/day | Therapeutic range: 4-15 mg/L. Half-life: 11-60 hours (depending if on inducer or inhibitor). | Rash or Stevens-Johnson syndrome more likely if increased rapidly. Nausea, lethargy, dizziness, headache. |
| **Topiramate.** Topamax by Ortho Biotech, 1996 | Blocks repetitive neuron firing. Blocks kainate and AMPA receptors. Improves GABA inhibition, carbonic anhydrase inhibitor. | Predominantly renal, but has enzyme-inducing effects. | Adults: start 25 mg daily, increase by 25-50 mg div b.i.d. weekly, target 100-200 mg b.i.d. Children: 1-3 mg/kg/day, increase by 1-3 mg/kg/day every 1-2 weeks div b.i.d., target 5-9 mg/kg/day | Therapeutic range: 4-10 mg/L. Half-life: 18-30 hours. | Nephrolithiasis, acute angle closure glaucoma, metabolic acidosis, hyperthermia, tingling, altered taste, anorexia/weight loss, lethargy, word finding problems, diarrhea, dizziness. |

| Drug | Mechanism | Metabolism | Dosing | Therapeutic range/Half-life | Side effects |
|---|---|---|---|---|---|
| **Tiagabine,** Gabitril by Cephalon, 1997 | Potentiates GABA by blocking glial uptake. | Hepatic > 90%. Protein bound. | Adults: start 4 mg daily, increase to 4 mg b.i.d. in 2 weeks, then increase by 4 mg day, div b.i.d. weekly, target 32–56 mg div b.i.d. Children: (12–16 years): start same as adult, but target 20–32 mg | Therapeutic range: 0.1–0.3 mg/L. Half-life: 4–9 hours. | Fatigue, weakness, poor attention, ataxia, nausea, tremor. |
| **Levetiracetam,** Keppra by UCB Pharma, 1999 | Decreased high-voltage $N^+$-type $Ca^{2+}$ channel current, reduces effects of Zn and beta-carbolines at GABA A and glycine receptors. | Renal > hepatic. Not enzyme inducing. <10% protein bound. | Adults: start 250 mg b.i.d. for 1 week, then target 500 mg b.i.d. May increase to 1500 b.i.d. | Therapeutic range: 5–40 mg/L. Half-life: 6–8 hours. | Personality changes, irritability, sedation, hallucinations. |
| **Oxcarbazepine,** Trileptal by Novartis, 2000 | Blocks $Na^+$ and $Ca^{2+}$ channels, stops high-frequency firing. | Hepatic = renal. Metabolized to active monohydroxy metabolite by cytosolic liver enzymes, then further glucuronidation and oxidation to other less active metabolites, then renal excretion. 40% protein bound. | Adults: start 300 mg b.i.d., increase by 300 mg every 3 days, to initial target 600 mg b.i.d. Max 2400 mg/day. Children (4–16 years): start 8–10 mg/kg every 2 weeks to target (all div b.i.d.). 20–29 kg: 900 mg/day, 29–39 kg: 1200 mg/day, >39 kg: 1800 mg/day. | Therapeutic range: 10-monohydroxyr metabolite 12–30 mg/L. Half-life: 8–12 hours. | Hyponatremia, fatigue, somnolence, ataxia, nausea, vomiting, diplopia, nystagmus. |
| **Zonisamide,** Zonegran by Elan, 2000 | Blocks $Na^+$ and $Ca^{2+}$ channels, stops high-frequency firing, interacts with $GABA_A$ channels, carbonic anhydrase inhibitor. | Hepatic > renal. | Adults: start 100 mg/day, increase by 100 mg every 2 weeks, target of 400 mg once daily (may div b.i.d.). Children: start 1.2 mg/kg/day, increase by 0.5–1 mg/kg/day every 2 weeks to target of 5–8 mg/kg/day. | Therapeutic range: 15–40 mg/L. Half-life: 63 hours. | Nephrolithiasis, tingling, altered taste, anorexia/weight loss, lethargy, word finding problems, visual field defects, dizziness. |

*(continued)*

## TABLE 20-6. MAJOR ANTIEPILEPTIC MEDICATIONS (continued)

| AED, Trade Name, Manufacturer, Year Released | Mechanism | Metabolism | Common Dosages | Therapeutic Level, Half-Life | Common or Significant Side Effects |
|---|---|---|---|---|---|
| **Pregabalin**, Lyrica by Pfizer, 2005 | Increases GABA and decreases glutamate, decreases influx through voltage-dependent $Ca^{2+}$ channels. | Renal. | Start 75 mg b.i.d., increase to 300 mg b.i.d. | Therapeutic range: variable. Half-life: 6 hours. | Dizziness, drowsiness. |
| **Vigabatrin**, Sabril by Ovaron Pharma, under FDA consideration in 2009 | Inhibits GABA transaminase to increase brain levels of GABA. | Renal. | Adults: start 500 mg b.i.d., increase by 500 mg/day every week up to 3 gm/day b.i.d. Infantile spasms: 50 mg/kg/day b.i.d, titrate by 25-50 mg/kg/day every 3 days to max of 150 mg/kg/day. | Therapeutic range: unknown. Half-life: 5-12 hours. | Peripheral visual field defects, behavioral changes. Requires informed consent because of the visual field effects. |
| **Vimpat**, (lacosamide) by Eisai, 2009 | Enhances slow inactivation of Na+ channel | Renal and Hepatic | Begin 25-50 mg BID and titrate by 50-100 mg/week to dose of 200 mg BID | 13 hours, therapeutic levels not established | Dizziness, headache, nausea, diplopia. May be increased with other AEDS that block sodium channels. |
| **Banzel**, (rufinamide) by Eisai, 2009 | Sodium Channel | Hepatic | Begin with 200-400 mg BID and increase weekly by 400-800 mg/day to target of 1600 mg BID | 6-10 hours, therapeutic levels not established | Somnolence, vomiting, headache, can shorten QT interval at higher doses and contraindicated in individuals with short QT interval. |

SIADH: syndrome of inappropriate antidiuretic hormone, LFT = liver function tests, AED = antiepileptic drug; TTP = thrombotic thrombocytopenic purpura

35. **What are the advantages of monotherapy?**
    1. In most situations, one drug controls seizures as well as two drugs.
    2. Monotherapy prevents interactions between antiepileptic medications.
    3. Monotherapy is less expensive.
    4. Monotherapy improves compliance.

36. **What are the main drug interactions among AEDs?**
    - Valproate decreases lamotrigine metabolism.
    - Felbamate, oxcarbazepine, and topiramate inhibit phenytoin metabolism via inhibition of hepatic enzymes.
    - The other main mechanism of drug interaction is protein binding. Phenytoin, valproate, and tiagabine are highly bound (>90%) to plasma proteins and can compete for binding sites.
    - Valproate protein binding displaces phenytoin or tiagabine so that free phenytoin and tiagabine levels increase.

37. **Summarize the main effects of add-on drugs on original drug levels.**
    See Table 20-7.

38. **When and how often should blood levels of AEDs be checked?**
    Monitoring of AED levels is indicated when the patient is initially loaded with the medication and when the drug reaches a steady-state concentration, usually after approximately 5 half-lives. Monitoring of drug levels is helpful in determining patient compliance and in documenting high levels when the patient has toxic symptoms.

39. **Which screening blood tests should be performed for patients taking AEDs? How often should they be done?**
    Many AEDs may affect the ability of the bone marrow to produce blood cells or may cause liver dysfunction. It is reasonable to use complete blood count (CBC) and liver function tests as baseline studies to identify predisposing problems. After this initial screening, it is usually not necessary to perform these studies routinely unless the patient is symptomatic. The exceptions are young children and mentally retarded patients who cannot communicate their toxic symptoms. Another special situation is the use of felbamate, which requires hematologic and hepatic function monitoring.

40. **What are the main side effects of commonly used antiepileptic medications?**
    Side effects may be dose-dependent or dose-independent. In general, most anticonvulsants can have sedative properties and interfere with motor performance in a dose-dependent manner (Table 20-8).

## WOMEN AND EPILEPSY

41. **Describe the differences between the effect of estrogen and progesterone on seizures.**
    Progesterone tends to decrease cortical excitability, increases seizure threshold, and decreases interictal spike frequency. Estrogen tends to have the opposite effects.

42. **In catamenial epilepsy, how do hormone changes predispose to seizures?**
    The rapid drop in the relatively protective progesterone levels occurs just prior to the onset of menses and lasts for the first few days of bleeding. Estrogen levels rise again just prior to ovulation and this may also increase seizure frequency in mid-cycle. The rising progesterone levels produced by the corpus luteum may then become protective again.

**TABLE 20-7. EFFECTS OF ADD-ON DRUGS ON ORIGINAL DRUG LEVELS**

| | Add-On Drug | | | | | | | | | |
|---|---|---|---|---|---|---|---|---|---|---|
| Original Drug | Carbamazepine | Felbamate | Lamotrigine | Oxcarbazepine | Phenobarbital/ Primidone | Phenytoin | Rufinamide | Topiramate | Valproate | Vigabatrin |
| Carbamazepine (CBZ) | N/A | Decrease CBZ, increase 10-11 epoxide | | Decrease CBZ, increase 10-11 epoxide | Decrease CBZ, increase 10-11 epoxide | | Decrease | Decrease CBZ, increase 10-11 epoxide | | |
| Ethosuximide | Decrease | | | | | Decrease | | Decrease | Increase or decrease (seldom significant) | |
| Felbamate | Decrease | N/A | | | Decrease | Decrease | | | | |
| Lacosamide | Decrease | | | | Decrease | Decrease | | | | |
| Lamotrigine | Decrease | Insignificant increase | N/A | Decrease | Decrease | Decrease | Decrease | | Increase | |
| Oxcarbazepine (active metabolite 10-OH-carbazepine) | Decrease | | | N/A | Decrease | Decrease | | Decrease | Decrease | |
| Phenobarbital/ Primidone | Insignificant decrease | Increase | | Increase | N/A | | Increase | | Increase | |

| Drug | | | | | | | | | |
|------|---|---|---|---|---|---|---|---|---|
| Phenytoin | Increase or decrease | Increase | Increase | Decrease | N/A | Increase | Increase | Increase, unbound fraction | Decrease |
| Rufinamide | Decrease | | | Decrease | Decrease | | | Increase | |
| Tiagabine | Decrease | Decrease | | Decrease | Decrease | | | Increase, unbound fraction | |
| Topiramate | Decrease | Decrease | | Decrease | Decrease | | N/A | Slight increase | |
| Valproate | Decrease | Increase | | Decrease | Decrease | | Slight decrease | N/A | |
| Zonisamide | Decrease | | | Decrease | Decrease | | | N/A | |

## TABLE 20-8.   SIDE EFFECTS OF ANTICONVULSANTS

| Concentration-Dependent | | Concentration-Independent | |
| --- | --- | --- | --- |
| Ataxia | Nausea, vomiting | Weight gain | Hirsutism |
| **Anorexia** | **Cognitive problems** | Carbamazepine | Phenytoin |
| Felbamate | Phenobarbital | Gabapentin | **Diarrhea** |
| Topiramate | Primidone | Pregabalin | Carbamazepine |
| Zonisamide | Topiramate | Valproate | Topiramate |
| **Ataxia** | **Headache** | Vigabatrin | **Dupuytren's** |
| Carbamazepine | Ethosuximide | **Behavioral** | **contractures** |
| Gabapentin | Felbamate | Ethosuximide | Phenobarbital |
| Lacosamide | Lacosamide | Gabapentin | **Edema** |
| Lamotrigine | Lamotrigine | Lacosamide | Gabapentin |
| Phenobarbital | Pregabalin | Levetiracetam | Valproate |
| Phenytoin | Vigabatrin | Phenobarbital | **Gingival** |
| Pregabalin | **Insomnia** | Pregabalin | **hyperplasia** |
| Primidone | Felbamate | Primidone | Phenytoin |
| Rufinamide | **Nausea** | Rufinamide | |
| Topiramate | Carbamazepine | Topiramate | |
| **Diplopia, blurred vision** | Ethosuximide | Vigabatrin | |
| Carbamazepine | Lacosamide | **Edema** | |
| Lacosamide | Phenytoin | Vigabatrin | |
| Lamotrigine | Pregabalin | **Hair loss** | |
| Phenytoin | Valproate | Valproate | |
| Pregabalin | **Paresthesias** | **Rash** | |
| Rufinamide | Topiramate | Carbamazepine | |
| Vigabatrin | Zonisamide | Lamotrigine | |
| **Hyponatremia** | **Renal stones** | Oxcarbazepine | |
| Carbamazepine | Topiramate | Phenobarbital | |
| Oxcarbazepine | Zonisamide | Phenytoin | |
| **Sedation** | **Thrombocytopenia** | Primidone | |
| Carbamazepine | Valproate | Zonisamide | |
| Gabapentin | **Tremor** | **Visual field loss** | |
| Lacosamide | Pregabalin | Vigabatrin | |
| Lamotrigine | Tiagabine | | |
| Levetiracetam | Valproate | | |
| Phenobarbital | Vigabatrin | | |
| Phenytoin | **Weight gain** | | |
| Pregabalin | Valproate | | |
| Rufinamide | | | |
| Topiramate | | | |
| Valproate | | | |
| Vigabatrin | | | |
| Zonisamide | | | |

43. **Compare the profile of the AEDs with regard to effects on oral contraceptives, and their teratogenicity.**
Because some AEDS cause neural tube defects, all sexually active and fertile women with epilepsy should be taking folate on a daily basis (0.4 to 5 mg/day) (Table 20-9).

Harden CL, Pennell PB, Koppel BS, et al.: Practice Paramater update: Management issues for women with epilepsy_Focus on pregnancy (an evidence-based review): Vitamin K, folic acid, blood levels, and breastfeeding: Report of the Quality Standards Subcommittee and Therapeutics and Technology Assessment Subcommittee of the American Academy of Neurology and American Epilepsy Society. Neurology 73:142-149, 2009.

**TABLE 20-9. ANTIEPILEPTIC DRUGS CONTRACEPTION AND PREGNANCY**

| AED | Oral Contraceptive Efficacy | Pregnancy Category | Known Teratogenicity Issues |
|---|---|---|---|
| Phenobarbital | Decrease | D | Cleft lip and palate and heart defects |
| Phenytoin | Decrease | D | Hypoplasia of the nails plus stiff joints, cleft lip and palate |
| Primidone | Decrease | D | Cleft lip and palate |
| Carbamazepine | Decrease | D | Neural tube defects 0.5-1%, other major malformations, microcephaly, and growth retardation |
| Valproic acid | None | D | Neural tube defects 1-2%, also cardiac anomalies, hypospadias, polydactyly, bilateral inguinal hernia, dysplastic kidney, and equinovarus club foot |
| Felbamate | None | C | Uncertain |
| Gabapentin | None | C | Uncertain |
| Lamotrigine | None | C | Uncertain |
| Topiramate | Decrease | C | Uncertain |
| Tiagabine | None | C | Uncertain |
| Levetiracetam | None | C | Uncertain |
| Oxcarbazepine | Decrease | C | May be more favorable than carbamazepine (no epoxide metabolite) |
| Zonisamide | None | C | Uncertain |
| Lacosamide | None | C | Uncertain |
| Pregabalin | None | C | Uncertain |
| Rufinamide | Decrease | C | Uncertain |
| Vigabatrine | None | C | Uncertain |

## SEIZURES AND EPILEPSY IN OLDER PATIENTS

44. **Are seizures in the elderly easily identified?**
Seizures in the elderly are notoriously underdiagnosed and misdiagnosed. The average delay to diagnosis in patients age 59 to 96 is about 1.7 years. These patients tend not to seek help initially, but even after medical evaluation, only 28% of elderly patients with complex

partial seizures and about 50% of the patients with generalized seizures are correctly diagnosed initially.

Pugh MJ, Knoefel JE, Mortensen EM, et al.: New onset epilepsy risk factors in older veterans. J Am Geriatr Soc 57:237-242, 2009.

45. **Discuss some of the age-related changes that can affect AED pharmacokinetics and pharmacodynamics.**
Elderly patients frequently have progressive decline in AED protein binding by albumin, increased volume of distribution, and slow elimination. They also appear to have increased sensitivity to the side effects of many AEDs, and they are also often on many other medications, which can lead to drug interactions. A recently completed VA Cooperative Study on epilepsy in the elderly demonstrated that lamotrigine and gabapentin were better tolerated than carbamazepine. More frequent monitoring of drug levels may be appropriate in this age group.

## ACUTE EPILEPSY TREATMENT

46. **What is status epilepticus?**
Status epilepticus is a state of continuous seizures without return of normal neurologic function between them. Any of the classified seizures types may progress to status epilepticus.

47. **How is status epilepticus classified?**
One way to classify status epilepticus is convulsive or nonconvulsive. Convulsive status epilepticus is a medical emergency that can be produced by either primary generalized or secondary generalized tonic-clonic seizures. Nonconvulsive status epilepticus refers to either absence or complex partial status epilepticus. In either case, the patient does not have major motor seizures but is abnormal cognitively and may appear to be in a fugue state. Absence status appears to have no morbidity (unless injuries occur during the status), but complex partial status may lead to permanent cognitive deficits.

48. **What are the most common causes of status epilepticus?**
1. AED noncompliance or withdrawal (most common in emergency department)
2. Alcohol withdrawal
3. Metabolic abnormalities
4. Intractable epilepsy
5. Brain tumors
6. Cerebral infarction
7. Cerebral hemorrhages
8. Meningitis
9. Undetermined (10% to 15% of patients)

49. **How is absence status epilepticus treated?**
Absence status is treated with intravenous diazepam or derivatives, not with phenytoin or the barbiturates. Intravenous valproate also can be an effective therapy.

50. **How is complex partial status epilepticus treated?**
Complex partial status is usually not associated with life-threatening systemic complications but may result in impairment of memory function and should be treated aggressively, similar to generalized tonic-clonic status.

51. **How is convulsive status epilepticus treated?**
Generalized tonic-clonic or convulsive status epilepticus is a medical emergency, and every effort should be made to stop the seizures within 1 hour. Initial therapy should use lorazepam, 0.1 mg/kg IV at 1 to 2 mg/minute. If seizures continue, intravenous fosphenytoin should be

given at a rate up to 150 mg/min. If the patient still continues to have seizures, phenobarbital should be given or anesthesia induced. Phenobarbital is likely to cause respiratory arrest in combination with lorazepam and the patient should be intubated. If the patient is resistant to phenytoin, phenobarbital, and lorazepam, anesthesia should be administered, preferably with propofol. An outline for the treatment of status epilepticus is presented in Table 20-10.

Millikan D, Rice B, Silbergleit R: Emergency treatment of status epilepticus: Current thinking. Emerg Med Clin North Am 27:101-113, 2009.

| TABLE 20-10. | PROTOCOL FOR TREATMENT OF GENERALIZED TONIC-CLONIC STATUS EPILEPTICUS |
|---|---|
| Time | Action |
| 0-5 min | Provide for maintenance of vital signs. Maintain airway. Give oxygen. Observe and examine patient. |
| 6-10 min | Obtain 50 mL of blood for glucose, calcium, magnesium, electrolytes, blood urea nitrogen, liver functions, anticonvulsant levels, CBC, and toxicology screen. Begin normal saline IV and give 50 mL of 50% glucose and 100 mg of thiamine. Monitor ECG, blood pressure, and, if possible, EEG. |
| 11-30 min | Use intravenous lorazepam to stop seizures, 0.1 mg/kg at 1-2 mg/min. |
| 11-30 min | If seizures continue, load with phenytoin using fosphenytoin 20 mg phenytoin equivalents (PE)/kg at 150 mg PE/min. If cardiac arrhythmia or hypotension occurs, slow the infusion rate. |
| 31-60 min | If seizures persist 10-20 min after administration of phenytoin, give an additional 10 PE/kg. If seizures continue, intubate patient. Consider phenobarbital at a rate of 50-100 mg/min until seizures stop or 20 mg/kg is given. Alternatively move to anesthetic agents. |
| After 60 min of status | Review laboratory results and correct abnormalities. Arrange for anesthesia, neuromuscular blockade, and EEG monitoring. Options include midazolam (0.15-0.2 mg/kg load, then 0.06-1.1 mg/kg/hr) or propofol (1-2 mg/kg load, then 3-10 mg/kg/hr), or barbiturate anesthesia (pentobarbital, 6-15 mg/kg loading dose, then 0.5-5 mg/kg/hr). Pentobarbital often causes circulatory collapse, so be prepared to administer a pressor agent such as dopamine. |

CBC, complete blood count; ECG, electrocardiogram; EEG, electroencephalography
From Lowenstein DH, Alldredge BK: Status epilepticus. N Engl J Med 338:970-976, 1998, and Treiman DM, Meyers PD, Walton NY, et al.: A comparison of four treatments for generalized convulsive status epilepticus. N Engl J Med 339:792-798, 1998.

52. **What is epilepsia partialis continua? How is it treated?**
Epilepsia partialis continua is simple partial motor status epilepticus, which consists of rhythmic contractions of a restricted region of the body, usually the face and hand or fingers. The patient is usually fully conscious during these seizures. The most common causes include nonketotic hyperglycemic states, cerebral infarction, encephalitis, and cerebral neoplasms. Treatment is directed at correcting metabolic abnormalities. AEDs are used, but epilepsia partialis continua may be resistant to drug therapy short of anesthesia.

**53. Does continuous seizure activity cause nervous system damage?**
Certain seizure types, such as absence seizures, are not known to have any significant sequelae. In other settings, after a certain duration of epileptiform activity, there is irreversible neuronal loss. A number of mechanisms probably mediate this neuronal death, including calcium loading of neurons and excitotoxicity produced by excessive glutamate release. Because continuous seizure activity can cause neuronal death, it is important to monitor the patient's EEG during the treatment of status, particularly if the patient is paralyzed by neuromuscular blockade. It is also important to try to prevent any neuronal death by controlling the patient's status within the first 60 minutes.

## EPILEPSY SURGERY

**54. Which patients are good candidates for epilepsy surgery?**
The actual criteria for choosing patients depend on a number of variables. First and foremost, the patient has seizures that are intractable to medical therapy. Second, the patient will derive significant benefit from becoming seizure-free. Third, seizure onset can be localized. Fourth, the potential morbidity of the surgery is acceptable and less than the morbidity of the seizures. In general, patients who have failed appropriate trials of two or three accepted antiseizure medications, and who suffer from debilitating focal-onset seizures should be considered for epilepsy surgery. Other cases, including some with generalized epilepsy, may also be appropriate for certain procedures such as corpus callosotomies.

Engle J Jr., Wiebe S, French J, et al.: Temporal lobe and localized neocortical resections for epilepsy. From AAN Guidelines Practice parameter. Neurology 60:538-547, 2003.

**55. At what point are epilepsy patients considered to be "refractory"?**
This remains somewhat controversial. After two to three generally effective AEDs have failed to render a patient seizure-free, the chances of that patient ever becoming seizure-free on any medication is only about 5% to 10%. In general, about 47% of patients will become seizure-free after the first AED. An additional 13% will become seizure-free after the second AED. On a third or multiple AEDs, the chance of seizure-freedom is about 1% to 3%.

Kwan P, Brodie MJ: Early identification of refractory epilepsy. N Engl J Med 342:314-319, 2000.

## KEY POINTS: SEIZURES AND EPILEPSY

1. Accurate seizure classification and if possible syndromic diagnosis guides therapeutic choices.

2. All partial seizures should be evaluated with an MRI scan.

3. A significant change in antiepileptic drug levels should alert you to either non-compliance or a new drug interaction.

4. The most common cause of antiepileptic drug treatment failure is drug side effects.

5. Patients whose seizures are refractory to two appropriate and tolerated antiepileptic drug trials should be evaluated at an epilepsy center for definitive diagnosis and surgical evaluation.

**56. What is hippocampal sclerosis? How is it diagnosed?**
Hippocampal sclerosis is a common disorder associated with complex partial seizures of temporal origin. The term describes the pathology of the hippocampus that includes a loss of neurons and associated gliosis. MRI scans may demonstrate hippocampal sclerosis. Unilateral hippocampal sclerosis associated with intractable complex partial seizures is important to identify because it is a surgically curable syndrome.

**57. What types of epilepsy surgery are available?**

The three basic types of epilepsy surgery are as follows: (1) focal resection of areas of epileptogenesis; (2) disconnecting procedures, usually corpus callosotomy; and (3) implanted stimulators. Corpus callosotomy may be indicated in severe generalized seizures, usually associated with atonic or tonic seizures that produce falling. Resective surgeries should be considered in partial seizures, particularly those that seem to begin exclusively from one circumscribed area of the brain. A new Food and Drug Administration (FDA)-approved treatment for refractory partial seizures is stimulation of the vagus nerve and should be considered if resective surgery is not an option.

**58. How effective is epilepsy surgery?**

For patients who undergo temporal lobectomies, about two-thirds are free of major seizures (other than focal seizures without alterations of consciousness). Between 10% to 15% are not improved. For patients with extra-temporal, neocortical epilepsy, about half are free from major seizures and about 15% are not improved. Patients seem to have better quality of life and better social function compared with their peers receiving only antiseizure medications.

## EPILEPSY AND DRIVING

**59. What recommendations about driving should a physician make to patients with epilepsy?**

It depends on the state where the physician is practicing. Basically, states either require the physician to report any patient with a seizure or require the patient to report any medical condition that may interfere with the ability to operate a motor vehicle. In general, physicians should caution against driving if the seizures are not controlled and involve impairment of consciousness or motor function. It is usually appropriate to have the patient's case evaluated by the state's driver-licensing authorities. Of interest, drivers with epilepsy have only a slightly increased risk of an accident.

Drazkowski J: An overview of epilepsy and driving. Epilepsia 48(Suppl): 10-12, 2007.

## ACKNOWLEDGEMENT

The authors thank Michael Collins and Barry Gidal for helpful comments and suggestions.

# WEBSITES

1. http://www.aesnet.org

2. http://www.efa.org

3. http://www.pslgroup.com/epilepsy.htm

4. http://epilepsy.org

5. http://ilae-epilepsy.org

## BIBLIOGRAPHY

1. Engle J, Pedley TA, Aicardi J, Dichter M: Epilepsy: A Comprehensive Textbook, 2nd ed. Hagerstown, MD, Lippincott Williams & Wilkins, 2007.
2. Wilner AN: Epilepsy in Clinical Practice. New York, Demos, 2004.
3. Wyllie E (ed): The Treatment of Epilepsy, 4th ed. Baltimore, Lippincott Williams & Wilkins, 2005.

# CHAPTER 21

# SLEEP DISORDERS

*Merrill S. Wise, MD*

## GENERAL PRINCIPLES

1. **What is sleep?**

   Sleep is a complex physiologic state that occurs periodically in most vertebrate species, and similar states are often observed in invertebrate organisms. It is characterized by relative quiescence, immobility, and greatly decreased responsiveness to external stimuli. In mammals, two distinct sleep states are recognized: rapid-eye-movement (REM) sleep and non-REM sleep.

2. **Describe the main features of REM sleep.**

   REM sleep is characterized by pronounced muscular atonia, phasic twitches, and bursts of rapid eye movements. During this state, the electroencephalogram (EEG) is relatively low in amplitude and often is similar to that seen during drowsiness, although people in REM sleep appear deeply asleep by behavioral criteria. Most dreaming apparently occurs during the REM stage.

3. **Is non-REM sleep a uniform state?**

   No. The Rechtschaffen and Kales (1968) sleep scoring manual subdivided non-REM sleep into stages 1, 2, 3, and 4, which are characterized by progressively increasing amplitude and decreasing frequency on EEG. Muscle tone tends to be higher than that seen during REM, and phasic movements are not typical. More recently, the American Academy of Sleep Medicine (AASM) Manual for the Scoring of Sleep and Associated Events (2007) subdivides non-REM sleep into three stages (N1, N2, and N3). N3 (deep non-REM) is equivalent to stages 3 and 4 in the older scoring method.

4. **Do the various stages of sleep occur randomly during the night?**

   No. People normally exhibit a fairly regular alternation of non-REM and REM sleep during the sleep period, with cycle times of approximately 90 min. There are usually few awakenings (typically fewer than 10 per night), and the various stages of sleep are present in consistent amounts. In the typical adult, the total sleep time is divided as follows: N1, less than 5%; N2, 40% to 60%; N3, 10% to 20%; and stage REM, 18% to 25%.

5. **Which areas of the brain control sleep?**

   Essentially every area of the brain is involved in sleep. Although no discrete "sleep center" exists, several regions appear to serve crucial roles that govern sleep timing and stage sequencing. The suprachiasmatic area of the hypothalamus is directly involved in the regulation of circadian cycles that determine when sleep occurs within the 24-hour day. On the other hand, a group of nuclei in the pontomesencephalic region (including locus ceruleus, dorsal raphe, and several cholinergic areas) are critical for the alternating sequence of REM and non-REM cycles. Neurons of the basal forebrain and anterior hypothalamus also appear to play a primary role in control of sleep onset.

6. **How many pathologic conditions are associated with disturbances of sleep?**
   The International Classification of Sleep Disorders, 2$^{nd}$ edition (2005), classifies several dozen
   sleep disorders into six broad categories: insomnia, sleep-related breathing disorders,
   hypersomnias of central origin, circadian rhythm sleep disorders, parasomnias, and sleep-
   related movement disorders. There is an additional category for isolated symptoms, apparently
   normal variants, and unresolved issues. Many other medical and psychiatric conditions may
   produce disturbed sleep as a secondary manifestation.

7. **What are the major symptoms of disturbed sleep?**
   Disordered sleep may be manifested in several ways: insomnia (difficulty with initiating or
   maintaining sleep), excessive and/or inappropriate sleepiness (hypersomnia), and atypical
   motor or behavioral events occurring in a particular relationship to sleep states or sleep-wake
   transitions.

8. **How are sleep disorders classified?**
   The **insomnias** are defined as chronic difficulty with sleep initiation, duration, consolidation, or
   quality that occurs despite adequate time and opportunity for sleep, and results in some form
   of daytime impairment. The **sleep-related breathing disorders** include central sleep apnea
   syndromes, obstructive sleep apnea syndromes, sleep-related hypoventilation/hypoxemic
   syndromes, and other sleep-related breathing disorders. The **hypersomnias of central origin**
   (not due to circadian rhythm sleep disorder, sleep-related breathing disorder, or other cause of
   disturbed nocturnal sleep) include a group of disorders in which the primary complaint is
   daytime sleepiness and in which the cause of the sleepiness is not disturbed nocturnal sleep or
   misaligned circadian rhythms. The **circadian rhythm sleep disorders** are characterized by a
   persistent or recurrent pattern of sleep disturbance due primarily to alterations of the
   circadian timing system or a misalignment between the timing of the individual's endogenous
   circadian rhythm of sleep propensity and exogenous factors that affect the duration or
   timing of sleep. The **parasomnias** are undesirable physical events or experiences that occur
   during entry into sleep, within sleep, or during arousals from sleep. **Sleep-related movement
   disorders** are conditions that are primarily characterized by relatively simple, usually
   stereotyped, movements that disturb sleep or by other sleep-related monophasic movement
   disorders such as sleep-related leg cramps. Representative examples of each category of sleep
   disorders are summarized in Tables 21-1 and 21-2.

9. **Are patient complaints of excessive daytime sleepiness reliable?**
   People with significant hypersomnia conditions are sometimes unaware of the fact that they
   fall asleep at inappropriate times. Motor vehicle accidents may be attributed to "blackouts" or
   seizures. Impaired job performance may be related to poor memory function. Patients with
   certain conditions (such as sleep apnea or periodic limb movements) may awaken literally
   dozens of times throughout the night and have both a low total sleep time and atypical
   sleep-stage distribution yet report to the physician that they fall asleep quickly every night
   and sleep soundly with few or no arousals.

10. **Can the physician rely on patient reports of insomnia?**
    Many people who report severe insomnia later prove (during sleep laboratory testing) to
    have normal sleep times and few awakenings. Because this phenomenon is common, the
    physician must be wary of all subjective reports of sleep characteristics and seek independent
    verification whenever evidence suggests a clinically significant condition.

11. **How much sleep is required for optimal daytime function?**
    Most normal people average between 6 and 8 hours of sleep per night, but there is a great deal
    of individual variability. As a general rule, if daytime performance is significantly impaired by

## TABLE 21-1. REPRESENTATIVE EXAMPLES OF SLEEP DISORDERS BY CATEGORY

| Insomnia | Sleep-Related Breathing Disorders |
|---|---|
| Adjustment | Obstructive sleep apnea syndrome |
| Psychophysiological | Central sleep apnea syndrome |
| Idiopathic | Sleep-related hypoventilation/hypoxemic syndromes |
| Behavioral insomnia of childhood | Other sleep-related breathing disorder |
| Insomnia due to mental disorder | **Hypersomnias of Central Origin** |
| Insomnia due to drug or substance | Narcolepsy with cataplexy |
| Insomnia due to medical disorder | Narcolepsy without cataplexy |
| Inadequate sleep hygiene | Narcolepsy due to medical condition |
| Circadian Rhythm Sleep Disorders | Recurrent hypersomnia (Kleine-Levin syndrome) |
| Delayed sleep phase type | Idiopathic hypersomnia |
| Advanced sleep phase type | Behaviorally induced insufficient sleep syndrome |
| Irregular sleep-wake type | Hypersomnia due to medical condition |
| Free-running type | Hypersomnia due to drug or substance |
| Jet lag type | **Sleep-Related Movement Disorders** |
| | Restless leg syndrome |
| | Periodic limb movement disorder |
| | Sleep-related leg cramps |
| | Sleep-related bruxism |
| | Sleep-related rhythmic movement disorder |

## TABLE 21-2. EXAMPLES OF PARASOMNIAS

**Disorders of Arousal (From NREM Sleep)**

Confusional arousals
Sleepwalking
Sleep terrors

**Parasomnias Usually Associated with REM Sleep**

REM sleep behavior disorder
Recurrent isolated sleep paralysis
Nightmare disorder

**Other Parasomnias**

Sleep enuresis
Sleep-related groaning (catathrenia)
Exploding head syndrome
Sleep-related eating disorder
Sleep-related dissociative disorders

NREM, non-rapid eye movement; REM, rapid eye movement

excessive sleepiness, and this condition persists despite adherence to a regularly scheduled nocturnal sleep period of at least 8 hours, more definitive diagnostic tests are indicated. In addition, a significant change in apparent sleep requirements may indicate an underlying sleep disorder.

12. **Is total sleep time the only determinant of the ability to maintain a normal level of daytime alertness?**
No. The structure, or architecture, of the sleep pattern is also crucial for normal waking function. When sleep is fragmented by frequent brief arousals or other factors disturb the normal distribution of stages, excessive daytime sleepiness may result, even if the total sleep time is not significantly reduced.

## KEY POINTS: MAJOR FACTORS INFLUENCING QUALITY OF SLEEP

1. Total sleep time
2. Number of awakenings and partial arousals
3. Distribution of sleep stages

## DIAGNOSTIC EVALUATIONS

13. **Can the physician obtain an objective assessment of sleep quality and quantity?**
The most important diagnostic tool available to the physician dealing with sleep disorders is the sleep study or polysomnogram. By monitoring sleep-wake state throughout the night, concurrently observing multiple physiologic parameters, and continuously documenting behavioral status, it is possible to obtain objective diagnostic information. (See Table 21-3 for a listing of polysomnographic parameters.) This test provides quantitative measures of total sleep time, number of awakenings, sleep-stage distribution, respiratory dysfunction, cardiac arrhythmias, atypical movements, nocturnal seizures, and character of parasomnias.

14. **How can daytime sleepiness be evaluated objectively?**
Both the multiple sleep latency test (MSLT) and the maintenance of wakefulness test (MWT) document the presence and degree of daytime sleepiness. These procedures both

| TABLE 21-3. PARAMETERS RECORDED DURING POLYSOMNOGRAPHY | |
| --- | --- |
| EEG | Respiratory effort (chest and abdomen) |
| EOG | Nasal and oral airflow |
| EMG, submental | Oxygen saturation |
| ECG | End-tidal $P_{CO_2}$ |
| Leg movement (EMG or accelerometer) | Body position |
| Snoring/vocalizations (audio monitoring) | Behavioral/motor events (video monitoring) |

EEG, electroencephalogram; EOG, electrooculogram; EMG, electromyogram; ECG, electrocardiogram

make use of polygraphic monitoring (EEG, electrooculogram [EOG], electromyogram [EMG], and electrocardiogram [ECG]) during a series of 4 or 5 sessions spaced at 2-hour intervals throughout the day. During the MSLT, the patient is asked to nap during each of the sessions, and quantitative information is provided about both average sleep latency and abnormalities of sleep-onset transition. During the MWT, the patient is asked to remain awake during each session, and the occurrence of any sleep episodes is documented. The MSLT must be performed the day after an overnight polysomnogram to permit meaningful analysis of the results. The MWT is performed after a typical night of sleep in the home environment or during polysomnography.

15. **What is the normal sleep latency during the MSLT?**
Normal people usually have a mean sleep latency (time from onset of a nap session until the first appearance of any stage of sleep) of 10 to 20 min when studied on their usual sleep/wake schedule.

16. **Can medications alter the results of polysomnography and MSLT?**
Many drugs (e.g., hypnotics, sedatives, tranquilizers, and stimulants) can significantly alter the results of these procedures. In particular, both periods of drug initiation and acute withdrawal are often associated with major alterations of sleep characteristics, and the resultant patterns may mimic other sleep disorders, including narcolepsy. If possible, discontinue central nervous system (CNS)-active drugs for 2 weeks or more before diagnostic studies. When this is not possible, such drugs should be continued at constant and stable levels for at least 2 weeks prior to testing. Patients should never be told simply to refrain from taking a medication on the night of a study or for several nights before the examination, and this approach may invalidate the results.

17. **What are the major indications for polysomnography?**
Polysomnography is required for the diagnosis of sleep-related breathing disorders such as obstructive sleep apnea syndrome, for titration of nasal continuous positive airway pressure (CPAP) as therapy of obstructive sleep apnea, to evaluate for possible narcolepsy or idiopathic hypersomnia (combined with the MSLT), and to evaluate sleep-related behaviors that are violent or otherwise potentially injurious to the patient or others. Polysomnography may also be indicated to evaluate patients with neuromuscular disorders who have sleep-related symptoms, to assist with the diagnosis of paroxysmal arousals, or to confirm a clinical suspicion of periodic limb movement disorder.

## HYPERSOMNIAS

18. **What is the most common medical condition associated with excessive daytime sleepiness and sleep at inappropriate times?**
The obstructive sleep apnea syndrome. Sleep onset is associated with increased upper airway resistance, and partial or complete airway obstruction occurs intermittently. The patient is usually aroused within a short time by ensuing hypoxia or hypercapnia, as well as by the increased effort associated with attempts to breathe. These events typically recur throughout the nocturnal sleep period causing repeated arousals, and the resultant sleep fragmentation is presumably the basis for the daytime sleepiness. Pronounced oxygen desaturation may occur during obstructive events, and cause potentially life-threatening cardiac arrhythmias. This condition affects 2% to 4% of the adult population, and is under-recognized. The polysomnographic characteristics permit a conclusive diagnosis of this condition and also provide a measure of its severity.

19. **How can obstructive sleep apnea be treated?**
Therapy must be directed toward correction of the airway obstruction (which can result from anatomic factors or abnormal relaxation of musculature in the oropharynx). Administration of CPAP by means of a nasal mask is currently the most frequently used therapeutic modality. Surgical procedures are effective in some cases, particularly when a discrete structural factor producing airway obstruction can be demonstrated. In some cases, significant improvement is achieved by preventing sleep in the supine position or by elevation of the head and trunk (positional therapy). Tongue-retaining devices and other dental appliances are beneficial in a small number of instances, particularly when the respiratory disturbance is mild. Weight loss is often beneficial in patients who are obese. Alcohol should be avoided because it may increase the degree of upper airway obstruction during sleep and it serves to fragment sleep.
    Sanders MH, Redline S: Obstructive sleep apnea/hypopnea syndrome. Curr Treat Options Neurol 1:279-290, 1999.

20. **How does the obstructive sleep apnea syndrome differ between adults and children?**
Most adults with obstructive sleep apnea syndrome experience daytime sleepiness, whereas children tend to experience behavioral changes such as inattentiveness, distractibility, irritability, and overactivity. The most common anatomic finding in children is enlarged tonsils and adenoids, while most adults have no tonsillar hypertrophy. Obesity is common among adults and adolescents with obstructive sleep apnea, but a significant number of young children have normal weight or even failure to thrive. Children most frequently have obstructive hypopnea or hypoventilation, whereas adults are more likely to have obstructive apnea. The nocturnal sleep pattern is typically highly fragmented in adults but children may have fewer respiratory-related arousals than adults.

21. **What conditions predispose a child to obstructive sleep apnea?**
Tonsillar and adenoidal hypertrophy are strong risk factors in children. A number of neurogenetic disorders also predispose children to obstructive sleep apnea including Down's syndrome, Prader-Willi syndrome, muscular dystrophy and other myopathies, Arnold-Chiari malformations and other structural abnormalities involving the brain stem, Pierre-Robin syndrome and other craniofacial malformations, and achondroplasia. As in adults, obesity also represents a risk factor for obstructive sleep apnea in children.

22. **What is the classic narcoleptic tetrad?**
Narcolepsy is the most familiar neurologic condition associated with episodes of sleep at inappropriate times, although it is probable that many people diagnosed with this condition in the past actually had obstructive sleep apnea or one of the other conditions associated with disturbed nocturnal sleep. The classic narcoleptic tetrad is: excessive sleepiness, cataplexy, sleep paralysis, and hypnagogic hallucinations. No more than 50% of patients meeting current criteria for the diagnosis of narcolepsy exhibit all the four symptoms, and 90% lack at least one symptom.

23. **How is cataplexy defined?**
Cataplexy is a condition characterized by sudden episodes of muscular weakness or paralysis, without loss of consciousness, precipitated by emotional changes such as laughter, excitement, or anger. Episodes typically last from a few seconds to several minutes and sometimes are terminated by a direct transition to sleep.

## KEY POINTS: SLEEP DISORDERS

1. A very common cause of excessive daytime sleepiness and/or episodes of sleep that occur at inappropriate times is the obstructive sleep apnea syndrome.

2. A patient's own assessment of sleep quantity and quality is often unreliable. Polysomnographic evaluation (sleep laboratory testing) is the only reliable means for obtaining objective information regarding a suspected sleep disturbance.

3. Objective confirmation of suspected excessive daytime sleepiness requires an MSLT conducted during the day following an overnight polysomnogram.

4. A definitive diagnosis of narcolepsy with cataplexy requires subjective and objective evidence of excessive daytime sleepiness, the presence of unequivocal cataplexy, demonstration of two or more sleep-onset stage REM episodes on the MSLT, and an absence of other conditions that produce severe disruption of the nocturnal sleep pattern.

5. Sleep disorders pose significantly elevated risks, including those for automobile-related and job-related accidents associated with hypersomnia conditions, and injuries related to falls and other trauma associated with parasomnias.

6. The classic narcoleptic tetrad is: excessive daytime sleepiness, cataplexy, sleep paralysis, and hypnagogic hallucinations.

24. **What are the features of sleep paralysis?**
It is characterized by a transient inability to move voluntarily, either near the time of sleep onset or during an arousal. Consciousness is maintained, and the person may experience severe anxiety as well as hallucinatory images or dream-like mentation. Eye and respiratory movements are not impaired. The condition disappears spontaneously within a few seconds to minutes but may be terminated immediately by external stimulation. A transition to sleep may occur during the event.

25. **Is the occurrence of sleep paralysis pathognomonic of narcolepsy?**
No. Although sleep paralysis is often a manifestation of narcolepsy, it is sometimes seen as an independent entity in the absence of other signs of narcolepsy. It may occur sporadically or in a familial form. In some people, this phenomenon may occur more frequently in the presence of sleep deprivation or other sleep disturbance. Although sleep paralysis is typically identified by its symptoms, a sleep study may be required to rule out narcolepsy or the presence of another sleep disorder that triggers sleep paralysis through sleep disruption. Treatment is usually not required, although if the condition is frequent or results in a high degree of anxiety, treatment may be indicated. Tricyclic antidepressant (TCA) medications and selective serotonin reuptake inhibitors (SSRIs) often are effective.

26. **Do hypnagogic hallucinations occur during REM sleep?**
No. They occur during sleep-wake transitions, either when falling asleep or during arousals, and can involve various sensory modalities (most commonly visual). Although this entity is typically observed in association with narcolepsy, it occasionally occurs in normal people.

27. **List the crucial diagnostic criteria for narcolepsy.**
The current ICSD (2005) diagnostic criteria for **narcolepsy with cataplexy** include the following: (1) a complaint of excessive daytime sleepiness occurring almost daily for at least three months; and (2) a definitive history of cataplexy (defined as sudden and transient loss of muscle tone triggered by emotions). The diagnosis of narcolepsy with cataplexy should be

confirmed whenever possible by nocturnal polysomnography followed by the MSLT. The mean sleep latency on the MSLT is less than or equal to eight minutes and two or more sleep onset REM periods are present. Alternatively, CSF hypocretin-1 levels less than 110 pg/mL or one third of mean normal control values are present.

The current ICSD (2005) diagnostic criteria for narcolepsy without cataplexy include the following: (1) a complaint of excessive daytime sleepiness occurring almost daily for at least three months; (2) typical cataplexy is not present (atypical or doubtful cataplexy may exist); and (3) diagnosis must be confirmed by nocturnal polysomnography followed by an MSLT. As with narcolepsy with cataplexy, the mean sleep latency must be eight minutes or less with two or more sleep onset REM episodes on the MSLT.

For both narcolepsy with cataplexy and narcolepsy without cataplexy, the hypersomnia is not better explained by another sleep disorder, medical or neurological disorder, mental disorder, medication use, or substance abuse disorder. Although often present, *HLA-DQB1*0602* or *HLA-DR2* positivity are not required diagnostic criteria for narcolepsy.

28. **Is the cause of narcolepsy known?**
Recent investigations suggest that dysfunction of the hypothalamic hypocretin/orexin system is involved in the pathophysiology of narcolepsy. Animal studies have demonstrated that gene abnormalities resulting in either a lack of the hypocretin/orexin peptide or its receptor result in narcolepsy. While analogous genetic abnormalities are apparently very rare in human cases, several studies have reported low or undetectable cerebrospinal fluid (CSF) levels of the peptide in the majority of patients with unambiguous narcolepsy. This suggests that narcolepsy could be a result of acquired cell death affecting hypocretin neurons within the hypothalamus.
   Nishino S: Narcolepsy. Biol Psychiatry 54:87-95, 2003.

29. **Can narcolepsy be treated successfully?**
Excessive daytime sleepiness can often be controlled with stimulant medications (e.g., methylphenidate, dextroamphetamine) and/or modafinil (a stimulant-like medication). The amount of medication required can sometimes be reduced by prescribing several (typically 2 or 3) regularly scheduled short naps during the day. Cataplexy and sleep paralysis are often treated successfully with tricyclic antidepressants (e.g., imipramine, protriptyline) or selective serotonin reuptake inhibitors (e.g., fluoxetine). Sodium oxybate (a derivative of gamma-hydroxybutyrate) is effective for treatment of daytime sleepiness and cataplexy. It is administered at night at sleep onset and again midway through the sleep period.
   Mahmood M, Black J: Narcolepsy-Cataplexy: How does recent understanding help us in evaluation and treatment? Curr Treat Options Neurol 7:363-371, 2005.

30. **Are any other conditions, besides narcolepsy and sleep apnea, typically associated with excessive daytime somnolence?**
Yes, as indicated in Table 21-4, a number of specific disorders can be associated with excessive sleepiness and episodes of sleep at inappropriate times. In addition, daytime somnolence can be a secondary manifestation of many other medical conditions.

31. **Is HLA typing useful in the diagnosis of narcolepsy?**
It is of very limited value. Nearly 100% of confirmed narcoleptic patients have been found to be HLA-DR2 and HLA-DQ1 (including DR15 and DQ6)-positive in several studies. The DQB1*0602 marker (a subtype of DQ6) has been reported to be the most specific such marker for narcolepsy among various ethnic populations, and patients with narcolepsy/cataplexy are nearly always positive. However, the HLA test is of limited diagnostic value because 10% to 35% of the general population is also positive for these markers. Conversely, negativity for these HLA subtypes, although rare, does not entirely exclude the presence of narcolepsy.
   Mignot E: Genetic and familial aspects of narcolepsy. Neurology 50:S16-S22, 1998.

| TABLE 21–4. DISORDERS OFTEN ASSOCIATED WITH EXCESSIVE DAYTIME SLEEPINESS | |
|---|---|
| Narcolepsy | Obstructive sleep apnea |
| Periodic limb movement disorder | Mood disorders (depression) |
| Central sleep apnea | Cerebral degenerative disorders |
| Insufficient nocturnal sleep syndrome | Dementia |
| Circadian rhythm disorders | Trypanosomiasis |
| Drug or alcohol dependency | Idiopathic hypersomnia |
| Toxin-induced sleep disorder | Posttraumatic hypersomnia |
| Diencephalic lesions | Hydrocephalus |
| Recurrent hypersomnia (e.g., Kleine-Levin syndrome) | |

32. **Identify the most significant risk factor common to all conditions associated with excessive daytime sleepiness.**
   People with hypersomnia conditions are at a significantly increased risk for death or serious injury as a result of motor vehicle-related and job-related accidents.

33. **Can individuals with hypersomnia conditions safely resume driving and other potentially dangerous activities?**
   The physician should recommend that such activities be avoided until there is evidence that the causative condition has been adequately controlled, and that there is proper compliance with treatment. This is especially important if the individual is employed in an area that affects public safety (e.g., pilots, air traffic controllers, bus and truck drivers, and those involved with nuclear power plants). In many cases, objective testing, including repeat polysomnography, MSLT, and/or the MWT may be necessary to assess response to treatment.

## INSOMNIAS

34. **How is insomnia defined?**
   Insomnia is a subjective symptom characterized by the perception that sleep is inadequate or nonrestorative. It includes complaints of a low total sleep time, difficulty in falling asleep, frequent awakenings, or unrefreshing sleep. It is a common symptom and is associated with a wide spectrum of underlying medical conditions as well as with specific sleep disorders.
   Sateia MJ, Doghramji K, Hauri PH, Morin CM: Evaluation of chronic insomnia: An American Academy of Sleep Medicine review. Sleep 23:243-308, 2000.

35. **Describe an appropriate treatment protocol for psychophysiologic insomnia.**
   1. Establish a regular and fixed sleep period, with a consistent bedtime and rise time. The sleep period should be long enough to permit adequate sleep time (typically 8 hours for an adult) but no longer.
   2. Avoid daytime napping.
   3. Minimize concern about inability to sleep.
   4. Establish a regular, daily program of exercise, but do not exercise immediately before bedtime.
   5. Avoid excessive consumption of caffeine and alcohol, and exclude these substances entirely during the evening before bedtime.

6. Ensure that the sleeping environment is optimal with regard to noise and temperature.
7. Avoid use of medication to induce sleep.
8. Obtain behavioral therapy (e.g., cognitive-behavioral or relaxation therapy) if indicated.
   Dundar Y, Dodd S, Strobl J, et al.: Comparative efficacy of newer hypnotic drugs for the short-term management of insomnia: A systematic review and meta-analysis. Hum Psychopharmacol 19:305-322, 2004.

## KEY POINTS: LEADING CAUSES OF INSOMNIA

1. Psychophysiological factors

2. Circadian rhythm disturbances (time zone change syndrome, shift work)

3. Underlying medical or psychiatric disorders (e.g., anxiety, depression)

4. Periodic limb movement disorder

5. Drug or alcohol dependency

6. Irregular or improper sleep habits (poor sleep hygiene)

7. Obstructive sleep apnea syndrome

36. **What is the time zone change syndrome?**
    This condition, commonly known as jet lag, is characterized by insomnia, associated with daytime fatigue and various somatic symptoms, and begins immediately after rapid travel across several time zones. It results from loss of proper synchronization between the endogenous circadian timing system of the brain and external environmental cues (primarily day and night cycles).

37. **Can the time zone change syndrome be prevented?**
    While some people adapt without difficulty, others (particularly those older than 50 years) experience a prolonged period of disturbed sleep. Symptoms can be prevented, or at least minimized, by doing the following:
    1. Immediately adopt a sleep-wake schedule appropriate for the new environment.
    2. Avoid prolonged napping immediately after arrival in a new location. A mild degree of sleep deprivation the first day facilitates adaptation to the new environment.
    3. Spend some time outdoors in bright light during the daytime on the first few days after arrival. This facilitates resetting of the circadian clock.
    4. Avoid excessive use of caffeine and alcohol.
    5. Avoid use of sleep medications.

## PARASOMNIAS

38. **Describe the major characteristics of sleep terrors.**
    Sleep terrors, also known as parvor nocturnus, are episodes of apparent intense fear, often associated with crying or screaming, that occur during arousal from non-REM (typically N3) sleep. These events are characteristically accompanied by elevated heart and respiratory rates, and the patient may exhibit confusion and disorientation. Amnesia is most common, although some people later recall brief dream-like images. This condition is very common in children between 4 and 12 years of age but may persist into the adult years. Episodes typically

end spontaneously after several minutes but attempts to awaken the person may prolong the duration of sleep terrors. Treatment is usually unnecessary, but is sometimes indicated when episodes become frequent or if risk of injury is high. Benzodiazepines are often effective for short-term use.

39. **What are the key features of the periodic limb movement disorder?**
The periodic limb movement disorder, formerly called nocturnal myoclonus, is characterized by frequent clusters of extremity movements (typically the legs, but occasionally the arms) that tend to recur periodically during sleep at intervals of 10 to 90 seconds for an extended time. When these events produce arousal, as they often do, the sleep pattern may be severely disrupted, and the patient may experience significant daytime sleepiness. The patient is typically unaware of the nocturnal limb movements, but this condition is readily apparent during sleep laboratory evaluation (polysomnography), and its severity can be quantitatively assessed.

40. **How would you manage a patient with the periodic limb movement disorder?**
This disorder is typically resistant to therapy, but pramipexole and certain other dopaminergics (e.g., ʟ-dopa, bromocriptine, and pergolide) have been demonstrated to decrease the number of abnormal limb movements and improve daytime symptoms in several studies, although side effects and loss of effectiveness are relatively common. Clonazepam may reduce the number of nocturnal arousals associated with the limb movements (even though the actual number of movements may remain essentially the same). Additional medications that have been reported to be useful include other benzodiazepines (e.g., diazepam, temazepam, and triazolam), opiates (e.g., codeine, propoxyphene, and oxycodone), carbamazepine, and clonidine.

41. **Which sleep disorders are associated with paroxysmal episodes of abnormal motor activity that might sometimes be confused with epileptic seizures?**
    1. REM sleep behavior disorder
    2. Sleepwalking and other arousal disorders
    3. Rhythmic movement disorder (head banging)

42. **Describe the key clinical and polysomnographic features of sleepwalking.**
Sleepwalking is a complex behavior (walking, sitting up in bed, talking, etc.) that occurs during non-REM sleep (typically beginning in stage N3). It occurs most frequently early in the night but may occur at other times. The patient is difficult to awaken, appears confused, and usually is amnesic for the event. It occurs most commonly in children (3 to 10 years) but may occur in older people. Some medications and medical conditions (such as febrile illness) can induce or potentiate sleepwalking. Because serious accidental injury may result during these episodes (especially when sleep running occurs), patients of all ages should be protected by appropriate safety precautions. Although drug treatment is usually not necessary, benzodiazepines (e.g., diazepam or clonazepam) are often effective, especially for short-term use.

43. **What is the cause of nocturnal paroxysmal dystonia?**
This is a disorder characterized by repeated dystonic or dyskinetic episodes during or immediately after arousal from non-REM sleep or, more rarely, during wakefulness. Episodes typically last less than 1 minute but can be prolonged (reportedly up to 1 hour). Movements are often relatively violent and may result in injury to the patient or bed partner. Patients typically do not recall these events after arousal. This condition has been reported in both children and adults. Although episodes may not be associated with abnormal EEG findings, this condition is now considered by many to represent a form of localization-related epilepsy. The possibility that this condition is of epileptic origin is supported by the observation that carbamazepine is efficacious in many instances.

44. **How can you distinguish the REM sleep behavior disorder from other conditions associated with atypical nocturnal events?**
This condition is typified by episodes of complex, often violent, and high amplitude motor activity during periods of REM sleep that appear to represent enactment of dream mentation as a result of loss of normal inhibitory mechanisms originating in the brain stem. Patients often kick or punch repeatedly and may jump from the bed and run through the bedroom, frequently colliding with furniture or walls. Injuries to the patient and bed partner are common. Although full-blown episodes may occur infrequently, atypical movements and abnormally increased EMG tonic activity are typically present during REM periods, as demonstrated during polysomnographic testing. Patients often recall the dream content after the event is over.

45. **Is the REM sleep behavior disorder responsive to medical therapy?**
Clonazepam is often efficacious in eliminating or significantly reducing the frequency of episodes. However, patients should be advised to take safety precautions to minimize injury if an occasional episode does occur. Some cases are idiopathic, but a significant number are associated with specific neurologic disorders (e.g., Parkinson's disease, ischemic cerebrovascular disease, olivopontocerebellar degeneration, multiple sclerosis, brain stem neoplasm), which may require other therapeutic interventions. REM sleep behavior disorder may also occur in association with use of certain medications including the SSRIs and TCAs, and alcohol withdrawal.

46. **Describe restless legs syndrome (RLS).**
It is characterized by unpleasant sensations in the lower (and occasionally the upper) extremities before sleep onset (and sometimes at other times as well) that produce a strong urge to move the limbs. This sensation is typically described as a "crawling" or "creeping" feeling, and it disappears temporarily when the involved extremities are moved, only to recur within a few seconds. The symptoms last from minutes to several hours and can significantly delay sleep onset, with resultant sleep deprivation. Many patients also experience periodic limb movements during sleep. The cause is unknown, and the condition is typically long-term, although gradual improvement is sometimes observed.

Ohayon MM, Caulet M, Priest RG: Violent behavior during sleep. J Clin Psychiatry 58:369-376, 1997.

47. **Can restless legs syndrome be successfully managed by medication?**
Medications reported to be beneficial include dopaminergics (e.g., L-dopa, bromocriptine, pramipexole, and pergolide), opiates (e.g., codeine, propoxyphene, and oxycodone), and benzodiazepines (clonazepam, diazepam, triazolam, temazepam, and nitrazepam). Both idiopathic (presumably genetic) and symptomatic forms of this disorder are recognized. Common symptomatic forms include those associated with iron deficiency, pregnancy, and metabolic dysfunction such as renal failure. Resolution of these latter conditions may also alleviate the associated symptoms of the restless legs syndrome. Avoidance of caffeine may help minimize the severity of symptoms due to RLS.

Mahowald MW: Restless leg syndrome and periodic limb movements of sleep. Curr Treat Options Neurol 5:251-260, 2003.

48. **What sleep disorders or problems occur with increased frequency during pregnancy?**
Restless legs syndrome and obstructive sleep apnea syndrome occur more frequently during pregnancy than in the nonpregnant state. Insomnia (difficulty initiating or maintaining sleep) and hypersomnia are also common during pregnancy. This latter disorder may be due to a variety of causes or contributing factors.

49. **What are the common medicolegal issues that arise in caring for patients with sleep disorders?**
Patients with hypersomnias, such as obstructive sleep apnea and narcolepsy, are at increased risk for accidents, and should be counseled about avoidance of driving and other potentially dangerous activities during periods of drowsiness. Patients and family members should be counseled regarding safety precautions for individuals with sleepwalking, REM sleep behavior disorder, and rhythmic movement disorders. In some cases, this may involve physical barriers and, in REM sleep behavior disorder, it may be necessary for the bed partner to sleep in a different bed. Individuals who receive zolpidem, especially in combination with alcohol, may experience prolonged sleepwalking and other complex behaviors such as driving an automobile during sleep.

# WEBSITE

1. http://www.aasmnet.org

# BIBLIOGRAPHY

1. Ambrogetti A, Hensley MJ, Olson LG (eds): Sleep Disorders: A Clinical Textbook. London, Quay Books, 2007

2. Iber C, Ancoli-Israel S, Chesson A, Quan SF for the American Academy of Sleep Medicine: The AASM MAnual for the Scoring of Sleep and Associated Events: Rules, Terminology, and Technical Specifications. Westchester Illinois, American Academy of Sleep Medicine, 2007.

3. International Classification of Sleep Disorders, Second Edition: Diagnostic and Coding Manual (ICSD-2). Westchester, Illinois, American Academy of Sleep Medicine, 2005.

4. Kryger MH, Roth T, Dement WC: Principles and Practice of Sleep Medicine, 4th ed. Philadelphia, W.B. Saunders, 2005.

5. Kushida CA: Sleep Deprivation: Basic Science, Physiology, and Behavior. New York, Marcel Dekker, 2005.

# CHAPTER 22

# NEUROLOGIC COMPLICATIONS OF SYSTEMIC DISEASE

*Ericka P. Simpson, MD*

## CARDIAC DISEASE

**1. What is the major neurologic complication of cardiac disease?**

Stroke is the most common neurologic sequela of cardiac disease. The risks for embolic, thrombotic, and hemorrhagic strokes are elevated in the presence of cardiac disease. Nonvalvular atrial fibrillation, followed by ischemic heart disease and valvular heart disease are the most common types of cardiac abnormalities causing embolic ischemic strokes. Infective endocarditis is most frequently associated with hemorrhagic strokes. The presence of a patent foramen ovale is a less common but noteworthy risk factor for thromboembolic stroke in patients of all ages.

> Vahedi K, Amarenco P: Cardiac causes of stroke. Curr Treat Options Neurol 2:305-318, 2000.

**2. What is the association between transient ischemic attack (TIA) and myocardial infarction (MI)?**

Patients who suffer a TIA are more likely to suffer a fatal MI than a stroke, although the stroke incidence is three times higher in those who suffer from a TIA. All patients who have suffered a mild stroke or TIA should undergo careful cardiac assessment as soon as possible.

> Atanassova PA, Chalakova NT, Dimitrov BD: Major vascular events after transient ischaemic attack and minor ischaemic stroke: Post hoc modelling of incidence dynamics. Cerebrovasc Dis 25:225-233, 2008.

**3. What is the association between sleep, MI, and stroke?**

In the stage of sleep associated with rapid eye movements (REM sleep), profound changes in centrally mediated sympathetic activity occur. These large changes in autonomic output are manifest by smaller increases in blood pressure and heart rate, skin conductance changes, momentary restorations in muscle tone, mesenteric and renal vasodilation, and skeletal muscle vasoconstriction. In the elderly, it is hypothesized that large fluctuations in sympathetic activity associated with REM sleep also cause increased rates of arrhythmia and increased risk for cardiac vasospasm and subsequent stroke and MI. The presence of heart rate abnormalities during sleep in normotensive patients is also reported as a predictor of future cardiovascular disease.

> Plante GE: Sleep and vascular disorders. Metabolism 55(10 Suppl 2):S45-S49, 2006.
> Somers VK, Dyken ME, Mark AL, Abboud FM: Sympathetic nerve activity during sleep in normal subjects. N Engl J Med 328:303-307, 1993.

**4. What are the non-stroke-related neurologic complications of cardiac disease?**

Cardiac arrhythmias (especially sick sinus syndrome) may produce decreased cardiac output, causing syncope, and, rarely, encephalopathy. Cerebral blood flow can be altered due to changes in cerebral autoregulation caused by abnormal autonomic vagal activity associated with cardiac disease. Persistent decreased brain perfusion, such as in the case of cardiac arrest or cardiogenic shock, may lead to laminar necrosis of the cerebral cortex or hippocampus.

## GASTROINTESTINAL DISEASE

5. **What is the major cause of neurologic symptoms associated with gastrointestinal (GI) disease?**
   Most known neurologic complications of GI disease are the consequence of malabsorption of essential nutrients and vitamins. The consequences of some nutrient deficiencies have been well described, including those involving thiamine, folate, cyanocobalamin, niacin, vitamin D, vitamin E, and copper.

   Henri-Bhargava A, Melmed C, Glikstein R, Schipper HM: Neurologic impairment due to vitamin E and copper deficiencies in celiac disease. Neurology 71:860-861, 2008.

6. **What are the neurologic manifestations of celiac disease?**
   Celiac disease, or gluten enteropathy, is an autoimmune disease of the small intestine that produces chronic small bowel malabsorption of nutrients and vitamins, often with iron deficiency anemia, osteoporosis and osteomalacia, and hypoalbuminemia. Individuals with the disease are intolerant to gluten proteins that are present in rye, wheat, barley, and in some adhesives, including that of stamps and envelopes. Ten percent of affected patients have neurologic complaints, the most notable being cerebellar dysfunction secondary to chronic fat malabsorption. Tremor, intranuclear ophthalmoplegia, encephalopathy, subacute combined degeneration, seizures, or myopathy are other features associated with the disease. The observed myopathy is often treatable by vitamin D replacement.

   Baldassarre M, Laneve AM, Grosso R, Laforgia N: Celiac disease: Pathogenesis and novel therapeutic strategies. Endocr Metab Immune Disord Drug Targets 8:152-158, 2008.

   Beyenburg S, Scheid B, Deckert-Schluter M, Lagreze HL: Chronic progressive leukoencephalopathy in adult celiac disease. Neurology 50:820-822, 1998.

7. **What is the triad of neurologic clinical features associated with Whipple's disease?**
   Whipple's disease is a multisystem granulomatous infection caused by *Tropheryma whippelii*. Neurologic complaints develop in 10% of afflicted patients. The common triad of findings includes ocular disturbance (often ophthalmoparesis), gait ataxia, and dementia. Other associated abnormalities include seizures, myelopathy, meningoencephalitis, autonomic dysfunction, and steroid-unresponsive myopathy. Effective treatment involves antibiotic therapy directed against the organism. Untreated, most patients die within 1 year of the onset of neurologic symptoms.

8. **What is the triad of neurologic complaints associated with Wernicke's encephalopathy?**
   Wernicke's encephalopathy is associated with thiamine deficiency. Clinical symptoms include a triad of ophthalmoparesis, gait ataxia, and disturbances of mental function. An axonal sensorimotor neuropathy appears in half of patients with this deficiency state, and Korsakoff's psychosis (dementia associated with profound amnesia and confabulation) is also variably present. The mortality associated with Wernicke's encephalopathy is still greater than 10%, although this is more due to concomitant infections and malnutrition than to the neurologic disorders.

9. **What is known about the etiology of nervous system impairment associated with $B_{12}$ malabsorption?**
   The deficiency of methionine synthetase activity secondary to absence of its cofactor ($B_{12}$) leads to accumulation of homocysteine. The resulting impairment in DNA synthesis is responsible for the megaloblastic anemia associated with $B_{12}$ deficiency, while neurologic abnormalities are the result of failure to maintain methionine biosynthesis.

10. **What are the neurologic manifestations of vitamin B$_{12}$ deficiency?**
Neurologic manifestations of B$_{12}$ deficiency include cognitive, behavioral dysfunction, myelopathy, and peripheral neuropathy. Patients may manifest slowed cerebration, dementia, or delirium (with or without delusion), while others exhibit depression, amnesia, or acute psychotic states. Rare cases of reversible manic or schizophreniform states have also been reported. B$_{12}$ deficiency also can result in subacute combined degeneration of the spinal cord due to dorsal and lateral column involvement, and sensorimotor neuropathy. Copper deficiency due to small bowel malabsorption or zinc overconsumption can produce a similar neurologic presentation.

So YT, Simon RP: Deficiency diseases of the nervous system. In Bradley WG, Daroff RB, Fenichel G, Jankovic J (eds): Neurology in Clinical Practice, 3rd ed. Boston, Butterworth-Heinemann, 2000, pp 1495-1509.

Winston GP, Jaiser SR: Copper deficiency myelopathy and subacute combined degeneration of the cord - why is the phenotype so similar? Med Hypotheses 71:229-236, 2008.

11. **Which vitamin deficiencies cause different neurologic syndromes in children than in adults?**
**Lack of absorption of vitamin D** from the intestinal tract leads to rickets in children and osteomalacia in adults. In children with rickets, neurologic sequelae include head shaking, nystagmus, and increased irritability that may evolve into tetany with a sufficient fall in serum calcium concentrations. **Malabsorption of folate** in infants leads to mental retardation, seizures, and athetotic movements, whereas in adults, polyneuropathy and depression are the primary complications. **Pyridoxine deficiency** leads to seizures in infants, but a sensory polyneuropathy in adults.

12. **Malabsorption of which vitamins will lead to an increased risk for subdural hematoma?**
Malabsorption of vitamin C or vitamin K results in an increased tendency for hemorrhage, especially following trauma. Lack of thiamine, vitamin B$_{12}$, or vitamin E all can result in ataxia, with an increased tendency for falls and head trauma.

13. **Besides thiamine, malabsorption or dietary lack of which vitamin may produce a syndrome resembling Korsakoff's dementia?**
Nicotinic acid deficiency results in pellagra, whose major and often sole manifestation is psychiatric disturbance, sometimes mimicking Korsakoff's psychosis.

## HEPATIC DISEASE

14. **What are the five major neurologic syndromes associated with hepatic dysfunction?**
   1. Encephalopathy
   2. Hepatocerebral degeneration
   3. Wilson's disease
   4. Reye's syndrome
   5. Intracranial hemorrhage (ICH)

15. **What causes hepatic encephalopathy?**
This complication may occur with hepatic failure or with portal or hepatic circulatory dysfunction, as caused by acute or chronic hepatitis, hepatic necrosis, cirrhosis, or portocaval anastomosis. The exact cause for neuropsychiatric features is unknown, but ammonia is considered an important toxin, precipitating encephalopathy by increasing glutamine and

gamma-aminobutyric acid (GABA), and playing a significant role in oxidative damage of RNA species in neuronal and astroglial cells. Other undefined endogenous toxins appear to affect central neurotransmission, especially of the dopaminergic and GABA-ergic systems. Reduction in the serum concentration of ammonia, or addition of centrally acting GABA antagonists may temporarily improve hepatic encephalopathy, although correction of the precipitating causes of hepatic dysfunction is necessary for ultimate recovery.

Görg B, Qvartskhava N, Keitel V, et al.: Ammonia induces RNA oxidation in cultured astrocytes and brain in vivo. Hepatology 48:567-579, 2008.

Lockwood AH: Hepatic encephalopathy. In Aminoff MJ (ed): Neurology and General Medicine, 2nd ed. New York, Churchill-Livingstone, 1995.

16. **How is hepatic encephalopathy treated?**
Acute therapy for hepatic encephalopathy requires removal or blockade of neurologically acting toxins produced in the gut. Reduction of protein intake with lactulose therapy to enhance ammonia excretion and reduce ammonia absorption is the mainstay of therapy. Oral antibiotics, such as neomycin, and amino acids L-ornithine and L-aspartate, are used as second-line agents to reduce gut bacterial levels and ammonia formation. Long-term treatment of hepatic encephalopathy by medical therapies has only limited success, depending on whether the hepatic damage is reversible, static, or progressive. Ultimately, the most effective therapy involves treatments directed at reversing the hepatic failure, including surgical shunting procedures and liver transplantation for selected individuals.

Dhiman RK, Chawla YK: Minimal hepatic encephalopathy: Time to recognise and treat. Trop Gastroenterol 29:6-12, 2008.

Lockwood AH, Weissenborn R, Butterworth RF: An image of the brain in patients with liver disease. Curr Opin Neurol 10:525-533, 1997.

17. **What is Reye's syndrome?**
Reye's syndrome is a rare acute noninflammatory encephalopathy that primarily affects children and adolescents. A correlation between the disease and a preceding viral infection (especially influenza and varicella) treated with salicylates has been reported, although other toxic, metabolic, or hypoxic insults may play roles in the pathogenesis. Hyperammonemia, hypoglycemia, coagulopathy, and cerebral edema with hypoxia may be associated. Treatment is supportive and includes administration of intravenous glucose to prevent hypoglycemia, and in severe cases, hyperventilation and intravenous mannitol to reduce intracranial pressure.

Defects in fatty acid oxidation, such as medium-chain acyl coenzyme A dehydrogenase deficiency, can also present as a Reye-like syndrome and may be more common than Reye's syndrome, warranting a work-up for inborn errors of metabolism in affected children.

Gosalakkal JA, Kamoji V: Reye syndrome and Reye-like syndrome. Pediatr Neurol 39:198-200, 2008.

Smith TC: Reye's syndrome and the use of aspirin. Scott Med J 41:4-9, 1996.

18. **In addition to hepatic encephalopathy, what other diseases cause asterixis?**
Asterixis, or flapping tremor, is best elicited by the extension of outstretched, opened hands. It results from the acute loss of muscle tone or contraction associated with passive or active hand/wrist extension, most likely induced by pathologic coupling of the thalamus and motor cortex. This sign is encountered in many metabolic encephalopathies, including uremia, malnutrition, severe pulmonary disease, and polycythemia rubra vera.

Timmerman L, Gross J, Butz M, et al.: Mini-asterixis in hepatic encephalopathy induced by pathologic thalamo-motor-cortical coupling. Neurology 61:689-692, 2003.

**19. What electroencephalographic (EEG) abnormality is associated with hepatic encephalopathy?**

Slow triphasic waves are the abnormal EEG pattern reported with hepatic encephalopathy and the pattern is commonly used to support the diagnosis. It can also be seen with encephalopathy associated with head trauma (especially with subdural hematoma), acute cerebral anoxia, uremia, electrolyte imbalance, and thyrotoxicosis.

**20. What are the neurologic manifestations of Wilson's disease?**

Wilson's disease is a rare disorder of copper metabolism resulting in accumulation of copper in the liver, kidneys, and central nervous system (CNS). In almost half of patients, neurologic manifestations are present, including tremors, dysarthria, clumsiness, drooling, and gait instability in order of decreasing frequency. Psychiatric symptoms, including those of dementia, mania, depression, or schizophrenia, may dominate the presentation in up to 20% of patients. Kaiser-Fleischer rings, copper deposits in Descemet's membrane of the cornea, are present in 98% of patients with neurologic manifestations and are visualized by slit-lamp examination. Neurologic manifestations invariably follow liver involvement, even in silent, unrecognized liver disease.

El-Youssef M: Wilson disease. Mayo Clin Proc 78:1126-1136, 2003.

**21. What is the treatment for Wilson's disease?**

Early diagnosis and copper chelation therapy are the mainstays of therapy. The chelation therapy of choice is oral D-penicillamine and is considered the gold standard of therapy. Penicillamine should be administered concomitantly with pyridoxine to prevent vitamin $B_6$ deficiency. Side effects include rash, fever, thrombocytopenia, relative eosinophilia with total leukopenia, and reversible lupus-like and myasthenia-gravis-like syndromes. Trientene and zinc acetate are alternative agents with fewer side effects. Liver transplantation is recommended in patients with fulminant hepatic failure and end-stage liver cirrhosis but is not generally recommended for patients with neurologic disease without pronounced liver involvement.

**22. What are the neurologic complications of hemochromatosis?**

Hemochromatosis is a disorder of iron overload resulting in multi-organ fibrosis and dysfunction. Acquired causes are usually because of excess total body iron due to multiple blood transfusions. Hereditary hemochromatosis is due to mutations in a gene (*HFE* gene), which encodes for a protein involved in the regulation of GI iron absorption and uptake. Encephalopathy, truncal ataxia, and rigidity may all complicate hemochromatosis and invariably are due to liver disease (liver cirrhosis and failure) resulting from massive iron deposition in the liver. Neuritis is either a complication of the diabetes mellitus (DM) that accompanies most cases of hemochromatosis, or is a result of local iron deposition.

Treatment requires serial phlebotomies four to six times per year. Lifetime treatment with phlebotomies is currently the treatment of choice, although newer therapies using growth factor control over red blood cell production are being tested.

**23. Which porphyrias are associated with primarily neurologic manifestations?**

Hepatic porphyrias, acute intermittent porphyria (AIP), and variegate (South African) porphyria can be distinguished from the rare "erythropoietic" forms that produce dermatologic symptoms without neurologic disease. In AIP, clinical symptoms develop during crises, most often precipitated by ingestion or administration of drugs that adversely affect porphyrin metabolism. These clinical symptoms include the following: (1) abdominal pain with vomiting, constipation or diarrhea, and often a previous history of exploratory abdominal surgery; (2) psychiatric disorder, with symptoms suggesting conversion reactions, delirium, or psychosis; (3) peripheral neuropathy, primarily motor, often with autonomic abnormalities, that may be severe or fatal and mimic Guillain-Barré syndrome; and (4) central abnormalities, such as syndrome of inappropriate antidiuretic hormone (SIADH) or convulsions.

Greer M: Neurologic manifestations of the porphyrias. In Samuels MA, Peske S (eds): Office Practice of Neurology, 2nd ed. New York, Churchill-Livingstone, 2001.

24. **Chronic ingestion of what substance may produce a condition similar to AIP?**
Lead poisoning produces a condition (termed saturnism) that closely resembles AIP clinically, and also appears to share heme synthetic dysfunction with accumulation of delta-aminolevulinic acid.

Graeme KA, Pollack CV Jr: Heavy metal toxicity. J Emerg Med 16:45-56, 1998.

25. **What is the treatment for neurologic crises in AIP?**
Therapy is directed at modifying the biochemical abnormalities found in the disease, including overproduction of the neurotoxin delta-aminolevulinic acid and heme deficiency. Intravenous administration of hematin increases available heme and downregulates the patient's abnormal heme biosynthetic pathway, thus reducing delta-aminolevulinic acid levels. Prevention of crises is the primary goal in treating patients with AIP. Education of patients to the many precipitants of acute attacks is necessary for their survival.

Anderson KE, Bloomer JR, Bonkovsky HL, et al.: Recommendations for the diagnosis and treatment of the acute porphyrias. Ann Intern Med 142:439-450, 2005. Erratum in Ann Intern Med 143:316, 2005.

## RENAL DISEASE

26. **What are the most common neurologic complications of renal disease?**
Typical neurologic complications of renal disease are peripheral neuropathy and metabolic encephalopathy.

27. **What are the characteristics of uremic neuropathy?**
Uremic neuropathy appears as a symmetric distal sensorimotor axonal neuropathy and is almost invariably present in patients by the time they require dialysis. Other conditions that predispose to renal failure (e.g., diabetes and vasculitis) may also produce neuropathy, thus symptoms can result from several different etiologies. Uremic neuropathy is at least partially reversible by repeated dialysis or by kidney transplantation.

28. **What are the characteristics of uremic encephalopathy?**
Patients with uremia often develop a metabolic encephalopathy. The mechanisms responsible for this encephalopathy remain unclear, but presumably involve the retention of inorganic and organic acids, fluid alterations among cerebral cellular compartments, and abnormalities caused by hypertension, hypocalcemia, hyperkalemia, hypernatremia, hyperphosphatemia, and hypochloremia. Uremic encephalopathy is unusual because of the coexistence of signs of neuronal depression (lethargy, coma) with those of neuronal excitation (agitation, muscle cramps, myoclonus, tetany, asterixis, and seizures).

29. **Name three neurologic complications associated with dialysis.**
Dialysis disequilibrium, dialysis dementia, and ICH.

30. **What is the dialysis disequilibrium syndrome?**
Dialysis disequilibrium is the name given to the cerebral edema produced by the rapid removal of urea and other osmoles, and fluid and electrolyte shifts associated with dialysis. Symptoms

may be mild, such as persistent headache or fatigue, or may be sufficiently severe to produce seizures, coma, and death. Recognition of this problem has led to newer protocols using more frequent, but less vigorous, dialysis.

## KEY POINTS: COMMON ASSOCIATIONS WITH TRIPHASIC WAVES

1. Hepatic encephalopathy

2. Uremic encephalopathy

3. Acute cerebral anoxia

4. Thyrotoxicosis

31. **What is dialysis dementia?**
Dialysis dementia refers to a rarer but much more serious syndrome of irreversible progressive dementia with apraxias, dysarthria, hyperreflexia, myoclonus, and multifocal seizures. Aluminum present in the dialysate is thought to be the primary agent causing CNS toxicity, and removal of aluminum with ion exchange resins prior to dialysis has significantly reduced the problem.

32. **What causes ICH in patients undergoing dialysis?**
Anticoagulation during dialysis and chronic hypertension associated with renal failure increases the incidence of ICH.

33. **What neurologic complications are associated with renal transplantation?**
Neurologic complications of renal transplantation are primarily the result of immunosuppression. Calcineurin inhibitors may cause tremors, paresthesia, or a severe disabling pain syndrome and leukoencephalopathy. Severe neurological syndromes may also be caused by monoclonal antibody OKT3. Stoke occurs in about 8% of renal transplant patients, likely due to existing hypertension, diabetes, and accelerated atherosclerosis. Guillain-Barré syndrome may also develop, triggered in some cases by cytomegalovirus (CMV) or *Campylobacter jejuni* infection. Infection represents the most frequent neurologic complication. Acute meningitis, usually caused by *Listeria monocytogenes*, and subacute and chronic meningitis, caused by *Cryptococcus neoformans*, account for more than 90% of nonviral CNS infections. Focal brain infection is caused by *Aspergillus fumigatus*, *Toxoplasma gondii*, or *Nocardia asteroids*, and progressive dementia caused by polyoma J virus or other viruses are the most frequent types of neurologic infections. Lymphomas are the most frequent brain tumors. They are usually associated with an Epstein-Barr virus (EBV) infection and are more frequent in patients who receive an aggressive immunosuppressive therapy. The overall risk of developing cancer following renal transplantation is approximately 6%, or about 100-fold greater than that expected for the general nonimmunosuppressed population.

Amato AA, Barohn RJ: Transplantation and immunosuppressive medication. In Rolak LA, Harati Y (eds): Neuro-Immunology for the Clinician. Boston, Butterworth-Heinemann, 1997, pp 341-376.

Ponticelli C, Campise MR: Neurological complications in kidney transplant recipients. J Nephrol 18:521-528, 2005.

## PULMONARY DISEASE

34. **What are the neurologic signs and symptoms of respiratory insufficiency?**
Neurologic features of this medical emergency result from hypoxemia and acute hypercapnia. Initial symptoms may be those of a nocturnal or early morning headache, associated with lethargy, drowsiness, inattentiveness, and irritability. Motor signs at this stage include tremor and twitching, caused by hypercapnia-induced stimulation of sympathetic nervous system output. More severe levels of hypoxia result in somnolence, confusion, and asterixis. Prolonged severe hypoxia results in coma and generalized seizures. Ocular findings include papilledema in 10% of patients, probably from hypercapnia-induced increases in intracranial pressure. However, isolated chronic hypercapnia with $Pco_2$ measurements of up to 110 mmHg may exist without apparent neurologic symptoms or signs.

## KEY POINTS: NEUROLOGIC DISEASES ASSOCIATED WITH RESPIRATORY INSUFFICIENCY

1. Brain/brain stem

2. Spinal cord

3. Peripheral nerve

4. Neuromuscular junction

5. Muscle

35. **What neurologic diseases may result in respiratory insufficiency?**
**Brain and brain stem**
   - Brain herniation
   - Muscular dystrophy (central apnea)

**Spinal cord**
   - Upper cervical cord injury, transection ($\leq$ C6)
   - Lower motor neuron disease (amyotrophic lateral sclerosis, postpolio syndrome, spinal muscular atrophy)

**Peripheral nerve**
   - Acute inflammatory polyradiculoneuropathy (Guillain-Barré syndrome)

**Neuromuscular junction**
   - Myasthenia gravis
   - Botulism
   - Congenital myasthenic syndromes

**Muscle**
   - Muscular dystrophy (peripheral/obstructive apnea)
   - Congenital myopathy
   - Inflammatory myopathies (polymyositis, inclusion body myositis)

36. **Describe the clinical features of prolonged hyperventilation.**
Anxious patients with acute psychogenic hyperventilation usually complain of lightheadedness, dyspnea, circumoral and acral paresthesias, and the presence of visual phosphenes. Visual blurring, tremor, muscle cramps, carpopedal spasm, and chest pain are found with prolonged hyperventilation. In addition to psychogenic etiologies, prolonged hyperventilation may be the result of drug effects, metabolic acidosis, CNS damage or edema, or response to heat stroke or overexercise.

37. **What causes high-altitude sickness? How is it treated?**
Cerebral hypoxia results from the lower partial pressure of oxygen at high altitudes. A shift of water and sodium into neurons may also occur as the result of the failure of glycolysis-dependent cellular enzymes and transporters, such as the $Na^+/K^+$ pump. Exercise in the cold temperatures encountered at high altitude worsens cerebral edema by further increasing cerebral blood flow. Treatment prophylactically with dexamethasone will prevent most cases of acute mountain sickness. The use of high-pressure oxygen, removal to lower altitudes, and acetazolamide therapy may reduce symptoms in patients with preexisting high-altitude sickness.
Aminoff MJ: Neurologic complications of systemic disease. In Bradley WG, Daroff RB, Fenichel G, Jankovic J (eds): Neurology in Clinical Practice, 3rd ed. Boston, Butterworth-Heinemann, 2000, p 1020.

## HEMATOLOGIC DISEASE

38. **Name the most common symptoms associated with anemia.**
Headache, lightheadedness, and fatigue are the most commonly reported neurologic complaints of the anemic patient.

## KEY POINTS: SYSTEMIC DISEASES ASSOCIATED WITH AN INCREASED RISK OF STROKE

1. Hematologic disease (sickle cell anemia, hemophilia, platelet disorders)

2. Diabetes

3. Cardiac disease

4. Vitamin C and K deficiencies

5. Connective tissue disease and central nervous system (CNS) vasculitides

6. Pregnancy

39. **What is the most serious neurologic complication of sickle cell anemia?**
Ischemic stroke, often affecting patients in childhood or adolescence, is the most frequent serious sequela of a vascular crisis in sickle cell disease. Intimal hyperplasia and stenosis of proximal cerebral vessels have been described in the pathogenesis for medium-vessel and large-vessel stroke in these patients. Hyperventilation (with associated vasoconstriction) is thus a common precipitating event for stroke in the young patient with sickle cell disease. Recurrence rates for stroke in patients with sickle cell disease exceed 67%. Intracranial hemorrhage may also be seen in patients with sickle cell disease. Rupture of intracranial aneurysms is the usual cause for ICH in affected individuals. Both clinical strokes and silent infarcts occur, affecting motor and cognitive function.
Adams RJ, McKie VC, Hsu L, et al.: Prevention of a first stroke by transfusions in children with sickle cell anemia and abnormal results on transcranial Doppler ultrasonography. N Engl J Med 339:5-11, 1998.
Prengler M, Pavlakis SG, Prohovnik I, Adams RJ: Sickle cell disease: The neurological complications. Annals of Neurology 51:543-552, 2002.

40. **What are the primary neurologic manifestations of hyperviscosity states?**
Hyperviscosity states are conditions in which red blood cells, white blood cells, or serum proteins are increased to a sufficient degree that impedance of blood flow and/or oxygen delivery results. Neurologic manifestations include symptoms of chronic or acute vertebrobasilar insufficiency (tinnitus, lightheadedness, and headache); paresthesias; and problems with mentation, visual/auditory disturbances, seizures, stroke, stupor, or coma.

41. **What red cell diseases can produce a hyperviscosity state?**
Polycythemia rubra vera and "secondary" or "relative" polycythemia increase the hematocrit or the red cell volume/plasma volume ratio, respectively. This increases blood viscosity, producing symptoms. Chronic reduction in hematocrit by phlebotomy or acute expansion of the plasma volume both reduce symptoms and may decrease the risk for serious sequelae.

42. **What diseases produce elevated serum proteins and cause hyperviscosity states?**
Paraproteinemias may be first detected by the onset of neurologic symptoms. Multiple myeloma and Waldenström's macroglobulinemia are the most common causes of increased serum viscosity, which appears to produce the complications of this state. In most cases, plasmapheresis is used in combination with corticosteroids and immunosuppressive drugs to prevent production of abnormal proteins or to treat the underlying disease.

43. **What are the neurologic complications of hemophilia?**
Intracranial hemorrhage is the most serious consequence of factor VIII deficiency. A history of head trauma is often obtained, preceding symptoms of a subdural hemorrhage by days. Subarachnoid and intraparenchymal hemorrhages cause more rapid progression of symptoms and carry an increased risk for mortality. Intraspinal hemorrhage, while rare, rapidly produces cord compression and paralysis, while soft-tissue hematomas may cause focal compressive neuropathies.

44. **Which platelet disorders produce neurologic disease?**
Primary acute or chronic immune thrombocytopenia purpura (ITP), disseminated intravascular coagulation (DIC), thrombotic thrombocytopenic purpura (TTP), dysimmune thrombocytopenia (DIT) secondary to rheumatic disease (associated with anticardiolipin antibodies) or hyperviscosity states, and heparin-associated thrombocytopenia (HAT) all are associated with neurologic disease due to thrombocytopenic states. TTP produces a microangiopathic hemolytic anemia with prominent neurologic symptoms of headache, encephalopathy, or seizures, whereas DIC and (less commonly) ITP may produce larger intracerebral hemorrhages. HAT and DIT more commonly cause stroke. Thrombocytosis usually results from essential thrombocythemia, which produces symptoms of a hyperviscosity state when platelet counts exceed 600,000 to 1,000,000 per microliter. Cerebrovascular complications—TIAs and stroke—are the serious consequences of this disease.

45. **How are antiphospholipid antibodies related to neurologic disease?**
Antibodies directed against phospholipids are associated with thrombotic states and are found with a high frequency in patients with retinal vascular thrombosis, amaurosis fugax, ischemic optic neuropathy, and stroke in the young. The most common antibodies, lupus anticoagulant and anticardiolipin antibody, probably induce thrombosis via multiple mechanisms. The presence of these antibodies has also been associated with migraine, chorea, myelopathy, and orthostatic hypotension. Non-neurologic features may include miscarriage, livedo reticularis, and pulmonary hypertension. The pathophysiology of these symptoms is poorly understood.
    Jacobs BS, Levine SR: Antiphospholipid antibody syndrome. Curr Treat Options Neurol 2:449-458, 2000.

**46. What is the treatment for the antiphospholipid antibody syndrome?**

Few controlled trials have been conducted, and there is no consensus about the optimal treatment for patients with antiphospholipid antibodies. Most authorities favor use of the antithrombotic agent warfarin, but plasmapheresis combined with immunosuppression and intravenous immunoglobulin (IVIG) increasingly is being used in severe cases. IVIG is the treatment of choice for pregnant women.

Valesini G, Pittoni V: Treatment of thrombosis associated with immunological risk factors. Ann Med 32(suppl 1):41-45, 2000.

## ENDOCRINE DISEASE

**47. Which endocrine diseases are commonly associated with neurologic complications?**

1. DM
2. Hyperthyroidism
3. Hypothyroidism
4. Hyperparathyroidism
5. Hypoparathyroidism
6. Acromegaly
7. Adrenal insufficiency
8. Glucocorticoid excess
9. Diabetes insipidus (DI)

**48. Which endocrine diseases are complicated by seizures?**

Seizures most commonly occur after an acute change in endocrine function and usually result from electrolyte imbalance. They occur in 50% or more of patients with hypoparathyroidism because of the hypocalcemia. Although seizures are usually generalized, partial or absence seizures may also complicate hypoparathyroidism. Seizures do not occur in hyperparathyroidism.

Seizures may be the presenting sign in 20% of all hypothyroid patients, and are nearly always generalized. In contrast, the incidence of seizures in thyrotoxicosis is only 5% to 10%.

In Addison's disease, seizures follow the rapid onset of serum hyponatremia ($<$115 mEq/L), and carry a subsequent mortality of greater than 50%. Seizures are seen in DI only with rapid elevation of serum sodium (usually to greater than 160 mEq/L). In DI, seizures are often partial and may occur as a result of brain shrinkage with focal hemorrhage, or during rehydration.

Seizures are observed with other endocrine causes of brain shrinkage, such as in nonketotic hyperosmolar states from DM. In this setting, up to 25% of patients develop partial or generalized motor seizures that may evolve into epilepsia partialis continua or generalized status epilepticus. Seizures may also be seen in DM as the result of hypoglycemia from insulin therapy but are distinctly uncommon in diabetic ketoacidosis. Seizures are not typically associated with Cushing's disease or acromegaly.

**49. Which endocrine diseases may cause coma?**

Coma is a rare and life-threatening complication of both hypothyroidism and hyperthyroidism. In the latter case, coma is almost always associated with thyroid storm. Coma is also found in hyperparathyroidism when serum calcium is greater than 19 mg/dL, in adrenal hypofunction with severe hyponatremia, and in DM associated with therapy-related hypoglycemia.

**50. What are the common neurologic features of hypothyroidism?**

Hypothyroidism causes headache, fatigue, slowness of speech and thought, apathy, and inattention in 90% of patients and are often mistaken for early dysthymia or depression.

Reversible sensorineural hearing loss, with or without tinnitus, develops in 75% of hypothyroid patients, and reversible ptosis occurs in 60% of patients as a result of diminished sympathetic tone. Sleep apnea occurs in up to half of hypothyroid patients and usually results from obstructive problems due to associated obesity and myxedema. Seizures are reported in 20% of patients, often as the presenting neurologic sign. Prolonged relaxation time for deep tendon reflexes can be elicited in many hypothyroid patients but is not specific for the disease.

Rarely, hypothyroidism is associated with limb ataxia, nystagmus, carpal tunnel syndrome, demyelinating polyneuropathy, optic neuropathy, ophthalmoparesis, pseudotumor cerebri, trigeminal neuralgia, Bell's palsy, reversible dementia, or overt psychosis (myxedema madness).

Myopathy in hypothyroidism is common and ranges between 30% to 80% of cases. The major symptoms related are weakness, muscular cramps, and myalgia. The pseudohypertrophic form is called Hoffman's syndrome. Laboratory investigation shows increased levels of muscle enzymes, low serum thyroid hormones, and elevated thyrotrophic-stimulating hormone (TSH).

Abend WK, Tyler HR: Thyroid disease and the nervous system. In Aminoff M (ed): Neurology and General Medicine. New York, Churchill-Livingstone, 1995, pp 333-348.

## 51. What are the most dangerous neurologic complications of hypothyroidism?

Although myxedema coma develops in only 1% of hypothyroid patients, its often rapid onset with associated bradycardia, ventricular arrhythmias, hypotension, hypopnea, hypothermia, hypoglycemia, electrolyte disturbance, and seizures makes it life-threatening. Treatment is supportive, with correction of metabolic abnormalities, rewarming, ventilatory and/or cardiovascular support, and adequate replacement of thyroxine and corticosteroids. In utero and in the newborn period, undiagnosed and untreated hypothyroidism leads to cretinism. Treatment requires early screening prior to the onset of symptoms and thyroid hormone replacement before permanent damage occurs.

## 52. What are the neurologic features of hyperthyroidism?

Thyrotoxicosis may manifest with reversible behavioral and cognitive changes, including emotional lability, euphoria, irritability, mania, and psychosis. Delirium may be observed as a manifestation of thyroid storm. Apathetic hyperthyroidism may appear as fatigue, with symptoms suggesting depression or dementia. Other features of thyrotoxicosis are tremor of the hands, eyelids or tongue, chorea, spasticity (sometimes with clonus and Babinski's signs), thyrotoxic periodic paralysis, and myopathy.

Neurologic problems usually resolve after treatment of the underlying thyrotoxicosis, but thyroid ophthalmopathy often requires surgical orbital decompression. Additionally, bulbar palsies and motor weakness may not recover following correction of hyperthyroidism secondary to coexistence of other dysimmune disease, such as acute myasthenia gravis.

## 53. What are the neurologic features of parathyroid dysfunction?

Up to 25% of patients with hyperparathyroidism have prominent psychiatric symptoms resembling mania, schizophrenia, or acute confusional state. An additional 50% of hyperparathyroid patients may have symptoms suggesting depression. Interestingly, 80% of patients with hypoparathyroidism also exhibit psychological manifestations of their disease, including symptoms resembling depression, pseudodementia, mania, schizophrenia, and toxic delirium.

In hyperparathyroidism, hypercalcemia-induced coma and spinal cord or root compression caused by collapse of decalcified vertebrae are the major nonpsychiatric symptoms. Myopathy is also a common finding in hyperparathyroidism. In contrast, hypocalcemia resulting from hypoparathyroidism is more closely associated with seizures and tetany. Seizures are often difficult to control with correction of the electrolyte imbalance. Latent tetany, which can present as laryngeal spasm, can be evoked by mechanical stimulation of the facial nerve (Chvostek's sign), by hyperventilation, or by occlusion of venous return from an arm resulting in carpopedal spasm (Trousseau's sign).

**54. How may adrenal insufficiency lead to weakness?**
Up to 50% of patients with Addison's disease have a glucocorticoid-sensitive myopathy with associated cramping. Adrenal insufficiency results in decreased blood flow to the muscle, reduced muscle carbohydrate metabolism, and altered $Na^+/K^+$ pump function and potassium homeostasis with resulting reduced muscle intracellular potassium and altered muscle contractility. Decreased adrenergic sensitivity in patients with Addison's disease also results in reduced exercise tolerance and exercise-related hypotension. Abnormalities in potassium homeostasis may additionally result in the episodic appearance of extreme weakness, resembling hyperkalemic periodic paralysis.

Horak HA, Pourmand R: Endocrine myopathies. Neurol Clin 18:203-213, 2000.

**55. How does prolonged glucocorticoid excess lead to weakness?**
Most patients with Cushing's disease have frank weakness and demonstrable myopathic findings on electromyography and selective type IIb muscle fiber atrophy on muscle biopsy. Chronic treatment with glucocorticoids, especially with the fluorinated steroids, will reproduce these effects on ectopic adrenocorticotropic hormone (ACTH) production in 10% to 20% of patients. Glucocorticoids produce an insulin-resistant state in myotubes, in which both glycolytic (nonoxidative) carbohydrate metabolism and protein synthesis are adversely affected. Type IIb fibers, which are least able to compensate for this reduction of glycolytic metabolism, are most affected.

**56. What neurologic disorders are associated with excess growth hormone?**
Sustained excessive growth hormone (GH) appears to directly produce myopathy. GH-induced changes in the myotube include impaired glycolytic carbohydrate metabolism, increased fatty acid oxidation, and increased protein synthesis with reduced protein degradation. The more highly oxidative type I and type IIa muscle fibers are typically most affected by GH. Myotube hypertrophy from abnormal protein synthesis produces weakness in the face of increased muscle size. Although central sleep apnea may also be caused directly by excessive GH production, the obstructive sleep apnea, basilar impression, myelopathy, and compressive neuropathies reported in this disease are all indirect effects of bony, ligamentous, and soft-tissue hyperplasia with secondary compression of neural tissue.

**57. How does DM affect the peripheral nervous system?**
Damage to the peripheral nervous system accounts for the main neurologic manifestations of diabetes. Initially, a symmetric distal stocking-and-glove sensory neuropathy involving small, unmyelinated or thinly myelinated fibers appears and is often associated with painful, burning paresthesias. In more severe cases, larger proprioceptive fibers are also affected, leading to Charcot joints. Autonomic nerve damage causes atrophic skin changes, impotence, orthostatic hypotension, arrhythmias, gastroparesis, and sphincter incontinence. Motor fibers may also be damaged, leading to symmetric distal weakness, especially of the lower extremities. Focal destruction of nerves may cause cranial nerve palsies, diabetic amyotrophy, and thoracoabdominal neuropathy.

## FLUID AND ELECTROLYTE DISORDERS

**58. What are the most common neurologic complications of hypokalemia and hyperkalemia?**
Myalgias and weakness can be found with serum potassium concentrations of 2.5 to 3.0 mEq/L. Prolonged hypokalemia of less than 2.5 mEq/L will lead to rhabdomyolysis, myoglobinuria, and cardiac arrhythmias.

Hyperkalemia (>6.0 mEq/L) likewise causes functional and structural muscle abnormalities, including weakness and cardiac arrhythmias. Ventricular asystole or fibrillation are life-threatening and occur long before neurologic symptoms are usually manifested. The few previous reports of drowsiness, lethargy, and coma in hypokalemia may actually be the result of acid-base disequilibrium.

59. **How do changes in serum sodium affect the nervous system?**
Because extracellular fluid volume changes as a direct function of total body sodium, patients who are hyponatremic are usually hyposmolar, whereas hypernatremic patients are hyperosmolar. Neurologic manifestations of sodium dysregulation mainly result from shrinkage or swelling of the brain, and the degree to which these changes occur depend both on the amount and the rapidity of the sodium changes.

60. **What are the most common neurologic complications of hyponatremia and hypernatremia?**
Alteration of mental status is the common neurologic alteration resulting from hyponatremia. This may occur after acute reduction of serum sodium to below 130 mEq/L, or with chronically depressed sodium concentrations of below 115 mEq/L. Seizures, seen in the presence of acute reduction of serum sodium to less than 125 mEq/L, are generalized in nature and prognostically signify mortality of greater than 50%. Therapy includes fluid restriction or sodium replacement in severe hyponatremia, which can result in myelinolysis throughout the brain due to rapid osmotic shifts (central pontine and extrapontine myelinolysis) in patients whose sodium is corrected too rapidly or in patients at particular risk for this complication (alcoholism, renal disease) despite slow, and carefully monitored sodium replacement.

Hypernatremia (serum sodium >160 mEq/L) may lead to an altered mental state, progressing to coma or to seizures. Focal cerebral hemorrhage resulting from the tearing of parenchymal vessels or bridging veins produces multiple neurologic symptoms, including hemiparesis, rigidity, tremor, myoclonus, cerebellar ataxia, and chorea, as well as signs of subarachnoid hemorrhage or subdural hematoma.

61. **What are the neurologic complications of hypercalcemia and hypocalcemia?**
Hypercalcemia (>12 mg/dL) leads commonly to symptoms of progressive encephalopathy and coma, and more rarely to seizures or signs of corticobulbar, corticospinal, or cerebellospinal tract dysfunction. Elevated serum calcium may also produce weakness with reduced membrane excitability at the level of the neuromuscular junction, and may possibly cause a reversible myopathy.

Hypocalcemia may present with seizures or with neurobehavioral changes and dementia. Some patients develop parkinsonism after prolonged hypocalcemia. Increased excitability at the neuromuscular junction with reduced serum calcium may manifest as tetany.

62. **What are the most common neurologic complications of hypomagnesemia and hypermagnesemia?**
Because, like potassium, magnesium is an intracellular ion whose intracellular concentrations are tightly controlled, the presence of neurologic complications may not directly correlate with extracellular magnesium concentrations. Hypomagnesemia, however, appears to present in patients with essentially the same findings as hypocalcemia. Because serum-ionized calcium concentrations are reduced in the presence of hypomagnesemia, some of these symptoms may, in fact, be the functional result of hypocalcemia.

Hypermagnesemia results in CNS depression and muscle paralysis. The mechanism of CNS depression is still being addressed; muscle paralysis occurs as a result of direct neuromuscular blockade.

## RHEUMATOLOGIC DISEASE

63. **What are the neurologic manifestations of systemic lupus erythematosus (SLE)?**
Neurologic symptoms and signs appear as manifestations of SLE in 50% of afflicted patients. Central dysfunction includes neuropsychiatric and behavioral changes, such as dementia, psychosis, and confusional states (the most common central manifestation of SLE). Localizing neurologic findings include hemiparesis, chorea, tremor, cerebellar ataxia, cranial neuropathies and optic neuritis, and transverse myelitis. Aseptic meningitis, seizures, and signs of increased intracranial pressure may also develop in patients with SLE. The mean 5-year survival for patients with neurologic symptoms is 30% less than that found in SLE patients without neurologic problems. Vasculitis with CNS hemorrhage accounts for a large portion of this difference.

    Peripheral neuropathy may appear in SLE as a vasculitis mononeuropathy or mononeuritis multiplex, or as an ischemic symmetric distal sensorimotor deficit. Myositis occurs in 25% of patients with SLE but is a serious complication only when the myocardium is involved.
    Boumpas DT, Austin HA 3rd, Fessler BJ, et al.: Systemic lupus erythematosus: Emerging concepts. Ann Intern Med 122:940-950, 1995.

64. **What are the major neurologic manifestations of rheumatoid arthritis (RA)?**
The major sequelae of RA are limited to the peripheral nervous system due to nerve entrapment near inflamed joints, perineural inflammation and demyelination of sensory nerves, and vasculitic destruction of large nerves giving rise to an asymmetric sensorimotor neuropathy. Diffuse nodular polymyositis may occur in 30% of patients with RA, although classic polymyositis is rare (5%). Focal ischemic myositis occurs as a result of vasculitis attack on the muscle vasculature.

    CNS manifestations are rare and include a polyarteritis–nodosa-like vasculitis affecting cerebral vasculature, hyperviscosity syndrome producing focal ischemic and hemorrhagic CNS lesions, and rheumatoid cervical spine disease with myelopathy most commonly occurring at C4-C5. Compression or laceration of the spinal cord may be the direct result of impaction or subluxation of one or more vertebral bodies or rings against the cord. Vascular compression syndromes may also be found in RA patients with cervical disease, especially involving the anterior spinal artery. These syndromes lead to ischemic central gray destruction and to necrosis of the dorsal columns and corticospinal tracts.
    Akil M, Amos RS: ABC of rheumatology. Rheumatoid arthritis: Clinical features and diagnosis. Brit Med J 310:587-590, 1995.

65. **Trigeminal neuropathy is found in which rheumatic diseases?**
Isolated trigeminal neuropathy may be the presenting sign in 10% of patients with neurologic manifestations of scleroderma and occurs in 4% to 5% of all patients with scleroderma. Fibrosis with nerve entrapment is the likely cause for this and other cranial neuropathies in progressive systemic sclerosis. Vasculitis damage to the trigeminal nerve is found in SLE and less commonly in mixed connective tissue disorder (MCTD).

66. **What is the most common neurologic manifestation of Behçet's disease?**
Central nervous system disease is found in 10% to 30% of patients afflicted with Behçet's disease. An initially relapsing and remitting focal meningoencephalitis that predominantly affects the brain stem is the most commonly finding. Cranial nerve and long tract signs may eventually lead to spastic quadriplegia and pseudobulbar palsy. Subcortical dementia, pseudotumor cerebri, vasculitis with cerebral infarction, and peripheral neuropathy have also been reported in this disease.
    Siva A, Fresko II: Behçet's disease. Curr Treat Options Neurol 2:435-448, 2000.

## VASCULITIDES

**67. Which vessels are affected by primary vasculitic disease?**

Although all vessels may be damaged in vasculitis, different vasculitides affect different vessel types. The aorta is selectively damaged in Takayasu's arteritis, whereas giant cell arteritis more commonly affects the temporal, vertebral, and carotid arteries. Medium-sized muscular intracerebral arteries are affected in polyarteritis nodosa (PAN), allergic granulomatosis, and granulomatous angiitis, whereas small muscular arteries are thrombosed in Wegener's granulomatosis. Hypersensitivity angiitis selectively involves capillaries and venules, sparing the arterial system.

**68. What are the neurologic manifestations of polyarteritis nodosa?**

Half of patients diagnosed with polyarteritis nodosa have evidence of peripheral neuropathy. The five following peripheral neuropathy syndromes have been identified: (1) mononeuritis multiplex of sensory and motor nerves; (2) extensive mononeuritis multiplex with severe, primarily distal weakness and sensory deficits; (3) isolated small cutaneous sensory nerve involvement; (4) distal symmetric sensorimotor neuropathy; and (5) radiculopathy. Myalgias have also been reported in 25% of patients with PAN, usually associated with weakness. Peripheral neuropathy is a common and early finding of PAN.

CNS manifestations of vasculitic disease can be found in 40% to 45% of patients with PAN, including encephalopathy, seizures (40%), and focal deficits related to infarction (50%). Cranial nerve palsies occur in 15% of patients, most commonly involving cranial nerves II, III, and VIII. Hypertensive CNS changes with papilledema and focal hemorrhages are observed in 10% of patients with an acute confusional state, and often signify a poorer prognosis. CNS sequelae are often late manifestations of this disease, occurring 2 to 3 years after the initial diagnosis.

**69. Does Churg-Strauss syndrome cause neurologic damage?**

Two-thirds of patients with allergic granulomatosis (Churg-Strauss syndrome) have CNS manifestations similar to those seen in PAN, including encephalopathy, seizures, and coma, and mononeuritis multiplex in the majority of patients. Hemorrhage is more common in this disorder than in PAN, but the clinical distinction between these two diseases rests on the almost invariable presence of pulmonary involvement with asthma in patients with Churg-Strauss syndrome, along with eosinophilia and elevated serum IgE levels.

**70. What are the neurologic effects of Wegener's granulomatosis?**

Wegener's granulomatosis presents as a triad of focal segmental glomerulonephritis, granulomas of the respiratory tract, and necrotizing vasculitis. Neurologic complications occur in 25% to 50% of affected individuals, with mononeuritis multiplex as the most common manifestation. CNS manifestations are commonly the result of granulomatous invasion from the sinuses or nasal passages, and may appear as exophthalmos, pituitary disease, or basilar meningitis with cranial neuropathies. Up to 5% of patients will have ICH secondary to either focal vasculitis or intragranulomatous hemorrhage.

Moore PM, Calabrese LH: Neurologic manifestations of systemic vasculitides. Semin Neurol 14:300-306, 1994.

Nishino H, Rubino FA, DeRemee RA, et al.: Neurological involvement in Wegener's granulomatosis: An analysis of 324 consecutive patients at the Mayo Clinic. Ann Neurol 33:4-8, 1993.

**71. What is the clinical triad associated with temporal arteritis?**

Headache, jaw claudication, and constitutional symptoms compose the triad of clinical symptoms often found in temporal arteritis. The headache is typically boring, throbbing, or lancinating, radiating from one or both temples to the neck, jaw, tongue, or back of the head.

Fever, malaise, night sweats, and anorexia with weight loss usually present early in the disease. Patients are usually older than 50 years of age, and 50% will have concomitant polyarthralgia rheumatica. Mononeuritis multiplex may occur in 10% of afflicted patients. Untreated, one-third of the patients will develop amaurosis fugax, monocular or binocular blindness, diplopia, or ophthalmoplegia. Cerebral infarctions or TIAs are common complications late in the disease.

**72. How is temporal arteritis diagnosed and treated?**
Evidence of an elevated sedimentation rate (>60 mm/h by the Westergren method) and characteristic findings of arteritis on biopsy of the temporal artery are helpful in making the diagnosis, but biopsy is frequently negative (70% diagnostic after bilateral biopsy). Treatment of temporal arteritis is with steroids and should not await biopsy (biopsy should be performed within the first few days of therapy). Treatment should continue at least 2 years with oral steroid therapy. Treatment effect is usually on the basis of sedimentation rates.

Nesher G, Nesher R, Mates M, et al.: Giant cell arteritis: Intensity of the initial systemic inflammatory response and the course of the disease. Clin Exp Rheumatol 26(3 Supple 49): S30-S34, 2008.

**73. What are four vasculitides whose effects are localized to the CNS?**
**Cogan's syndrome** produces vestibular and/or auditory dysfunction with episodic acute interstitial keratitis, scleritis, or episcleritis. **Eales' syndrome** is an isolated peripheral retinal vasculitis. Both of these rare syndromes tend to afflict young adults. **Spinal cord arteritis** is a diagnosis of exclusion, because many diseases may present with myelopathy. Among these diseases is **granulomatous angiitis of the nervous system (GANS)**, the most severe isolated CNS vasculitic syndrome.

**74. What are the nervous system manifestations of granulomatous angiitis?**
Granulomatous angiitis of the nervous system is also called isolated angiitis of the CNS. Thirty percent of patients have elevated opening pressure on spinal tap with associated cerebrospinal fluid (CSF) pleocytosis in 65% of patients, and increased protein in 80% of patients. Cerebral angiography and brain biopsy may each be diagnostic in 50% of cases. The differential diagnosis includes other vasculitides, tuberculosis, multiple sclerosis (MS), strokes due to emboli, sarcoidosis, syphilis, Lyme disease, drug abuse associated CNS vasculopathy, neoplasm, and lymphomatoid granulomatosis.

Goldberg JW: Primary angiitis of the central nervous system. In Rolak LA, Harati Y (eds): Neuro-Immunology for the Clinician. Boston, Butterworth-Heinemann, 1997, pp 177-186.

West SG: Central nervous system vasculitis. Curr Rheumatol Rep 5:116-127, 2003.

## PREGNANCY

**75. What is the most common neurologic symptom found during pregnancy?**
Headache is the most common neurologic symptom reported in pregnancy. Headaches beginning during pregnancy are a cause for concern for serious underlying illnesses that occur with higher frequency in pregnant women. These include subarachnoid hemorrhage, rapid expansion of a tumor, cortical venous thrombosis, pseudotumor cerebri, L. *monocytogenes* meningitis, or preeclampsia and eclampsia. History and physical examination can usually exclude serious problems. Other headaches that may begin during pregnancy include migraines, even though the majority of female migraineurs improve during pregnancy. Onset of benign bifrontal nonmigranous headaches is also seen in pregnancy and is most common during the first trimester. Postpartum headache is the most common self-limited headache of the puerperium and occurs in up to 40% of all women.

Shaner DM: Neurological problems of pregnancy. In Bradley WG, Daroff RB, Fenichel G, Jankovic J (eds): Neurology in Clinical Practice, 3rd ed. Boston, Butterworth-Heinemann, 2000 pp 2257-2268.

76. **What is eclampsia?**
Eclampsia, which means "to shine forth," is a state characterized by the neurologic complications o' seizures and/or coma, presenting in a pregnant patient with preeclampsia (i.e., with signs of hypertension and proteinuria with or without edema). It occurs in 0.05% to 0.2% of all pregnancies extending beyond the 20th week of gestation. Seizures or coma develop in 50% of eclamptic patients prior to the onset of labor, with an additional 25% becoming symptomatic during labor. The remaining 25% of eclamptic patients have onset of symptoms after delivery, usually within the firs' 24 hours postpartum. The differential diagnosis for eclampsia includes cerebrovascular accidents hypertensive encephalopathy, epilepsy, brain neoplasms and abscesses, meningitis/encephalitis, and metabolic diseases such as hypoglycemia or hypocalcemia.

Fox MW, Harms RW, Davis DH: Selected neurologic complications of pregnancy. Mayo Clin Proc 65:1595-1618, 1990.

77. **What is the cause of associated mortality in eclampsia?**
If present, eclampsia results in a maternal mortality of up to 14%, with associated fetal mortality of up to 28%. Maternal death from eclampsia is caused by complications of sustained intracranial and systemic hypertension. Death can be due to intracerebral hemorrhage, vasospasm, pulmonary edema, DIC, abruptio placentae, the HELLP syndrome (hemolysis, elevated liver enzymes, and low platelet count), or renal or hepatic failure from decreased organ perfusion. Fetal mortality results from decreased uteroplacental perfusion.

78. **How is eclampsia treated?**
The primary objective of treatment is to reduce blood pressure without compromising uteroplacental or maternal renal perfusion. Intracranial hypertension is usually present in patients with encephalopathy or coma, and thus intracranial pressure (ICP) should be monitored in such persons and managed with intubation and hyperventilation. These patients should also be imaged by computed tomography (CT) to assess for ICH and cerebral edema.

Eclamptic seizures must be aggressively controlled due to increased fetal mortality and increased intracranial pressure in the mother. Diazepam with concomitant phenytoin or phenobarbital is usually given for seizure prophylaxis. Intravenous administration of magnesium sulfate is effective as well.

The definitive treatment for eclampsia occurring before birth is termination of the pregnancy by delivery of the fetus. The risk of recurrent seizures decreases within 24 hours following delivery, and long-term prophylaxis of eclampsia-induced seizures is unnecessary. Although hypertension resolves more slowly, normalization of blood pressure occurs in the first postpartum week.

79. **Is the risk for stroke altered in pregnancy?**
Cerebrovascular ischemic events occur 13 times more frequently in pregnant patients than in age-matched nonpregnant women, with an overall stroke risk of 1 in 3000 pregnancies. Stroke accounts for 10% of all maternal deaths during pregnancy, and 35% of all strokes in female patients aged 15 to 45 years occur during pregnancy or in the puerperium. Atherosclerotic disease is less commonly a cause for stroke in this population than is arterial embolus or cerebral venous thrombosis (Figure 22-1).

80. **How does the physician clinically distinguish puerperal cerebral venous thrombosis from arterial thrombosis?**
Central venous thrombosis usually occurs in the first three postpartum weeks and commonly presents with headache, focal or generalized seizures, stupor or coma, transient focal deficits, and/ or signs of increased intracranial pressure. Rare thromboses include superior sagittal sinus

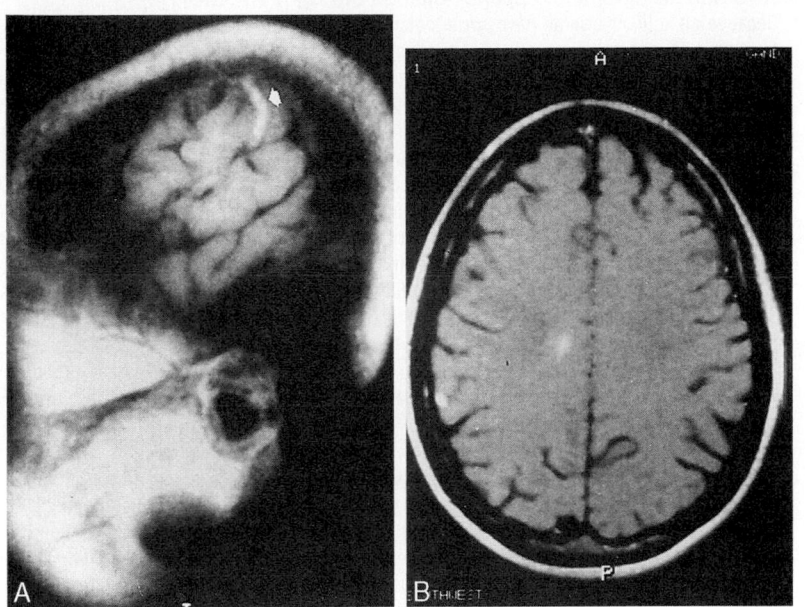

**Figure 22-1.** T1-weighted sagittal view of the superficial cerebral cortex of the parietal lobe, showing a cerebral vein thrombosis (A, *arrow*). The axial T1 view, (B) shows the small hemorrhagic infarction caused by the venous thrombosis.

thrombosis, with paraplegia and sensory deficits of the leg and bladder dysfunction, and rolandic vein thrombosis, with sensory and motor deficits of the leg, hip, and shoulder, sparing the face and arm. Mortality in sagittal sinus thrombosis approaches 40% but may be reduced to 20% with intensive care and, in some cases, anticoagulants. Recovery of survivors is usually complete.

Arterial thrombosis is more rare than arterial embolus or venous thrombosis, is more likely to occur in the second or third trimester than in the puerperium, and commonly presents with persistent focal deficit, such as hemiparesis, without alteration of consciousness, seizures, or signs of increased intracranial pressure.

Recently an immune mechanism has been hypothesized for a significant percentage of pregnancy-related venous and arterial thromboses. The presence of antiphospholipid antibodies should be sought, especially when a history of previous miscarriages or preeclampsia is obtained.

81. **What is the differential diagnosis for seizures during childbirth?**
As cause for seizures, **eclampsia**, **HELLP syndrome**, and **TTP** are most commonly observed during the third trimester. **Amniotic fluid embolism, water intoxication, autonomic stress in patients with upper spinal cord injury**, and **toxicity from local anesthetics** are all intrapartum causes for seizures. **Cerebral vein thrombosis** usually occurs postpartum and may present with seizures.

**Subarachnoid hemorrhage** may occur at any time during pregnancy to produce seizures, although aneurysms most commonly rupture during the third trimester, with greatest risk for rebleeding in the postpartum period. Arteriovenous malformations are more likely to rupture in the second trimester and rebleed during delivery or with subsequent pregnancies. **Epilepsy** may manifest at any time before, during, or after pregnancy, and may require lifelong therapy. However, such patients must be distinguished from those with **gestational epilepsy**, which requires therapy only during pregnancy.

82. **How should therapy of epilepsy change during pregnancy?**
Because all anticonvulsants have some potential to be teratogenic or harmful to the fetus, treatment should be aimed toward monotherapy at the lowest functionally effective dose.

Due to physiologic changes that occur in pregnancy the pharmacokinetics of anticonvulsants are usually altered. Effective prepregnancy anticonvulsant levels should be used as the target levels during pregnancy. Drug levels should be measured as soon as pregnancy is diagnosed because blood concentrations of anticonvulsants may drop precipitously during the first trimester, as a result of alterations in drug absorption, metabolism, or protein binding. This is especially true for phenytoin, with its nonlinear kinetics, in which doses may need to be increased by 50% to 100% during pregnancy to maintain prepregnancy levels. Routine drug levels should be measured each trimester, and more frequently if seizure control worsens, or if patients have a history of previous alterations in drug levels during pregnancy. Because drug clearance returns to prepregnancy norms within 3 to 6 weeks postpartum, prepregnancy anticonvulsant doses should be gradually introduced during this period.

All patients of childbearing age should take folic acid to lower risks of neural tube defects, which have a higher incidence in this population. Doses up to 4 mg should be prescribed as soon as pregnancy is suspected.

83. **What neuropathies are commonly associated with pregnancy and childbirth?**
Prior to birth, **carpal tunnel syndrome** is the most commonly associated neuropathy. Treatment is conservative with wrist splinting and it commonly resolves within 3 months postpartum. **Meralgia paresthetica** (numbness or dysesthesia of the anterolateral thigh due to compression of the lateral femoral cutaneous nerve along the pelvic wall or obturator canal) occurs as the fetus enlarges, and also typically resolves within 3 months of delivery. Bell's palsy is seen with increased frequency in pregnant women. Treatment with corticosteroids during pregnancy for the treatment of Bell's palsy is still controversial.

Traumatic mononeuropathy usually occurs during childbirth. Trauma involving the obturator nerve may result from compression by the fetal head, from misplaced forceps, or from hyperflexion in the lithotomy position. Compression injuries during delivery have also been reported involving the femoral, saphenous, common peroneal, or sciatic nerves. Postpartum foot drop is an interesting example of traumatic mononeuropathy with generally excellent prognosis, most typically observed in short primigravid women with large infants.

## IATROGENIC (DRUG-INDUCED)

84. **What factors are important with regard to an increased risk for seizures due to drug therapy?**
High-dose intrathecal or intravenous administration, blood-brain barrier (BBB) permeability, prior history or family history of epilepsy, preexisting cerebral or systemic disease (renal, liver disease), abrupt withdrawal.

85. **What drugs are associated with increased seizure risk at therapeutic dose and serum levels?**
Tricyclic antidepressants (1%), aliphatic (chlorpromazine, promazine, prochlorperazine) phenothiazines (1% to 2%), tetracyclic antidepressants.

86. **What drugs are associated with the development of pseudotumor cerebri?**
Pseudotumor cerebri is characterized by headache, papilledema, diplopia and impaired vision due to raised intracranial pressure possibly due to CSF malabsorption. Drugs associated with its development include oral contraceptives, estrogens, tetracyclines, nalidixic acid, nitrofurantoin, ketamine, nitrous oxide, vitamin A, minocycline, danazol, ampicillin, amiodarone, etretinate, and thyroxine. Abrupt withdrawal of corticosteroids has been associated with its development in children.

87. **What drugs induce movement disorders?**
Major classes of psychotropic drugs, antiparkinsonian agents, and tricyclic antidepressants may induce involuntary movements or changes in muscle tone and posture associated with action on dopaminergic neurotransmission.

88. **What extrapyramidal disorders can be induced by drugs?**
Acute dystonic-dyskinetic reactions, akathisia, tardive dyskinesia, chorea and choreoathetosis, drug-induced parkinsonism, neuroleptic malignant syndrome, tremor, tic, and myoclonus.

89. **What category of drugs affects or induces neuromuscular disorders?**
Peripheral neuropathy
    Antimicrobial (isoniazid, ethambutol, dapsone)
    Antineoplastic (vincristine, vinca alkaloids)
    Antirheumatic (chloroquine, gold treatment, D-penicillamine)
    Cardiovascular (amiodarone)
    Other: colchicine
Neuromuscular junction (*aggravation or unmasking of myasthenia gravis)
    Antimicrobial (aminoglycosides)*
    Anticonvulsants (phenytoin)
    Antirheumatic (D-penicillamine, chloroquine)
    Cardiovascular (quinidine, propranolol)*
    Psychotropic (lithium, chlorpromazine)*
    Muscle relaxants*
Muscle (rhabdomyolysis,* neuroleptic malignant syndrome,** cramps/myalgias,[†] myopathy[‡])
    Amphotericin B*
    Antirheumatic (gold[†], D-penicillamine[†], steroid*)
    Psychotropic (lithium*, haloperidol**, fluphenazine**)
    Sedatives (barbiturates, diazepam)*
    Analgesics (heroine, morphine, salicylates, codeine)*
    Cardiovascular (statins[‡], clofibrate*, labetalol[†], captopril[†])
    Anesthetics (suxamethonium*)

# WEBSITES

1. http://www.wilsonsdisease.org

2. http://www.sjogrens.com

3. http://www.neuropathy.org

# BIBLIOGRAPHY

1. Aminoff MJ: Neurology and General Medicine, 2nd ed. New York, Churchill-Livingstone, 1995.
2. Bradley WG, Daroff RB, Fenichel GM, Marsden CD: Neurology in Clinical Practice, 3rd ed. Boston, Butterworth-Heinemann, 2000.
3. Rosenbaum RB, Campbell SM, Rosenbaum JT: Clinical Neurology of Rheumatic Diseases. Boston: Butterworth-Heinemann, 1996.
4. Samuels MA, Feske S (eds): Office Practice of Neurology. New York, Churchill-Livingstone, 1996.

# CHAPTER 23

# INFECTIOUS DISEASES, INCLUDING AIDS

*Maria E. Carlini, MD, and Richard L. Harris, MD*

## BACTERIAL INFECTIONS

1. **What clinical findings differentiate meningitis from encephalitis?**
   Patients with meningitis have nuchal rigidity, headache, photophobia, and fever. Patients with encephalitis have disruption of cognitive function that may include altered consciousness, disorientation, behavioral or speech difficulties, and focal neurologic signs such as seizures or hemiparesis. In reality, the majority of infections cause a combination of symptoms and thus lead to meningoencephalitis. In classic presentations, however, bacterial meningitis leads to predominantly meningeal symptoms and processes, whereas herpes encephalitis produces predominantly cerebral symptoms.

   Greenberg BM: Central nervous system infections in the intensive care unit. Semin Neurol 28:682-689, 2008.

2. **When may a bacterial infection produce cerebrospinal fluid (CSF) results identical to aseptic meningitis?**
   Aseptic meningitis is often a viral infection and typically produces lymphocytic pleocytosis, normal glucose, mildly elevated protein, negative Gram stain, and sterile bacterial cultures. Similar CSF findings may occur in partially treated bacterial meningitis or parameningeal foci such as epidural, subdural, or brain abscesses.

3. **Bacterial meningitis is the most common cause of hypoglycorrhachia (low CSF glucose). What are the other common causes?**
   1. Cryptococcal meningitis
   2. Tuberculous meningitis
   3. Syphilitic meningitis
   4. Neurosarcoidosis
   5. Meningeal carcinomatosis

4. **A patient presents with probable acute bacterial meningitis, but you are unable to obtain informed consent for lumbar puncture until after a computed tomography (CT) scan. You wisely decide to start antibiotics immediately and not wait for the lumbar puncture. What tests can you still perform that might identify the etiologic agent?**
   1. Blood cultures should be obtained before antibiotics are given. Approximately 50% of patients with bacterial meningitis have a positive blood culture.
   2. Serologic studies, such as latex agglutination or counterimmunoelectrophoresis (CIE), for *Streptococcus pneumoniae, Neisseria meningitidis, Hemophilus influenzae,* and *Listeria monocytogenes* may be positive in blood, urine, and CSF (even after antibiotics).
   3. Culture of CSF, even after antibiotics are given, will probably be positive for hours.

5. **Who should receive prophylaxis after contact with a patient with meningitis?**
   Prophylaxis depends on the organism and the age of the exposed person:

1. *H. influenzae*, **type B**—all children who have close contact with the patient and who have not been vaccinated.
2. *N. meningitidis*—all close contacts, regardless of age.
   Rifampin is usually considered the drug of choice for prophylaxis. Quinolones such as ciprofloxacin are also effective.

6. **What are the most common gram-negative bacilli causing meningitis after the neonatal period?**
   *Klebsiella* spp., *Escherichia coli*, and *Pseudomonas* spp. account for 75% to 90% of gram-negative bacillary meningitis after the neonatal period. Eighty percent of gram-negative meningitis occurs in conjunction with head trauma or neurosurgical procedures.

7. **Which organisms are most likely to cause meningitis after neurosurgical procedures?**
   Gram-negative bacilli and staphylococci are the most common organisms, but virtually any kind of bacteria and even fungi such as *Candida* spp. can gain access to the subarachnoid region.
   Morris A, Low DE: Nosocomial bacterial meningitis, including central nervous system shunt infections. Infect Dis Clin North Am 13:735-750, 1999.

8. **In a patient with a ventriculoatrial or ventriculoperitoneal shunt, what is the most common cause of bacterial meningitis?**
   Coagulase-negative staphylococci account for more than 50% of cases of meningitis in patients with ventricular shunts, followed by *Staphylococcus aureus*, *Propionibacterium acnes*, gram-negative bacilli, and enterococci.

9. **What bacteria is the most common cause of meningitis in patients with a CSF leak?**
   *S. pneumoniae.*

10. **What is the most common cause of meningitis after blunt head trauma?**
    *S. pneumoniae.*

11. **What are the most common clinical settings in which brain abscesses develop?**
    1. Contiguous suppurative foci such as otitis media or sinusitis
    2. Hematogenous spread from a distant focus
    3. Penetrating cranial injuries or neurosurgical procedures
    4. Cryptogenic (20% of cases)
       Menon S, Bharadwaj R, Chowdhary A, et al.: Current epidemiology of intracranial abscesses. J Med Microbiol 57:1259-1268, 2008.

12. **Describe the presentation of a brain abscess.**
    A patient with brain abscess often presents with symptoms similar to those of a brain tumor, but they are more rapidly progressive. Headache, focal neurologic signs dependent on the site of the lesion, and signs of increased intracranial pressure are present. Fever and elevated white blood cell (WBC) count are *not* common.

13. **How does an abscess appear on CT scan?**
    An abscess appears as a hypodense lesion surrounded by a contrast-enhancing ring. A thin-walled ring is more common in an abscess, whereas a thick-walled, irregular ring is more characteristic of tumor.

14. **What is the most common bacterial agent involved in spinal epidural abscess?**
    *S. aureus* accounts for approximately 62% of cases, aerobic gram-negative rods for 18%, aerobic streptococci for 8%, and *Staphylococcus epidermidis* and anaerobes for about 2% each. Unknown or other organisms (1%) cause the remainder. Empirical antibiotics must include an antistaphylococcal agent. Gram-negative coverage may be warranted in patients with a history of a spinal procedure, intravenous drug abuse, or recent gastrointestinal (GI) or genitourinary infection. Antibiotic therapy is required for 4 to 6 weeks, and prompt surgical drainage may be needed.

    Pradilla G, Ardila GP, Hsu W, Rigamonti D: Epidural abscesses of the CNS. Lancet Neurol 8:292-300, 2009.

15. **Describe the clinical course of an untreated spinal epidural abscess.**
    The first symptom noted is usually focal vertebral pain, followed by root pain, then deficits of motor, sensory, or sphincter function, and finally paralysis.

16. **What conditions predispose to recurrent bacterial meningitis?**
    1. Anatomic communications with paranasal sinuses, nasopharynx, middle ear, skin (such as congenital midline dermal sinus tracts), or prosthetic devices such as ventriculoperitoneal shunts.
    2. Parameningeal foci may either drain into the meninges or lead to repeated inflammatory reactions and meningeal signs or symptoms.
    3. Immunologic defects such as hypogammaglobulinemia, splenectomy, leukemia and lymphoma, sickle cell anemia, and other hemoglobinopathies, or complement deficiencies.

17. **Name conditions that predispose to polymicrobial meningitis.**
    1. Infections at contiguous foci
    2. Tumors in close proximity to the central nervous system (CNS)
    3. Fistulous communications
    4. Disseminated strongyloidiasis (enteric organisms carried "piggy-back" from the gut through the bloodstream to the subarachnoid space)

18. **A 72-year-old man was hospitalized 1 week ago for stroke. He has dense right hemiplegia and is incontinent of bowel and bladder. Today he developed a fever of 101° F, along with shaking chills. What sources are most likely responsible?**
    The cause of fever is probably a nosocomial infection. A lower urinary tract infection is most likely—whether he has a Foley catheter, a condom catheter, or a neurogenic bladder that does not fully empty. Other good possibilities include pneumonia (especially aspiration pneumonia) or venous catheter-related infection.

19. **An elderly man taking steroids chronically for lung disease presents with a history and physical examination consistent with meningitis and new-onset seizures. The laboratory tells you that the "preliminary" examination of the CSF shows "diphtheroids" on the Gram stain. What organism is probably responsible for the infection?**
    *Listeria* may be mistaken for diphtheroids on Gram stain; both are gram-positive bacilli. Listerial infection often occurs in immunocompromised patients. Risk factors include cirrhosis, neoplastic disease, renal failure, pregnancy, chronic steroid therapy, and extremes of age (i.e., very young and elderly). Some outbreaks have been traced to food-borne sources, and the disease has been classically associated with animal exposure. CSF cell counts, protein, and glucose are variable and do not distinguish listerial infection from other forms of meningitis. Monocytosis is not common. Common treatment is with ampicillin and an aminoglycoside. Cephalosporins are not effective.

    Clauss HE, Lorber B: Central nervous system infection with *Listeria monocytogenes*. Curr Infect Dis Rep 10:300-306, 2008.

20. **A 14-year-old boy whose only medical problem is acne presents with diplopia, photophobia, and right periorbital edema. His neurologic examination reveals a midposition, fixed right pupil, decreased sensation over the upper face, right ophthalmoplegia, and papilledema on the right. What is wrong?**
The symptoms and signs are consistent with an infectious cavernous sinus thrombosis on the right, most likely from squeezing a pimple. Untreated, he may develop progressive exophthalmos, loss of corneal reflex, retinal hemorrhage, and visual loss. As the infection spreads to the contralateral cavernous sinus, similar findings appear in the opposite eye. Cranial nerves III, IV, V, and VI are affected as they pass through the cavernous sinuses.

21. **A 57-year-old diabetic man presents with a right facial nerve palsy, otalgia, and otorrhea. What is the most likely organism?**
The condition is most often due to *Pseudomonas aeruginosa,* producing the syndrome of necrotizing or "malignant" external otitis.
    Franco-Vidal V, Blanchet H, Bebear C, et al.: Necrotizing external otitis. Otol Neurotol 28:771-773, 2007.

22. **In what clinical situations does a CNS infection merit the use of systemic steroids?**
    1. An infant with *H. influenzae* meningitis
    2. A severely ill adult with tuberculous meningitis
    3. A patient with neurocysticercosis and increased intracranial pressure

## ANTIBIOTIC TOXICITY

23. **What is the clinical presentation of a patient receiving excessive doses of beta-lactam antibiotics?**
Toxicity may cause confusion, jitteriness, myoclonic jerks, and seizures.

24. **In addition to aminoglycosides, what other drugs cause ototoxicity?**
    1. Ethacrynic acid—probably the highest risk
    2. Furosemide
    3. Erythromycin—usually reversible hearing loss with high-dose therapy
    4. Vancomycin—listed as ototoxic, but if so, rarely

25. **Which conditions predispose to peripheral neuropathy in patients who take isoniazid?**
Peripheral neuropathy is especially likely to occur in patients who are slow acetylators, are poorly nourished, or have an underlying neuropathy secondary to diabetes, uremia, or alcoholism. Concomitant administration of pyridoxine (vitamin $B_6$) may prevent the neuropathy.

## TOXINS

26. **What three bacteria produce exotoxins that affect peripheral nerves either directly or indirectly?**
    1. The B subunit of diphtheria toxin binds to cell membranes and allows the A subunit to enter nerves, where it inhibits protein synthesis and causes a noninflammatory demyelination. Cranial nerves are affected more frequently than peripheral nerves.
    2. Tetanus toxin is transported up the axon and binds to the presynaptic endings on motor neurons in the anterior horns of the spinal cord. Inhibitory input is blocked, resulting in muscle spasms.
    3. Botulinum toxin binds to the presynaptic axon terminal of the neuromuscular junction, preventing acetylcholine release and producing a flaccid paralysis.

27. **What are the manifestations of ciguatera? How does one acquire this illness?**
Patients ingest ciguatoxin, produced by the dinoflagellate *Gambierdiscus toxicus,* when they eat large, carnivorous reef fish such as grouper or snapper. Within about 6 hours, GI symptoms of nausea, vomiting, diarrhea, and cramps begin. Bizarre neurologic symptoms may appear early or after the GI complaints and resolve in 24 to 48 hours. Neurologic manifestations include numbness and tingling of lips and extremities, reversal of hot-cold sensation, and tooth pain. Paresthesias may not follow dermatomal patterns. Vertigo, hypersalivation, blurred vision, tremor, ataxia, and coma may occur.

28. **What illness is caused by eating puffer fish?**
Tetrodotoxication occurs within 3 hours of eating a tetrodotoxic fish such as puffer fish, porcupine fish, ocean sunfish, blue-ringed octopus, and some species of newts and salamanders. Symptoms include lethargy, paresthesias, hyperemesis, salivation, weakness, ataxia, and dysphagia. Ascending paralysis, respiratory failure, hypotension, and bradycardia may occur. Diagnosis is clinical, and treatment is supportive. Gastric lavage, activated charcoal, and anticholinesterase inhibitors may be helpful.

29. **What are the symptoms of scombroid poisoning?**
Symptoms of scombroid poisoning begin within minutes to hours of ingestion of toxic fish. The fish are usually of the family Scombroidea, which includes tuna, mackerel, and jacks, but cases are also reported from nonscombroid fish. Victims experience flushing and a hot sensation of the skin, headache, dizziness, burning sensation in the mouth and throat, and palpitations. Nausea, diarrhea, and occasionally vomiting occur. A sunburn-like skin rash appears. In severe case, bronchospasm, palpitations, supraventricular arrhythmias, and occasionally mild hypotension may occur. The diagnosis is clinical. Treatment is supportive. Deaths have not been reported.

30. **What is the scombrotoxin?**
The scombrotoxin is formed when surface bacteria (*Proteus* and *Klebsiella* spp.) proliferate on the flesh of the fish because of improper refrigeration. Free histidine, present in increased quantities in dark meat fish, is degraded to histamine by the bacteria. The exact role of histamine is unclear because orally ingested histamine is degraded in the gastrointestinal tract, but a histamine-like substance such as saurine produces the clinical effects. Another substance in the fish may prevent degradation or increase absorption of histamine.

    Fusetani N, Kem W: Marine toxins: An overview. Prog Mol Subcell Biol 46:1-44, 2009.


## SPIROCHETAL INFECTIONS

31. **What serologic laboratory tests are used to assist in the diagnosis of syphilis? How should they be interpreted?**
Two general classes of laboratory tests are used: nontreponemal antigen tests and treponemal tests. The nontreponemal tests use extract of normal tissues (i.e., beef cardiolipin) as antigens to measure antibodies formed in the blood. The commonly used nontreponemal tests are the rapid plasma reagin (RPR) and Venereal Disease Research Laboratory (VDRL) tests. Both become positive in the early stages of the primary lesion and are almost always positive by the secondary stage. They decline in later stages of the disease. False-positive results occur in autoimmune illness, malaria, mononucleosis, and pregnancy, among others. The nontreponemal tests, therefore, should be used as a screening test for the more specific treponemal tests. They also may be used to follow response to treatment because they decline with time after successful treatment.

The treponemal tests use live or killed *Treponema pallidum* as antigen to detect treponemal antibody directly. The commonly used treponemal tests are the microhemagglutination test for antibody to *T. pallidum* (MHA-TP) and the fluorescent treponemal antibody absorption test (FTA-ABS). These tests remain positive even after appropriate treatment.

If a patient has strongly positive serum RPR or VDRL and MHA-TP or FTA-ABS tests and symptoms consistent with neurosyphilis, most experts agree that the patient should undergo a lumbar puncture, if feasible, to look for a positive VDRL and/or MHA-TP in the CSF, which helps to confirm the need for treatment for neurosyphilis. These tests may be falsely negative even in CSF. If clinical suspicion is high enough, most clinicians treat for neurosyphilis. Obtaining documentation of prior treatment for syphilis is important because it can obviously shorten the evaluation considerably.

32. **How frequent are abnormalities in the CSF of patients with primary or secondary syphilis?**
    Abnormalities in the CSF are found in 15% to 40% of patients who have primary or secondary syphilis and are usually asymptomatic.

33. **At what stage of syphilis (primary, secondary, or tertiary) does neurosyphilis occur?**
    Neurosyphilis may occur in any stage of syphilis. CNS invasion by *T. pallidum* occurs in nearly one-third of patients with primary and secondary syphilis.
    Marra CM: Update on neurosyphilis. Curr Infect Dis Rep 11:127-134, 2009.

34. **What circumstances predispose to early neurosyphilis?**
    Inadequate treatment of early syphilis and human immunodeficiency virus (HIV) infection predisposes to early neurosyphilis.

35. **Which cranial nerves are most often involved in syphilitic meningitis?**
    Syphilis affects the seventh and eighth cranial nerves most often (40%) and the second, third, and fourth cranial nerves less frequently (25%).

36. **What are the neurologic complications of Lyme disease?**
    Early in the course, meningitis, cranial neuritis, Bell's palsy, motor or sensory radiculoneuritis, subtle encephalitis, mononeuritis multiplex, myelitis, chorea, or cerebellar ataxia may occur. Chronically, patients may develop encephalitis, spastic paraparesis, ataxic gait, subtle mental disorders, chronic axonal polyradiculography, or dementia.
    Halperin JJ: Nervous system Lyme disease: Diagnosis and Treatment. Rev Neurol Dis 6:4-12, 2009.

37. **What is the most likely clinical presentation of infection with *Borrelia burgdorferi* (Lyme disease)?**
    A 10-cm erythematous lesion with central clearing on the patient's back. The presence of the typical tick-bite wound is a more reliable guide to infection than serologic titers or (often vague) clinical symptoms.

38. **What is the clinical presentation of leptospirosis?**
    Leptospirosis often develops after a camping trip and may present as aseptic meningitis (with normal CSF glucose), bulbar conjunctivitis, erythematous rash, adenopathy, hepatosplenomegaly, and renal insufficiency.
    Panicker JN, Mammachan R, Jayakumar RV: Primary neuroleptospirosis. Postgrad Med J 77:589-590, 2001.

## FUNGAL, PARASITIC, AND OTHER PROCESSES

39. **Describe the clinical presentation of infection with *Acanthamoeba* or *Naegleria* spp.**

    Both infections usually present as severe persistent frontal headache after swimming in a freshwater lake.

40. **What neurologic abnormalities occur with cerebral malaria? What does the spinal fluid show?**

    Neurologic abnormalities include disturbances of consciousness, acute organic brain syndromes, seizures, meningismus, and, rarely, focal neurologic signs. A lumbar puncture usually reveals an elevated opening pressure with normal CSF. Occasionally CSF protein is elevated. Low-level pleocytosis occurs, but hypoglycorrhachia does not. Therapy is with quinine, chloroquine, and dexamethasone.

41. **What is the epidemiology of neurocysticercosis?**

    Infection with eggs of the pork tapeworm, *Taenia solium*, can lead to neurocysticercosis. In the intermediate stage, it is referred to as *Cysticercus cellulosae*, but *T. solium* and *C. cellulosae* are the same parasite. Ingestion of infected pork → intestinal tapeworm (often asymptomatic) → fecal excretion → human fecal-oral contamination → egg ingestion and penetration of intestinal wall → onchospheres → larvae that encyst → neurocysticercosis. Therapy is with praziquantel, 50 mg/kg for 15 to 30 days.

    The clinical presentation of neurocysticercosis depends on the number and location of the cysts but usually includes seizures. Headache, altered mental status, or symptoms of hydrocephalus may occur. Disease may be active or inactive; this distinction guides further evaluation and treatment.

    Sinha S, Sharma BS: Neurocysticercosis: A review of current status and management. J Clin Neurosci 16:867-876, 2009.

42. **A 21-year-old archeology student complains of headache, fever, lethargy, and difficulty with concentrating in class. He had been well until 2 months previously, when he had a brief illness with fever, arthralgia, cough, and sputum production just after he returned from a dig in Arizona. He was again well until his current symptoms began 2 weeks ago. What is his probable diagnosis? How should he be treated?**

    The most likely diagnosis is coccidioidomycosis meningitis, a fungus found in the soil in hot, arid climates. He needs intrathecal amphotericin B as well as small doses of systemic amphotericin. Treatment will be long-term and relapses are common. Other drugs that may have a role are fluconazole and itraconazole.

43. **Which antifungal agents are most useful in CNS infections because of their good spinal fluid penetration?**

    Amphotericin B and fluconazole enter the CSF adequately. Ketoconazole has poor penetration.

44. **What are the side effects of treatment with amphotericin?**

    Amphotericin may produce fever, chills, hypotension, nausea, headache, and tachypnea during or shortly after administration. Premedication with antipyretics and supplemental intravenous hydration may reduce these effects. Meperidine has been used to reduce discomfort secondary to severe chills. Renal impairment may occur, chiefly in the form of decreased glomerular filtration rate and increased blood urea nitrogen and creatinine. But hypokalemia and hypomagnesemia also result from renal wastage and renal tubular acidosis. Hydration may lessen renal side effects.

**45. Describe the presentation of tuberculous meningitis.**

The onset of symptoms is usually gradual, and behavioral changes may precede more classic symptoms of headache, vomiting, seizures, and cranial nerve abnormalities. A focus of tuberculosis may be found in another organ system. Meningitis follows rupture of subependymal lesions (Rich foci) into the subarachnoid space. Basilar inflammation with cranial nerve entrapment and severe arteriolitis with subsequent thrombosis (commonly of middle and anterior cerebral artery territory) is characteristic.

CSF shows increased protein, decreased glucose, increased opening pressure, and 50 to 1000 WBC (polymorphonuclear cells predominate early, lymphocytes predominate late). Acid-fast stains and cultures are often negative in the presence of disease. Treatment with antituberculous drugs should be initiated if clinical suspicion is high. Initial concurrent treatment with steroids is controversial.

**46. A patient in whom you are about to begin high-dose steroids has a purified protein derivative (PPD) test that is positive at 17 mm with a known negative PPD 1 year ago. What should you do before beginning steroids?**

The patient should have a chest radiograph to exclude evidence of active pulmonary tuberculosis. If the chest radiograph is positive, the patient needs treatment for pulmonary tuberculosis. If no evidence of active infection is found, the patient needs isoniazid prophylaxis for tuberculosis because of the recent and strongly positive conversion and immunosuppression by steroids.

**47. An 82-year-old woman presents with fever, sweats, generalized body aches, weakness, severe headache, and weight loss. She describes intermittent cough and painful jaw muscles while chewing food. Her laboratory studies show anemia, elevated alkaline phosphatase, and sedimentation rate of 92 mm/h. What is the diagnosis?**

Temporal arteritis. This granulomatous arteritis often mimics an infectious disease.

**48. A patient whom you diagnosed 1 year previously with temporal arteritis has done well on her therapy. She returns for an office visit and complains of dysphagia and weight loss. What do you suspect?**

Infectious esophagitis. *Candida* spp. or perhaps herpes simplex virus (HSV) is the most likely pathogen in a patient who has taken long-term steroids.

**49. What is Vogt-Koyanagi-Harada syndrome?**

This syndrome consists of subacute meningoencephalitis with severe, protracted granulomatous uveitis and depigmentary skin changes. The cause is unknown, but it is noninfectious. Other noninfectious lymphocytic meningitides include Behçet's disease and CNS vasculitides.

**50. What is neuroleptic malignant syndrome (NMS)?**

NMS is a noninfectious cause of fever characterized by autonomic and extrapyramidal dysfunction as a consequence of neuroleptic drug use (e.g., haloperidol, chlorpromazine, fluphenazine). Major clinical findings include fever, hyperreflexia, tachypnea, diaphoresis, altered mental status, labile blood pressure, tremor, and rigidity. Laboratory findings include elevated creatine phosphokinase (CPK), leukocytosis, myoglobinuria, and metabolic acidosis. Therapy involves immediate discontinuation of neuroleptics and treatment with dantrolene and bromocriptine.

Haddad PM, Dursun SM: Neurological complications of psychiatric drugs. Hum Psychopharmacol 23:15-26, 2008.

Seitz DP, Gill SS: Neuroleptic malignant syndrome complicating antipsychotic treatment of delirium or agitation in medical and surgical patients. Psychosomatics 50:8-15, 2009.

51. **What is Whipple's disease? Describe the CNS manifestations.**
Whipple's disease is a systemic illness caused by *Tropheryma whippelii,* a gram-positive bacillus. Gastrointestinal signs and symptoms are usually primary components of the illness and include weight loss, diarrhea, and malabsorption. Arthralgias, pleural effusions, and fever also may be present. CNS involvement can include upper motor neuron signs, hypothalamic dysfunction, supranuclear gaze palsy, and cognitive and psychiatric aberrations. CNS findings are rare in the absence of systemic illness but have been reported.
   Panegyres PK: Diagnosis and management of Whipple's disease of the brain. Pract Neurol 8:311-317, 2008.

## PRIONS

52. **What is a prion? Why is it important in neurologic disease?**
A prion is a small proteinaceous infectious particle that resists inactivation by procedures that modify nucleic acids. The concept of an infectious agent that does not require DNA or RNA is novel. This type of agent is thought to be responsible for scrapie, Creutzfeldt-Jakob disease, and kuru.
   Cobb NJ, Surewicz WK: Prion diseases and their biochemical mechanisms. Biochemistry 48:2574-2585, 2009.

53. **A 45-year-old man presents with myoclonus and dementia that have progressed rapidly over the past 6 months. CSF is normal. What is the likely diagnosis? What does his electroencephalogram (EEG) show?**
The patient has findings characteristic of Creutzfeldt-Jakob disease. Dementia progresses rapidly over months, and death usually occurs in less than 1 year. The EEG characteristically (but not always) has periodic-appearing, biphasic or triphasic, high-amplitude sharp waves. CSF is usually normal, although a mild elevation in protein is occasionally found.

54. **What is the pathologic lesion in Creutzfeldt-Jakob disease?**
The pathologic lesion is spongiform encephalopathy characterized by loss of neurons, with astrocytic proliferation and gliosis, swelling, and intracytoplasmic vacuolization of neuronal and astroglial processes.

55. **What infection-control measures should be observed for a patient with Creutzfeldt-Jakob disease?**
Blood, brain, cornea, visceral organs, and CSF are infectious. Autoclaving for 1 hour at 250° F and 15 psi, exposure to 1 or 0.1 N sodium hydroxide for 1 hour at room temperature, or exposure to 0.5% sodium hydrochlorite will kill the causative agent. Of note, the agent is not destroyed by boiling, ultraviolet radiation, ionizing radiation, 70% ethyl alcohol, formaldehyde, glutaraldehyde, or 10% formalin. The patient need not be isolated, but blood and body fluid precautions should be observed.

56. **What is "mad cow" disease?**
Mad cow disease is the sobriquet of bovine spongiform encephalopathy (BSE), a variant of Creutzfeldt-Jakob disease recently described in a series of young patients in the United Kingdom. It is believed to be transmissible by consumption of contaminated beef. Studies are under way to determine the scope of the problem and measures needed for containment.
   Harman JL, Silva CJ: Bovine spongiform encephalopathy. J Am Vet Med Assoc 234:59-72, 2009.
   Weihl CC, Ross RP: Creutzfeldt-Jakob disease, new variant Creutzfeldt-Jakob disease, and bovine spongiform encephalopathy. Neurol Clin 17:835-859, 1999.

57. **What is kuru? How is it transmitted?**
    Kuru, another disease caused by prions, is transmitted by cannibalism. New Guinea natives practicing ritualistic consumption of dead kinsmen (including their brains) as a rite of mourning developed this illness. Clinically, kuru presents as a progressive fatal dementia with severe ataxia.

## VIRAL INFECTIONS

58. **When may aseptic meningitis be confused with bacterial meningitis? How do you resolve the confusion?**
    Early in viral meningitis, the spinal fluid may have a predominance of polymorphonuclear (PMN) leukocytes. The Gram stain is negative, and CSF glucose is normal. Because the PMN predominance quickly changes to a mononuclear cell predominance, a repeat lumbar puncture 6 to 12 hours later will clarify the issue.

59. **Other than culture results, which of the routine studies performed on CSF is the most useful for distinguishing between meningitis due to tuberculosis and that due to a virus, such as ECHO 9? What does ECHO stand for?**
    The glucose test is most useful. Glucose is usually low in tuberculous infection, but normal in viral infections. ECHO stands for enteric cytopathic human orphan [virus]. ECHO viruses are among the most common causes of viral meningitis.

60. **Worldwide, what is the most common cause of epidemic encephalitis?**
    Japanese B encephalitis is the most common epidemic infection outside North America. It is a major medical problem in China, Southwest Asia, and India.

61. **What is the most common sporadic encephalitis in the United States?**
    Herpes simplex causes encephalitis most frequently.

62. **What are the common arthropod-borne viral encephalitides in the United States?**
    1. **St. Louis encephalitis** occurs in the central, western, and southern United States and affects older adults.
    2. **La Crosse encephalitis:** La Crosse, a type of California encephalitis, is a common arthropod-borne encephalitis in the United States. It occurs in the central and eastern United States and primarily affects children. It has a mortality of less than 1%, and sequelae are rare.
    3. **Venezuelan equine encephalitis** occurs in the South, affects adults, and has low mortality and sequelae rates.
    4. **Western equine encephalitis** occurs in the West and Midwest, affecting people at extremes of age. Mortality is 5% to 15%, and sequelae are more common in infants than in older survivors.
    5. **Eastern equine encephalitis** affects children in the East, South, and Gulf Coast. Mortality is 50% to 75%, and 80% of survivors have sequelae.

63. **What are the major differences between Western, Eastern, and Venezuelan equine encephalitis?**
    1. **Eastern** is a summertime disease that causes less than 15 human cases per year but has a 50% to 75% mortality rate. It strikes mainly in the Gulf and Atlantic states.
    2. **Venezuelan** occurs in epidemics that have caused tens of thousands of cases but with a fatality rate of only 0.6%; mainly in Central and South America.
    3. **Western** occurs in the summer months also, usually in states west of the Mississippi river. It causes 0 to 200 cases/year, and infants are most susceptible. The risk is greatest in rural areas. The case fatality rate is 3% to 5%.

64. **What is West Nile encephalitis?**
West Nile encephalitis is caused by a flavivirus endemic in Africa, West Asia, and the Middle East. It is related to St. Louis encephalitis. Recently cases of West Nile encephalitis have been reported throughout the United States, and the virus has been isolated in local mosquito populations. Symptoms are usually mild and include headache, fever, and myalgias, but severe forms of the illness also occur.
   Madden K: West Nile virus and its neurological manifestations. Clin Med Res 1:145-150, 2003.
   Petersen LR, Hayes EB: West Nile virus in the Americas. Med Clin North Am 92:1307-1322, 2008.

65. **A patient presents with aphasia, right-sided weakness, fever, and confusion. A lumbar puncture reveals CSF with 400 RBC/mm$^3$, 30 WBC/mm$^3$ (predominantly mononuclear cells), glucose of 70 mg/dL, and protein of 60 mg/dL. EEG shows periodic high-voltage spike wave activity from the left temporal region. What is the most likely causative agent?**
Herpes simplex encephalitis. The main clue to herpes versus other causes of viral encephalitis is focality, especially to the temporal lobe.
   Baringer JR: Herpes simplex infections of the nervous system. Neurol Clin 26:657-674, 2008.

66. **What are typical CSF findings in herpes encephalitis?**
Normal CSF cell counts and chemistries are occasionally seen in HSV encephalitis. Typical CSF findings are lymphocytic predominance, elevated protein, and the presence of RBCs. In most cases, HSV cannot be cultured from the CSF. Diagnosis may be made with polymerase chain reaction (PCR) for herpes DNA in CSF.

67. **What histopathologic finding is pathognomonic for herpes encephalitis?**
The Cowdry type A inclusion body, an eosinophilic, intranuclear particle.

68. **What is the recommended therapy for HSV encephalitis?**
Treatment requires acyclovir, 10 mg/kg every 8 hours for at least 14 days. Because acyclovir is cleared by the kidney, the dose requires adjustment for renal insufficiency, and patients with normal renal function should be encouraged to drink generous amounts of free water each day.

## KEY POINTS: INFECTIOUS DISEASES

1. Antibiotics should be given immediately in patients with meningitis, and not delayed while other tests are performed.

2. Syphilis can affect the nervous system at any time in its course. It is now rarely seen except in HIV-positive patients.

3. Mad cow disease is a variant of Creutzfeldt-Jakob disease caused by a prion—a protein that does not require DNA or RNA to replicate and produce infection.

4. Herpes simplex, the most common sporadic encephalitis, often produces focal neurologic damage and must be aggressively treated with acyclovir.

5. Acquired immune deficiency syndrome (AIDS) patients may develop neurologic problems from the virus itself, the drugs used to treat it, or opportunistic infections.

69. **A 32-year-old woman presents with painful genital vesicular lesions, urinary retention, and severe headache. CSF shows lymphocytic pleocytosis. The neurologic examination is otherwise unremarkable. What is the probable diagnosis?**
Herpes simplex virus II meningitis. Genital lesions usually recur, but the meningitis usually does not. It has an excellent prognosis neurologically. This benign form of "aseptic" meningitis should not be confused with the potentially fatal, necrotizing form of HSV 1 encephalitis.

70. **What is Ramsay Hunt syndrome?**
Herpes zoster infection involving cranial nerves VII and VIII. Patients present with vertigo, ipsilateral hearing deficit, and facial palsy plus vesicles in the external auditory canal.

71. **What are the most important neurologic complications of primary varicella infections?**
1. Reye's syndrome. This acute, noninflammatory encephalopathy is characterized by fatty destruction of the liver, hypoglycemia, and increased intracranial pressure. It has a 20% fatality rate. Aspirin use with varicella and influenza has been associated with Reye's syndrome in children, and it has become rare since aspirin is now seldom given.
2. Aseptic meningitis
3. Transverse myelitis
4. Guillain-Barré syndrome
5. Cerebellar encephalitis. In children, it results in ataxia, nausea, and rigidity, but most make a full recovery. In adults, it results in altered sensorium, seizures, focal signs, and a mortality rate up to 35%.

72. **Which two viruses enter the CNS by peripheral intraneural routes to cause encephalitis?**
Herpes simplex and rabies viruses enter the nervous system by peripheral intraneuronal routes. One route for HSV may be the olfactory tract.

73. **Who should receive postexposure rabies prophylaxis?**
Postexposure prophylaxis for rabies is recommended for all persons bitten or scratched by wild or domestic animals that may be carrying the disease, or who have an open wound or mucous membrane contaminated with saliva or other potentially infectious material from a rabid animal. It is also recommended for persons who report a possibly infectious exposure to a human with rabies. Potentially rabid animals include (but are not limited to) dogs, cats, skunks, raccoons, foxes, and bats.

74. **Which infections may lead to a postinfectious encephalomyelitis?**
Immune-mediated inflammation following an infection, sometimes called *acute disseminated encephalomyelitis,* usually presents with multifocal lesions of the brain and spinal cord that may closely resemble multiple sclerosis. This demyelinating syndrome is most common after infections with varicella, influenza, and measles virus.

75. **What clinical features characterize postpolio syndrome?**
The main symptoms of postpolio syndrome are the new onset of weakness, pain, and fatigue years after acute poliomyelitis. About 25% of survivors of polio are affected. EMG and muscle biopsy show evidence of both chronic and recent denervation, although these changes are nonspecific; asymptomatic survivors of polio also exhibit these changes.

76. **What virus appears to be the most common cause of Bell's palsy?**
Recent studies implicate herpes simplex as one cause of Bell's palsy. A benefit for steroids or acyclovir has not been established, however, either or both are sometimes given.

Grogan PM, Gronseth GS: Steroids, acyclovir, and surgery for Bell's palsy (an evidence-based review): Report of the Quality Standards Subcommittee of the American Academy of Neurology. Neurology 56:830-836, 2001.

## AIDS

77. **Which antiretroviral drug may cause myopathy and myositis?**
Zidovudine (AZT) may cause both myopathy and myositis, especially with long-term therapy. It is often difficult to distinguish this entity from myopathy due to HIV itself, but a drug holiday usually makes the distinction. In addition, muscle biopsy shows abnormal mitochondria in AZT-induced myopathy.

78. **Which medications used to treat HIV may cause peripheral neuropathy?**
D4T (Zerit), ddI (Videx), ddC (Hivid), and 3TC (lamivudine) have been shown to cause neuropathy. The first three medications may have added toxicity when combined.

79. **What is the most common type of peripheral neuropathy in patients with HIV infection?**
A chronic, distal, symmetric polyneuropathy is most common. It is predominantly sensory with painful dysesthesias, numbness, and paresthesias. Weakness or autonomic dysfunction is less frequent. Occasionally, a chronic or acute inflammatory demyelinating polyneuropathy is seen.

80. **How is the acute, inflammatory, demyelinating neuropathy of HIV infection distinguished from Guillain-Barré syndrome?**
In the HIV-related disorder, CSF pleocytosis ranges between 10 to 50 cells/mm$^3$ along with CSF protein elevation. In Guillain-Barré syndrome, pleocytosis generally does not occur.

81. **What CSF findings do you expect in a patient with HIV-associated aseptic meningitis?**
Like other causes of viral meningitis, HIV infection may produce a mononuclear pleocytosis with 20 to 300 cells/mm$^3$ and a protein elevation in the range of 50 to 100 mg/dL. Meningeal signs, headache, fever, and cranial nerve palsies, especially of the fifth, seventh, and eighth cranial nerves, also occur.

82. **What are the most common causes of new-onset seizures in patients with HIV infection?**
Toxoplasmosis, HIV encephalopathy, *Cryptococcus,* and lymphoma.
Modi M, Mochan A, Modi G: New onset seizures in HIV. Epilepsia 50:1266-1269, 2009.

83. **A patient treated with phenytoin for many years was seizure-free until initiation of treatment of HIV. What medication may the patient be taking?**
Zidovudine may decrease serum phenytoin levels so that the patient now requires a higher dose to achieve therapeutic levels.

84. **What clinical feature distinguishes AIDS dementia complex from Creutzfeldt-Jakob disease?**
In AIDS dementia, a normal level of consciousness is usually maintained, even late in the disease, unless some other systemic disease intervenes. This is not true in Creutzfeldt-Jakob disease, which otherwise is clinically similar to AIDS dementia.
Ances BM, Clifford DB: HIV-associated neurocognitive disorders and the impact of combination antiretroviral therapies. Curr Neurol Neurosci Rep 8:455-461, 2008.

35. **A patient with known AIDS complains of decreased visual acuity. What infectious agents are most likely responsible?**
Cytomegalovirus (CMV) retinitis is most common, occurring in about 30% of patients with AIDS. Toxoplasmosis is probably the second most common retinal infection, accounting for only 4% of retinitis cases. Ocular syphilis may manifest as iridocyclitis, neuroretinitis, optic perineuritis, and retrobulbar neuritis. HIV infection itself may cause cotton-wool spots that usually are not visually significant. A rare cause of retinitis is tuberculosis.

36. **What are the diagnostic features of toxoplasma encephalitis in patients with AIDS?**
Most patients have elevated IgG antibodies to toxoplasma. The absence of toxoplasma IgG in a patient with suspected toxoplasma encephalitis militates strongly against the diagnosis. Routine analyses of the CSF may be normal. Contrast-enhanced CT scans demonstrate nodular or ring-enhancing lesions in more than 90% of patients. The treatment of choice is high-dose pyrimethamine and sulfadiazine.

37. **What is PML? How does it present?**
Progressive multifocal leukoencephalopathy (PML) is an opportunistic infection caused by a polyomavirus called the JC virus (JCV). It occurs in HIV-infected patients and other immunocompromised hosts. It is characterized by patchy areas of demyelination in the white matter of the cerebral hemispheres. The clinical presentation is diverse, reflects the scattered areas of demyelination, and progresses rapidly. Motor weakness, personality changes, dementia, ataxia, and cortical blindness occur and may culminate in coma. Survival after diagnosis is often less than 6 months.
   Epker JL, van Biezen P, van Daele PL, et al.: Progressive multifocal leukoencephalopathy. Eur J Intern Med 20:261-267, 2009.

38. **How does cryptococcal meningitis present in an HIV-positive patient?**
The common presentation includes fever, altered mentation, headache, and meningismus. Papilledema may result from increased intracranial pressure. CSF cell counts and chemistries may be minimally altered. Cryptococcal antigen is the most sensitive marker of infection. India ink stain may be positive but has a high rate of false negatives. Initial treatment is with amphotericin B with or without flucytosine. Chronic suppressive treatment must be continued with fluconazole, and relapses are common.

39. **What are the most common presentations of neurosyphilis in patients with HIV infection?**
1. Acute meningitis
2. Cranial neuropathy
   Optic neuritis
   Eighth cranial nerve palsy
3. Meningovascular, causing strokes

# BIBLIOGRAPHY

1. Mandell GI, Douglas RG, Bennett JE: Principles and Practice of Infectious Disease, 6th ed. New York, Churchill Livingstone, 2009.
2. Hammer SM, Eron JJ Jr, Reiss P, et al.: Antiretroviral treatment of adult HIV infection: 2008 recommendations of the International AIDS Society. JAMA 300:555-570, 2008.
3. Scheld WM, Marra CM: Infections of the Central Nervous System, 3rd ed. Lippincott Williams & Wilkins, 2004.
4. Tyler KL: Neurological infections: Advances in therapy, outcome, and prediction. Lancet Neurol 8:19-21, 2009.

# CHAPTER 24

# PEDIATRIC NEUROLOGY

*Angus A. Wilfong, MD, and James Owens, MD, PhD*

## NORMAL NEUROLOGIC GROWTH AND DEVELOPMENT

1. **In addition to the routine questions asked during a neurologic interview, what additional questions are important for a complete pediatric neurology history?**
   1. Antenatal history and risk factors
   2. Perinatal history and risk factors
   3. Neonatal history and complications
   4. History of developmental milestones

2. **List important features of the physical examination of infants and young children that may not be included in the examination of adults.**
   1. Measurement of the fronto-occipital circumference (FOC)
   2. Palpation of cranial sutures and fontanelles if open
   3. Cranial and ocular auscultation
   4. Limb asymmetries and malformations (including dermatoglyphics)
   5. Abnormal skin lesions
   6. Developmental reflexes

3. **List the common developmental reflexes. When do you expect them to be present?**
   See Table 24-1.

| TABLE 24-1. COMMON DEVELOPMENTAL REFLEXES | | |
|---|---|---|
| **Reflex** | **Appears** | **Disappears** |
| Lateral incurvation of trunk | Birth | 1-2 months |
| Rooting | Birth | 3 months |
| Moro | Birth | 5-6 months |
| Tonic neck reflex | Birth | 5-6 months |
| Palmar grasp | Birth | 6 months |
| Crossed adduction | Birth | 7-8 months |
| Plantar grasp | Birth | 9-10 months |
| Extensor plantar responses | Birth | 6-12 months |
| Parachute response | 8-9 months | Persists |
| Landau reflex | 10 months | 24 months |

4. **What is the average FOC for a term newborn? What is the rate of growth over the first year?**
   Average FOC of a term newborn in 35 cm. Average FOC growth is 2 cm per month for the first 3 months, 1 cm per month for the next 3 months, and 0.5 cm per month for the last 6 months. Adult head size averages approximately 57 cm.

## PRENATAL DISEASES AND DEVELOPMENTAL DEFECTS

5. **What is the Apgar score?**
   The Apgar score is a clinical vitality rating scale applied to newborn infants in an attempt to identify those at risk for certain neonatal complications. Apgar is an eponym (Virginia Apgar, U.S. anesthesiologist), although it is often used as an acronym (Table 24-2).
   Infants are routinely scored at 1 and 5 minutes after birth. Further scores may be made at 10 and 20 minutes if the infant appears to have been compromised.

### TABLE 24-2. APGAR SCORE

| Sign | | Score | | |
| --- | --- | --- | --- | --- |
| | | 0 | 1 | 2 |
| A | Appearance (color) | Blue, pale | Acrocyanosis | Pink |
| P | Pulse (heart rate) | Absent | < 100 | > 100 |
| G | Grimace (reflex irritability in response to nasal suctioning) | No response | Grimace | Cry |
| A | Activity (muscle tone) | Limp | Some flexion | Active motion |
| R | Respiration (respiratory effort) | Absent | Slow and irregular | Strong crying |

6. **How is neonatal intraventricular hemorrhage (IVH) classified?**
   See Figure 24-1.
   - Grade I: Localized subependymal hemorrhage into the germinal matrix
   - Grade II: Subependymal hemorrhage with extension into the ventricles (less than 50% of the ventricular volume filled with blood)
   - Grade III: Subependymal hemorrhage with extension into the ventricles and acute ventricular dilatation (greater than 50% of the ventricular volume filled with blood) (see Figure 24-1)
   - Grade IV: Subependymal, intraventricular, and extension into the surrounding cerebral parenchyma

7. **What risk factors are thought to play a role in the genesis of IVH?**
   The most important risk factor for the development of an IVH is prematurity. Approximately 40% to 50% of neonates weighing less than 1500 gm experience an IVH. Other risk factors include

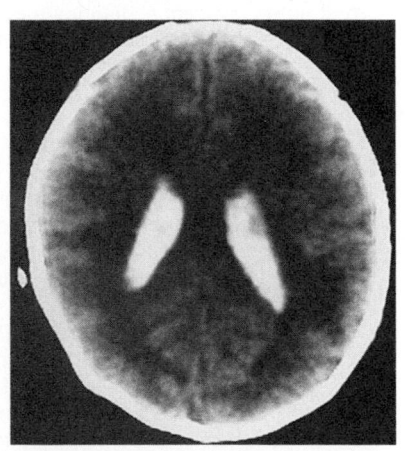

**Figure 24-1.** Unenhanced axial computed tomography (CT): grade III, intraventricular hemorrhage (IVH) in a premature newborn (32 weeks' gestation). Note acute ventricular distention with blood filling more than 50% of the ventricular volume. There is no parenchymal extension of the hemorrhage.

mechanical ventilation, pneumothoraces, rapid expansion of intravascular volume (large or rapid IV infusions), rapid or wide fluctuations in blood pressure, hypoxic-ischemic injury, hypernatremia and hyperosmolality, and administration of certain medications such as indomethacin.

8. **What complications may arise secondary to an IVH?**
   The most common complications of IVH include posthemorrhagic hydrocephalus, seizures, and the parenchymal cerebral injury associated with grade IV bleeds.

9. **Does the neurologic prognosis correlate with the different IVHs?**
   Long-term follow-up studies of neonates grouped with all grades of IVH who reached kindergarten age revealed that 40% survived and 60% were neurologically abnormal. Approximately 30% now have a static encephalopathy (cerebral palsy); 30% have hydrocephalus, most of which required a shunting procedure; and 30% are multihandicapped with combinations of blindness, paresis, spasticity, delayed fine motor and language skill, hydrocephalus, hearing loss, and seizures. Generally, grades I and II IVH are relatively benign, grade III has more significant hydrocephalus and seizures, and grade IV has by far the greatest likelihood of severe neurologic sequelae such as spastic quadriparesis, blindness, and mental retardation. Unilateral hemorrhages are associated with better neurodevelopmental outcomes than bilateral hemorrhages.

10. **What are the most common causes of a floppy baby? What are the least common?**
    By far the most frequent are the central causes involving the cerebellum, brain stem, basal ganglia, and cerebral hemispheres. The least common causes of infantile hypotonia afflict the peripheral nerves.

11. **What is the difference between macrocephaly and megalencephaly?**
    Macrocephaly refers to a large head, whereas megalencephaly refers specifically to a large brain.

12. **What is the differential diagnosis of macrocephaly in an infant?**
    1. Hydrocephalus—obstructive or communicating
    2. Extra-axial fluid collections
    3. Thickened skull
    4. Megalencephaly

13. **What is the differential diagnosis of megalencephaly?**
    1. Toxic: cerebral edema from lead poisoning
    2. White matter diseases: Canavan's disease and Alexander's disease
    3. Neurocutaneous: neurofibromatosis (NF) and tuberous sclerosis
    4. Genetic: cerebral gigantism (Sotos' syndrome) and fragile X
    5. Familial megalencephaly

14. **What is hemimegalancephaly? What clinical manifestations are commonly associated with hemimegalancephaly?**
    Hemimegalancephaly is a rare brain malformation associated with cortical overgrowth on one hemisphere. It is commonly associated with intractable partial seizures, significant developmental delay, and progressive hemiparesis. Surgical removal of the malformed hemisphere (hemispherectomy) may be necessary to achieve seizure control.

15. **In evaluating a child with microcephaly, what are the most important questions to ask in the history?**
    Is the microcephaly congenital or acquired? Serial measurements of FOC are helpful. Is the FOC getting progressively worse (Rett's syndrome in girls), returning to normal (catch-up growth after a serious illness or prematurity), or remaining on the same percentile line (static process)? Review the antenatal history carefully for evidence of intrauterine infection. Did the infant appear healthy at birth? Any postnatal central nervous system (CNS) infections or trauma? Family history of microcephaly?

16. **Which laboratory tests, if any, would you order in a child with microcephaly?**
Plain skull x-ray studies evaluate premature closure of the cranial sutures. A head computed tomography (CT) scan or cranial ultrasound (before closure of the fontanelles) surveys for evidence of CNS malformations, abnormal calcification (which may indicate infection with a toxoplasmosis, other agents, rubella, cytomegalovirus, herpes simplex [TORCH] agent or earlier hypoxic-ischemic injury), or massive destruction of the cerebrum as in hydranencephaly. Magnetic resonance imaging (MRI) gives greater anatomic detail of the brain but is rarely needed in this circumstance. In addition, TORCH titers may be measured if such an infection is suspected, or a chromosomal analysis—particularly chromosomal microarray—may be used to evaluate genetic causes.

## KEY POINTS: CAUSES OF INTRAUTERINE INFECTION

1. **TO** = Toxoplasmosis, other agents

2. **R** = Rubella

3. **C** = Cytomegalovirus

4. **H** = Herpes simplex virus

17. **How would you evaluate and manage a newborn with spina bifida?**
Perform a careful neurologic examination to estimate the level of spinal cord and nerve root involvement, including assessment of bowel and bladder function. Cranial neuroimaging (ultrasound, CT, MRI) is essential to determine the presence of other CNS conditions that are frequently present. Plain spine x-rays evaluate the bony extent of the lesion. Immediately following birth, sterile saline-soaked gauze pads must be gently applied to the myelomeningocele membrane and all attempts should be made to keep the membrane intact during transfer to a tertiary center.

18. **What are the most common complications of a lumbosacral myelomeningocele?**
See Figure 24-2.
1. Type II Arnold-Chiari malformation resulting in hydrocephalus
2. CNS infectious complications are common and devastating
3. Renal failure due to chronic and repeated urinary tract infections and obstructive uropathy
4. Seizures
5. Progressive spasticity and weakness in the legs, worsening bladder and bowel function, progressive scoliosis, or increasing low back pain and stiffness due to a "tethered cord"

19. **Classify the Arnold-Chiari malformations.**
Type I: Downward displacement of the cerebellum with elongation of the medulla such that the cerebellar tonsils egress through the foramen.
Type II: Associated with lumbosacral myelomeningocele and numerous other nervous system malformations.
1. Posterior fossa is small
2. Cerebellar tonsil herniation through the foramen magnum
3. Medulla is elongated and thinned
4. Characteristic beaking appearance of the quadrigeminal plate is present
5. Hydrocephalus
6. Syringomyelia and occasionally syringobulbia
7. Interdigitation of gyri along the interhemispheric fissure

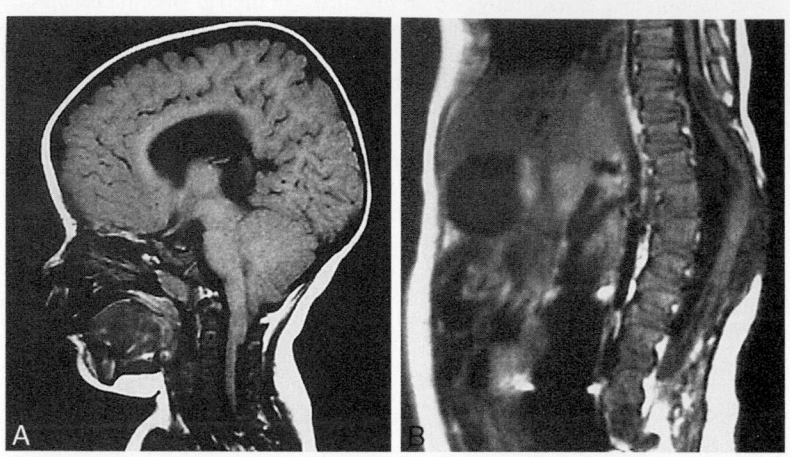

**Figure 24-2.** (A) Unenhanced midsagittal T1-weighted magnetic resonance image (MRI) in a 6-month-old boy with type II Arnold-Chiari malformation. Note "herniation" or downward displacement of the cerebellar tonsils through the foramen magnum to the level of C2 and the associated obstructive hydrocephalus. (B) Unenhanced midsagittal T1-weighted MRI lumbosacral spine: extensive thoracolumbar myelomeningocele associated with the Arnold-Chiari malformation in (A). Note the dorsal kyphosis, absence of posterior elements of the vertebrae, and the malformed spinal cord at the level of the defect. A small syrinx in the cord is present above the defect.

Type III: An occipital encephalocele with protrusion of cerebellar remnants into the overlying sac
Type IV: Isolated hypoplasia of the cerebellum not associated with other nervous system malformations

**20. List the major developmental abnormalities of cortical development.**
1. Lissencephaly
2. Holoprosencephaly
3. Schizencephaly
4. Polymicrogyria
5. Pachygyria
6. Double cortex syndrome (laminar heterotopia)
7. Periventricular nodular heterotopia
8. Focal cortical dysplasia

**21. What is Down syndrome?**
A chromosomal anomaly with trisomy 21 characterized by marked infantile hypotonia with hyperflexibility of joints, cognitive impairment, brachycephaly with flat occiput, up-slanting palpebral fissures, late closure of fontanelles, flattened nasal bridge, epicanthal folds, speckling of iris (Brushfield's spots), fine lens opacities, small ears, hypoplastic teeth, short neck, brachydactyly with clinodactyly of fifth fingers, simian creases, wide space between first and second toes, congenital heart disease (in 40%), and hypogonadism.

**22. What is meant by the term "learning disability"?**
A learning disability is present when a child with overall normal intellect has a deficit in acquiring the skills needed to perform a specific cognitive task. For example, the most common learning disability is dyslexia, a disorder manifested by difficulty in learning to read despite conventional instruction, adequate intelligence, and sociocultural opportunity.

23. **A school-aged child is referred for evaluation of possible absence epilepsy because of constant "day-dreaming" and worsening grades. The mother and teachers relate a history of short attention span for schoolwork but not for television or video games, easy distractibility, impulsiveness, constant supervision needed to complete homework and chores, adventurous and risk-taking behavior, and constant physical activity (as if driven by a motor). What is the most likely diagnosis?**
    This is the usual presentation of a child with attention-deficit/hyperactivity disorder (ADHD). Some children have the attention deficit without the hyperactivity. Affected children have unusually short attention spans and are simply unable to concentrate for more than a few minutes for all but the most stimulating and enjoyable activities. Their constant distractibility and day-dreaming may be confused with the seizures of absence epilepsy.

24. **What are the clinical manifestations of infantile autism?**
    1. Onset usually occurs by the end of the first year of life
    2. Social and language developmental regression and a relative lack of communication
    3. Motor development is generally not affected
    4. Very limited, if any interpersonal interactions
    5. Easily disturbed by even the slightest change in their environment, such as rearranging the furniture or books on a shelf
    6. Repetitive self-stimulation behaviors are common and consist of rocking, head banging, whirling, and flapping of hands in front of face
    7. Limited repertoire of interests and activities.
       Zwaigenbaum L, Bryson S, Lord C, et al.: Clinical assessment and management of toddlers with suspected autism spectrum disorder. Pediatrics 123:1383-1391, 2009.

## NEURODEGENERATIVE DISORDERS

25. **In general terms, how does a neurodegenerative disease affecting white matter present?**
    Loss of motor skills, spasticity, and ataxia. A disorder affecting the white matter is referred to as a leukodystrophy.

26. **In general terms, how does a neurodegenerative disease affecting gray matter present?**
    Loss of intellectual skills (dementia), seizures, and blindness. A disorder affecting gray matter was once called a poliodystrophy.

27. **Name a neurodegenerative disorder that affects both the central nervous system and the peripheral nervous system.**
    Krabbe's disease (globoid cell leukodystrophy) is an autosomal recessive enzyme defect in galactosylceramide beta-galactosidase that results in irritability, increased tone, optic atrophy, cortical blindness, and peripheral nerve segmental demyelination. Metachromatic leukodystrophy is an autosomal recessive disorder that also affects both central and peripheral myelin.

28. **Which leukodystrophy is virtually always associated with a particular endocrinologic deficiency?**
    See Figure 24-3. Adrenoleukodystrophy, an X-linked recessive disorder, is one of the peroxisomal disorders. It is characterized by impaired beta-oxidation of the very long-chain (C26) fatty acids, leading to their accumulation. In addition, patients also have adrenocortical insufficiency. Onset is usually between 4 and 6 years of age. An adult form of the disease called adrenomyeloneuropathy is characterized by progressive spastic paraparesis and peripheral neuropathy.

29. **How often does multiple sclerosis present in children?**
Approximately, 3% to 5% of all patients with multiple sclerosis (MS) have onset of symptoms in childhood. The majority of affected children (more than 90%) are older than 10 years of age, but MS cases have been described in patients younger than 3 years old.
   Waubant E, Chabas D: Pediatric multiple sclerosis. Curr Treat Options Neurol 11:203-210, 2009.

30. **What is a cherry-red spot?**
It is the bright red appearance of the fovea centralis of the eye as seen by funduscopy in children with certain gray-matter storage diseases, classically Tay-Sachs disease. As the storage material accumulates in the nerve fiber layer, the retina takes on a grayish-white appearance. Because there are very few fibers traversing the fovea, it retains its normal color and continues to reflect the bright red vascular choroid underneath.

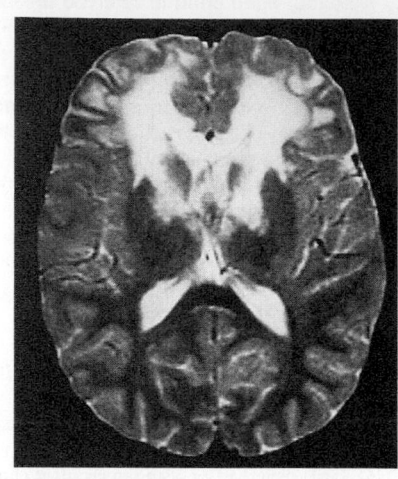

**Figure 24-3.** Unenhanced axial T2-weighted magnetic resonance image (MRI) in a 9-year-old boy with adrenoleukodystrophy. Note extensive dysmyelination involving the anterior centrum semiovale, subcortical white matter, genu of the corpus callosum, and internal capsule. The cerebral cortex, basal ganglia, and thalami are unaffected.

31. **What are the neuronal ceroid lipofuscinoses (NCL)?**
Neuronal ceroid lipofuscinoses is a group of autosomal recessively inherited disorders characterized by excessive neuronal accumulations of the lipid pigments, ceroid, and lipofuscin. They present as classic gray matter diseases with intractable seizures, progressive dementia, and blindness.

32. **Which endocrinologic disorder may present as a gray matter neurodegenerative disease if it is missed on the newborn screening?**
Congenital hypothyroidism (cretinism) is extremely difficult to detect clinically at birth and the diagnosis may not be suspected until it is too late for replacement therapy to be maximally efficacious. Left untreated, these children develop prolonged jaundice, abdominal distention with umbilical hernia, large fontanelles, hypotonia, impaired bony development, large tongue, psychomotor retardation, seizures, spasticity, ataxia, and deafness.

33. **What are ragged-red fibers?**
In some of the mitochondrial cytopathies, mitochondria become clumped beneath the skeletal muscle sarcolemmal membrane. When the muscle biopsy specimen is prepared with modified Gomori's trichrome stain and viewed by light microscopy, the clumps of mitochondria stain red and give the muscle fibers a ragged appearance—hence the term ragged red fibers.

## NEUROCUTANEOUS SYNDROMES

34. **What is the most common neurocutaneous syndrome?**
Neurofibromatosis (NF) type I has an incidence of 1/3000 to 4000 population. Inheritance is autosomal dominant and the spontaneous mutation rate (chromosome 17) is very high (30%

to 50%). Clinical characteristics include café-au-lait spots, neurofibromas, axillary/inguinal freckling, optic gliomas, megalencephaly, mental retardation, seizures, and characteristic bony lesions.

Kandit RS: Tuberous sclerosis complex and neurofibromatosis type 1: The two most common neurocutaneous diseases. Neurol Clin 20:941-964, 2002.

35. **Which neurocutaneous syndrome is associated with infantile spasms and a hypsarrhythmia pattern on electroencephalogram (EEG)?**
Tuberous sclerosis (TS), an autosomal dominant disorder with genetic heterogeneity (similar phenotype with mutation on either chromosome 9 or 16). Incidence is 1/10,000 with a high-spontaneous mutation rate. Clinical features include mental retardation, seizures, adenoma sebaceum, ash-leaf spots, shagreen patches, café au lait spots, subungual and periungual fibromas (Koenen's tumors), gingival fibromas, dental enamel pits, retinal tumors (mulberry tumor of the optic disc), cardiac rhabdomyomata, renal angiomyolipomata, and CNS cortical tubers and subependymal hamartomas that calcify.

36. **Of the more common neurocutaneous syndromes, which has no clear pattern of inheritance?**
Sturge-Weber syndrome (encephalofacial angiomatosis), which is less common than NF or TS. Patients have a facial port-wine stain (nevus) that is usually unilateral involving the $V_1$ segment of the trigeminal nerve. The nevus may involve the ocular choroidal membrane, causing glaucoma. Arteriography reveals extensive arteriovenous malformation involving the ipsilateral cerebral hemispheric dura.

37. **In addition to brain and skin involvement, which other neurocutaneous syndrome has an immune disorder and a high propensity for malignancy?**
Ataxia-telangiectasia is an autosomal recessive disorder with an incidence of 1/100,000. Affected individuals develop telangiectasias by 2 to 4 years of age on exposed areas of skin and conjunctiva. Progressive cerebellar ataxia begins within the first few years of life. Patients have decreased or absent IgA and IgE and decreased $IgG_2$ and $IgG_4$. Defective cellular DNA repair leads to increased spontaneous and radiation-induced chromosomal aberrations, inducing various neoplasia.

Spacey SO, Gatti RA, Bebb G: The molecular basis and clinical management of ataxia-telangiectasia. Can J Neurol Sci 27:184-191, 2000.

## INFECTIONS AND INFESTATIONS

38. **What are the most common bacterial pathogens for meningitis at different ages?**
Neonatal
1. Group B beta-hemolytic streptococci
2. *Escherichia coli*
3. *Listeria monocytogenes*
4. *Klebsiella pneumoniae*
Childhood
1. *Haemophilus influenzae* type B
2. *Streptococcus pneumoniae*
3. *Neisseria meningitides*

39. **What are the usual signs and symptoms of neonatal meningitis?**
1. Lethargy
2. Irritability

3. Hypothermia or hyperthermia
4. Poor feeding
5. Bulging fontanelle
6. Seizures

40. **What are the usual signs and symptoms of an older infant or child with meningitis?**
    1. Fever
    2. Headache
    3. Altered mental status
    4. Stiff neck
    5. Nausea and vomiting
    6. Seizures

41. **A child from Central America presents with a prolonged partial motor seizure. Neurologic examination reveals no focal or lateralizing findings; however, funduscopic examination reveals early papilledema. CT scanning of the brain discloses a number of small, densely calcified lesions scattered along the gray-white junction of the cerebral hemispheres. What is the most likely diagnosis and how might you confirm your suspicions?**

    The pork tapeworm, *Taenia solium*, is endemic in Central America. When a human becomes the intermediate host (rather than the pig), he may develop neurocysticercosis. This occurs when the ingested *T. solium* ova become partially digested, releasing onchospheres that gain access to the circulation and are carried throughout the body. They then become larvae (cysticerci) in subcutaneous tissue, muscle, and brain where the majority die and become densely calcified. The diagnosis can be confirmed by serum or cerebrospinal fluid (CSF) antibody and antigen detection methods and in certain cases by tissue biopsy (Figure 24-4).

    Carpio A: Neurocysticercosis: An update. Lancet Infect Dis 2:751-762, 2002.

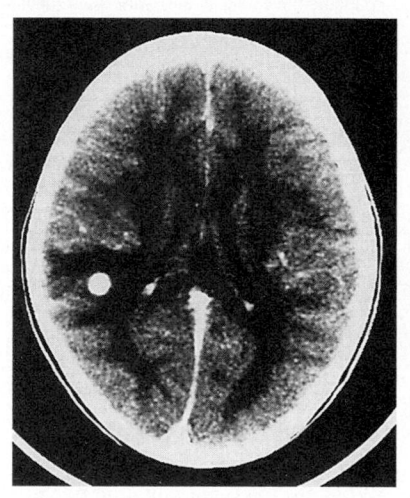

**Figure 24-4.** Enhanced axial computed tomography (CT): neurocysticercosis in a 7-year-old girl. Note the solitary, densely enhancing lesion with surrounding edema.

## VASCULAR DISORDERS

42. **What is the most common hemoglobinopathy associated with cerebrovascular disease?**

    Approximately one-fourth of all patients with sickle cell disease experience cerebrovascular complications; the vast majority are children. When strokes occur in adults, they are more likely to be intracerebral hemorrhages as opposed to the infarctions that affect children. In addition to small vessel occlusion by sickled red cells, endothelial proliferation is also thought to be an important mechanism in the genesis of these strokes.

## NEOPLASMS

43. **Where are brain tumors most common in infants, children, and adults?**
In infants less than 1 year of age, supratentorial brain tumors predominate. In children older than 1 year, infratentorial tumors are more common. In adults, supratentorial tumors are again more frequently encountered.

Mainprize TG, Taylor MD, Rutka JT: Pediatric brain tumors: A contemporary prospectus. Clin Neurosurg 47:259-302, 2000.

44. **What is a primitive neuroectodermal tumor (PNET)?**
These are highly malignant, small, blue cell tumors. If a PNET is completely undifferentiated and is in the midline posterior fossa, it is often referred to as a medulloblastoma. PNET may show varying degrees of differentiation along different cell lines, including glial, ependymal, pineal, and neuronal (Figure 24-5).

45. **A school-aged child complains of recurrent headaches and recent onset of marked polyuria and polydipsia. Examination reveals bitemporal homonymous hemianopsia and papilledema. Laboratory tests are consistent with diabetes insipidus. Where is the lesion?**
The anatomic location of this lesion must be in the parasellar region. The visual field defect is produced by compression of the optic chiasm. The diabetes insipidus is produced by compression of the pituitary stalk (Figure 24-6).

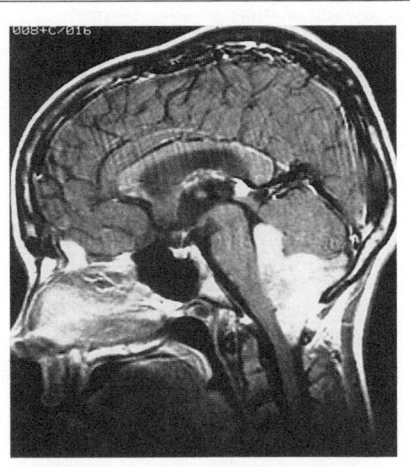

**Figure 24-5.** Enhanced midsagittal T1-weighted magnetic resonance image (MRI) reveals a posterior fossa primitive neuroectodermal tumor (PNET) in a 5-year-old boy. Note the brightly enhancing tumor mass extending upward through the fourth ventricle into the cerebral aqueduct and downward through the foramen magnum. There is compression of the medulla and marked displacement of the cerebellum. Early obstructive hydrocephalus is developing.

46. **What is the differential diagnosis of parasellar tumors in children?**
   1. Craniopharyngioma
   2. Germ-cell tumor, including teratoma
   3. Pituitary adenoma
   4. Optic glioma
   5. Hypothalamic glioma
   6. Chordoma of the clivus

47. **Most posterior fossa tumors in children have a poor prognosis except for one, which has an excellent prognosis. What is it?**
Juvenile cerebellar pilocystic astrocytoma has virtually a 100% 50-year survival rate. This tumor develops in the cerebellar hemispheres of school-aged children. Histologically, the tumor cells are hair-like (pilocystic). The tumor is well circumscribed without local invasiveness. Neurosurgical resection is usually complete and recurrence is very uncommon.

48. **An older child with medically intractable complex partial seizures has an MRI scan performed. The scan reveals a partially calcified mass in the right mesial temporal lobe without associated edema. What is the most likely diagnosis?**
Gangliogliomas, oligodendroglioma, and dysembryoplastic neuroepithelial tumors (DNETs) are slow-growing benign neoplasms whose only clinical signs may be intractable seizures.

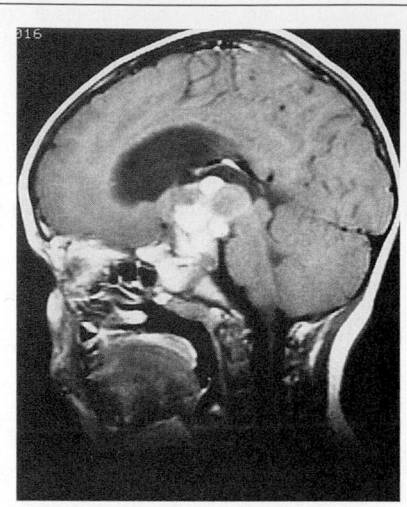

**Figure 24-6.** Enhanced midsagittal T1-weighted magnetic resonance image (MRI) demonstrates a craniopharyngioma in a 3-year-old girl. Note the large, multilobulated tumor extending from the parasellar region through the midbrain. The tumor has brightly enhancing solid areas and fluid-filled cysts. There is associated obstructive hydrocephalus.

Duchowny M: Recent advances in candidate selection for pediatric epilepsy surgery. Semin Pediatr Neurol 7:178-186, 2000.

## INJURY BY PHYSICAL AGENTS AND TRAUMA

49. **Does age have any effect on whether or not cranial irradiation would be considered as treatment for cancer?**
Children who received cranial x-ray therapy (XRT) prior to 3 years of age have significantly reduced intelligence quotients.

50. **What are some of the other adverse effects that may be encountered in children who receive cranial XRT?**
    1. Transient somnolence, headaches, and anorexia 6 to 8 weeks after initiation of XRT is common
    2. Radiation necrosis (radionecrosis) may occur 1 to 3 years post-XRT and can mimic a mass effect; making it difficult to distinguish tumor recurrence from radionecrosis. Pathologically the lesion involves hyalinization of blood vessels with infarction and necrosis of brain tissue.
    3. Hypothalamic-pituitary dysfunction, which usually involves decreased production of growth hormone and thyroid-stimulating hormone
    4. Formation of cataracts if the ocular globes were exposed to irradiation
    5. Induction of a second malignancy that may appear years later

51. **A 6-month-old infant presents with obtundation and recent seizures. Examination reveals no fever, anterior fontanelle slightly bulging, depressed level of consciousness, and hypotonia. On funduscopic examination, extensive, bilateral retinal hemorrhages and mild papilledema are observed. What is your leading diagnosis?**
    Child abuse, specifically the shaken-baby syndrome, needs to be first on the list of diagnostic possibilities. Because of the violent shaking of the body and head, these infants sustain subarachnoid hemorrhages and associated retinal hemorrhages. This commonly leads to seizures and may cause cortical infarctions as the cerebral vessels spasm.

52. **What is a growing skull fracture?**
    This is a rather rare complication of linear skull fractures, usually occurring in children younger than 3 years of age. Because of brain and CSF pulsations, the opposing edges of bone along the fracture do not fuse. Resorption of bone along the edges occurs so that the fracture opening progressively enlarges, producing a "growing skull fracture."

## SEIZURES AND OTHER PAROXYSMAL DISORDERS

53. **What is a complex febrile seizure?**
    The seizure has focal features, lasts longer than 15 min or recurs within 24 hours, or occurs in a child younger than 6 months or older than 5 years of age.

## KEY POINTS: SIMPLE FEBRILE SEIZURE

1. A generalized tonic or tonic-clonic seizure

2. Between 6 months and 5 years of age

3. Fever greater than 38° C, but not in the presence of a CNS infection

4. Lasting less than 15 min, no focal features, does not recur within 24 hours

5. No postictal neurologic abnormalities

54. **Does having had a simple febrile convulsion increase the risk for later development of epilepsy (recurrent nonfebrile seizures)?**
    If there is increased risk for later development of epilepsy, it is only slightly elevated.
    Knudson FU: Febrile seizures: Treatment and prognosis. Epilepsia 41:2-9, 2000.

55. **An 18-month-old child is referred for possible epilepsy. The mother relates a history of paroxysmal spells that have occurred over the past month. Each spell consists of the child turning red, then blue in the face, and then passing out with a few clonic jerks of the extremities. Immediately preceding each spell, the child had been startled, frightened, or frustrated and began crying. What is the probable diagnosis?**
    This is a typical history of blue breath-holding spells, a form of infantile syncope. Breath-holding spells occur in 4% to 5% of children; there is a positive family history in 25% of cases. Two-thirds have cyanotic or blue breath-holding spells, 20% have pallid breath-holding spells, and the remainder has a mixture of the two. The peak incidence

is between 1 and 2 years of age and resolution occurs by 6 years of age. The spells follow minor injuries, fright, or frustration.

Kolkiran A, Tutar E, Atalay S, et al.: Autonomic nervous system functions in children with breath-holding spells and effects of iron deficiency. Acta Paediatr 94:1227-1231, 2005.

## HEAD PAIN

56. **What are the clinical features of childhood migraine headaches?**
   1. Migraine headaches in children are common.
   2. Fifty percent of all individuals who develop migraine had the onset of their attacks before 20 years of age.
   3. Boys are more frequently affected until puberty, after which time the incidence is considerably higher in girls.
   4. Younger children usually complain of a generalized or bifrontal or bitemporal headache, rather than the hemicranial pain characteristically present in the older child or adult.
   5. Abdominal distress with nausea and sometimes vomiting is prominent.
   6. The child often appears pale and frequently stops all activities and lies down.
   7. Photophobia and phonophobia are usually present.
   8. If the child is able to fall asleep, the headache is virtually always gone on awakening.
   9. Family history for migraine is positive in 70% to 90% of cases.

   Maytal J, Young M, Shechter A, Lipton RB: Pediatric migraine and the International Headache Society Criteria. Neurology 48:602-607, 1997.

57. **What are the different types of migraine headaches in children?**
   1. **Migraine without aura** (formerly common migraine): accounts for up to three-quarters of all migraine attacks. Clinical manifestations are those listed in the preceding answer.
   2. **Migraine with aura** (formerly classic migraine): same as above except these individuals experience an aura just before the onset of the headache.
   3. **Complicated migraine**: migraine headache associated with various transient neurologic phenomena. These include hemiplegic migraine, ophthalmoplegic migraine, vertebrobasilar migraine, and acute confusional migraine.
   4. **Migraine variants or equivalents**: benign paroxysmal vertigo of childhood, paroxysmal torticollis, and cyclical vomiting of childhood are syndromes thought to be related to migraine.

58. **What are some of the therapeutic strategies used in treating migraines?**
   Biofeedback and relaxation techniques seem to work well for some individuals. In addition, avoidance of particular foods that appear to precipitate migraines in a small percentage of patients is helpful. Foods that have been implicated include chocolate, caffeine, nitrites, monosodium glutamate, and sharp cheeses. However, the mainstay of treatment is medication.

59. **What are the most important pharmacologic agents used in treating migraine?**
   1. **Symptomatic treatments:** Analgesics that have no action on the underlying cause of the migraine headache. Examples include aspirin, ibuprofen, acetaminophen, codeine, and meperidine. It is usually best to avoid narcotic preparations in the treatment of chronic illnesses if at all possible.
   2. **Abortive therapies:** Vasoactive agents that modify the vasculature so that the migraine headache is aborted before becoming fully developed. Examples include ergotamine preparations, isometheptene mucate, and serotonin receptor agonists (triptans).
   3. **Prophylactic medications:** Drugs that prevent the migraine headaches from occurring. Examples include nonsteroidal anti-inflammatory agents (aspirin), beta-blockers, calcium channel blockers, antiepileptic medications (sodium valproate), tricyclic antidepressants

(amitriptyline), the serotonin antagonists (cyproheptadine and methysergide), and the selective serotonin reuptake inhibitor antidepressants (sertraline).

Goadsby PJ, Lipton RB, Ferrari MD: Migraine - Current understanding and treatment. N Engl J Med 346:257-270, 2002.

## KEY POINTS: HEADACHES FROM INTRACRANIAL MASS LESION

1. Recent onset of headaches or change in character of chronic headaches

2. Headaches that awaken the patient from sleep or are present on awakening in the morning

3. Association with altered mental status, vomiting, constriction of visual fields, or focal neurologic deficits

## NEUROMUSCULAR DISORDERS

60. **What is the gene product of the Xp21 portion of the X chromosome?**
The gene product is a protein called dystrophin. Dystrophin is a structural protein that is important in several tissues, including skeletal muscle, cardiac muscle, and brain. Certain mutations of the dystrophin gene lead to essentially no dystrophin production and result in Duchenne muscular dystrophy (DMD). Other mutations allow for the production of some dystrophin and cause the less severe and late-onset Becker muscular dystrophy.

61. **What are the clinical manifestations of DMD?**
Affected children are normal through the first year of life. The first clue is that the child may walk later than expected, but detectable weakness is not present until 3 to 4 years of age. The pelvic girdle weakens first and gives rise to the characteristic Gowers' sign. Soon widespread weakness is apparent and relentless progression ensues. Most children become unable to walk by the end of their first decade. Once the patient is wheelchair bound there is development of flexion contractures and progressive scoliosis. Cardiac involvement is invariable. Mild intellectual impairment is also common in these patients. Death from pulmonary infection, respiratory failure, or cardiac failure usually occurs by age 30 years.

62. **What treatment is available for children with DMD?**
Treatment with daily oral corticosteroids from the time of diagnosis until the time the child requires a wheelchair appears to slow the course of DMD.

63. **What are the most common congenital myopathies?**
    1. Central core disease
    2. Centronuclear myopathy
    3. Nemaline myopathy
    4. Minimal change myopathy
    5. Congenital fiber type disproportion.
    Sharma MC, Jain D, Sarkar C, Goebel HH: Congenital myopathies - A comprehensive update of recent advancements. Acta Neurol Scand 119:281-292, 2009.

64. **What are the clinical manifestations of myotonic muscular dystrophy?**
    1. Autosomal dominant with mutation on chromosome 19
    2. Clinical manifestations usually begin in adolescence or early adult life with distal muscle weakness and myotonia

3. Muscle wasting about the face and sternocleidomastoids, in combination with facial weakness, leads to the distinctive "hatchet-face" appearance

4. Partial ptosis, swan-like posture of the neck, enlarged paranasal sinuses, early prominent male-pattern balding in both sexes

5. Cataracts, cardiac conduction abnormalities, hypogonadism with testicular atrophy, and abnormal glucose tolerance.
Miller TM: Differential diagnosis of myotonic disorders. Muscle Nerve 37:293-299, 2007.

65. **What is a common complication of neonates born to mothers with myotonic muscular dystrophy?**
Some newborns who have inherited the myotonic dystrophy gene from their mothers experience profound weakness, with respiratory failure and bulbar insufficiency requiring endotracheal intubation and mechanical ventilation. The mortality rate may be as high as 30% to 40%. Should the neonate survive, the weakness resolves spontaneously. The occurrence of the neonatal syndrome has no effect on the severity of the adult expression of the disease.

66. **What are the two types of myasthenia that may affect the newborn or young infant?**
1. **Transient neonatal myasthenia gravis**. Affected neonates are born to mothers with autoimmune myasthenia gravis. The newborns experience transient weakness and hypotonia, which may be severe and life-threatening, due to the transplacental transfer of maternal antiacetylcholine receptor antibodies.
2. **Nonautoimmune congenital myasthenia syndromes**.

67. **Which types of myasthenia are not due to autoimmune production of antibodies against the acetylcholine (ACh) receptor?**
1. Defects in ACh synthesis or mobilization
2. End-plate acetylcholinesterase deficiency
3. Slow-channel syndrome
4. End-plate ACh receptor deficiency

68. **A school-aged child presents with a few days' history of progressive weakness in his legs. This "ascending paralysis" was first noted at his ankles and now has spread to involve his hips. List the differential diagnoses.**
1. Guillain-Barré syndrome
2. Acute spinal cord lesion
3. Tick bite paralysis
4. West Nile virus
5. Poliomyelitis (usually asymmetrical weakness)
6. Periodic paralysis
7. Acute cerebellar ataxia
8. Myasthenia gravis
9. Botulism

## BIBLIOGRAPHY

1. Dubowitz V: Muscle Disorders in Childhood, 3rd ed. Philadelphia, W.B. Saunders, 2001.

2. Fenichel GM: Clinical Pediatric Neurology: A Signs and Symptoms Approach, 6th ed. Philadelphia, W.B. Saunders, 2009.

3. McMillan JA, Feigin RD, DeAngelis CD, Jones MD (eds): Oski's Pediatrics, 4th ed. Philadelphia, Lippincott Williams & Wilkins, 2006.

4. Menkes JH, Sarnat HB (eds): Child Neurology, 7th ed. Philadelphia, Lippincott Williams & Wilkins, 2005.

5. Swaimann KF, Ashwal S, Ferriero DM, (eds): Pediatric Neurology: Principles and Practice, 4th ed. St. Louis, Mosby, 2006.

6. Volpe JJ: Neurology of the Newborn, 5th ed. Philadelphia, W.B. Saunders, 2008.

# CHAPTER 25

# ELECTROENCEPHALOGRAPHY

*Richard A. Hrachovy, MD*

1. **What is believed to be the source of the electrical activity recorded by scalp electrodes in the electroencephalogram (EEG)?**
   The best available evidence indicates that surface-recorded and scalp-recorded electrical activity results from extracellular current flow associated with summation of excitatory postsynaptic potentials and inhibitory postsynaptic potentials.

2. **What are the different frequencies recorded on an EEG?**
   Four frequency bands are recorded: delta, $\leq 4$ Hz; theta, 4 to 7 Hz; alpha, 8 to 13 Hz; and beta, $\geq 13$ Hz.

3. **What are the features of an EEG in an awake, normal adult?**
   The EEG reveals a dominant rhythm in the occipital leads bilaterally. The frequency of this rhythm in most adult individuals is between 9 and 11 Hz. This rhythm is variously referred to as the occipital dominant rhythm, the occipital dominant alpha rhythm, or simply the alpha rhythm. The occipital dominant rhythm is best seen when the individual has his or her eyes closed and is relaxed. This rhythm usually attenuates when the eyes are opened. In the anterior regions, alpha frequency activity is also present but is lower in voltage and generally less continuous than that in the posterior regions. There is also low-voltage 18-22 Hz activity present in the anterior leads (Figure 25-1).

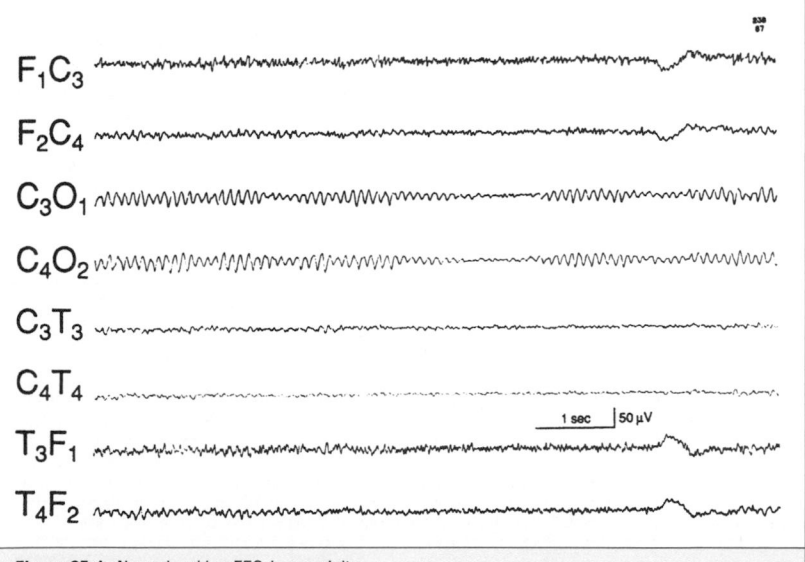

**Figure 25-1.** Normal waking EEG in an adult.

## 4. What are the EEG features of the various sleep stages in the adult?

### NON–RAPID EYE MOVEMENT (NREM) SLEEP

**Stage 1**: The first change in the EEG as an individual becomes drowsy is the disappearance of the occipital dominant alpha rhythm, followed by increasing amounts of theta frequency activity in all regions. During stage 1, diphasic sharp waves also appear in the EEG, occurring maximally at the vertex. These sharp waves are referred to as vertex transients (Figure 25-2A).

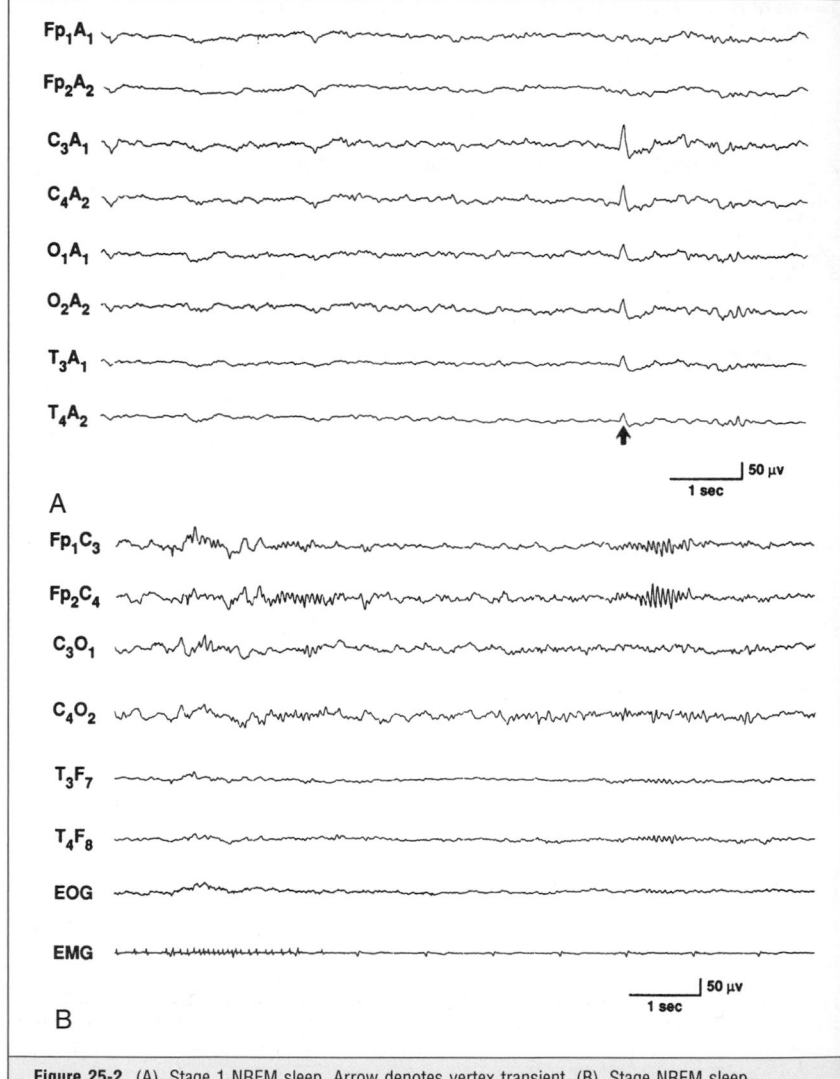

**Figure 25-2.** (A), Stage 1 NREM sleep. Arrow denotes vertex transient. (B), Stage NREM sleep.

*(continued)*

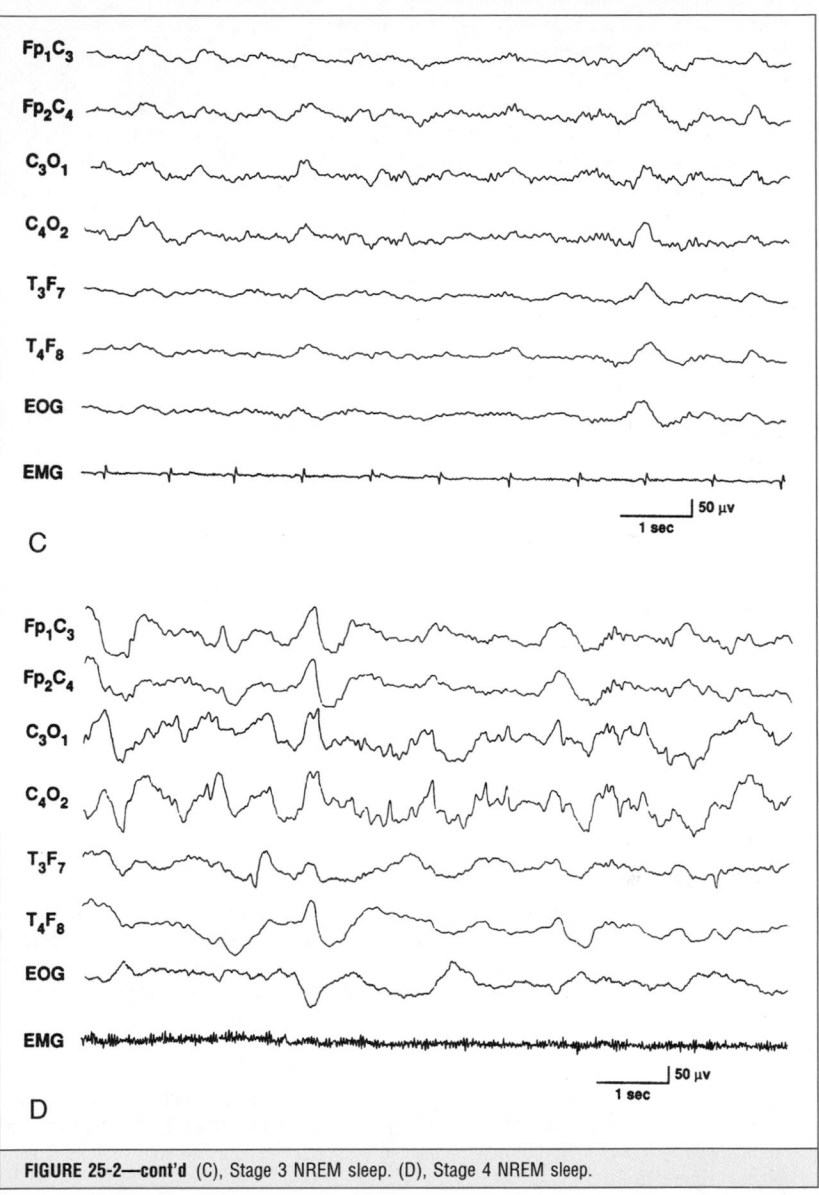

FIGURE 25-2—cont'd (C), Stage 3 NREM sleep. (D), Stage 4 NREM sleep.

(continued)

**Stage 2**: The onset of stage 2 NREM sleep is characterized by the appearance of sleep spindles. Sleep spindles consist of bursts of 12 to 14 Hz activity, maximally expressed over the central regions of the head. These bursts generally last less than 2 seconds in the adult. The background activity during stage 2 sleep consists of relatively low-voltage, mixed frequency EEG background activity, with delta activity comprising less than 20% of the sleep period (Figure 25-2B).

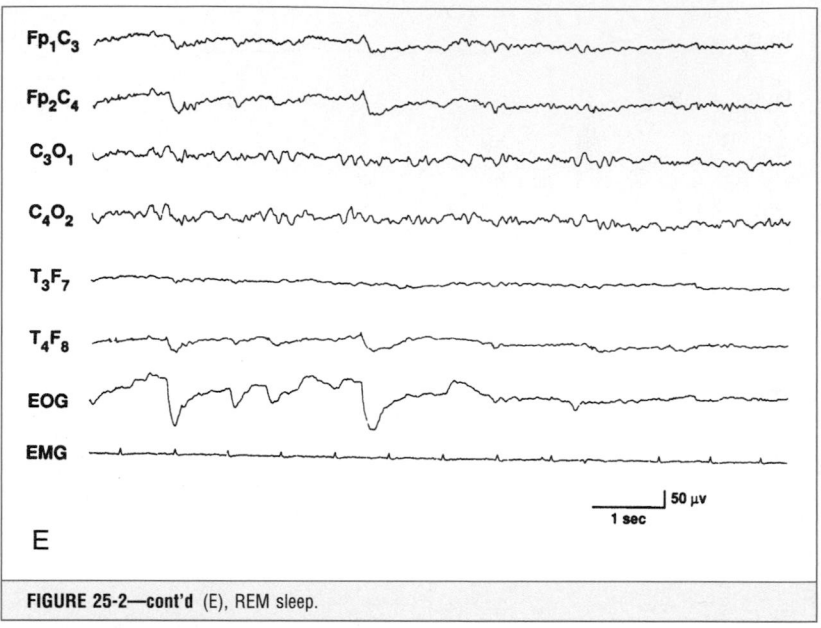

FIGURE 25-2—cont'd (E), REM sleep.

**Stage 3**: As the patient enters deeper NREM sleep, the amount of delta activity increases in voltage and quantity. During stage 3 NREM sleep, the amount of delta activity comprising the record varies between 20% and 50%. Sleep spindles persist into stage 3 sleep (Figure 25-2C).

**Stage 4**: During stage 4 NREM sleep, the amount of delta activity comprises more than 50% of the record. Spindles persist into stage 4 NREM sleep (Figure 25-2D).

## RAPID EYE MOVEMENT (REM) SLEEP

This state is also referred to as paradoxical sleep. The EEG during REM sleep reveals a generally lower voltage record similar in appearance to stage 1. However, in some individuals, runs of alpha frequency activity may appear in the occipital leads identical to the alpha rhythm in the awake tracing. During this stage of sleep, the individual has spontaneous rapid eye movements and tonic motor activity is suppressed (Figure 25-2E).

5. **What is a K complex?**
A K complex is a high-voltage diphasic slow wave that may be preceded or followed by a spindle burst, maximally expressed in the frontocentral regions bilaterally. K complexes occur spontaneously during sleep but may be elicited by sudden sensory stimuli, such as loud noises (Figure 25-3).

6. **What is the *tracé discontinu* pattern?**
*Tracé discontinu* refers to the EEG pattern seen in premature infants. When the brain's electrical activity first appears, it is discontinuous, with long periods of quiescence or flattening. Initially, it is present in all states of waking and sleep. In early prematurity (26 to 28 weeks), the periods of flattening may last up to 20 to 30 seconds. As age increases, the periods of inactivity shorten, and at 30 weeks' conceptional age, the EEG activity becomes continuous during REM sleep. At about 34 weeks, the EEG activity becomes continuous in the awake state. Continuity appears last in NREM, or quiet sleep, at about 37 to 38 weeks (Figure 25-4).

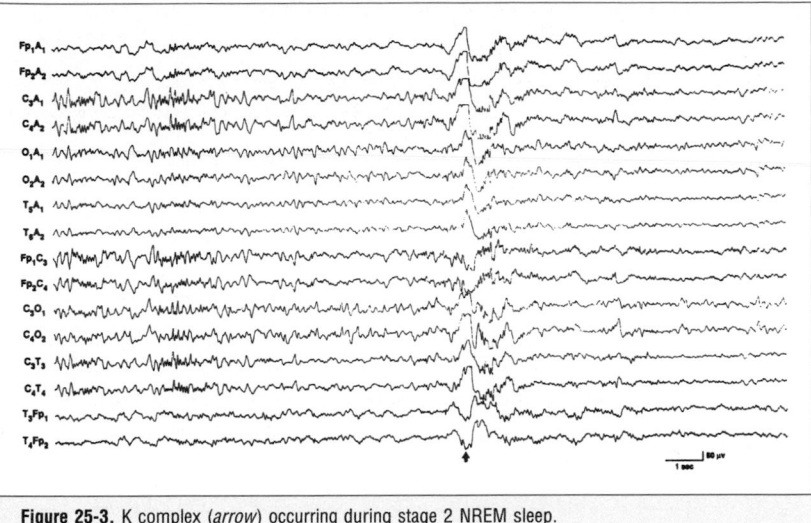

**Figure 25-3.** K complex (*arrow*) occurring during stage 2 NREM sleep.

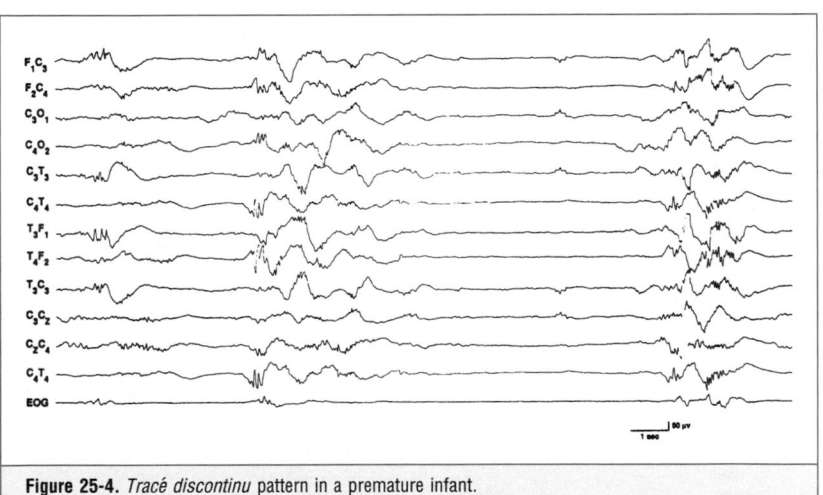

**Figure 25-4.** *Tracé discontinu* pattern in a premature infant.

7. **What does the EEG show in an awake term infant?**
The typical awake pattern in a term infant is characterized by a mixture of alpha, beta, theta, and delta frequencies, and is often referred to as a poly frequency record (Figure 25-5).

8. **What is the *tracé alternant* pattern? At what age is it seen?**
The *tracé alternant* pattern is seen from about 37 to 38 weeks' conceptional age to about 5 to 6 weeks post-term. This pattern occurs during NREM sleep and is characterized by bursts of slow waves mixed with low-voltage sharp activity, separated by episodes of generalized voltage attenuation lasting from 3 to 15 seconds but not absolute quiescence (Figure 25-6).

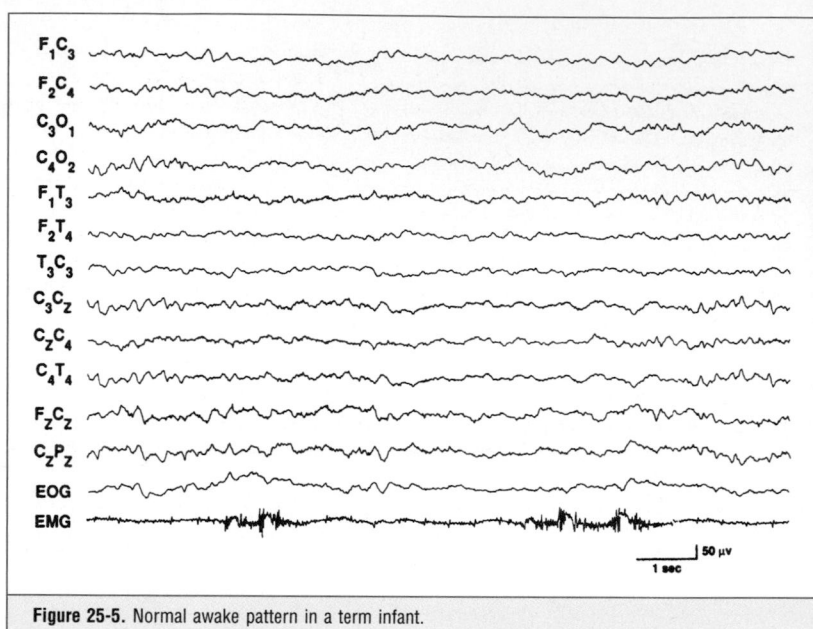

**Figure 25-5.** Normal awake pattern in a term infant.

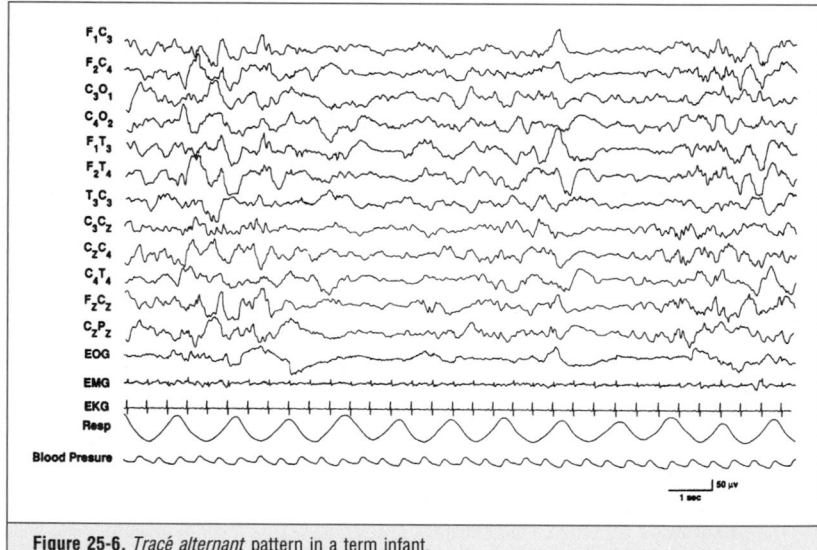

**Figure 25-6.** *Tracé alternant* pattern in a term infant.

9. **At what age do vertex transients appear in the EEG? At what age are these transients synchronous? At what age are they symmetrical?**
Vertex transients first appear in the EEG at 6 to 8 weeks post-term. They are synchronous and symmetrical from the time they first appear.

10. **At what age do sleep spindles first appear in the EEG? At what age are they synchronous? At what age are they symmetrical?**
    Like vertex transients, sleep spindles first appear in the EEG at 6 to 8 weeks post-term. From the time they first appear, they are symmetrical on the two sides; however, spindle synchrony does not occur until about 12 months of age.

11. **At what age does the occipital dominant rhythm first appear? At what age does the occipital dominant rhythm attain a frequency of 8 Hz?**
    At approximately 3 months of age, a rhythm that blocks with eye opening and disappears with drowsiness appears in the occipital leads bilaterally. The frequency of this rhythm when it first appears is 3 to 4 Hz. At 1 year of age, the occipital dominant rhythm is approximately 6 Hz. It does not reach 8 Hz until the age of 3 years.

12. **What are the differences in the EEG of an awake child or young adolescent compared with an adult?**
    - The background activity in the child's EEG is usually higher in voltage.
    - The occipital dominant rhythm in children is mixed, with slower fused waveforms referred to as slow waves of youth.
    - There is more theta frequency activity in the anterior leads of a child's EEG (Figure 25-7).

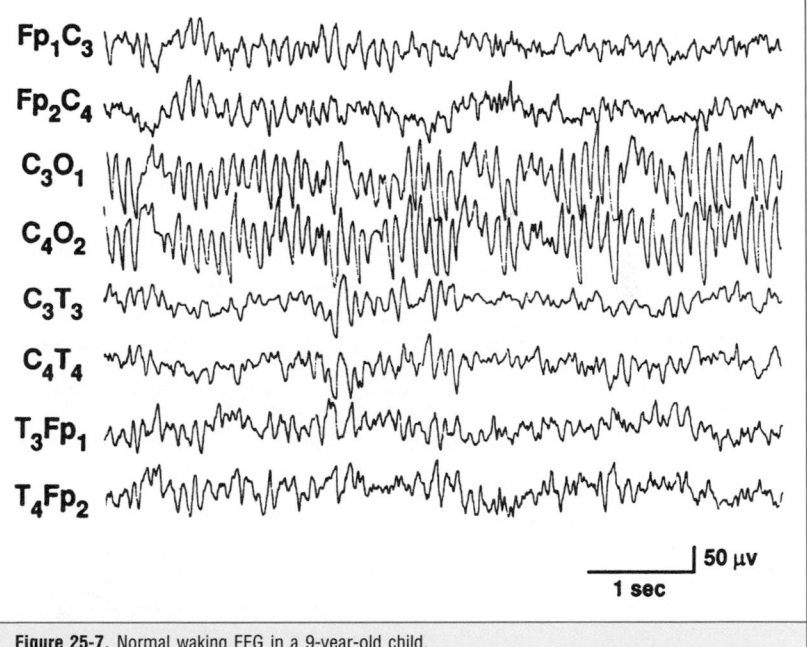

**Figure 25-7.** Normal waking EEG in a 9-year-old child.

13. **What is the mu rhythm?**
    The mu rhythm is a normal central rhythm of alpha-activity frequency, usually in the range of 8 to 10 Hz, that occurs during wakefulness. This rhythm is detectable in about 20% of young adults but is less common in older individuals and children. The mu rhythm is blocked or attenuated by movement, or thought of movement, of the contralateral extremity (Figure 25-8).

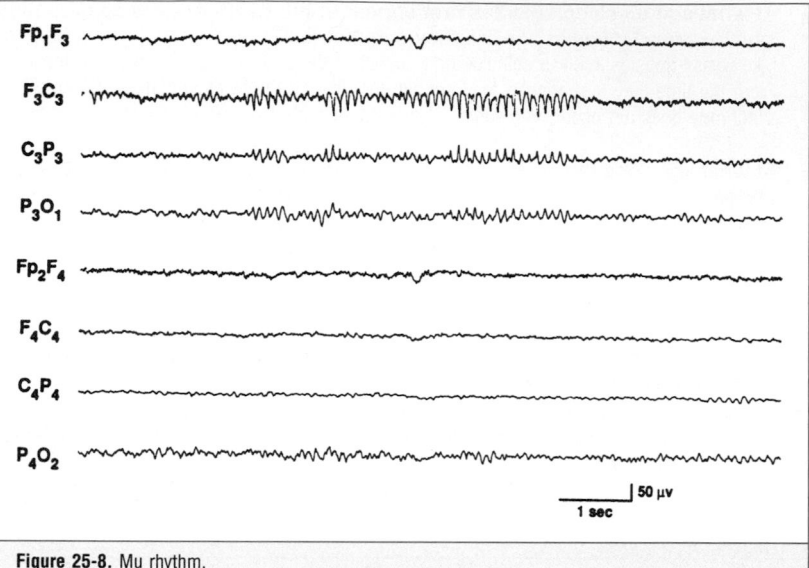

**Figure 25-8.** Mu rhythm.

14. **What is a breach rhythm?**

A breach rhythm typically refers to a high-voltage, sharply contoured rhythm appearing over an area of a skull defect. It is important to realize that this is an accentuated normal rhythm and should not be reported as a focal abnormality (Figure 25-9).

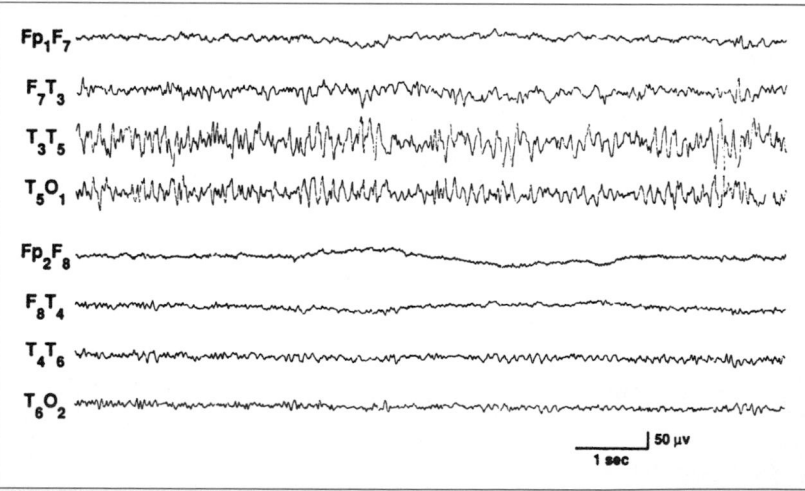

**Figure 25-9.** Breach rhythm in the left posterior temporal ($T_5$) region.

15. **What is the most common finding in pseudotumor cerebri?**
    Although there may be a variety of nonspecific findings in patients with pseudotumor cerebri, the EEG is usually normal.

16. **If you were recording the EEG at the time a patient experienced a middle cerebral artery infarction, what would be the sequence of EEG changes you would expect to see?**
    The initial change following an ischemic episode is depression of the background rhythms over the ipsilateral hemisphere, followed by the appearance of continuous polymorphic slow activity over this hemisphere, maximally expressed in the temporofrontal region (Figure 25-10).

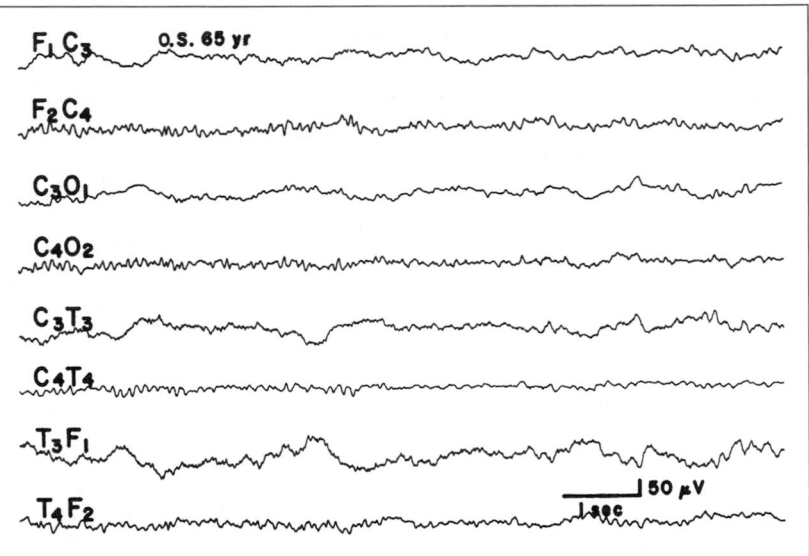

**Figure 25-10.** EEG of a patient with a left middle cerebral artery infarction. Note depression of activity over the left hemispheric leads and left temporal slowing.

17. **An EEG is obtained 3 years after a person has experienced a hemispheric infarction. What EEG findings may be seen in this patient?**
    As in the acute state, the EEG recorded years after a hemispheric infarction may continue to show depression of background activity over the ipsilateral hemisphere. Focal slow-wave activity may also continue ipsilaterally. However, the focal slow-wave activity is not as continuous as it is in the acute state. The patient may continue to show depression of the occipital dominant rhythm on the side of the infarct. However, in many patients, the amplitude of the occipital dominant rhythm returns to normal ipsilaterally, and in some patients, the occipital dominant rhythm becomes enhanced on the side of the infarction (so-called paradoxical enhancement of the alpha rhythm). A small number of patients may reveal a spike focus ipsilaterally. Finally, a large percentage of patients will show a normal EEG years after a hemispheric infarction.

18. **What are the typical EEG changes seen with a small lacunar infarct?**
    Small lacunar infarcts usually produce no change in the background EEG activity; the EEG in such infarcts is usually normal.

19. **What types of EEG findings may be seen with a subdural hematoma?**
Depression of background activity over the ipsilateral hemisphere or focal slow-wave activity over the ipsilateral hemisphere are the findings most frequently seen with a subdural hematoma. Episodic bifrontal slow activity may also occur. However, it is important to remember that the EEG may be normal.

20. **A 6-year-old child presents with headache and ataxia. A posterior fossa tumor is suspected. What EEG findings suggest this diagnosis?**
The most common EEG finding associated with posterior fossa tumors in children is paroxysmal bioccipital delta activity (Figure 25-11).

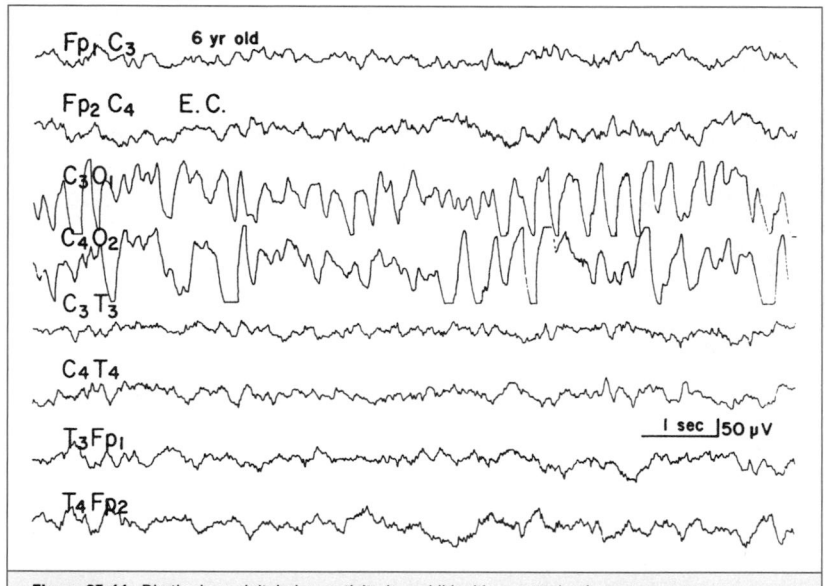

**Figure 25-11.** Rhythmic occipital slow activity in a child with a posterior fossa tumor.

21. **What is the significance of triphasic waves in the EEG?**
Triphasic waves usually appear in the EEG when there has been diffuse slowing of background rhythms. Although triphasic waves may be seen with a variety of encephalopathies (e.g., infectious, toxic, postanoxic), they most often are associated with metabolic encephalopathies, most commonly hepatic or renal (Figure 25-12).

22. **What is the relationship between clinical improvement and EEG improvement in children with various encephalopathies?**
Although in older individuals with various types of encephalopathies, clinical and EEG improvement usually occur simultaneously, in children the clinical status of the patient may improve more rapidly than the EEG.

23. **What is the usual progression of EEG changes in Alzheimer's disease (AD)?**
During the early stages of AD, the EEG may be normal. As the disease progresses, the EEG initially shows slowing of the occipital dominant rhythm, which, in turn, is followed by increasing amounts of theta-frequency activity and then by the appearance of bifrontal and, in some patients, bioccipital delta activity. Occasional sharp waves may appear in the frontal and

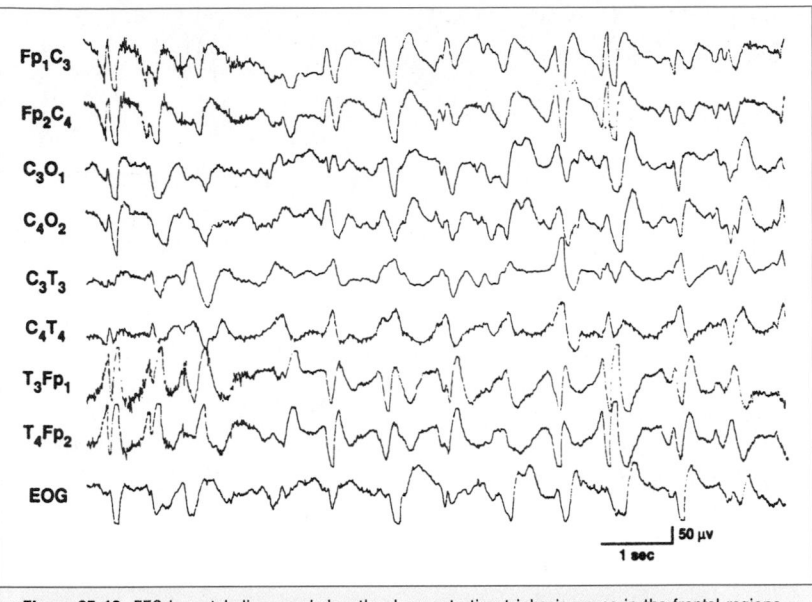

**Figure 25-12.** EEG in metabolic encephalopathy demonstrating triphasic waves in the frontal regions.

posterior head regions in severely demented patients; however, these sharp waves never develop the periodic character of the sharp waves seen with Creutzfeldt-Jakob disease. Marked asymmetries of the background activity and focal slow wave activity are not features of AD.

24. **What are the major differences between the periodic pattern seen with Creutzfeldt-Jakob disease and that seen with subacute sclerosing panencephalitis (SSPE)?**
   See Table 25-1 and Figure 25-13A and B.

| TABLE 25-1. CREUTZFELDT-JAKOB DISEASE VERSUS SUBACUTE SCLEROSING PANENCEPHALITIS | | |
|---|---|---|
| | **CJD** | **SSPE** |
| Complex morphology | Diphasic or triphasic sharp waves | Slow waves or groups of slow waves; may have sharp component |
| Period | Classically, 1 sec | 4-14 sec |
| Distribution | Generalized, but may begin focally or lateralized to one hemisphere | Usually generalized but maximal in frontocentral leads |
| Background activity | Diffusely slow when complexes first appear | May be normal when complexes first appear |
| CJD = Creutzfeldt-Jakob disease; SSPE = subacute sclerosing panencephalitis | | |

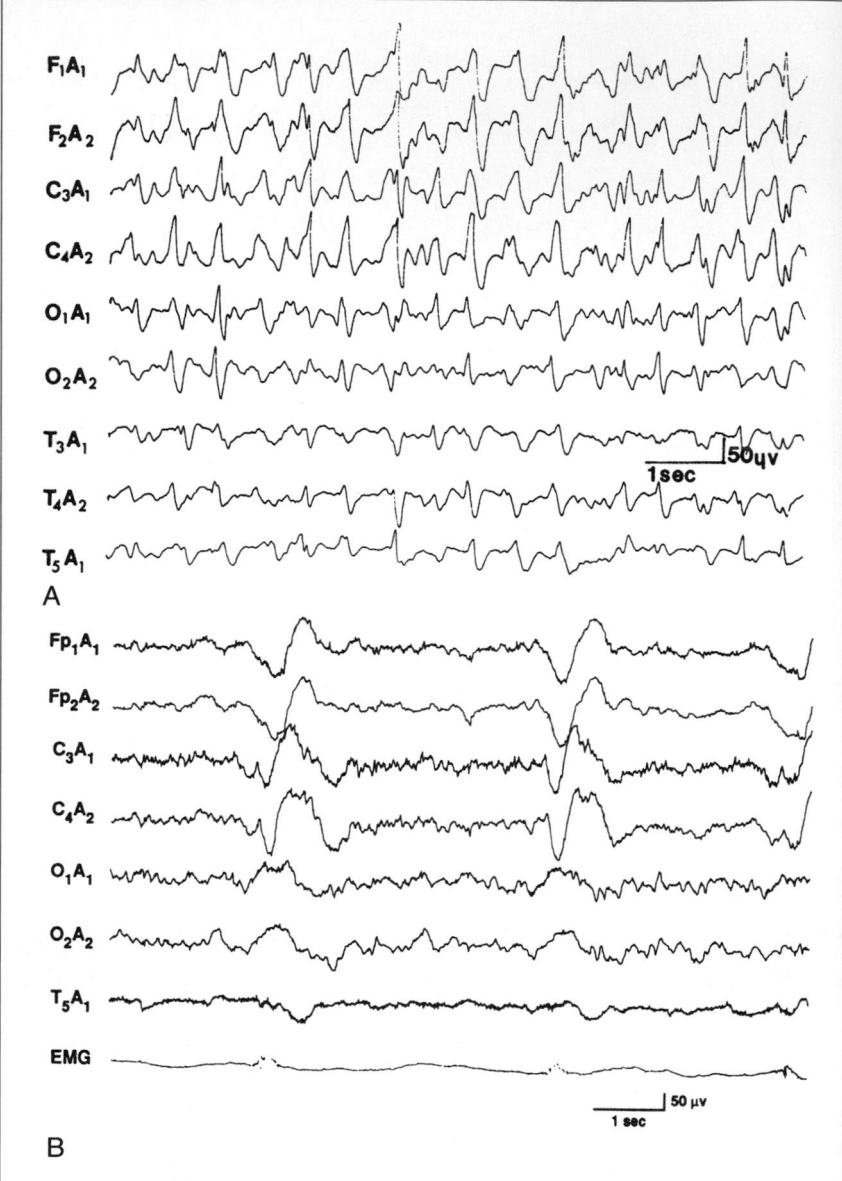

**Figure 25-13.** (A), Periodic pattern in Creutzfeldt-Jakob disease. (B), Periodic pattern in subacute sclerosing panencephalitis (SSPE).

25. **What other disease processes may produce a periodic pattern similar to that seen with Creutzfeldt-Jakob disease?**
The periodic pattern consisting of generalized, high-voltage diphasic and triphasic sharp waves recurring with a period of 1 second is highly suggestive of Creutzfeldt-Jakob disease. However, a pattern indistinguishable from that seen in Creutzfeldt-Jakob disease may occur in the postanoxic state. Also, a similar type of pattern may be seen with lithium intoxication.

26. **What is the significance of periodic lateralizing epileptiform discharges (PLEDs)? What is the most common etiology?**
Periodic lateralizing epileptiform discharges signify the presence of a large destructive lesion involving one hemisphere. They may be seen with a variety of lesions, including tumors, abscesses, hematomas, and herpes encephalitis. However, the most common cause of PLEDs is acute cerebral infarction (Figure 25-14).

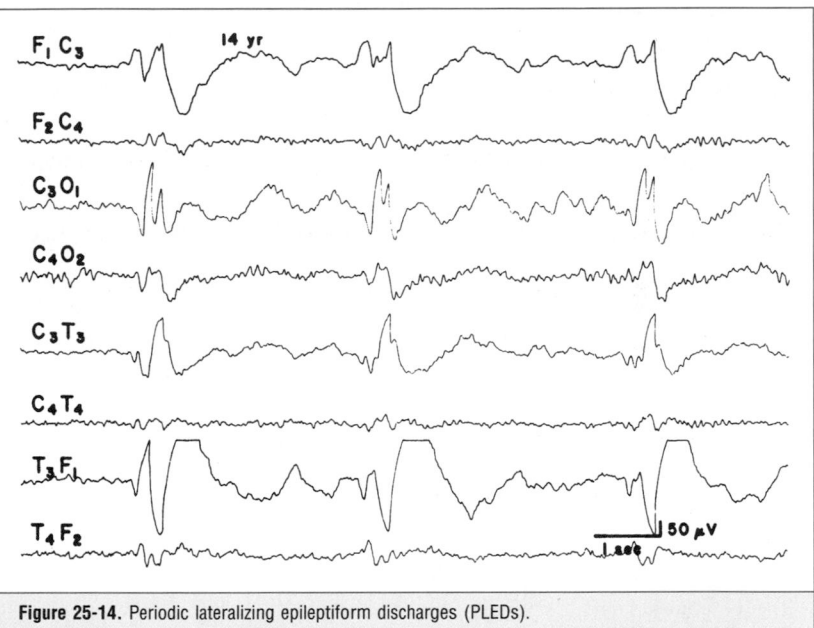

**Figure 25-14.** Periodic lateralizing epileptiform discharges (PLEDs).

27. **What classes of drugs produce increased amounts of voltages of beta activity in the EEG at therapeutic doses?**
The most common classes of drugs that produce increased fast activity in the EEG are the sedatives, anxiolytic agents, central nervous system (CNS) stimulants, and antihistamines. Antidepressants may increase the amount of beta activity in the EEG at therapeutic doses but also result in an increase in the amount of theta-frequency activity (Figure 25-15).

28. **What is hypsarrhythmia?**
Hypsarrhythmia is the interictal EEG pattern usually seen in infants who experience infantile spasms. The pattern consists of random, high-voltage slow waves mixed with high-voltage, multifocal spike and sharp waves arising from all cortical regions. The triad of infantile spasms, hypsarrhythmia, and mental retardation is often referred to as West's syndrome (Figure 25-16).

29. **What are the characteristics of the 3 per second spike and slow-wave pattern?**
This pattern is bilateral, symmetrical, and usually maximally expressed in the frontocentral regions. In some patients, however, the bursts of 3 per second spike and wave activity may be restricted to or maximally expressed in the occipital regions. The discharges appear and disappear suddenly. The frequency of the spike and wave complexes may vary slightly during

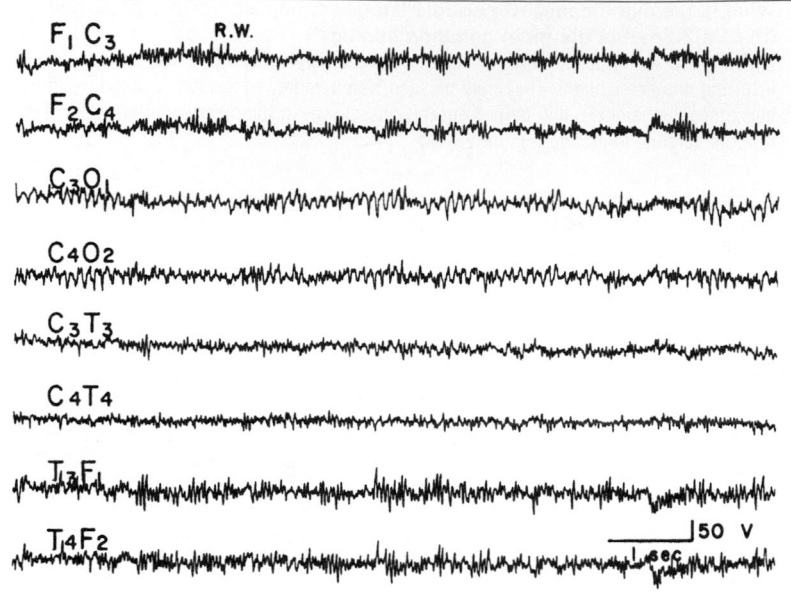

**Figure 25-15.** Excessive beta activity in a patient receiving a benzodiazepine.

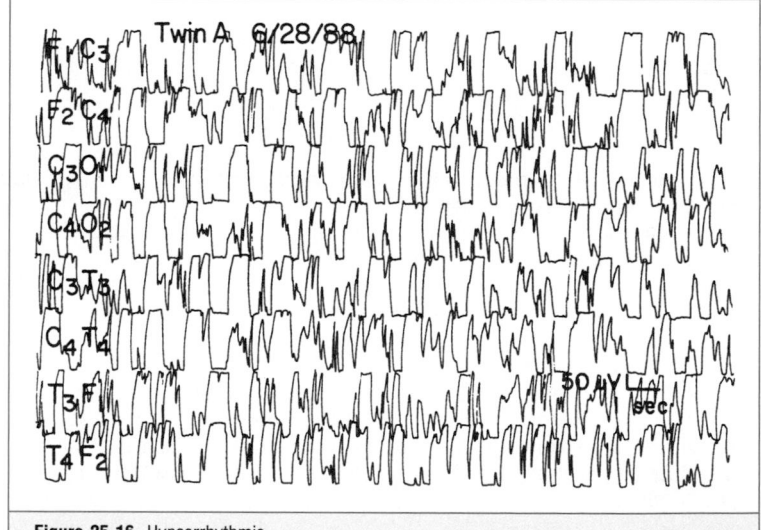

**Figure 25-16.** Hypsarrhythmia.

the bursts. The first few complexes of the bursts may occur at a frequency of 3.5 to 4.0 Hz, whereas the last few may slow to 2.5 Hz. As soon as the 3-Hz spike and wave bursts stop, the EEG returns to its interictal state immediately with no postictal depression or slowing (Figure 25-17).

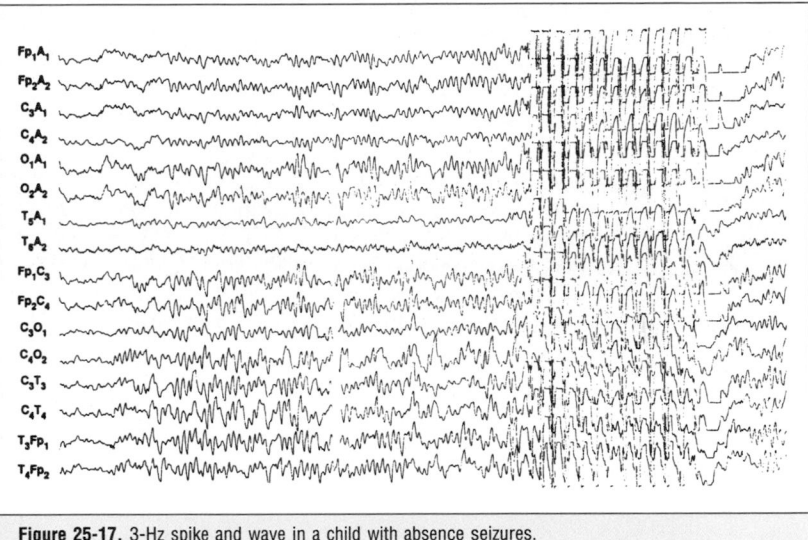

**Figure 25-17.** 3-Hz spike and wave in a child with absence seizures.

30. **A 10-year-old girl with staring spells is referred for an EEG. What routine activating procedures should be performed on this patient?**
The common activating procedures usually performed on patients with suspected seizures are hyperventilation, photic stimulation, and sleep. Generalized spike and wave activity may be activated by any of these three activating procedures, whereas focal spikes are usually activated only by sleep.

31. **Which two normal patterns are frequently confused with generalized spike and wave activity in children?**
The first is hypnagogic hypersynchrony. This pattern appears at 3 to 4 months of age and persists until 10 to 12 years of age. It consists of paroxysmal rhythmic 3 to 5 Hz activity, maximally expressed in the central and centrofrontal regions. This activity may occur in long runs; however, it may also appear in brief paroxysms. Faster components may be mixed with the paroxysmal slower activity. The second pattern often confused with generalized spike and slow-wave activity is the normal hyperventilation response. Children, particularly between the ages of 5 and 15 years, often show a buildup of high-voltage, frontal dominant, generalized 3 to 4 Hz activity. This high-voltage, rhythmic slow activity may be continuous or occur in a paroxysmal fashion while the child is deep-breathing. This pattern may be easily confused by the novice electroencephalographer with the 3-Hz spike and slow-wave pattern, which may also occur during hyperventilation in children (Figure 25-18A and B).

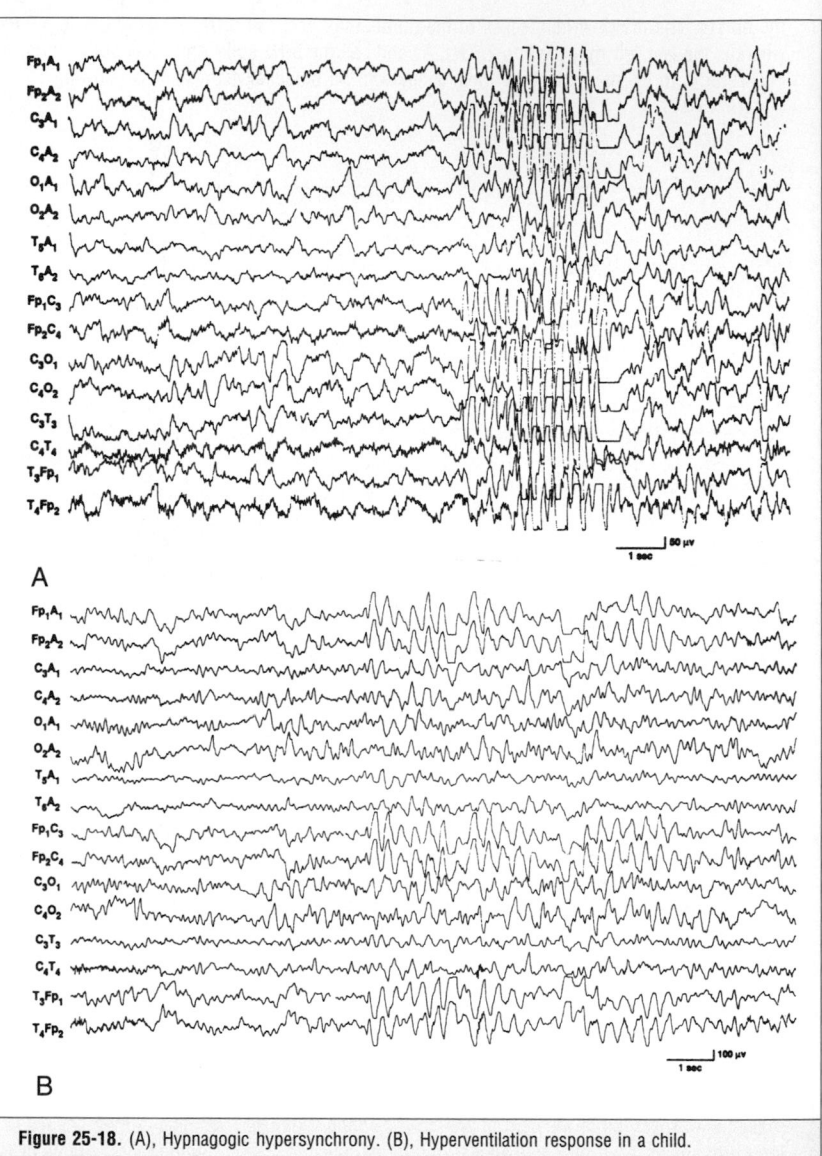

**Figure 25-18.** (A), Hypnagogic hypersynchrony. (B), Hyperventilation response in a child.

32. **What are the characteristics of focal epileptiform spikes?**
A spike is an EEG transient with a duration of less than 70 msec. The transient may occur alone, but frequently a slow wave follows, forming a spike and slow-wave complex. The duration of the slow wave may last from 150 to 350 msec. The spike transient may be monophasic or polyphasic. The polarity of most focal epileptiform spikes recorded at the scalp is surface negative. Surface positive spikes rarely occur in patients with epilepsy (Figure 25-19).

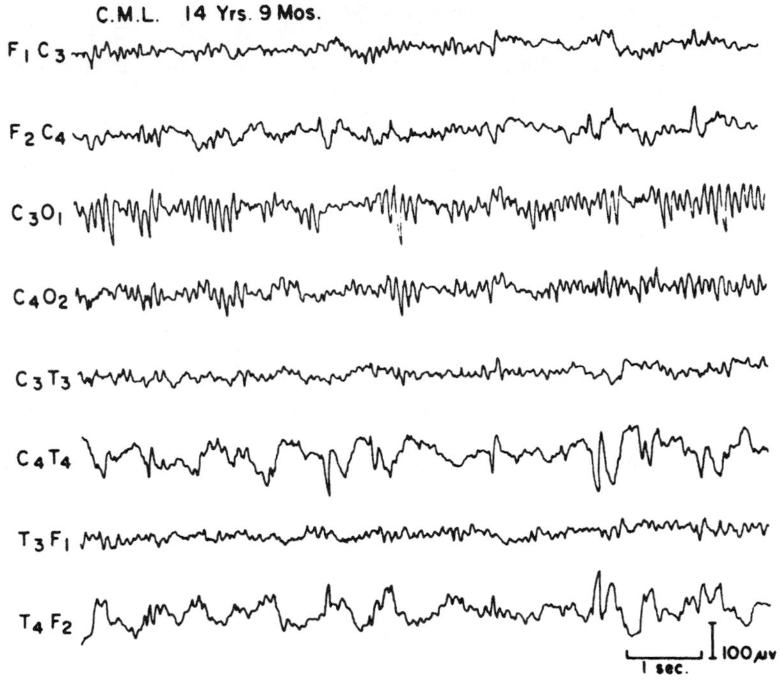

C.M.L.  14 Yrs. 9 Mos.

F₁ C₃

F₂ C₄

C₃ O₁

C₄ O₂

C₃ T₃

C₄ T₄

T₃ F₁

T₄ F₂

I sec.    100 μv

**Figure 25-19.** Right temporal spikes mixed with slow waves in a child with complex partial seizures.

## KEY POINTS: ELECTROENCEPHALOGRAPHY

1. The normal adult EEG, relaxed with eyes closed, is characterized by 9 to 11 cycles per second activity in the back of the brain (occipital lobes) called the alpha rhythm.

2. Each stage of sleep has a very characteristic EEG pattern.

3. Periodic lateralizing epileptiform discharges (PLEDs) on an EEG imply an acute, large lesion involving one hemisphere, such as a stroke or focal encephalitis.

4. The 3 per second spike and wave pattern on an EEG is usually seen in patients with absence seizures.

5. The finding on an EEG that is most suggestive of focal epilepsy is a very brief (less than 70 msec) transient deflection called a spike.

6. The EEG is one of the most important tests to confirm brain death.

33. **Which three normal EEG patterns may be confused with focal epileptiform spikes in the EEG?**
    A. Vertex transients—synchronous diphasic sharp waves that appear at the vertex.
    B. Lambda waves—multiphasic spikes that appear in the occipital leads, with eyes open, and are associated with saccadic eye movements when looking at geometric patterns.

C. Positive occipital sharp transients of sleep—positive sharp waves that appear in the occipital leads during NREM sleep (Figure 25-20A-C).

34. **What are the typical clinical characteristics of a patient whose EEG shows bursts of generalized 2-Hz spike and slow-wave activity?**
They have varying degrees of developmental and mental retardation. These patients experience multiple types of seizures, most commonly atonic, tonic, atypical absence, and generalized tonic-clonic. Partial seizures may also occur. These seizures are generally refractory to

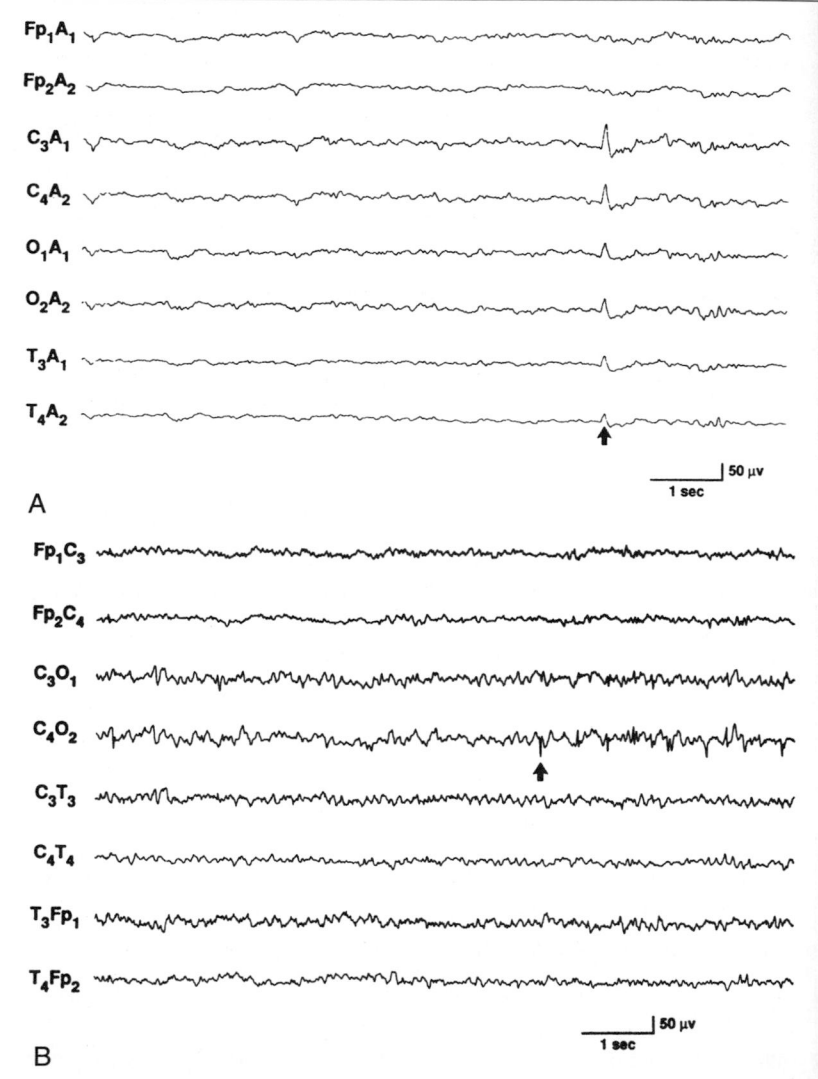

**Figure 25-20.** (A), Stage 1 NREM sleep. Arrow denotes vertex transient. (B), Lambda waves (*arrow*) in the occipital leads in an individual looking at a geometric design.

*(continued)*

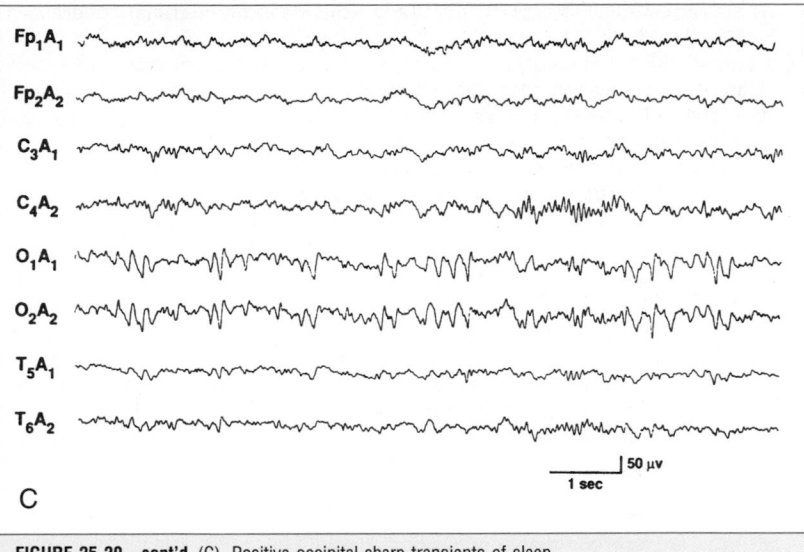

FIGURE 25-20—cont'd (C), Positive occipital sharp transients of sleep.

anticonvulsant therapy, and such patients will often be treated with polytherapy. This constellation of clinical and EEG features is often referred to as the Lennox-Gastaut syndrome, or slow-spike and slow-wave syndrome (Figure 25-21).

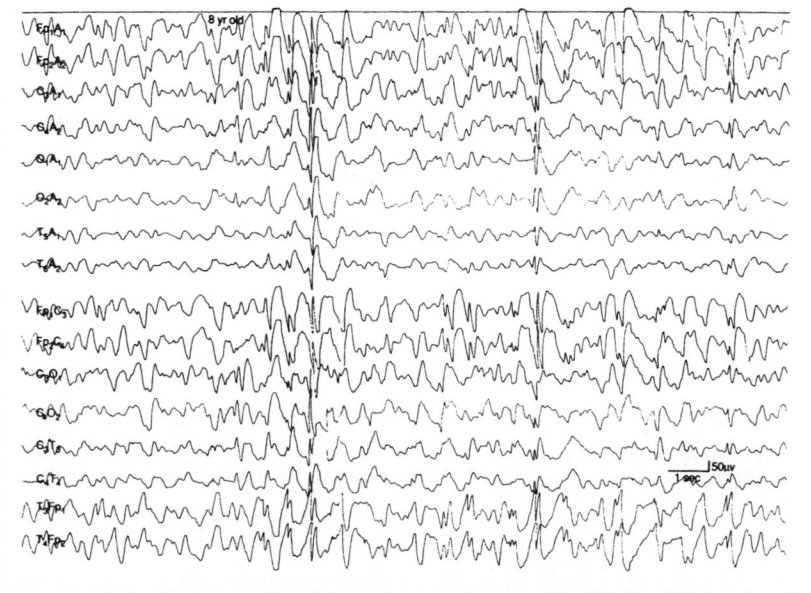

Figure 25-21. 2-Hz spike and slow-wave activity in a patient with Lennox-Gastaut syndrome.

35. **What are the usual effects of NREM and REM sleep on interictal generalized or focal epileptiform discharges?**
In general, NREM sleep greatly enhances the frequency of interictal generalized spike and wave or focal spike activity, particularly the first NREM sleep episode of nocturnal sleep. On the other hand, REM sleep is usually associated with a marked attenuation or total abolishment of epileptiform activity.

36. **What types of EEG changes may be seen postictally?**
Immediately after a generalized tonic-clonic seizure, there is marked depression of background activity in all regions, followed by an increase in the voltage and frequency of the background activity, and a gradual return to the baseline state. Focal slowing may also occur postictally in a patient who has experienced a generalized tonic-clonic seizure. Following a partial seizure, the EEG frequently shows regional or hemispheric depression of the background activity over the ipsilateral hemisphere and/or focal slow-wave activity over the ipsilateral hemisphere. The duration that the postictal changes will persist in the EEG is highly variable. In general, the longer the duration of the seizure, the longer the postictal changes persist. This is particularly true in children, who may show diffuse or focal postictal changes for days following a prolonged seizure or an episode of status epilepticus.

37. **What four EEG patterns with an epileptiform morphology are classified as patterns of uncertain diagnostic significance?**
1. The 14- and 6-Hz positive bursts (14 and 6 per second positive spikes)
2. The rhythmic temporal theta bursts of drowsiness (psychomotor variant pattern)
3. The 6-Hz spike and wave pattern (phantom spike and wave pattern)
4. The small, sharp spike pattern (benign epileptiform transients of sleep)
   The 14 and 6 per second positive burst pattern is a pattern of childhood and adolescence, whereas the remaining three patterns are usually seen in adulthood (Figure 25-22A-D).

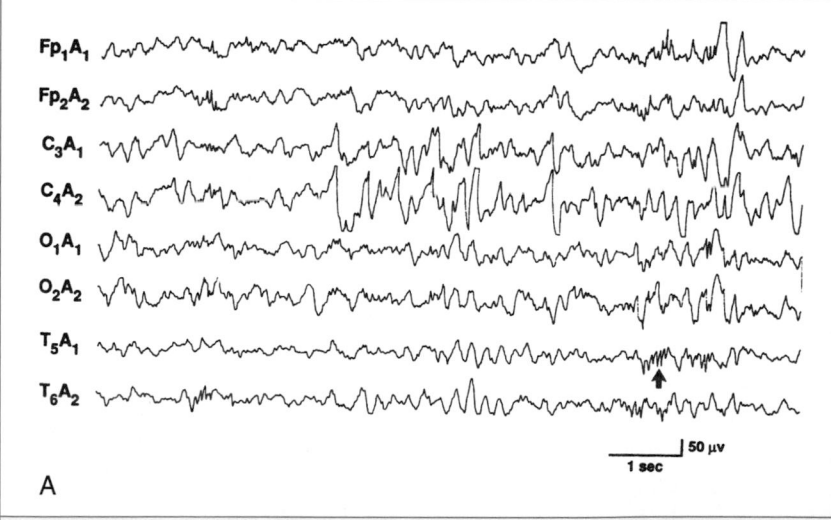

A

**Figure 25-22.** (A), 14 and 6 per second positive spike pattern.

(continued)

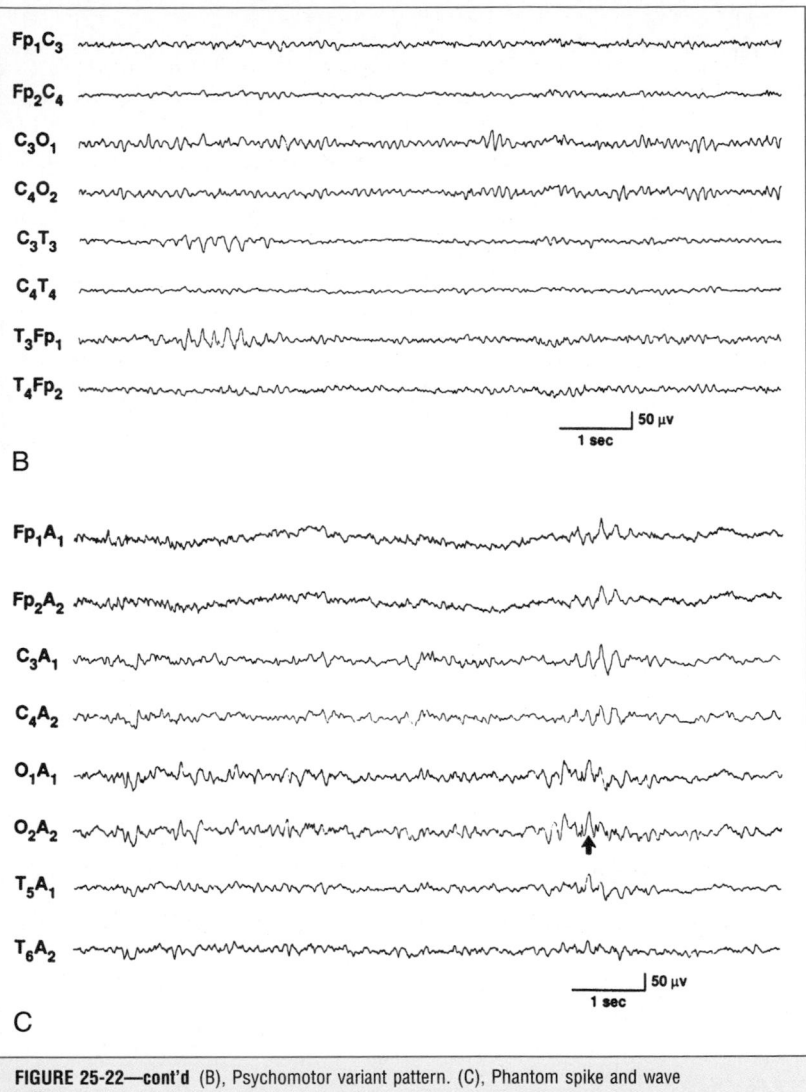

**FIGURE 25-22—cont'd** (B), Psychomotor variant pattern. (C), Phantom spike and wave pattern.

*(continued)*

38. **What is the significance of a suppression-burst pattern? Which conditions may produce this pattern?**

The suppression-burst pattern consists of brief paroxysms of activity occurring between periods of little or no discernible electrical activity. The activity during the bursts may consist of alpha, theta, or delta frequencies and/or sharp waves. The suppression-burst pattern indicates the presence of a severe diffuse disturbance in brain function. It may be seen in a variety of conditions, including anoxic insult, drug overdose, and severe head injury (Figure 25-23).

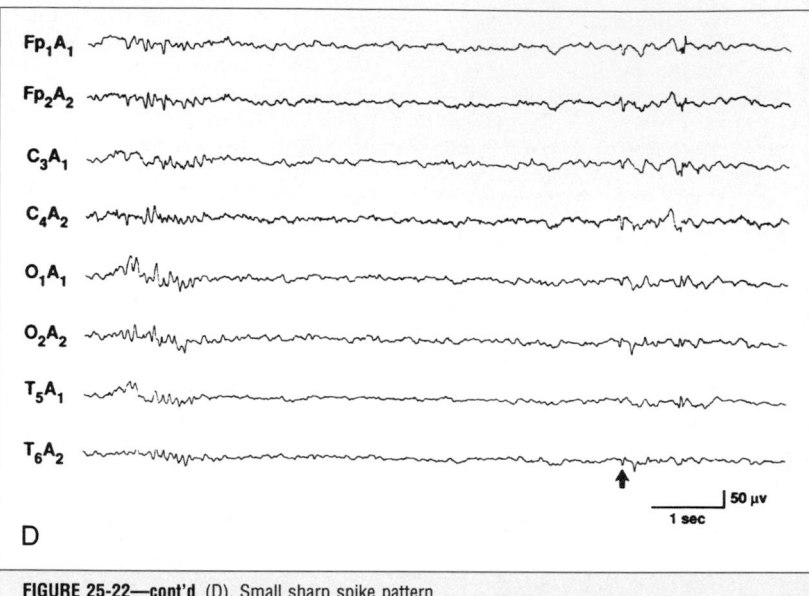

**FIGURE 25-22—cont'd** (D), Small sharp spike pattern.

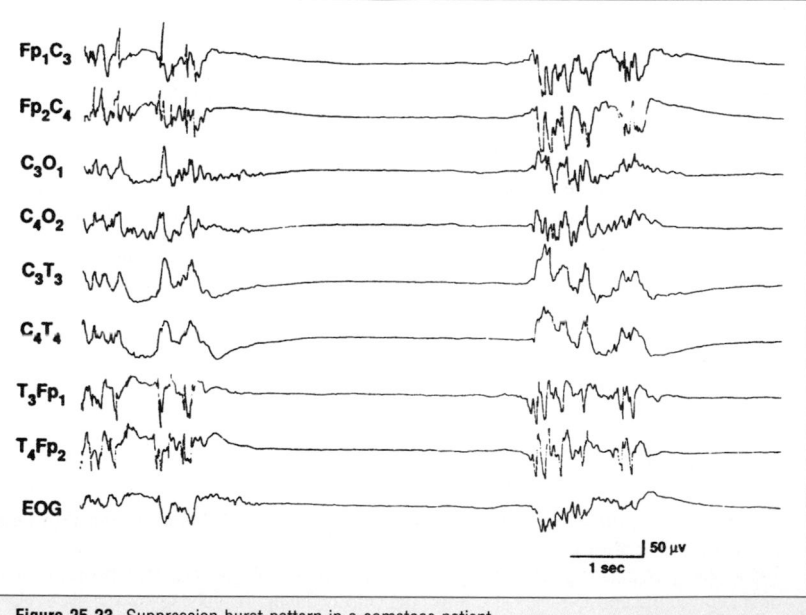

**Figure 25-23.** Suppression burst pattern in a comatose patient.

**39. What are some of the patterns that may be seen following an anoxic insult?**
Depending on the degree of the anoxic insult and the timing from the insult to the EEG, a variety of patterns may be seen. With mild insults, the EEG may be normal or show only slight diffuse slowing. As the severity of the insult increases, so does the degree of slowing of the background rhythms. In addition, periodic diphasic and triphasic sharp waves, superimposed upon a slow-background, alpha coma pattern, and suppression-burst patterns may all occur in the postanoxic state.

**40. What are the three brain stem coma patterns? Which pattern generally has the best prognosis?**
Alpha coma, spindle coma, and theta coma. Of these, spindle coma usually carries the best prognosis (Figure 25-24A-C).

**41. What are the major criteria for recording a case of suspected brain death?**
- A minimum of eight scalp electrodes and earlobe reference electrodes should be used.
- The interelectrode impedances should be under 10,000 ohms but over 100 ohms.
- The interelectrode distances should be at least 10 cm.
- The sensitivity should be changed from 7 to 2 mV/mm during most of the recording with inclusion of appropriate calibrations.
- A time constant of 0.3 to 0.4 seconds should be used during part of the recording.
- The integrity of the entire recording system should be tested.
- Monitoring techniques (e.g., electrocardiogram [ECG], ambient noise, respiratory) should be used as needed to identify other physiologic signals and artifacts as not being of brain origin.
- The EEG should be tested for reactivity by intense stimulation such as pain and loud sound.
- The EEG should be recorded for at least 30 min.
- The recording should be made only by qualified technologists.

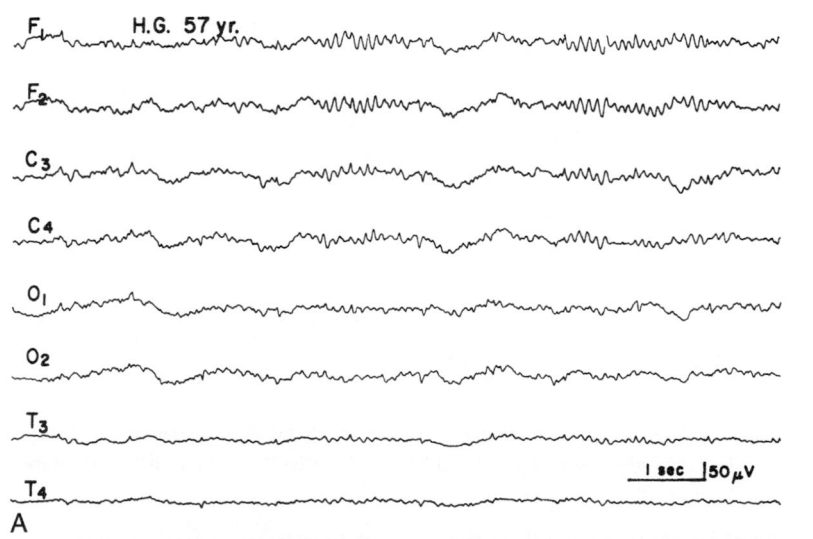

**Figure 25-24.** (A), Alpha coma pattern in a comatose patient following a brain stem infarction. Note alpha-frequency activity in frontal deviations.

*(continued)*

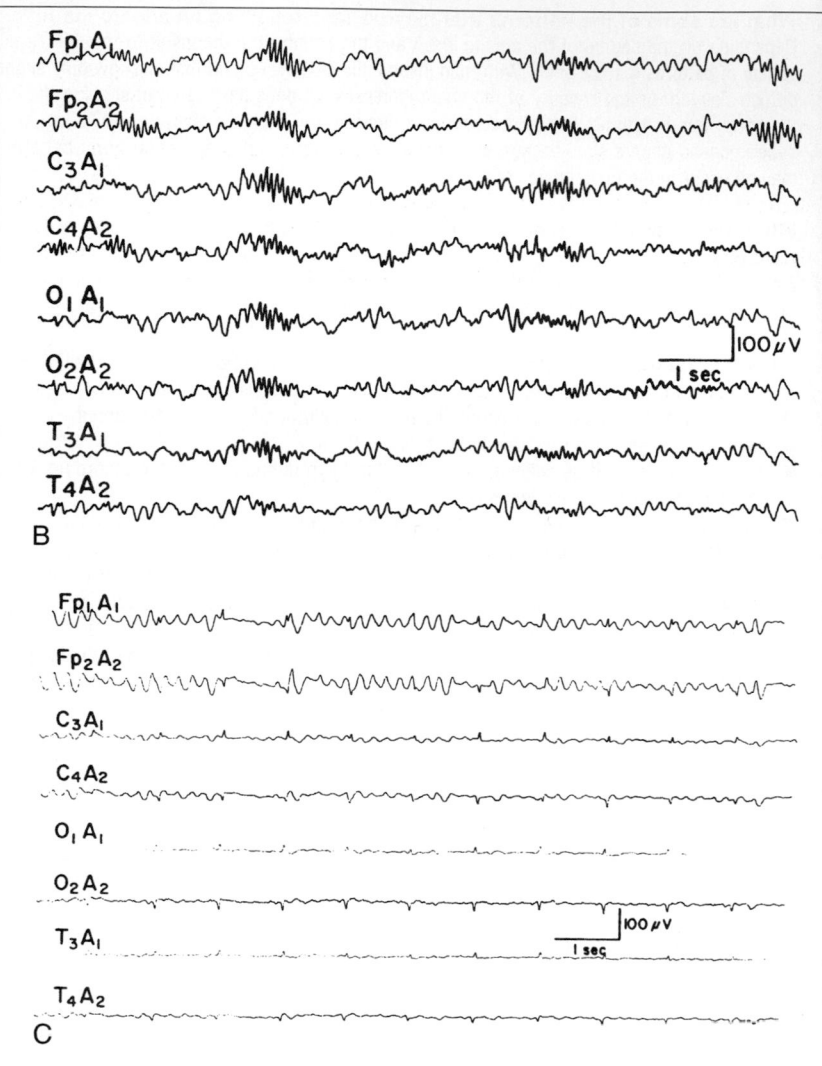

**FIGURE 25-24—cont'd** (B), Spindle coma pattern in a comatose patient following a midbrain contusion. (C), Theta coma pattern in a comatose patient following a cardiorespiratory arrest. Periodic low-voltage sharp waves represent electrocardiograph (ECG) artifact.

- A repeat EEG should be performed if there is any doubt about electrocerebral silence.
- Telephone transmission of an EEG should not be used for determination of electrocerebral silence.

42. **What are the two conditions that may produce temporary, reversible, electrocerebral inactivity?**
   The two conditions that may result in reversible electrocerebral inactivity are overdoses with CNS depressants and hypothermia.

# BIBLIOGRAPHY

1. Blume WT, Kaibara M: Atlas of Adult Electroencephalopathy, Philadelphia, Lippincott-Raven, 1995.
2. Ebersole JS, Pedley TA (eds): Current Practice of Clinical Electroencephalography, 3rd ed. New York, Lippincott, Williams & Wilkins, 2003.
3. Fisch B, editor: Fisch and Spehlman's EEG Primer: Basic Principles of Digital and Analog EEG, New York, Elsevier, 2006.
4. Hrachovy RA: Development of the normal electroencephalogram. In Levin KH, Lüders HO (eds): Comprehensive Clinical Neurophysiology, Philadelphia, W.B. Saunders, 2000, pp 387-413.
5. Niedermeyer E, Lopes da Silva F (eds): Electroencephalography: Basic Principles, Clinical Application, and Related Fields, 5th ed. Philadelphia, Lippincott Williams & Wilkins, 2004.

# CHAPTER 26

# ELECTROMYOGRAPHY

*James M. Killian, MD*

1. **What is an electromyogram (EMG)? How is it recorded?**

   An EMG is an electrical recording of resting and voluntary muscle activity transmitted from a needle electrode through a preamplifier and amplifier to a loudspeaker and digital visual display. When an EMG is ordered, motor and sensory nerve conduction studies are included with the needle recording as part of the overall electrodiagnostic examination.

2. **What are the clinical indications for ordering an EMG?**

   An EMG is usually ordered to determine the localization and severity of neurogenic disorders and to differentiate them from myogenic disorders. Focal neurogenic lesions are localized using the same logic used in the clinical muscle examination, but important subclinical information can be determined, especially in muscles with variable weakness. Myogenic disorders are separated into inflammatory (myositis) and noninflammatory (myopathy).

3. **What are the characteristics of normal voluntary motor unit potentials?**

   Normal muscle potentials appear as waveforms with a duration of 5 to 15 msec, 2 to 4 phases, and amplitudes of 0.5 to 3 mV (depending on the size of the unit and type of recording needle electrodes).

4. **What are polyphasic units? When are they seen on EMG?**

   These are voluntary motor units with more than four phases. They are seen in both myogenic and neurogenic disorders.

5. **What are the characteristics of abnormal voluntary motor unit potentials?**

   Abnormal motor unit potentials are classified as either neurogenic or myogenic. Neurogenic motor units appear of longer duration and higher amplitude than normal potentials and are usually polyphasic. Myopathic potentials are just the opposite, with shorter durations and smaller amplitudes than normal potentials. They are also usually polyphasic.

6. **What are the EMG characteristics of fasciculation potentials?**

   A fasciculation is an involuntary firing of a single motor neuron and all its innervated muscle fibers. It is displayed by EMG as a single motor unit and, if close to the surface, is visible as a brief irregular undulation of muscle.

7. **What is the significance of fasciculations? When are they nonpathologic?**

   Fasciculations may be associated with pathology in the anterior horn cells, motor roots, or the cramp-fasciculation syndrome. However, fasciculations may be present with no evidence of any nerve or muscle disease and then are termed "benign fasciculations."

8. **What are the EMG characteristics of fibrillation potentials?**

   Fibrillations are involuntary contractions of single muscle fibers and cannot be seen through the skin. Electrically, they appear as regular or irregular, short, small action potentials that sound like static or cooking bacon. Fibrillations are always abnormal and indicate loss of innervation of a single muscle fiber from a variety of causes.

9. **What is the importance of insertional activity?**
Insertional activity is the discharge of single muscle fibers during insertion of an EMG needle and does not indicate abnormality. The discharges look like fibrillations on the EMG. Increased insertional activity may indicate irritable muscle fibers, such as in early denervation, but it is often nonspecific.

0. **What are positive sharp waves?**
Positive sharp waves are spontaneous discharges from groups of denervated muscle fibers. They are larger than fibrillation potentials but have the same pathologic implication (i.e., denervation). They appear on the EMG screen as downward monophasic wave formations that indicate a positive polarity—hence the name.

1. **What electrical activity can be measured from the end plate?**
High-frequency, short-duration potentials can be seen when the EMG needle is close to or in the motor end plate. They are called end-plate activity or end-plate noise. This activity is not pathologic but may be confused with fibrillation potentials.

2. **What are the two types of myotonia? Describe their appearance on an EMG.**
Myotonia refers to a delayed relaxation of muscle after contraction or needle insertion. The two types of myotonia are true and pseudo. True myotonia occurs in the myotonic dystrophies and myotonia congenita and is seen as muscle action potentials that vary in amplitude and frequency with gradual termination and are heard on the loud speaker as "dive bombers." Pseudomyotonia has a more stable firing frequency that resembles an airplane in steady flight, with abrupt termination. Pseudomyotonia occurs in both muscle and nerve disorders, including myositis, glycogen storage diseases, hyperkalemic periodic paralysis, root disease, and anterior horn cell disorders.

3. **What are the EMG characteristics recorded in a myopathy?**
In myopathy, the individual motor unit potentials are smaller and shorter because of a reduction in the size of the muscle fibers. The discharging motor unit-firing rate is unchanged; therefore, a full pattern of muscle activity on effort ("interference pattern") is still seen on the EMG screen.

4. **What are the EMG characteristics of activity recorded from a denervated muscle?**
Fibrillations and positive sharp waves begin in resting muscles 7 to 14 days after the onset of axonal denervation. When partially denervated muscle is voluntarily contracted, clinical weakness from axonal loss is seen on the EMG as a reduction in motor unit firing patterns proportional to the amount of axonal loss.

5. **How soon do electrical changes develop after a nerve is transected?**
Transection of a nerve is followed immediately by loss of voluntary activity; therefore, no electrical motor units are seen with attempted contraction. Spontaneous abnormal EMG activity consisting of fibrillation and positive sharp waves begins 7 to 10 days later and reaches maximum level at about 14 to 21 days.

6. **After nerve transection, what happens to nerve conduction in the distal segment?**
Nerve conduction in the distal segment is retained for 3 days after proximal transection of the nerve. Wallerian degeneration rapidly interferes with nerve conduction, and after 3 to 5 days, all conductibility is lost.

17. **How do recruitment patterns differ in normal muscles, myopathies, and neurogenic disorders?**
The pattern of motor activity on effort does not differ between normal muscles and those with myopathic abnormalities because all motor units are intact and fire normally. However, neurogenic abnormalities show a dropout of motor units, which reduces the recruitment pattern according to the severity of axonal loss.

18. **What are the clinical indications for ordering nerve conduction velocities?**
Nerve conduction velocities (NCV) are ordered to demonstrate presence or absence of focal or generalized abnormalities of the peripheral motor and sensory nerves, to assess the severity of any abnormalities, and to determine whether the nerve pathology is axonal or demyelinative.

19. **What is the normal NCV?**
Normal motor NCV in the arm is above 50 m/s and in the leg above 42 meters/second. Distal latencies vary with the nerve studied, as do sensory nerve conduction (SCV) measurements.

20. **What is a normal compound motor action potential (CMAP)?**
A CMAP is the muscle contraction resulting from stimulation of a motor nerve and is a measure of the functioning motor axons in that nerve. The amplitude varies with the muscle that is stimulated, but in the hand, it is above 6 mV, and in the foot, it is above 1 mV.

21. **What is a normal sensory nerve action potential (SNAP)?**
A SNAP measures the conducting sensory axons after nerve stimulation with proximal velocities similar to motor conduction in the arms (50 meters/second) but slower than motor conduction in the legs (35 m/s). The SNAP amplitude depends on the size of the nerve studied but may range from 10 to 100 μV, which is small compared with the amplitude of CMAPs.

22. **What is the H reflex? How is it used clinically?**
The H-reflex is the electrical counterpart of the ankle jerk; it gives clinical information about any pathology in the S1 afferent–efferent reflex arc. The H may be prolonged or absent in neuropathies, S1 radiculopathies, or sciatic mononeuropathies. The H reflex in the arm can also be measured in the median nerve.

23. **What is the F wave? How is it useful clinically?**
After motor nerve stimulation, the F wave is seen as a late motor action potential that follows the initial compound muscles' action potential (M wave). Retrograde (antidromic) transmission of stimulated motor axons causes a discharge of the motor neurons in the spinal cord, resulting in a late discharge of the distal muscle. An F wave usually is tested on the median, ulnar, peroneal, and tibial motor nerves. The F wave gives information about abnormal conductibility across both proximal and distal nerve segments and is useful in acute and chronic demyelinating neuropathies.

24. **What is repetitive nerve stimulation? How is it used clinically?**
Repetitive nerve stimulation (RNS) measures the motor responses to slow rates of motor nerve stimulation. RNS is used as a diagnostic test for myasthenia gravis (MG) and Lambert-Eaton myasthenic syndrome (LEMS).

25. **What does repetitive nerve stimulation show in a patient with MG?**
About 65% to 85% of patients with MG show an abnormal (>10%) decremental motor response to slow repetitive stimulation of a motor nerve at 2 to 3 Hz. The highest yield is in the proximal muscles, such as the trapezius, when the spinal accessory nerve is stimulated in the neck. The facial nerve may also be tested and has a higher yield in MG, but the results are often technically unsatisfactory because of patient discomfort. Prolonged neuromuscular blockade in intensive care patients may show findings similar to MG.

26. **What does repetitive nerve stimulation show in a patient with LEMS?**
Repetitive stimulation in LEMS shows pre-exercise low-amplitude compound muscle action potentials in distal muscles because of reduced release of acetylcholine (ACh) at the motor nerve terminal. The muscle potentials double or triple in size after exercise because of increased release of ACh at the motor nerve terminal (postexercise facilitation). Decremental responses similar to MG often are superimposed on the facilitated motor units. Botulism may show findings similar to LEMS.

27. **What is the clinical utility of single-fiber EMG?**
Single-fiber EMG measures the difference in transmission time (jitter) between two individual muscle fibers from the same motor unit. A delay beyond normal, known as prolonged jitter, indicates an abnormality in neuromuscular transmission at the motor end plate. Special needles and recording equipment are necessary for the procedure. Single-fiber EMG is used mainly in the diagnosis of early cases of MG, for which its accuracy is 90% to 95%. However, it is a nonspecific measurement and may show abnormal results in motor neuron disease and other neurogenic disorders.

28. **Define neurapraxia and conduction block. How do they differ from axonal damage?**
Neurapraxia is a reversible diffuse or focal physiologic nerve lesion seen after trauma. If the lesion is focal, motor conduction distal to the lesion is normal but conduction proximal to the lesion is absent or slowed for up to 4 to 6 weeks but always recovers because there is no axonal loss. Focal axonal lesions have a long recovery because of wallerian degeneration of fibers, which requires reinnervation. Conduction block is a non-traumatic pathologic focal lesion of myelin. In early stages, conduction block shows up only as decreased proximal motor amplitude compared with distal conduction amplitude with normal motor velocities. Conduction block is seen in demyelinating neuropathies of various causes and may lead to marked slowing of motor nerve conductions.

29. **How can the EMG and nerve conduction studies help differentiate a demyelinating peripheral neuropathy from an axonal peripheral neuropathy?**
Demyelinating neuropathies show moderate to severe slowing of motor conduction, with temporal dispersion of the CMAP, normal distal and reduced proximal stimulation amplitudes (conduction block), and delayed distal latencies. Axonal neuropathies show a milder or borderline slowing in conduction velocity, with generally low CMAP amplitudes at both proximal and distal sites of stimulation because of axonal loss. The EMG shows denervation abnormalities early in axonal neuropathies and only late in demyelinating neuropathies, when axons begin to degenerate from loss of myelin.

30. **What does the EMG show in polymyositis?**
Myopathic motor units, fibrillations, and pseudomyotonia are the classic triad of EMG findings in polymyositis.

31. **Can inclusion body myositis (IBM) be differentiated from polymyositis by EMG?**

Proximal myositic abnormalities may be seen in both conditions, but the EMG findings in IBM may show a concentration of focal myositic abnormalities in the forearm flexors and quadriceps muscles, similar to the clinical weakness.

32. **Describe the EMG findings in spastic (upper motor neuron) paresis.**

No abnormal findings are noted if the anterior horn cells and roots are normal. EMG patterns on attempted maximum effort are reduced by lack of upper motor neuron control, but the patterns per se are nondiagnostic.

33. **What EMG findings confirm the diagnosis of amyotrophic lateral sclerosis (motor neuron disease)?**

The EMG should show widespread proximal and distal denervation with fasciculations and/or giant units in at least two extremities, plus denervation in either the tongue or thoracic paraspinous muscles. Cervical and lumbar spondylosis may show similar abnormalities in the extremities but normal tongue and thoracic paraspinous muscles.

34. **What do EMG and nerve conduction studies show in Guillain-Barré syndrome? What is their prognostic utility?**

In early Guillain-Barré syndrome, the EMG simply shows reduction in motor unit firing patterns, depending on the degree of paralysis. After 14 to 21 days, the development of spontaneous denervation activity (fibrillations and positive sharp waves) indicates wallerian degeneration (axonal loss). The EMG is useful prognostically because greater axonal loss generally implies longer recovery time. Motor conduction velocities show marked slowing in proximal and distal motor conduction, delayed distal latencies, and other changes of demyelination, beginning 3 to 5 days after onset. Severe slowing may be delayed for 7 to 14 days. Sensory conduction studies often show normal results, but an early sign may be a reduction in amplitude of the median sensory potential compared with that of the sural sensory potential as well as absent H reflexes.

35. **How is EMG useful in brachial plexus lesions?**

The main value of the EMG is in delineating the presence and degree of denervation in the appropriate arm muscles and thus localizing damage to the roots, trunks, cords, or distal branches of the brachial plexus. When the plexopathy is diffuse, motor and sensory conduction studies in the arm can be severely abnormal but may be relatively spared in many cases.

36. **What is the role of EMG and nerve conduction studies in evaluating a patient with a suspected radiculopathy from cervical or lumbar disc disease?**

EMG can confirm the root distribution of muscle weakness noted on clinical examination and give information about muscles that were not examined completely because of pain or lack of full effort. Nerve conduction studies have limited value unless multiple cervical or lumbar roots are involved, but such studies can identify or exclude other focal peripheral nerve lesions.

37. **Define carpal tunnel syndrome (CTS).**

Carpal tunnel syndrome (CTS) consists of nocturnal hand paresthesias caused by compression of the median nerve at the wrist from thickening of the flexor retinaculum, possibly in conjunction with congenital narrowing of the carpal tunnel or, rarely, in association with other conditions that cause thickening or pressure on the median nerve.

## KEY POINTS: ELECTROMYOGRAPHY

1. Fasciculations (the involuntary firing of a single motor unit) are often benign.

2. Myotonia, a delayed relaxation after muscle contraction, is most common in muscular dystrophies but can be seen in a host of other conditions.

3. On an EMG, muscle disease shows full contraction of all muscles but with short small units.

4. On an EMG, nerve disease shows a drop-out and reduction in muscle contraction, with prolonged, large motor units and fibrillations.

5. Patients with myasthenia gravis show a decremental response (fatigue) with repetitive stimulation of their muscles.

6. The most common compression neuropathy is the carpal tunnel syndrome of median nerve compression at the wrist.

---

38. **What is the best test for an electrical diagnosis of CTS?**
Sensory nerve action potential latencies of the median nerve are delayed twice as often as motor latencies. CTS is diagnosed electrically by a delay in sensory conduction latencies from the index finger or mid-palmar area to the wrist. The most sensitive is the palmar latency. Needle EMG is of limited value but can indicate denervation of the thenar muscles in more advanced cases.

39. **What other conditions are associated with median nerve entrapment at the wrist?**
The differential diagnosis of CTS includes the following: (1) fluid retention secondary to pregnancy, (2) hypothyroidism, (3) diabetes, (4) amyloid deposits, and (5) hereditary hypertrophic neuropathies (Charcot-Marie-Tooth type IA and hereditary neuropathy with liability to pressure palsies).

40. **How is CTS treated?**
Wrist splints at night may be helpful for mild to moderate cases that show mainly sensory abnormalities on nerve conduction studies. More severe or persistent cases require surgical sectioning of the transverse carpal ligament (flexor retinaculum), which should be decompressed from the wrist to the distal margin of the ligament in the upper palm region.

41. **What are the most common causes of ulnar nerve entrapment at the elbow (cubital tunnel syndrome)?**
External pressure over the flexed nerve in a shallow groove, repeated flexion dislocation of the nerve over the medial epicondyle, and compression of the nerve as it enters the aponeurosis of the flexor carpi ulnaris (cubital tunnel syndrome) may cause ulnar nerve lesions at the elbow. Arthritis from an old fracture (tardy ulnar palsy) and rheumatoid arthritis are less common causes.

42. **Describe the role of EMG and nerve conduction studies in diagnosing ulnar nerve entrapment at the elbow.**
Motor and sensory conduction studies can confirm ulnar nerve entrapment at the elbow in 60% to 80% of cases, with the EMG indicating the distribution and degree of denervation in the ulnar-innervated hand and forearm muscles.

43. **Which is the best conduction test for diagnosis of ulnar nerve entrapment at the elbow?**
Both motor and sensory conduction studies are helpful. The motor conduction across the elbow segment may show the earliest motor delay or conduction block. The proximal elbow amplitude and velocity of ulnar sensory conduction may be affected more than motor slowing. In early cases, studies may be normal.

44. **What is the best therapy for ulnar nerve entrapment at the elbow?**
Therapy varies according to the underlying mechanism of entrapment. Elbow protectors are helpful for mild or early moderate pressure lesions, but surgery is indicated for more persistent or severe entrapments. Surgery may involve sectioning of the flexor digitorum aponeurosis in cubital tunnel syndromes or medial epicondylectomy in flexion nerve dislocations and tardy ulnar palsies. Translocation of the nerve to the forearm muscles may be necessary in some cases.

45. **How is a lesion in the C8 root differentiated from a plexus or ulnar nerve lesion?**
   1. For a lesion in the C8 root, the EMG may show denervation in the following muscles: (1) extensor carpi ulnaris (radial), (2) abductor pollicis brevis (median), (3) first dorsal interosseous, abductor digiti quinti, and flexor carpi ulnaris (ulnar), and (4) C8 paraspinous muscles. Motor and sensory conductions are normal in the ulnar and median nerves unless multiple roots are involved.
   2. A lesion in the plexus (lower trunk or medial cord) involves denervation in all of the above muscles, except for normal C8 paraspinous muscles. Sensory conduction studies are abnormal in the ulnar and medial antebrachial cutaneous forearm nerves. Motor conduction is normal or minimally slow unless atrophy is severe.
   3. In ulnar nerve lesions, the EMG is normal in the radial and median-innervated C8 muscles but shows denervation in the ulnar-innervated muscles of the forearm and hand. Motor and sensory ulnar conduction studies also are abnormal, but the medial antebrachial cutaneous nerve is normal.

46. **What is the key muscle in differentiating a radial nerve palsy from a C7 radiculopathy?**
Flexor carpi radialis, which is a C7–C8 muscle innervated by the median nerve.

47. **How is a radial nerve palsy differentiated from a brachial plexus posterior cord lesion?**
Abnormalities in the deltoid muscle (axillary nerve) in addition to radial-innervated muscles indicate a lesion in the posterior cord of the brachial plexus.

48. **How is a suprascapular nerve lesion differentiated from a C5–C6 radiculopathy?**
Preservation of the deltoid, biceps, and rhomboid muscles, with abnormalities in the supraspinatus and infraspinatus muscles, indicates a suprascapular nerve lesion. A rotator cuff tear will show normal EMG of all the shoulder muscles.

49. **Describe the difference between a long thoracic nerve palsy and a C5–C6 radiculopathy.**
A long thoracic nerve palsy causes winging of the scapula with the arms outstretched from weakness of the serratus anterior muscle, with normal C5–C6 shoulder and arm muscles (e.g., deltoid, biceps supraspinatus). The serratus anterior muscle is not routinely studied by EMG. Long thoracic nerve conduction is slow or nonconductible when performed 3 days after onset.

50. **How is a peroneal nerve palsy differentiated from an L4–L5 radiculopathy?**
The invertors of the foot (posterior tibial muscle) are abnormal in L4–L5 radiculopathies and spared in peroneal nerve lesions.

51. **How does a femoral nerve lesion differ from an L3 radiculopathy?**
Abnormalities in the hip adductors in addition to the quadriceps muscles are present in L3 radiculopathies.

52. **How does a femoral nerve lesion in the pelvis differ from a lesion at the inguinal level?**
Weakness and denervation in the iliopsoas in addition to the quadriceps muscle indicate a femoral nerve lesion in the pelvis.

53. **What is the value of motor conduction velocities in Bell's palsy?**
Facial nerve conduction studies 3 to 5 days after the onset of Bell's palsy may indicate the prognosis. Normal latencies and amplitudes at 5 days indicate an excellent prognosis for recovery. In proximal lesions, loss of nerve conductibility as the nerve emerges from the angle of the jaw indicates the onset of wallerian degeneration with a prognosis of incomplete or non-recovery.

54. **Describe the role of EMG and nerve conduction studies in critical care patients who develop neuromuscular weakness.**
These studies help to distinguish critical illness polyneuropathy (CIP) from critical illness myopathy (CIM) and prolonged neuromuscular blockade.

55. **How does CIP differ from CIM (acute quadriplegic myopathy)?**
Critical illness polyneuropathy is an axonal polyneuropathy associated with sepsis. Nerve testing shows abnormal motor and sensory conduction. EMG shows distal denervation, more in the legs than arms. Results of direct muscle stimulation and repetitive nerve stimulation are normal. CIM is a muscle membrane disorder usually seen with use of nondepolarizing blocking agents and corticosteroids. EMG findings are limited by profound weakness, but motor nerve conduction studies and direct muscle stimulation are nonconductible and some cases may show spontaneous fibrillations from fiber necrosis.

56. **Which tests are used to diagnose neuromuscular blockade in the intensive care unit?**
Prolonged neuromuscular blockade occurs in patients with abnormal renal function who have been treated with nondepolarizing blocking agents. Repetitive nerve stimulation shows decrement similar to MG and distinguishes these patients from patients with polyneuropathy or myopathy.

57. **Which drugs can cause myopathic EMG changes with chronic use?**
Myopathic EMG abnormalities can be seen with long-term use of steroids, statin drugs and other cholesterol-lowering agents, chloroquine, amiodarone, and colchicine. The findings are usually mild but indistinguishable from other types of myopathies and are slowly reversible after cessation of the drug.

## BIBLIOGRAPHY

1. Pease WS, Lew HL, Johnson E: Practical Electromyography, 4th ed. Philadelphia, Lippincott Williams & Wilkins, 2006.
2. Preston DC, Shapiro BF: Electromyography and Neuromuscular Disorders, 2nd ed. Boston, Butterworth-Heinemann, 2005.

# CHAPTER 27

# NEURORADIOLOGY

*Jonathan N. Levine, MD*

1. **How is the image generated on a computed tomography (CT) scan?**
   The CT image depends on how much of the original x-ray beam reaches the detector. The CT measures the attenuation of the x-ray beam in units called Hounsfield units, and presents them in a gray scale. High-density tissue (more attenuation) appears brighter, and low-density tissue (less attenuation) appears darker.

2. **What are the normal tissue densities on CT?**
   Normal white matter is usually 25 to 30 Hounsfield units and normal gray matter is slightly brighter at 35 to 40 units. Tissue darker (blacker) than the brain includes cerebral spinal fluid (about 0 units) and fat (about -100 units). Tissue brighter (whiter) than normal brain includes acute blood (80 to 85 units) and bone (100+ units).

3. **How are the images created on magnetic resonance imaging (MRI)?**
   The interaction of magnetic field gradients with hydrogen atoms (protons) is manipulated to get an image. This is done by a radiofrequency pulse that causes the hydrogen atoms to emit energy.

4. **How is the energy from protons manipulated to obtain an MR image?**
   1. Echo time (TE): the image is created by altering the interval between initiating the radiofrequency pulse and measuring the emitted signal. Short TE has an interval of 10 to 40 msec, and long TE has an interval of 30 to 200 msec.
   2. Repetition time (TR): the image is created by altering the interval between repeated sequences. Short TR has an interval of 300 to 600 msec, and long TR has an interval of 2000 to 4000 msec.

5. **What are the most commonly used MRI sequences?**
   1. T1-weighted images: short TR and short TE signal. Good for showing anatomic detail.
   2. T2-weighted images: long TR and long TE. Good for detecting most types of pathology.
   3. Proton-density weighted images: long TR and short TE.
   4. Fluid-attenuated inversion recovery (FLAIR): this is essentially a T2-weighted image, which is manipulated to suppress water (cerebrospinal fluid) and make it appear darker. Such images are very sensitive for detecting tissue abnormalities and most types of pathology.
   5. Diffusion-weighted images: this technique is particularly sensitive for water diffusion and thus for detecting edema.
   6. Gradient echo: these sequences are very sensitive to flow and hence are used for MR angiography.

6. **What is the value of contrast enhancement?**
   Contrast enhancement accentuates areas of blood-brain barrier breakdown. It is thus particularly useful for identifying tumors, infections, inflammatory disease, and late changes following a stroke or hematoma.
   Enhancement also accentuates blood vessels and hence is useful in identifying vascular malformations and aneurysms.

7. **What normal structures usually enhance on a postcontrast CT scan?**
   1. Pituitary gland
   2. Midline structures of the infundibulum, tuber cinereum, and area postrema
   3. Sinus and nasal mucosa
   4. Extraocular muscles
   5. Blood vessels including venous sinuses
   6. Choroid plexus

8. **When should CT scan be used before MRI?**
   1. CT scans generate images much more quickly than MR scans and it is generally physically easier to place patients in the scanner. For very rapid neurologic assessments, the CT scan is thus often preferable. It should be considered instead of or prior to an MRI, therefore, to assess acute stroke, subarachnoid hemorrhage, and head trauma or mass effects.
   2. If the primary purpose is to evaluate ventricular size (hydrocephalus), the CT is quite adequate and much quicker and cheaper.
   3. Bone pathology. Skull fractures and other bone pathology are often seen best on a CT scan.
   4. Sinus disease

9. **When is an MRI scan contraindicated?**
   There are some patients who cannot obtain an MRI scan. These include patients who:
   1. Have a pacemaker or other implanted device that would be reprogrammed or reset by strong magnetic fields,
   2. Have a metal object in their body that would be moved by the magnetic fields,
   3. Are severely claustrophobic and so unable to tolerate the tight quarters of the MRI scanner,
   4. Are extremely obese (generally more than 300 pounds) and whose weight therefore physically prevents them from sliding into the scanning tube.

10. **What is "Gaussian carditis"?**
    It is the amusing term for the phenomenon of the magnetic strip on your credit card being erased when you accidentally bring it too close to the MRI's powerful magnetic field. (Carl Gauss, a German mathematician who died in 1855, did much of the theoretical work on magnetism that ultimately led to the invention of the MRI.)

## COMMON RADIOGRAPHS

Care has been taken to include in this book representative examples of the most common radiographs and images that appear on examinations and boards. These are located in their appropriate place in the text, but they are specifically indexed here to facilitate a neuroradiologic review. The radiographs in this book, representing the major areas of neuroradiology, are cross-referenced below by chapter and page number.

### Vascular disease

## BIBLIOGRAPHY

1. Hathout GM, Ferguson T: Clinical Neuroradiology: A Case-Based Approach. London, Cambridge University Press, 2008.
2. Kornienko VN, Pronin IN: Diagnostic Neuroradiology. Berlin, Springer, 2009.

# CHAPTER 28

# NEUROLOGIC EMERGENCIES

*Loren A. Rolak, MD*

A number of conditions affecting the nervous system may have a crippling or even fatal outcome. They often present abruptly and require rapid medical intervention. These illnesses have been discussed in their appropriate place in the text, but they are specifically indexed here to facilitate easy access and rapid review of neurologic emergencies. These particularly important conditions are cross-referenced below by chapter and page number.

## BIBLIOGRAPHY

1. Henry GL, Jagoda A, Little N, Pellegrino TR: Neurologic Emergencies: A Symptom-Oriented Approach. New York, McGraw-Hill, 2003.
2. Wijdicks EFM: Catastrophic Neurologic Disorders in the Emergency Department, 2nd ed. London, Oxford University Press, 2004.

# CHAPTER 29

# NEUROLOGY TRIVIA

*Loren A. Rolak, MD*

**QUESTIONS YOU WILL OFTEN BE ASKED BY ATTENDING PHYSICIANS, THAT ARE NOT IMPORTANT FOR UNDERSTANDING SCIENCE OR TAKING CARE OF PATIENTS, AND YOU SHOULD NOT HAVE TO ANSWER THEM**

1. **Who performed the first spinal tap?**
   Probably Dr. E. Wynter, in 1891, to drain cerebrospinal fluid from children with tuberculous meningitis. Dr. H. Quinke in the same year developed the instruments and technique still used today.
   Frederiks JA, Koehler PJ: The first lumbar puncture. J Hist Neurosci 6:147-153, 1997.
   Gorelick PB, Zych D: James Leonard Corning and the early history of spinal puncture. Neurology 37:672-674, 1987.

2. **Who suffered the first spinal tap headache?**
   The first postspinal tap headache was reported in 1899 by Dr. August Bier, who described it as a consequence of a spinal tap performed on himself by his laboratory assistant in the course of studies on spinal anesthesia. The fate of the assistant is unknown.

3. **How do you pronounce the last name of Dr. Georges Guillain, the French neurologist who helped to describe the Guillain-Barré syndrome?**
   According to Dr. Joseph Rogoff, writing in the *Journal of the American Medical Association*, "The mispronunciation of Dr. George Guillain's name by English-speaking physicians has bothered me for many years. Even the medical dictionaries (e.g., Dorland's) give the pronunciation as "ge-yan," which is incorrect. I was Dr. Guillain's extern in 1939, and I never heard him called anything but "ghee-lain" (with the final 'ain' nasalized). If Guillain wanted his name pronounced thus, why should we insist on changing it?"

4. **What is the smallest amount of light the human eye can detect?**
   The human eye has 125 million rods, each one containing 1000 folds in its photoreceptor membrane, with each fold containing 1 million molecules of photoceptor. This extraordinary light-sensing array can detect one single photon, which is $10^{-11}$ watts. (Wow!)

5. **What does the word *myelin* mean?**
   *Myelin* is the Greek word for "marrow" and comes from the belief that the white matter was the marrow of the brain, much as the central portion of the bone is the marrow of the bone.

6. **What is Baltic myoclonus?**
   It is another name for Unverricht-Lundborg disease. Does that help? (It is a type of progressive myoclonic epilepsy.)

7. **Why are the zigzag, scintillating, shimmering lights that often precede classic migraine headaches referred to as fortification spectra?**
   They are called fortification spectra because of their resemblance to the star-shaped, zigzag fortifications constructed in Europe during the Renaissance to protect cities and military compounds (Figure 29-1).

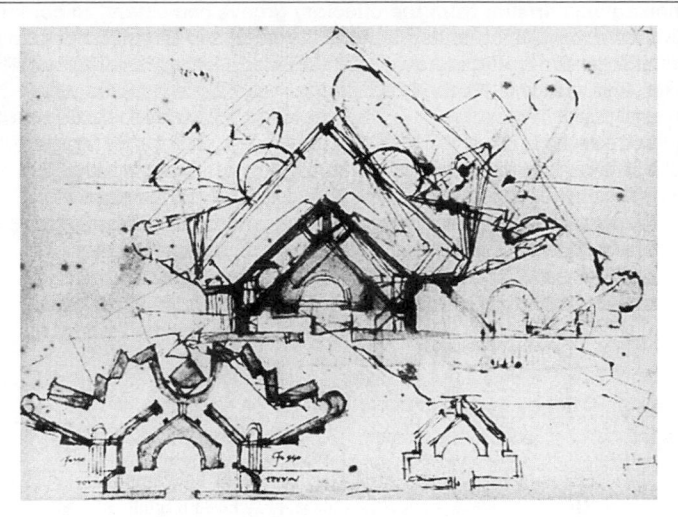

**Figure 29-1.** A drawing by Michelangelo for a proposed fortification, showing the triangular, zigzag defensive plan.

8. **A lesion that transects the lateral half of the spinal cord will produce a Brown-Sequard syndrome of weakness and loss of proprioception ipsilaterally, with contralateral numbness. Who was Brown, and who was Sequard?**
   This is a trick question. Brown-Sequard was only one person, Charles Edward Brown-Sequard. His father was an American sailor, and his mother was of French descent, from the island of Mauritius. He took the unusual course of combining his mother's and his father's last names. He became one of the preeminent neurologists of the 19th century, holding professorships, at various times, in America, England, and France.

9. **What happened to Charles Edward Brown-Sequard when he ate chocolate?**
   He developed gustatory perspiration and broke into a sweat.
   Gooddy W: Charles Edward Brown-Sequard. In Rose FC, Bynum WF (eds): Historical Aspects of the Neurosciences. New York, Raven Press, 1985, pp 371-378.

10. **Jules Dejerine was a brilliant contemporary of the great French neurologist Charcot and ultimately succeeded him at the Salpêtrière. He described Dejerine's syndrome (medial medullary infarction) and collaborated with other colleagues of Charcot's to describe the syndromes of Dejerine-Landouzy (muscular atrophy), Dejerine-Roussy (thalamic pain), Dejerine-Thomas (cerebellar-brain stem atrophy), and Dejerine-Sottas (neuropathy and tremor). But who was Klumpke of Dejerine-Klumpke (lower brachial plexopathy)?**
    Sorry, wrong Dejerine. When Augusta Klumpke married Jules Dejerine, she hyphenated her last name, in a fashion now popular with some modern women. An accomplished physician herself, the syndrome of brachial plexus injury is named after her, not her husband. Like Brown-Sequard (sort of), Dejerine-Klumpke is one person.

11. **A meningioma arising from the olfactory groove can extend to compress the optic nerve, producing anosmia, optic atrophy, and unilateral papilledema, a constellation of findings known as the Foster Kennedy syndrome. Who was Foster, and who was Kennedy?**

    This is another trick question. Dr. Foster (first name) Kennedy (last name) was a prominent American neurologist in the first part of the 20th century, at one time president of the American Neurological Association. (To muddle things further, his real first name was Robert, although he never used it.) This use of first names is rare, but it gets even more confusing—the famous eponymic Marcus Gunn pupil comes from the *middle* name of the Scottish physician Robert Marcus Gunn. Exactly how names are applied to diseases is one of medicine's great unsolved mysteries.

12. **Who first used the word *neurology*?**

    The word first appears in Pordage's English translation of Thomas Willis's book *Cerebri Anatome* in 1664. Incidentally, Willis assembled a collaborative research team composed of the greatest minds of his time: Christopher Wren, Robert Hooke, Robert Boyle, Isaac Newton, and William Harvey. In a sense, these men formed the first "Circle of Willis."

13. **What was the first description of a neurologic disease?**

    The first description of a neurologic disease appears in the Smith papyrus, which is the oldest known medical text. This ancient papyrus, translated by Edward Smith, consists of a number of "case reports" of different diseases, presented and discussed by an unknown Egyptian author, written about 3300 BC. One of the cases is a person with a traumatic head injury, which is the earliest known description of a neurologic problem.

14. **Neurology, more than most other specialties, abounds with eponyms and mellifluous phrases that roll off the tongue. For example, what is the torcular Herophili?**

    It is the confluence of the straight, lateral, and sagittal sinuses, where much of the venous drainage occurs in the brain. A torcula is a cistern or well, sometimes used to collect liquor from a wine press, and Herophilus (335 to 280 BC) was the ancient Greek anatomist who described this region of the brain (Figure 29-2).

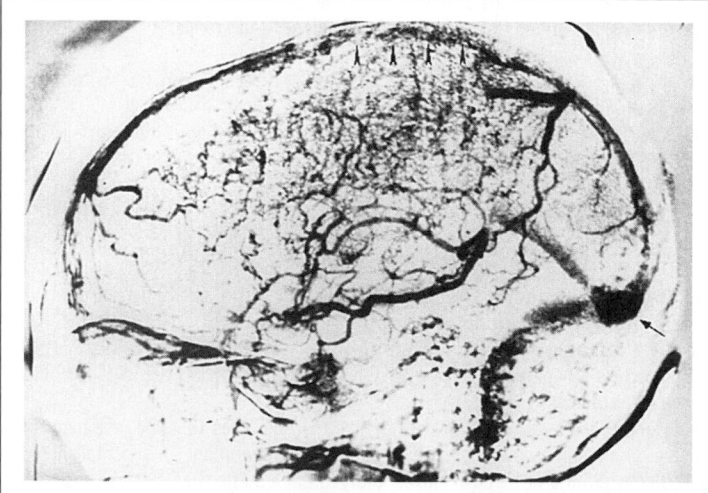

**Figure 29-2.** Venous phase of a cerebral angiogram, showing the venous drainage into the torcular Herophili (*arrow at the right of photo*). This patient also has a thrombosis of his superior sagittal sinus (*small arrowheads*).

15. **Refsum's disease is an inherited peripheral neuropathy with ataxia and accompanying retinitis pigmentosa, characterized by accumulation of phytanic acid. What is phytanic acid?**
    Phytanic acid is 3,7,11,15-tetramethyl-hexadecanoic acid.

16. **If you place a human skull on the ground and begin piling weight on top of it, how much weight can be added before it cracks?**
    If the weight is applied slowly, the human skull can support 3 tons. (Wow!)

17. **What does the word *carotid* mean?**
    It is derived from a Greek word meaning "to put to sleep" because pressure on the carotid arteries can cause loss of consciousness (as any fan of the World Wrestling Entertainment is aware).

18. **What did Aristotle say was the function of the brain?**
    To cool the heart.

19. **In 1909, Korbinian Brodmann divided the human cerebral cortex into 47 cytoarchitecturally distinct regions and gave each one a "Brodmann's number." What is found in Brodmann's areas 13 to 16?**
    Nothing. For some reason, Brodmann left out numbers 13 to 16, which do not appear anywhere on his cortical maps (see Figures 2-12 and 2-13). The reason for the omission has never been discovered.
    Gorman DG, Unutzer J: Brodmann's missing numbers. Neurology 43:226-227, 1993.

20. **Who first described transient ischemic attacks (TIAs) and noted that they were warning signs of a future stroke?**
    Hippocrates first described TIAs, noting that "unaccustomed attacks of numbness and anesthesia are signs of impending apoplexy."

21. **What are the five diagnoses neurologists most dread telling a patient (according to a recent survey of practicing clinical neurologists)?**
    The most distressing diagnoses to tell a patient, in order, are:
    1. Amyotrophic lateral sclerosis
    2. Malignant brain tumor
    3. Traumatic paraplegia
    4. Multiple sclerosis
    5. Epilepsy

22. **What are the top ten drugs most commonly prescribed by neurologists in America?**
    1. Topiramate (Topamax)
    2. Gabapentin (Neurontin)
    3. Levetiracetam (Keppra)
    4. Hydrocodone with acetaminophen (Vicodin)
    5. Lamotrigine (Lamictal)
    6. Carbidopa with levodopa (Sinemet)
    7. Clonazepam (Klonopin)
    8. Pregabalin (Lyrica)
    9. Amitriptyline (Elavil)
    10. Donepezil (Aricept)

23. **How many pounds of aspirin are consumed each year in the United States?**
    Americans ingest 30 million pounds of aspirin per year.

24. **Why did René Descartes choose the pineal gland as the seat of the soul?**
    He believed it was the only unpaired structure in the brain and occupied the brain's exact center.

25. **What was Gilles de la Tourette's first name?**
    George.

26. **Who did Gilles de la Tourette believe was the greatest neurologist of the century?**
    Himself. He died of general paresis, at age 47, in a state of grandiose megalomania.
    Guilly P: Gilles de la Tourette. In Rose FC, Bynum WF (eds): Historical Aspects of the Neurosciences. New York, Raven Press, 1985, pp 397-413.

27. **What percentage of all visits to a doctor are visits to a neurologist?**
    One percent of all doctors' visits are to a neurologist, which is reasonable because 1% of all doctors in America are neurologists.

28. **Who described the first reflex, and what was it?**
    In 1662, Rene Descartes described the blink reflex, where a blow aimed at the eyes causes a person to blink. The word reflex derives from the sight of an approaching object causing a "reflection" in the brain.

29. **Why are cerebral infarctions called strokes?**
    According to the *Oxford English Dictionary*, a sudden, inexplicable cerebrovascular accident was first likened to a "stroke of God's hand" in 1599. The relationship of a cerebral infarction to an act of God exists in other cultures as well: the Greek verb *plesso* means to "stroke, hit, or beat," and the derivative *plegia* gives us our term hemiplegia.
    Dirckx JH: Stroke. Stroke 17:559, 1986.

30. **The Babinski sign is produced by stroking the lateral aspect of the foot with a noxious stimulus and observing whether the great toe dorsiflexes. What did Babinski call the Babinski sign?**
    There is no more pompous figure in medicine than the posturing attending physician on rounds expounding pedantically on the supposed oxymoron of a "negative Babinski sign" and extolling the "extensor plantar reflex." In fact, in his original papers, Babinski referred to his sign as "the phenomenon of the toes," but on rounds with his pupils he always insisted it be called "the great toe sign." By the way, Babinski referred to the failure of the platysma to contract on the side of a hemiparesis as the "Babinski sign."
    Babinski J: Sur le reflexe cutane plantaire dans certaines affections organiques du system nerveux central. C R Soc Biol (Paris) 48:207-208, 1896.
    Babinski J: Du phenomene des orteils et de sa valeur semiologique. Semaine Medicale 18:321-322, 1898.

31. **There are many minor, generally useless variations of the Babinski sign, most of them with eponymic names bestowed by egotistical neurologists (e.g., Chaddock, Oppenheim). But sometimes pyramidal tract lesions cause hyperactive plantar flexion of the toes, a movement opposite to the Babinski sign. How many variations of this reflex can you name?**
    See Figure 29-3.

32. **What are crocodile tears?**
    After damage to the facial nerve, such as from Bell's palsy, regenerating fibers may become misdirected such that impulses to mouth and lip muscles instead stimulate the lacrimal gland.

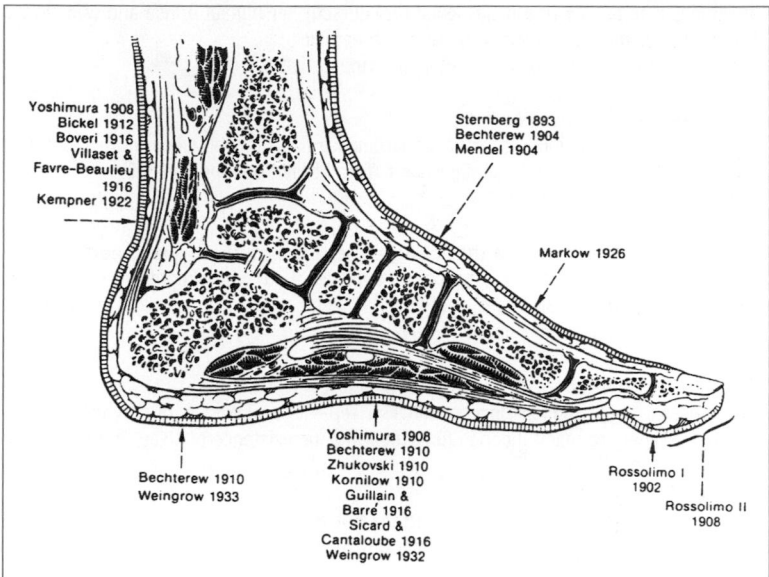

**Figure 29-3.** Some variations of the Rossolimo sign of toe flexion ("grasp reflex of the foot") with pyramidal tract disease. (From DeJong RN: The Neurologic Examination, 4th ed. Hagerstown, MD, Harper & Row, 1979, p 462, with permission.)

As a result, chewing food will cause the patient to weep. The expression comes from old African folklore that crocodiles felt compassion and remorse for their prey and wept with sorrow whenever they ate.

33. **The first successful treatment for epilepsy was bromides. Why was an obstetrician the first person to recommend their use?**
It was believed in the mid-19th century that excessive sexual activity, especially masturbation, contributed greatly to epilepsy. Because bromides are known to cause impotence, Sir Charles Locock, personal obstetrician to Queen Victoria, proposed in 1857 that their suppression of sexual function (and menstruation) would result in suppression of seizure activity. He was right, for the wrong reason.
    Scott DF: The discovery of anti-epileptic drugs. J Hist Neurosci 1:111-118, 1992.

34. **Ondine's curse refers to a neurologic lesion, usually in the medulla or high cervical cord that destroys the pathways for automatic, rhythmic breathing, thus forcing the patient to breathe voluntarily. Who was Ondine, and what was his curse?**
Nobody, and nothing. Ondine is simply the French word for mermaid and refers to the (unnamed) mermaid in the French version of Hans Christian Andersen's fairy tale, "The Little Mermaid." In this story, based on old Germanic legends, a mermaid can assume human form, but only as part of a pact or bargain (not a curse) that requires her to return to the ocean if her human lover is unfaithful to her. The mangled approbation of Ondine's curse, referring to a neurologic deficit that interrupts automatic breathing, is derived from the 1939 play Ondine by the French author Jean Giraudoux, who embellished the story by having the mermaid's hapless knight punished for his infidelity by the cessation of all his automatic functions (not just

breathing). The ondine (mermaid) loved (not cursed) her human prince and was always faithful. No Ondine, no curse, no one stops breathing.

Giraudoux J: Ondine. New York, Random House, 1954.

35. **What are Finnish snowballs?**
These are osmophilic, globular, intracellular inclusions seen with electron microscopy in patients with neuronal ceroid lipofuscinosis. They really don't look anything like Finnish snowballs.

36. **What is the softest sound that can be detected by the human ear?**
The decibel scale is set at 0 for the softest audible sound, which represents vibratory energy striking the eardrum at an intensity of 0.0002 $Dy/cm^2$, which is a range of vibration scarcely larger than the width of several atoms. (Wow!)

37. **What is the lowest form of life that sleeps?**
Some insects sleep. The reason why animals sleep—its evolutionary or survival advantage—is unknown. There are many theories to account for the existence of sleep, but none of them really makes much sense.

38. **Most humans have a clearly dominant hand (usually the right one). What is the lowest form of life that shows such a preference or dominance? Why are most people right-handed?**
Birds, which have neuronal populations in the left hemisphere that regulate their song production, are the lowest phylum with a convincing laterality or dominance. The reason for dominance—its evolutionary or survival advantage—is unknown. There are many theories to account for the existence of dominance, but none of them really makes much sense.

39. **What is the smallest concentration of a substance that can be smelled by the human nose?**
The more than 10 million specialized neuroepithelial cells that make up the olfactory sensory receptors can detect some substances, such as musks, in concentrations of $10^{-12}$ moles, which is scarcely more than a few molecules. (Wow!)

40. **What are the most common movements seen in dead people?**
The Lazarus sign is a quick flexion of both arms up over the chest, beneath the chin, observed in brain-dead patients. It may represent spontaneous firing of hypoxic cervical spinal cord neurons.

Ropper AH: Unusual spontaneous movements in brain-dead patients. Neurology 34:1089-1092, 1984.

# INDEX

Page numbers followed by *t* indicates tables; *f*, figures.